Memorizing Medicine

A Revision Guide

Second Edition

Memorizing Medicine

A Revision Guide

Second Edition

Paul Bentley &
Ben Lovell

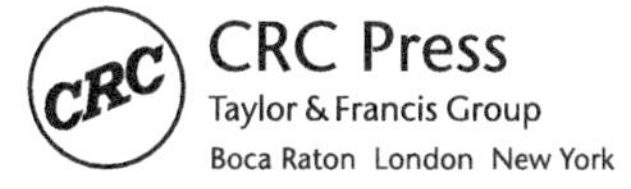

CRC Press
Taylor & Francis Group
Boca Raton London New York

CRC Press is an imprint of the
Taylor & Francis Group, an **informa** business

CRC Press
Taylor & Francis Group
6000 Broken Sound Parkway NW, Suite 300
Boca Raton, FL 33487-2742

Printed on acid-free paper

International Standard Book Number-13: 978-1-138-33271-3 (Hardback)
978-1-138-33269-0 (Paperback)

Library of Congress Cataloging-in-Publication Data

Names: Bentley, Paul, Dr., author. | Lovell, Ben, author.
Title: Memorizing medicine / Ben Lovell and Paul Bentley.
Description: Second edition. | Boca Raton, FL : Taylor & Francis Group, [2019] | Only Paul Bentley's name appears in the previous edition. | Includes bibliographical references and index.
Identifiers: LCCN 2019015648| ISBN 9781138332690 (pbk. : alk. paper) | ISBN 9781138332713 (hardbook : alk. paper) | ISBN 9780429185939 (e-book)
Subjects: | MESH: Clinical Medicine | Outline
Classification: LCC R834.5 | NLM WB 18.2 | DDC 610.76--dc23
LC record available at https://lccn.loc.gov/2019015648

Visit the Taylor & Francis Web site at
http://www.taylorandfrancis.com

and the CRC Press Web site at
http://www.crcpress.com

CONTENTS

Renal Medicine 401

Haematology 431

Abbreviations 493

Index 503

ACKNOWLEDGEMENTS AND DEDICATION

Thanks to Jo and Paul for inviting me onto this project, and thanks to Mark for his support.

Ben Lovell

To Annie, Mia, Tess and Noah

Paul Bentley

INTRODUCTION

The purpose of this book is two-fold: firstly, to inject an air of amusement and refreshing jollity into one's academic studies; secondly, to highlight an important point about how (rather than what) we should be studying.

With hope, the light-hearted aspect of the book will be immediately appreciated – punchy and practical mnemonics, entertaining pictures, sprinklings of humour and a general feeling of novelty and variety – at least relative to the average medical textbook. At the same time, weighty, wearisome text has been dispensed with as far as possible, to enable the salient points of each subject to stand out.

The serious side of the book, however, begins with the question, 'What does it take to memorize medicine?' A large part of what it takes to be a good doctor undoubtedly depends on the skill of being able to recall large quantities of information. Hence the training of doctors should not merely involve exposing students to knowledge in a passive manner, but should actively incorporate methods that engender efficient memorization. Medical textbooks should not simply be catalogues of facts, or even distillers of information, but should potentiate factual recall at a later date.

There are three reasons why a book such as this needs to be written, and they all seem to grow increasingly more compelling as each year goes by:

- The amount of medical knowledge increases exponentially with time.
- Technological advances, e.g. the internet, expose us to an increasing amount of data despite our brains being fixed in the rate at which we can 'input' it.
- Neuropsychological advances increasingly inform us on the nature of memory. A sharp mind is cultivated not so much by 'sheer hard work' or 'burning the midnight oil' as opposed to adopting optimal strategies of learning.

The manner in which we are exposed to knowledge assumes that our brains are built in a simple, sequential fashion, like home computers: read a new fact, listen to a lecture – and this information gets stored as easily as one's own name. Yet, it is clear from each of our own experiences that human memory does not work this way. Facts are most efficiently memorized as visual images, chunks, acronyms, rhymes, webs, etc. and as we update our knowledge, we must first recall our pre-existing schema of the topic, and then peg the new data onto this internal structure.

Enlightened with basic psychological truths about what it takes to memorize efficiently, this book aims to 'rewrite' the classical medical textbook by taking the same information as before but setting it out in an original style that lends itself to effective learning. We hope it succeeds in leaving an imprint in your mind while at the same time not taking itself too seriously.

EXAMPLES OF EFFECTIVE MEMORIZING

Consider SF, an ordinary undergraduate who set himself the task of learning long lists of arbitrary numbers. Starting with the average person's digit recall of 7 numbers, he was able to build up his memory to a staggering 80, albeit over one-and-a-half years of regular training sessions. He was not explicitly given formal mnemonic strategies but simply devised his own as he went along. The methods he stumbled upon just so happened to be similar to those utilized by world memory champions, as well as, coincidentally, pigeons trained on a picture task.

When SF was read the numbers 34928931944, he recalled this as short 'chunks' and made real-life associations, e.g. 3 minutes 49 seconds point 2 – 'near world-record mile time'; 89.3 years old – 'very old man'; 1944 – 'near the end of World War II'. Furthermore, whether he used a 3- or a 4-digit chunk was based upon a higher order of structure – the chunks were themselves chunked into blocks e.g. 444 444 333 333 444 333. This way he could remember the order in which the chunks were arranged.

Learning medicine is not quite like learning random number sequences – and not just for the obvious reason of the relative utility that distinguishes the two. Factual knowledge, unlike number lists, is structured with interconnections and hierarchies. This enables each topic to be naturally fragmented into a few elementary chunks, each possessing a core fact surrounded by details; the first-order of details may themselves be subsequently chunked, etc., repeating the structure at different scales.

That this sort of structuring actually occurs in the accumulation of expert knowledge has been demonstrated in chess masters in their recall of game positions. By measuring the time interval between the recall of particular positions, it has been found that masters chunk their memory of positions into meaningful groups. The maximum number of chunks that can be stored at any one time (into short-term memory) is about 4, but cumulatively the total number of chunks that can be stored in long-term memory can reach 100,000 or so – similar to the vocabulary span of the average adult!

In a more recent experiment, world memory champions performed a memory task while the metabolic activity of the brain was observed using functional magnetic resonance imaging. Not only did these experts utilize methods that involved chunking and ordering chunks according to a spatial plan (the 'method of loci'), but the activated parts of the brain were those recognized to be involved in spatial memory and navigation. The experts were no more intelligent and had no differences in the structural appearance of their brains, relative to control subjects. The results suggest that skilled memory can be learnt through efficient methods rather than necessarily being a quality that one is born with.

References

Science 1980; **208**: 1181; *Nature* 1987; **325**: 149; *Memory* 2004; **12**: 232;
Nature Neurosci 2003; **6**: 90

BOOK GUIDE

Sample page explained:

ASTHMA

Def

Definition

Episodic, reversible COAD, due to bronchial hyper-reactivity to various stimuli

Epi

Epidemiology

The order of facts is best remembered by recourse to the old mnemonic

'In A Surgeon's Gown A Physician Might Make Progress'

Incidence – and prevalence, **A**ge, **S**ex, **G**eographical (and ethnicity), **A**etiology, **P**redisposing factors, **M**acroscopic and **M**icroscopic pathology, **P**rognosis

Inc: Prevalence – Children 5%; Adults 2%
Age: Peaks at 5 years; most outgrow in adolescence
Sex: M:F =1:1, except under 5, when boys predominate (3:2)
Geo: Western world
Aet: Acute phase: mast cell–Ag interaction; Late phase: T_{H2} cell → IL-3, 4 , 5
Micro: Sputum contains mucus casts, eosinophils, Curschmann spirals

Causes

A.S.T.H.M.A^2.

Atopy, **S**tress, **T**oxins, **H**elminths, **M**alignancy – carcinoid, **A**utoimmune/**A**spergillosis

PC

Presenting complaint

For the purpose of memorization, this is sometimes meant loosely so as to include symptoms, signs and abnormal investigations, e.g. LFT derangement

- Cough: Often at night, tenacious yellow sputum
- Wheeze: Often post-exercise, early morning; relieved by empirical salbutamol Rx
- SOB, or 'chest tightness'

O/E

On examination

If there are multiple key signs, picture the order in which the examination is normally performed

General
Underweight
(hypermetabolic)

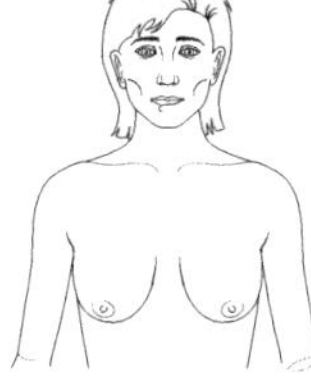

Chest
Inspection
Hyperexpanded, Harrison's sulci
Auscultation
Widespread, polyphonic wheeze
often normal – as often episodic

Ix

INVESTIGATIONS

If there are more than three crucial tests, use the mnemonic – **B.U.M.M.E^3.R.S^3.**

Bloods if there are multiple blood tests, split into the different departments

- Chemistry **R.E.A.L.M.S.**
  Renal, **E**lectrolytes, **A**BGs, **L**FTs, **M**etabolic (glucose, lipids, TFT), **S**pecial
- Haematology
- Immunology

Urine

Microbiology

- Blood: Culture, serology
- Excretions: Sputum, stool, urine, discharge
- Collections: CSF, joint, pleural or ascitic effusion, abscess, lymph node

Monitor: e.g. PEFR ('peak flow'); oxygen; cardiac monitor

Electro: **E**CG (± Echo), **E**EG

Radiology

- Plain X-rays, e.g. CXR
- CT/MRI
- Radionuclide scanning

Surgical/'**S**cope/**S**pecial

- Surgical, e.g. biopsy
- 'Scope, e.g. bronchosopy
- Special, e.g. respiratory function tests

Rx

TREATMENT

- Divide into 3-4 main category types: Conservative; Medical (supportive/disease-modifying), Surgical
- For emergencies, picture the patient lying in bed with the various investigation/treatments surrounding him/her in order of priority

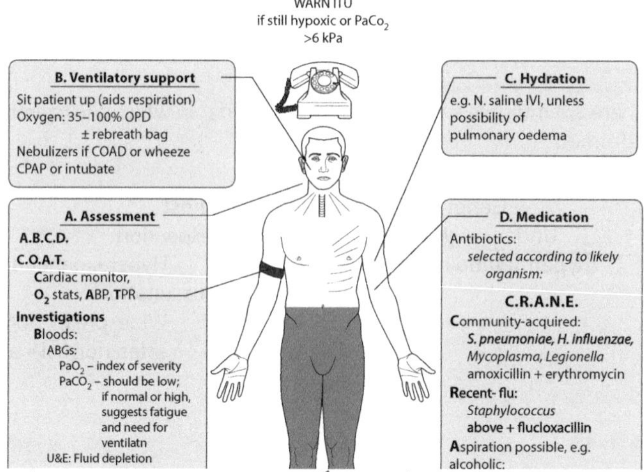

WARN ITU
if still hypoxic or $PaCo_2$
>6 kPa
B. Ventilatory support
Sit patient up (aids respiration)
Oxygen: 35–100% OPD
± rebreath bag
Nebulizers if COAD or wheeze
CPAP or intubate
C. Hydration
e.g. N. saline IVI, unless possibility of pulmonary oedema
A. Assessment
A.B.C.D.
C.O.A.T.
Cardiac monitor,
O_2 stats, ABP, TPR
Investigations
Bloods:
ABGs:
PaO_2 – index of severity
$PaCO_2$ – should be low; if normal or high, suggests fatigue and need for ventilatn
U&E: Fluid depletion
D. Medication
Antibiotics:
selected according to likely organism:
C.R.A.N.E.
Community-acquired:
S. pneumoniae, H. Influenzae, Mycoplasma, Legionella
amoxicillin + erythromycin
Recent- flu:
Staphylococcus
above + flucloxacillin
Aspiration possible, e.g. alcoholic:

MEMORIZING MEDICINE – 6 TIPS

One subject - one page

Have you ever tried to work out the route between two places using a map-book when the two places are on different pages? Similarly, if you sit down to learn a medical subject plot all the main headings on one piece of paper. It will also show you how much relative time to spend on each subheading. Never let a list run over 2 pages – you'll never remember it!

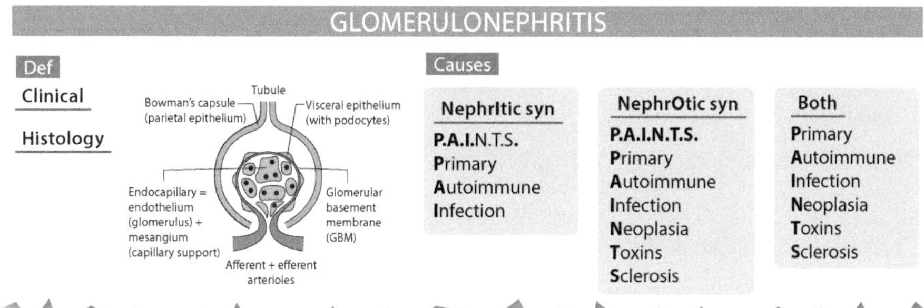

Hierarchy

Every doctor should know that glomerulonephritis can result in nephritic syndrome, nephrotic syndrome or both. Every general physician should know the main categories of causes. Every renal specialist should know the causes of each type of primary nephrotic syndrome. Therefore learning should proceed in this order.

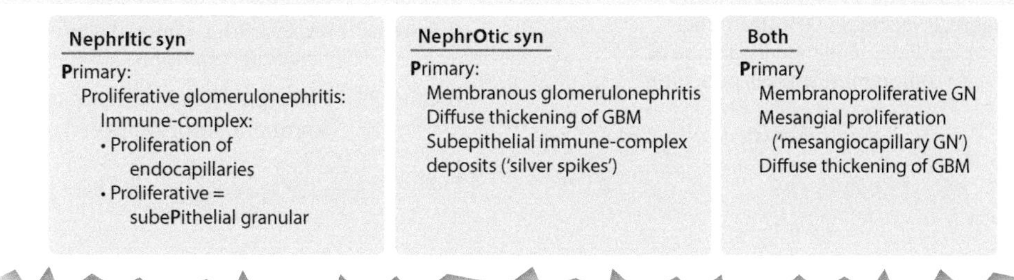

NephrItic syn
Primary:
Proliferative glomerulonephritis:
Immune-complex:
• Proliferation of endocapillaries
• Proliferative = subePithelial granular
NephrOtic syn
Primary:
Membranous glomerulonephritis
Diffuse thickening of GBM
Subepithelial immune-complex deposits ('silver spikes')
Both
Primary
Membranoproliferative GN
Mesangial proliferation ('mesangiocapillary GN')
Diffuse thickening of GBM

Nesting

As you learn finer and finer details of each subject, you'll need to move onto another page – but this needs to be done without breaking down the overall structure. The solution? Take those sub-headings with the greatest amount of extra information and cross-refer them to a new double page.

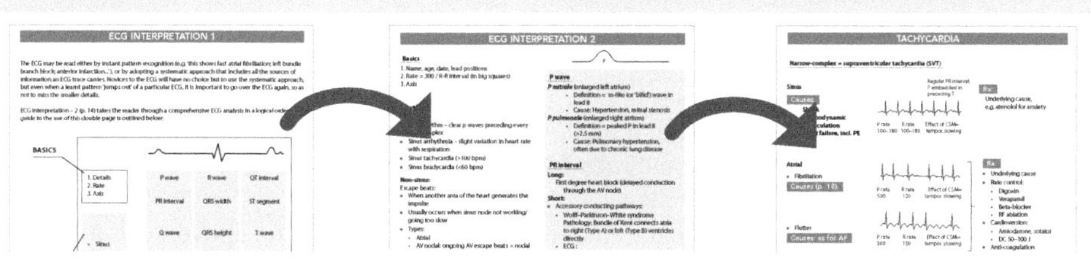

Logic

The first thing when learning a long list is to try breaking it down into categories that respect the underlying physiology or anatomy of the subject matter

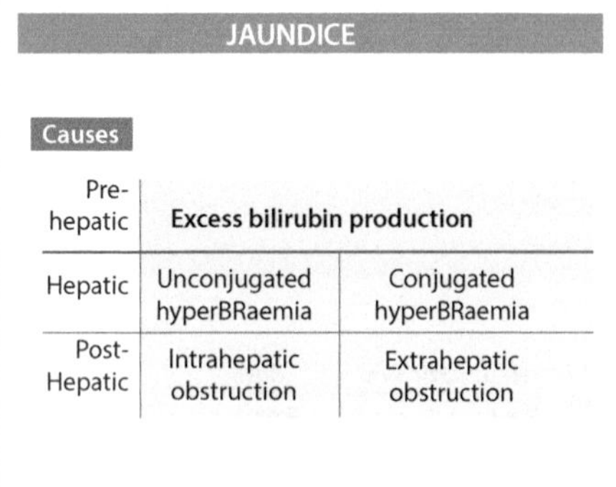

JAUNDICE

Causes

Pre-hepatic	**Excess bilirubin production**	
Hepatic	Unconjugated hyperBRaemia	Conjugated hyperBRaemia
Post-Hepatic	Intrahepatic obstruction	Extrahepatic obstruction

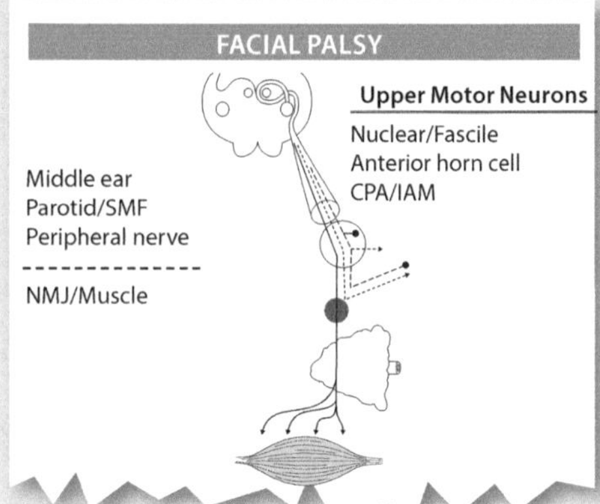

Chunking

If a list doesn't easily lend itself to logical breakdown, then arbitrarily break the list down into bite-size chunks of 3, or possibly 4. This seems to be the maximum number of items the brain can remember at any one time. For example, in 'Facial palsy' above, see how the anatomical list of 8 is more easily remembered as 1 + 3 + 3 + 1 (conveniently, symmetric). Also –

Pneumonia – clinical features

chest pain, cough, dyspnoea, malaise, myalgia, fever, rigors, D+V, headache, confusion; PMH of pulmonary disease or immunocompromise, smoker, pets, travel

(extract from standard textbook)

Pneumonia – clinical features

1. Specific – chest pain, cough, dyspnoea
2. Systemic – myalgia, fever + rigors, D+V; headache, confusion
3. Other PC – PMH (pulmonary disease or immunocompromise)

Mnemonics

1. Link

One of the main faults with mnemonics is remembering which mnemonic goes with which disease – so try to create ones with some meaningful connection

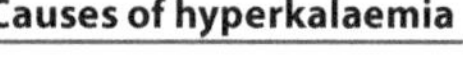

C.A.R.D.I².A.C².

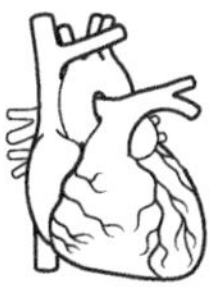

2. Order

Try to make the order of the items within the mnemonic approximate the order of importance or the frequency of occurrence

3. Consistency

Try to keep the same names between mnemonics to assist recalling what each letter stands for, e.g. use **T**oxins only, rather than sometimes **T**oxins and sometimes **D**rugs

4. Bend rules

Let's face it – you can't always make mnemonics that adhere to all of the above, so you will need to exercise artistic licence ... e.g. the '**B**' for 'hepatitis **B**' in **T.A.B.O².O².S².** (p. 152) and multiple entries for the same letter (denoted by a superscript number)

Cardiology

CHEST PAIN

Causes

C.A.R.N.A.G.E.

	Acute	Chronic
Cardiothoracic	**C**ardiac • Ischaemia: ACS • Pericarditis, myocarditis **A**ortic Dissection **R**espiratory • Pneumonia with pleuritis, TB • Pneumothorax • Pulmonary embolism • Pleural effusion	**C**ardiac • Ischaemia: Angina • Structural: Severe AS, HOCM **A**ortic Aortitis **R**espiratory • Bronchogenic carcinoma • Mesothelioma
Chest wall **Mediastinal**	**N**euromuscular • Herpes zoster **A**rthritic/musculoskeletal • Costochondritis	**N**euromuscular • Radiculopathic pain **A**rthritic/musculoskeletal • Chronic costochondritis • Fibromyalgia
Abdominal	**G**astrointestinal • Oesophageal spasm • GORD • Oesophagitis	**G**astrointestinal • GORD • Oesophagitis
Psychogenic	**E**xcitement • Anxiety attack	**E**xcitement • Psychogenic chronic chest pain

History Any symptom can be categorized exhaustively according to the following 4 logical categories, each of which has 2 convenient subdivisions:

- **When:**

  F.O.P.P.:
  First occurred (when + what were you doing then?)
  Onset (rapid/slowly?)
  Persistent (until present, or has now gone?)
  Pattern (continuous/episodic?)
  Ever had before? (first time or recurrent?)
- **Where:** Location
  Radiation
- **Character:** Type: e.g. pleuritic (sharp, localized, worse on inspiration); pressing; ache; burning
  Severity
- **Extra:** Aggravating/relieving factors
  Associated symptoms

Other history: PMH, e.g. arteriopathy (angina); immunodeficiency (pneumonia); SLE (PE)
DH: Thyroxine (angina), NSAIDs (gastritis). PH: Smoking (angina)
FH: Angina. SH: Travel abroad (pneumonia)

O/E

General: e.g. xanthelasma, fever, shingles, anxiety

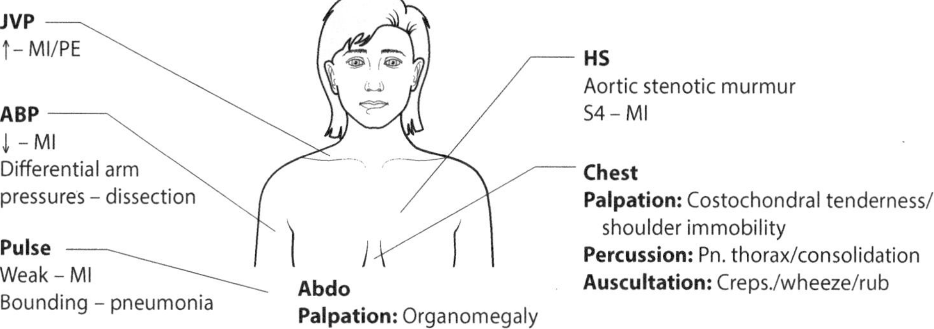

Ix

Bloods: WCC (pneumonia, cholecystitis)
Troponin (MI, myocarditis)
D-dimer (PE)
Urine: Glucose (diabetes – angina); blood (SBE)
Micro: Blood, sputum cultures, incl. for AFB
ECG: Angina/MI/pericarditis
Radiol: CXR: Pneumothorax/consolidation/dissection/pleural effusion/cancer
CT pulmonary angiogram or V/Q scan: PE
CT aortogram: Aortic dissection
ECHO: Pericardial effusion
Special: Looking for ischaemia:
Percutaneous or CT coronary angiogram
Myocardial perfusion scan
Stress echo
Looking for oesophagitis/GORD:
Upper GJ endoscopy
Oesophageal manometry

CARDIOLOGY EXAMINATION

4. Neck
Carotid pulse: Both; separately
JVP: Level + character
Other:
- Goitre; SVCO (distended veins)

3. Face – General
Eyes:
- Conjunctivae: Pallor, petechiae
- Sciera: Jaundice (CCF)
- Cholesterol: Xanthelasma, arcus

Mouth:
- Central cyanosis, dental caries

Cheeks:
- Flush (polycythaemia, SVCO, MS)
- Wasted (CCF)
- Plump (RSH failure)

Congenital syndromes:
- Chromosomal (Down, Turner)
- Connective tissue (Marfan, etc.)
- Myopathy (e.g. DMD, myotonia)

5. Precordium
Inspection:
- Scars (CABG, PPM, mitral valvotomy)
- Chest wall:
  - Ankylosing spondylitis (AR)
  - Pectus excavatum (ESM, R BBB)
  - Shield chest, wide nipples (Turner)
- Pulsation:
  - Apex = LV
  - L parasternal = RV

Palpation
Auscultation

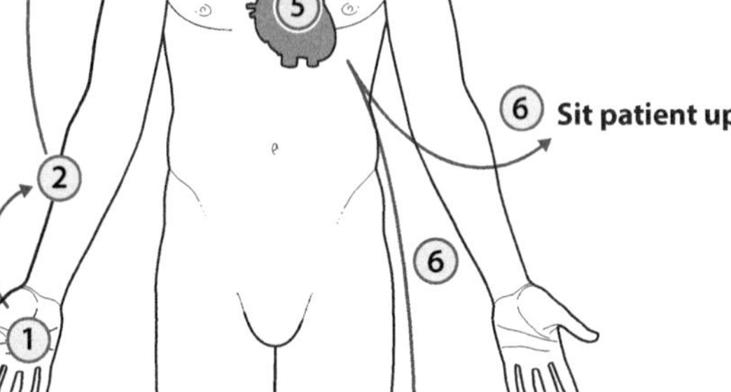

2. Pulse, ABP, RR
Pulse: Both radials; femorals; pedal x 4
ABP:
- Lying + standing
- R+L arm
- Pulsus paradoxus:
  > 10 mmHg ↓ on inspiration (cardiac tamponade)

RR: ↑ with CCF

1. Hands
Nails:
- Clubbing (SBE, CCHO)
- Splinter haemorrhages (SBE, vasculitis, trauma)
- Ouincke's sign (AR)

Fingers:
- Capillary refill
- Digital infarcts, Osier's nodes (SBE)
- Arachnodactyly

Palms:
- Temperature (CCF – cold)
- Erythema (Janeway lesions, polycythaemia, AR)

6. Other systems
Lung auscultation:
- Pulmonary oedema
- Pulmonary fibrosis

(ankylosing spondylitis, pulmonary hypertension)
Abdomen:
- Ascites, liver edge (RSH failure)
- Pulsatile liver (T R)
- Abdominal aortic aneurysm
- Renal bruits

Feet: Peripheral oedema
+
Fundi: OM, HT, Roth spots

7. AND FINALLY...
Temperature chart
Urine dipstick
BM stick (diabetes, SBE)

Pulse

Rate: Tachycardia (>100); bradycardia (<60)
Rhythm:

- Regular
- Reg. irregular: Bigeminy, Mobitz II AV block
- Irreg. irregular: AF, frequent ectopics

Volume (felt at brachial or carotid):

- ↑Bounding: Hyperdynamic circulation (fever, pregnancy, thyrotoxicosis, CO_2 narcosis, collapsing pulse of AR)
- ↓Thready: Hypovol. shock, LVF, AS, MS, MR
- Differential volume of R vs. L brachial: Dissection, stenosis, atheroma

Character:

- Slow-rising: AS
- Collapsing: AR, PDA, bradycardia
- Double:
  - Bisferiens = Mixed AR+AS
  - Bigeminy = Regular VEs
  - Jerky = HOCM
- Variable:
  - Paradoxus (↓a lot on inspiration) = cardiac tamponade
  - Alternans = LVF

p
d wave

Delay: R vs. L; radio vs. femoral = coarctation

JVP

Level: Normal: <3 cm above sternal notch. Causes of raised JVP may be classified according to the response to inspiration:

- ↓ on inspiration (normal response):
  - RSH failure/fluid overload
  - Bradycardia
  - Cardiac tamponade
- ↑ (Kussmaul's sign):
  - Constrictive pericarditis
  - Restrictive cardiomyopathy
  - Tricuspid stenosis
- None: SVCO

Character:

Waves: a c v
Descent: x y

a: Atrial systole
c: TV closure
v: Ventricular filling
x: Ventricular systole
y: TV opening

- **CAN**non waves: Big a wave + big x descent = atrial systole against closed TV
  Complete heart block
  Atrial flutter
  Nodal/ventricular rhythm (incl. pacemaker)
- Big a waves = RV filling ↓
  Pulmonary hypertension, tricuspid stenosis
- Giant a (single) waves = tricuspid regurgitation

Precordium – Palpation

Apex beat position:

- Normal = midclavicular line
- Displaced:
  - RV or LV enlargement
  - Mediastinal shift
  - Pectus excavatum, absent pericardium
  - Dextrocardia

Apex beat character:

- Heaving: Pressure overload = LVH, incl. AS, HT
- Thrusting: Volume overload = AR, MR, VSD
- Knocking: MS (palpable S1)
- Dyskinetic, rocking: LV aneurysm
- Double or triple ripple: HOCM
- Impalpable: Fat, fluid (effusion), air (COPD); CCF; dextrocardia

Heave: At either sternal edge = RVH or severe LA dilation, e.g. MS
Thrill: Palpable murmur over affected valve area

Precordium – Ausculation

Heart sounds

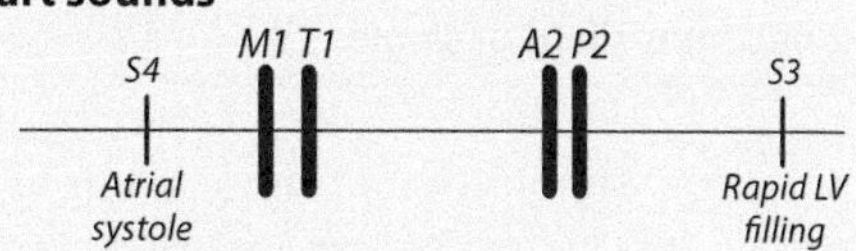

- S1: Loud (MS); soft (MR, heart block); wide split (normal at apex, heart block, VT)
- S2: Loud (HT, PHT); soft (aortic sclerosis, PS); wide split (ASD – fixed; VSD, MR – variable)
- S3: Volume overload: AR, MR, acute MJ
- S4: Pressure overload: AS, HT, HOCM; heart block

Added sounds

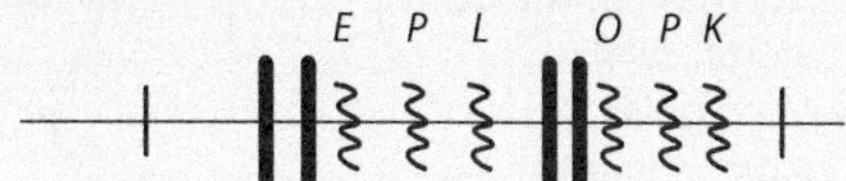

E: Ejection click (bicuspid AV – non-calcific)
P: Pericardial rub/click (pericarditis)
L: Late systolic click (mitral valve prolapse)
O: Opening snap: (MS, prosthetic MV, TS, ASD)
P: Plop (atrial myxoma)
K: Knock (constrictive pericarditis)

Murmurs (p. 6)

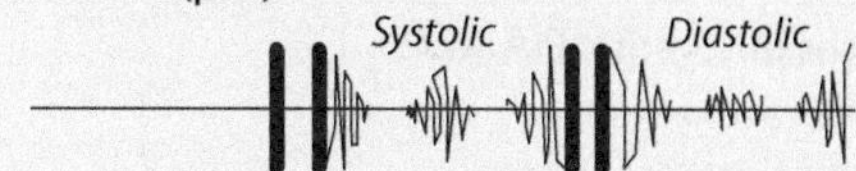

Early Sys: VSD, Ebstein's anomaly (TR)
Mid Sys (ESM): AS, PS, HOCM, coarc., ASD (flow)
Pan Sys: MR; late sys: MVP with regurgitation
Early Dias: AR, PR, Graham Steele (PR 2° to MS)
Mid Dias: MS, Austin Flint (aortic incomp.), MR (flow)
Late Dias: MS (pre-systolic accentuation) murmurs

MURMURS

Aortic stenosis

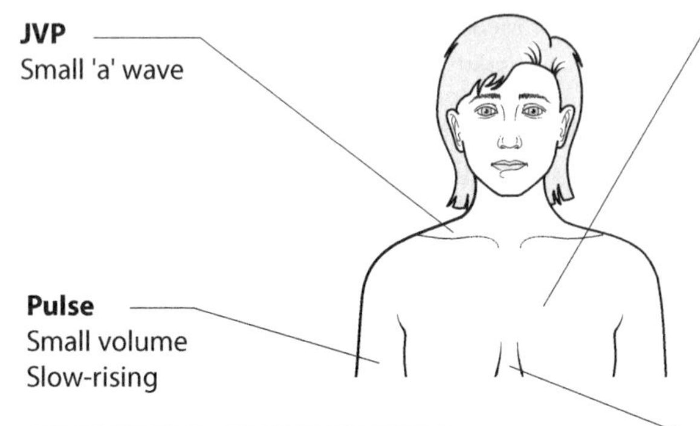

JVP
Small 'a' wave

Pulse
Small volume
Slow-rising

Auscultation
Ejection systolic murmer:
- Aortic area → carotids
- On sitting forward, on expiration
- Harsh

Ejection click: If pliable valves, e.g. bicuspid
S2:
- Single or reversed splitting S2 (due to delayed AV closure)
- Silent A2: If calcified valve

S4

Palpation
APB (apex beat):
Heaving, sustained, non-displaced
= pressure-overload
Systolic thrill at aortic area:
- On leaning forward, on expiration

Signs of severity: **P.A.M.S.**
Pulse pressure ↓/ABP ↓
Apex beat: Volume overload
Murmur: Loud (thrill) or soft (CCF)
S2 becomes silent or single

Aortic regurgitation

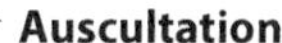

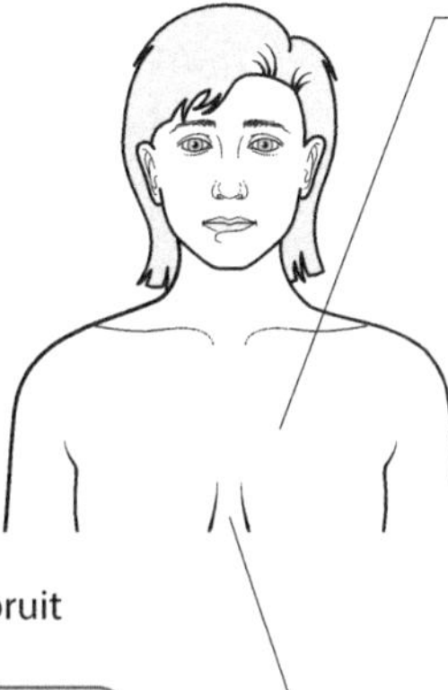

Pulse
Wide volume
(except in acute AR, CCF, or if hypertensive)
Collapsing pulse
or carotid shudder
Eponymous signs:
- Ouincke: Nail-bed pulsation
- Corrigan: Carotid pulsation
- DeMusset: Head nodding
- Traub: Pistol-shot femorals
- Duroziez: To-and-fro femoral bruit

Auscultation
Early diastolic murmur:
- LSE 3rd-4th ICS + tricuspid area (or RSE with dilated aortic root)
- On sitting forward, on expiration
- Blowing = chronic; musical = perforation

Other murmurs: Aortic incompetence
- Mid-diastolic murmur: 'Austin Flint' = anterior cusp of mitral valve hit by regurgitant stream
- Forward-flow systolic murmur

S1: Soft
S2: Soft, single
(cf. pulmo. regurg. = S2 + loud P2)
S3: ↑ LVEDP

Palpation
APB: Thrusting, non-sustained, displaced
= volume-overload
Diastolic thrill at LSE = acute AR

Signs of severity**: P.A.M.P.**
Pulse pressure ↑
Apex beat displacement
Murmur: length ↑
Pulmonary or peripheral oedema

Mitral stenosis

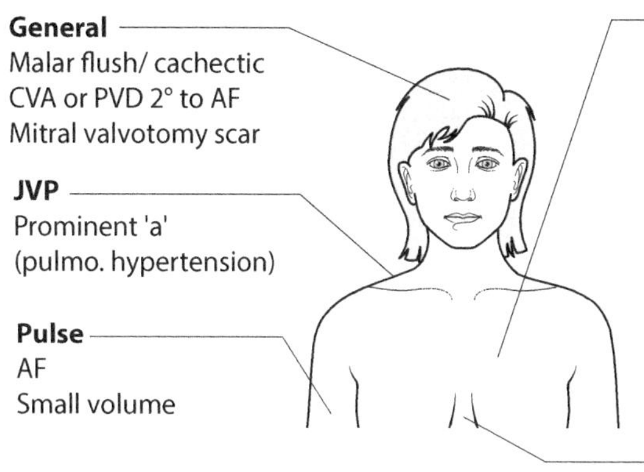

General
Malar flush/ cachectic
CVA or PVD 2° to AF
Mitral valvotomy scar

JVP
Prominent 'a'
(pulmo. hypertension)

Pulse
AF
Small volume

Auscultation
Mid-diastolic murmur:
- Apex
- Lean to left, on expiration., after exercise
- Rumble

Other murmurs
- Early diastolic murmur: 'Graham-Steele'
  = Pulmo. regurgitation loudest on inspiration
- Pre-systolic accentuation: If sinus rhythm

Opening snap: If pliable valves
S1: If pliable valves
S3: Always absent

Palpation
APB Tapping S1, undisplaced
Parasternal heave (LAD/PHT)

Signs of severity: **P.O.M.P.**
Pulse = AF, or systemic emboli
Opening snap – severity inversely prop. to time between S2 and OS
Murmur – length ↑ (except in CCF)
Pulmonary oedema or pulmonary hypertension (RSH failure)

Mitral regurgitation

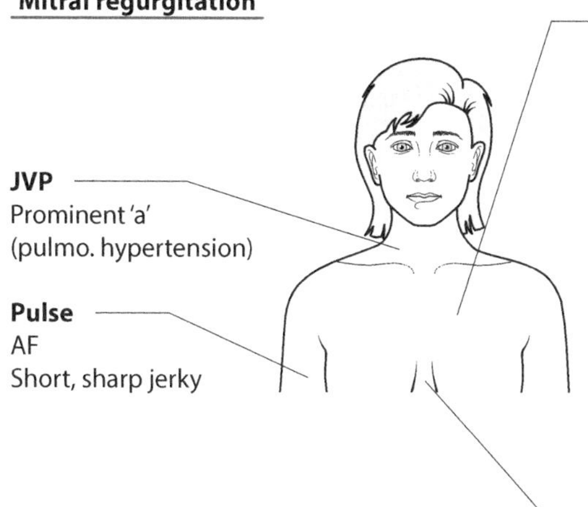

JVP
Prominent 'a'
(pulmo. hypertension)

Pulse
AF
Short, sharp jerky

Auscultation
Pan-systolic murmur:
- Blowing
- Apex → axilla (may be aortic area or spine)
- Lean to left, on expiration

Other murmurs: Forward-flow diastolic murmur
Mitral valve prolapse:
= late systolic click + subsequent crescendo decresc. murmur at LSE; make click louder + earlier by standing or Valsalva
S2: Wide splitting
S1: Soft,
S3: (↑ LADP)

Palpation
APB: Volume-overload
Parasternal heave:
= atrial dilation or pulmo. hypertension
Apical thrill

Signs of severity: **P.A.M.P.S.**
Pulse = AF
Apex beat displacement ↑
Murmur – becomes softer
Pulmonary oedema, or pulmonary hypertension (RSH failure)
S3 + soft S1; S2 = widely split

NB: Other murmurs:
Pulmonary hypertension (p. 98)
Congenital heart disease (p. 46)

AORTIC STENOSIS

Causes

Increasing age ↓

Congenital:
Presents in childhood; M:F = 4:1
- Valvular: 3, 2 or 1 cusp
- Subvalvular: Congenital ring or HOCM
- Supravalvular: William syn. = AS, Ca^{2+} ↑, elfin-like face ↓ IQ

Rheumatic fever
esp. females (*'tight-lipped' females*)
Rheumatoid arthritis: (Rare) due to nodular thickening

Atherosclerosis
esp. FH homozygotes

Bicuspid AV calcification (40–60 y):
EPI: Commonest congenital anomaly (1%)
PATH: Progressive mechanical stress leads to premature calcification
PC: Stenosis (1/3) + mixed (1/3) + asymptomatic (1/3)
ASSOC: Dissection; coarctation; Turner

Senile calcific degeneration (60+ y)
PATH:
- Initially, aortic sclerosis: Haemodynamically insignificant ring calcification
  O/E: ESM only, no radiation
- Later: Cusp calcification, renders them immobile

C.R.A.B.S.

PC

Angina
PROG: Survival = 2–3 y
AET: Due to O_2 demand ↑ but O_2 supply ↓

Arrhythmias
- Stokes-Adams
- Sudden death (8%)

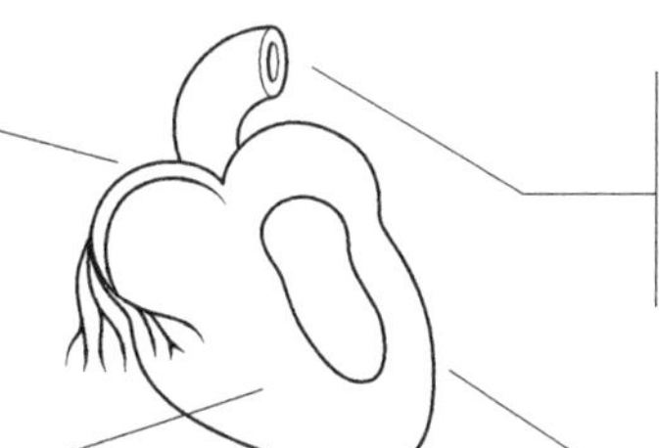

Exertional syncope
- Peripheral vasodilation
- Cardiac reflex
- Bradcardia/3° HB

Emboli, from calcified valve – TIA/CVA

Concentric LVH
LVF/RVF: Prognosis = 1–2 y

Ix

ECG:
- Pressure-overload: LVH, lateral strain, LAD
- P mitrale
- Heart block: Aortic valve calcification may spread to AV node

Radiol: CXR
- Calcified aortic valve
- Post-stenotic dilation
- LV prominence/LVF

ECHO:
- M-Mode: Thickened cusps; LVH
- 2D: Valve area reduced
- Doppler: High pressure gradient across valve

Rx

Medical:
Vasodilators contraindicated in severe AS (reduce preload)

Surgical:
Valve replacement – indications are:
- Symptomatic, esp. syncope or chest pain
- Valve area <0.5 cm^2
- Peak systolic gradient > 64 mmHg

Trans-catheter aortic valve implantation:
- For those not fit enough for open heart surgery

AORTIC REGURGITATION

Causes

Ring dilation

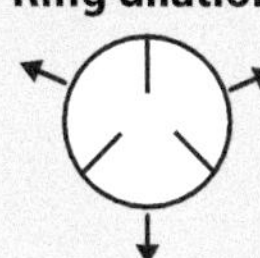

Ring dilation	Pressure	Hypertension, aortic dissection, dilated LV (e.g. dilated cardiomyopathy)
	Weak connective tissue	Hereditary: Marfan, Ehlers–Danlos syndromes Infective: Syphilis
Cusp contraction	Infection	Infective endocarditis
	Autoimmune	Seronegative arthropathies (ank. spond. reactive arthritis) SLE (Libman–Sacks endocarditis), RA
Poor fitting	Biscuspid valve	

Cusp contraction

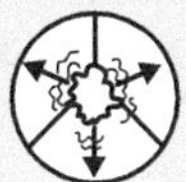

Poor fitting

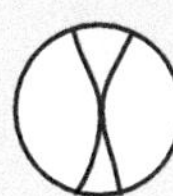

PC

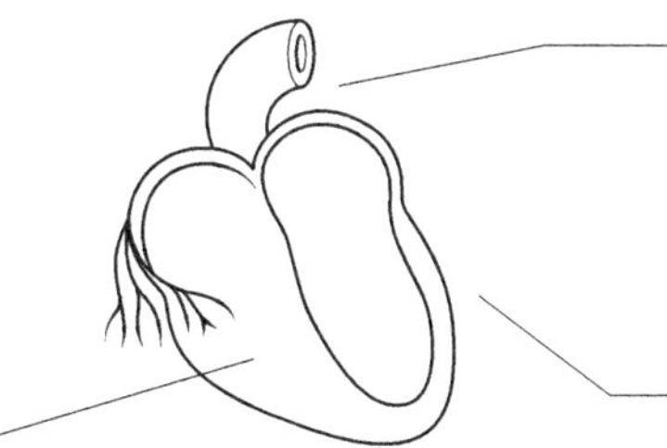

Emboli, from vegetation
- TIA: Amaurosis fugax
- CVA

Arrhythmias
- Sinus tachycardia
- Extrasystoles/AF
- Sudden death

Eccentric LVH
LVF, due to ↑ **LVEDP**
RVF

Ix

Radiol: CXR:
- Proximal aorta dilation
- LV → LA dilation
- LVF

ECHO:
- M-Mode: Dilated LV; flutter of anterior MV
- Doppler: Pressure half-time across the valve falls

Rx

Medical:
Nifedipine recommended, but avoid in heart failure
ACE inhibitors

Surgical:
Valve replacement – indications:
- Symptoms of heart failure
- Pulse pressure >100 mmHg
- Heart size on CXR >17 cm
- ECG: Lateral T inv: ST depression
- LV end-sys. volume >5.5 cm
- Ejection fraction <50%

Contraindication: Dilated heart (as irreversible)

MITRAL STENOSIS

Causes

Congenital: Rare
Rheumatic fever (esp. females)

PC

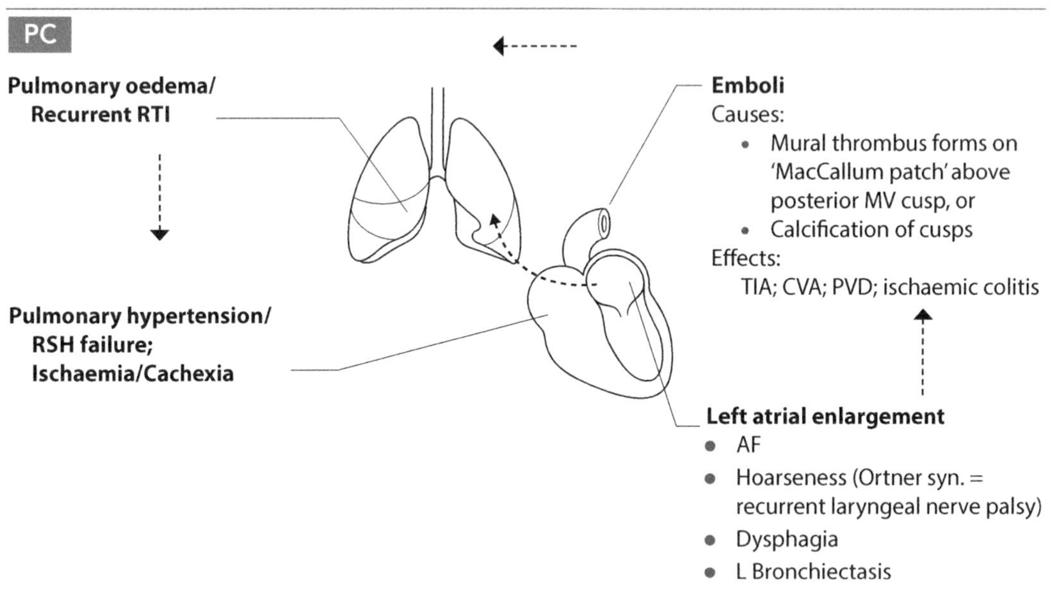

Ix

ECG:

- P mitrale (with sinus rhythm), AF
- RV strain (with RV hypertrophy)

Radiol: CXR:

- LA enlargement:
  - Loss of aorto-pulmonary concavity
  - Double R wall shadow
  - Splayed carina
- Pulmonary oedema → RV enlargement
- Calcified MV

2D-**E**CHO:

- Valve area: <1 cm = severe
- LA dilation ± thrombus
- RVH/RV enlargement
- Doppler: High pressure half-time across the valve

Rx

Medical:
Anticoagulate if in AF or LA thrombus present

Surgical:

- Closed valvotomy:
  - Intercostal
  - Percutaneous transluminal catheter balloon dilation
- Open valvotomy:
  - Median sternotomy
  - Allows ring insertion
- Valve replacement: Indicated if co-existing mitral regurgitation

MITRAL REGURGITATION

Causes

Ring dilation
- LV dilation ('functional MR')
- Connective tissue disorders: Marfan, RA, Ehlers–Danlos

Cusp degeneration
- Senile calcification of valve
- Immune-mediated cusp destruction
- Rheumatic heart disease
- Bacterial endocarditis

Subvalvular dysfunction
- Mitral valve prolapse

(C.R.U.M.P.L.E.)

Chordae tendonae rupture: Acute MI
Rheumatic heart disease
Unknown
Marfan
Polycystic kidney disease
Low BMI
Ehlers–Danlos syndrome

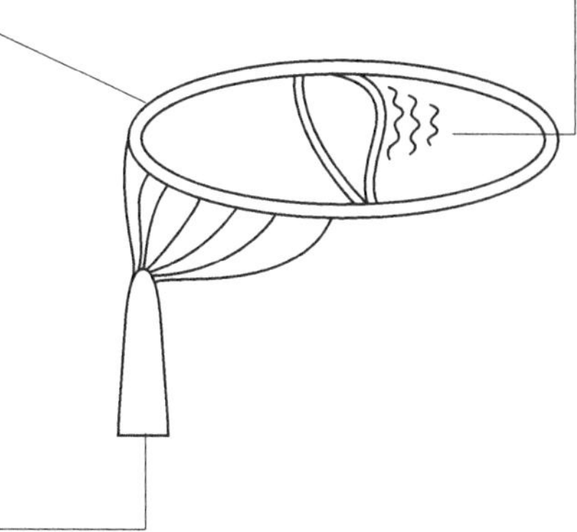

PC

Pulmonary oedema due to pulmonary hypertension
MVP:
- Palpitations
- Breathlessness
- Sudden death (due to VT)

Ix

ECG:
- P mitrale (with sinus rhythm)/AF
- LV strain (with RV hypertrophy)
- MVP: Inferior T wave inversion

Radiol: CXR:
- LA and LV enlargement
- Pulmonary oedema

2D-**E**CHO:
- Cause: Thickened/flail valves/MVP
- Volume overload of LV + LA

Rx

Medical:
Anti-coagulate if in AF

Surgical:
Valve replacement
IND: Deteriorating LV function (not asymptomatic patients, as the condition progresses slowly)

ECG INTERPRETATION 1

The ECG may be read either by instant pattern recognition (e.g. 'this shows fast atrial fibrillation; left bundle branch block; anterior infarction...'), or by adopting a systematic approach that includes all the sources of information an ECG trace carries. Novices to the ECG will have no choice but to use the systematic approach, but even when a learnt pattern 'jumps out' of a particular ECG, it is important to go over the ECG again, so as not to miss the smaller details.

ECG interpretation – 2 (p. 14) takes the reader through a comprehensive ECG analysis in a logical order. A guide to the use of this double page is outlined below:

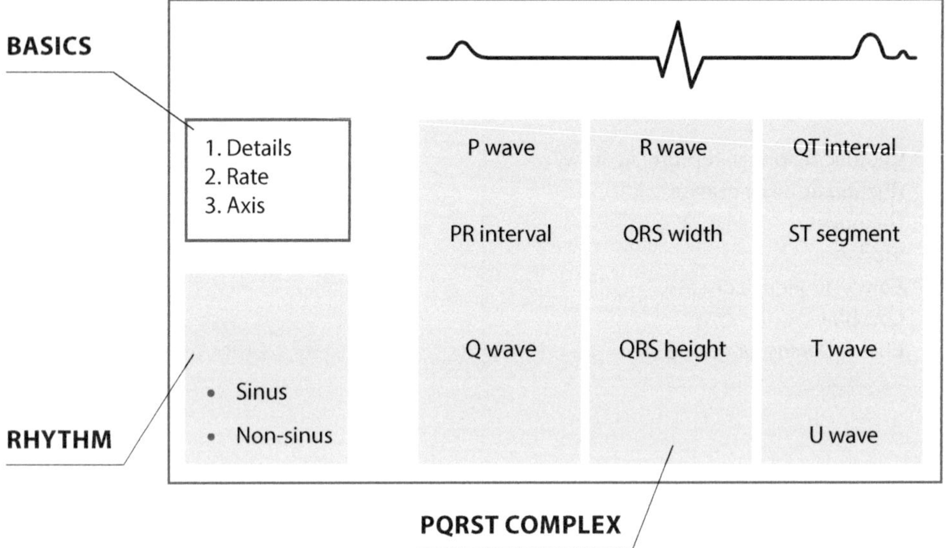

Tachycardias and bradycardias (pp. 14–23) provide an overview of most ectopics and dysrhythmias. Ectopics are beats that are interspersed randomly within a background rhythm. When frequent, ectopics may degenerate into an abnormal rhythm of their own.

Normal variants

Mostly 'to the right':
- R axis deviation
- R bundle branch block

Rhythm:
- Sinus arrhythmia
- Sinus bradycardia esp. in the young/athletes
- Extrasystoles: Ventricular or supraventricular

Other
- LVH voltage criteria (if very thin or Afro-Caribbean)
- T wave inversion in Afro-Caribbeans

Lead positions

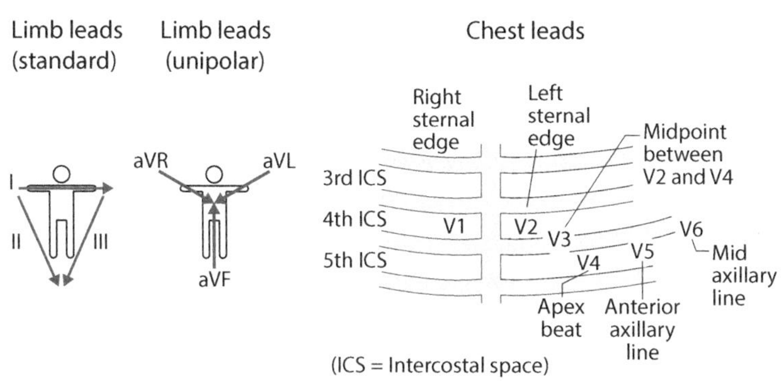

The 6 limb leads are 'virtual leads'

- Calculated by the ECG machine based on 4 actual leads placed on the 4 limbs, which are colour-coded
- **R**ide **Y**our **G**reen **B**ike (going clockwise round body)
  - Red – right arm
  - Yellow – left arm
  - Green – left leg
  - Black – right leg

Axis

The 6 limbs leads can be arranged as vectors. Lead I is designated as 0 degrees.

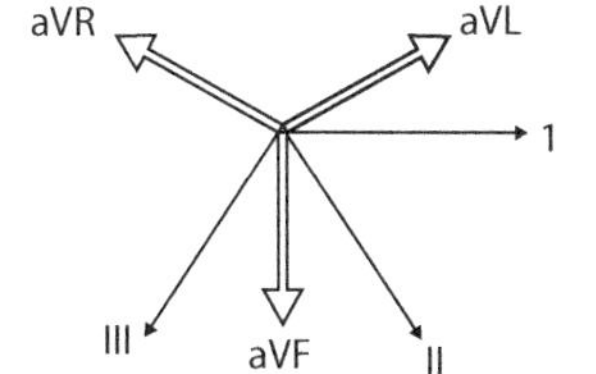

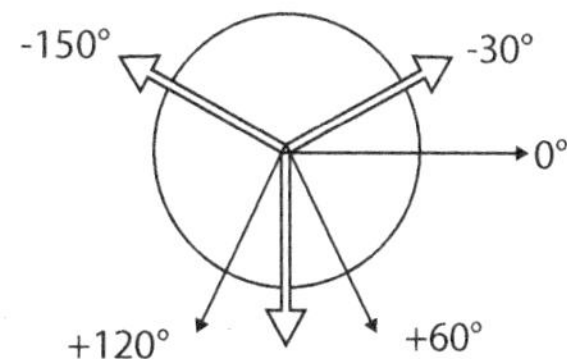

The axis is the general direction of depolarisation of the heart, from the sinus node to the Purkinje fibres. The vector diagram can be used to calculate the QRS axis. This can be estimated by noting the limb lead with the most positive complex, and reading off its 'viewing angle' as shown below. When two leads show equally positive vectors, average their corresponding angles. Leads with the smallest complexes lie at 90° to the axis, and leads showing negative complexes point 180° away from the axis.

A normal axis lies between -30° and 60°. A right axis is greater than 60° and a left axis is less than -30°.

Causes of right axis deviation = think 'R'

- **R**ight-sided heart (dextrocardia)
- **R**V hypertrophy
- **R**espiratory disease, e.g. COPD
- **R**ight bundle branch block
- **R**e-entry rhythm (Wolff–Parkinson–White)
- **R**elax! it's a normal variant

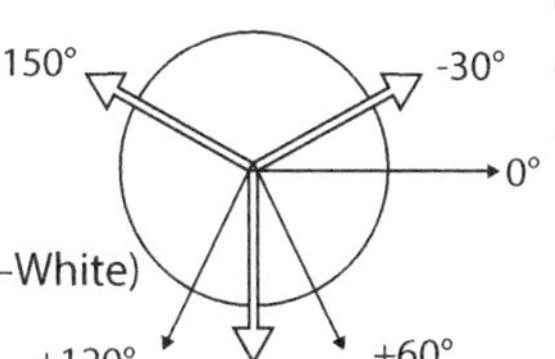

Causes of left axis deviation = think 'L'

- **L**eft anterior hemiblock
- **L**eft bundle branch block
- **L**V hypertrophy

PQRST complex

Normal ranges shown

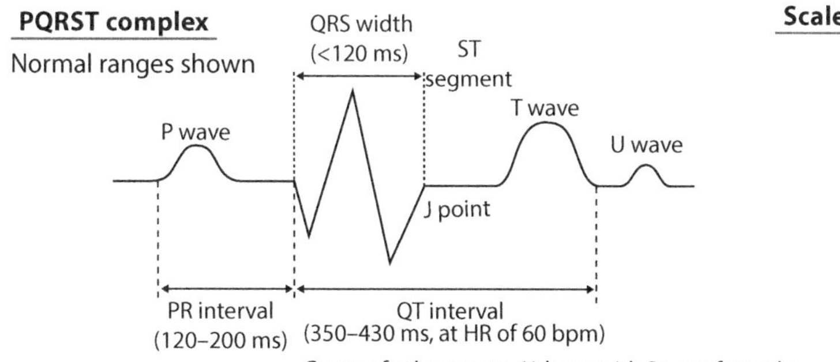

Correct for heart rate 60 bpm with Bazett formula:

$$\text{Corrected Q-T int.} = \frac{\text{Actual Q-T int.}}{\sqrt{\text{R-R interval}}}$$

Scale

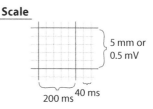

5 mm or 0.5 mV

200 ms

40 ms

ECG INTERPRETATION 2

Basics

1. Name, age, date, lead positions
2. Rate = 300/R-R interval (in big squares)
3. Axis

Rhythm

Sinus

- Sinus rhythm – clear p waves preceding every QRS complex
- Sinus arrhythmia – slight variation in heart rate with respiration
- Sinus tachycardia (>100 bpm)
- Sinus bradycardia (<60 bpm)

Non-sinus:

Escape beats:

- When another area of the heart generates the impulse
- Usually occurs when sinus node not working/ going too slow
- Types:
  - Atrial
  - AV nodal: Ongoing AV escape beats = nodal or 'junctional' rhythm
  - Ventricular:
    - Fast ventricular rhythm = ventricular tachycardia (VT)
    - Slow rhythm = idioventricular rhythms (occurs in complete HB)

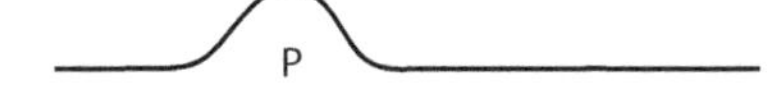

P wave

P mitrale (enlarged left atrium)

- Definition = m-like (or 'bifid') wave in lead II
- Cause: Hypertension, mitral stenosis

P pulmonale (enlarged right atrium)

- Definition = peaked P in lead II (>2.5 mm)
- Cause: Pulmonary hypertension, often due to chronic lung disease

PR interval

Long:

First degree heart block (delayed conduction through the AV node)

Short:

- Accessory conducting pathways:
  - Wolff–Parkinson–White syndrome
    Pathology: Bundle of Kent connects atria to right (Type A) or left (Type B) ventricles directly
  - ECG :
    - Short PR interval
    - Slurred upstroke of R wave = δ wave
    - R in V1; Q in III (Type A)
    - Paroxysmal SVT, esp. AVRT, AF

δ waves = slurred upstroke

broad QRS

inverted T

- DANGER! Rapid ventricular rate

Q waves

Significant Q waves =
>25% height of successive R (or >2 mm), or
>40 ms wide (i.e. >1 mm wide)

Causes: **I.N.C.H.E.S.**

Infarction, **I**nfection (myocarditis)
Normal: Septal Q, or disappear on inspiration
Conduction defect: LBBB, WPW
Hypertrophy: LVH/RVH/HOCM
Electrolytes: ↑ K^+
Sarcoid + other infiltration

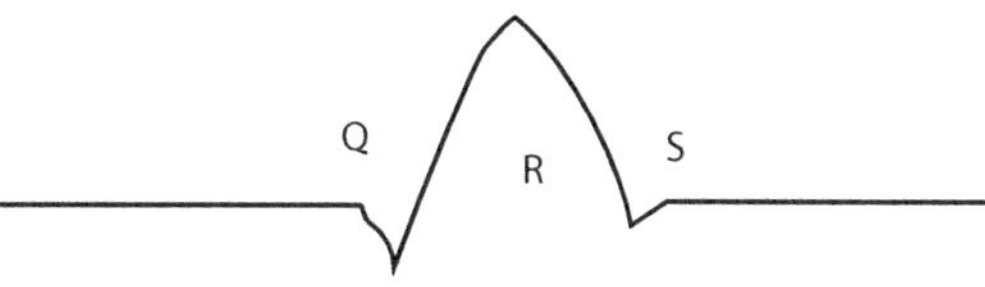

R wave

The (negative) S wave in V1 gradually transitions to a (positive) R wave across the chest leads from V1 to V3 – 'R wave progression'

Poor R wave progression = S wave dominant in ALL chest leads: Sign of chronic ischaemia or previous anterior MI

Causes of a dominant R wave in V1:

- R BBB (+ WPW Type A)
- RVH (+ myotonic dystrophy)
- Posterior MI

QRS width

The causes of a WIDE QRS are:

- Ventricular initiation: An impulse originating from the ventricle, e.g. VT, ventricular ectopic, idioventricular rhythm
- Wolff–Parkinson–White syndrome: Due to the delta wave
- Intraventricular conduction defect: Either right or left bundle branch block

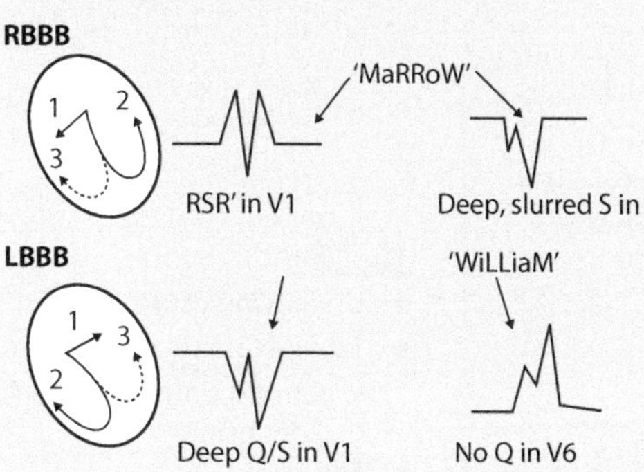

Fascicular block:

- Unifascicular: most common = Left anterior hemiblock = L axis deviation
- Bifascicular = unifascicular + R BBB
- Trifascicular = bifascic./LBBB + 1° HB

QRS height

↑Voltage (very tall/deep):

- LVH if S wave in V1 + R in V5/6 >35 mm
- RVH: Dominant R in V1 (normal QRS width)

↓ Voltage (very small complexes):

- Intervening tissue: Obesity, COPD, pericardial effusion
- Heart muscle weakening: Dilated cardiomyopathy, myxoedema

QT interval

LONG (>460 ms): → danger of developing VT

Causes = **T.I.M.E.**

Toxins:

- Anti-arrhythmics: Type Ia/III
- Antibiotics: Erythromycin, chloroquine
- Antidepressants: TCA, phenothiazines

Inherited:

- Romano Ward syndrome (autosomal dominant)
- Jervell–Lange–Nielsen syndrome (autosomal recessive) + deaf!

Mitral valve prolapse

Electrolytes: Hyp**O** = pr**O**long

- HypOcalcaemia
- HypOkalaemia
- HypOmagnesaemia

SHORT (<350 ms)

Causes: Digoxin, beta-blockers, phenytoin

ST segment

ELEVATION:

Infarction/ischaemia

- Acute MI:
  - >1 mm in 2 adjacent leads
  - Convex upwards
  - ST ↑ for <24 h; T inverts EARLY
- Vasospasm
- Ventricular aneurysm

Peri-, myocarditis:

- Concave upwards ('saddle-shaped')
- ST↑ for >24 h; T inverts LATE

LBBB/LVH in V1–2 ('high take off')

Brugada syn. = blackouts or sudden death, due to inherited Na channelopathy

DEPRESSION: (ST segment tries to **H.I.D.E.**)

Hypertrophy ('LVH strain pattern')

Ischaemia

Digoxin ('reversed tick' pattern)

Electrolytes: Hypokalaemia

T and U waves

Tented T: Hyperkalaemia

Flattened inverted T:

- As for ST depression (H.I.D.E.)
- Ventricular rhythm or WPW

U waves: Hypokalaemia

TACHYCARDIA

Narrow-complex = supraventricular tachycardia (SVT)

Sinus

Causes:

Shock
Haemodynamic circulation
Heart failure, incl. PE

Regular PR interval; P embedded in preceding T

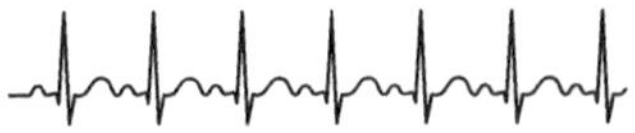

P rate 100–180 R rate 100–180 Effect of CSM= tempor. slowing

Rx:

Underlying cause, e.g. atenolol for anxiety

Atrial

- Fibrillation

Causes (p. 18)

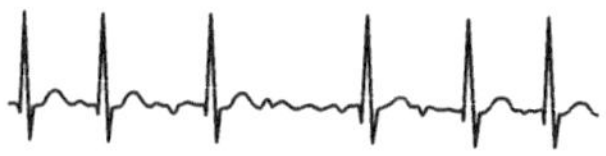

P rate 500 R rate 120 Effect of CSM= tempor. slowing

- Flutter

Causes – as for AF

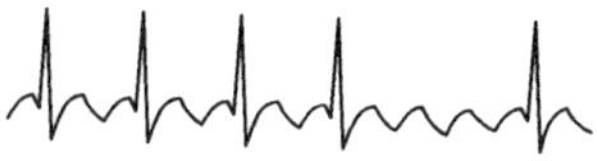

P rate 300 R rate 150 Effect of CSM= tempor. slowing

Rx:

- Underlying cause
- Rate control:
  - Digoxin
  - Verapamil
  - Beta-blocker
  - RF ablation
- Cardioversion:
  - Amiodarone, sotalol
  - DC 50–100 J
- Anti-coagulation

- Tachycardia

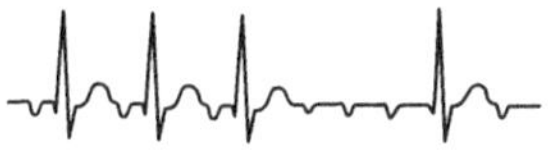

P rate 200 R rate 100 Effect of CSM= slows/terminates

Nodal

- AVNRE

Causes:

Idiopathic (majority)
+ as for AF

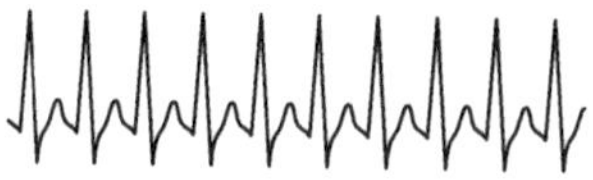

P rate 200 R rate 200 Effect of CSM= slows/terminates

P waves within/just after QRS
PR > RP′ (slow anterograde-quick retrograde)

- AVRE

Causes:

Wolff–Parkinson–White syn. (75% of SVTs in WPW)

- Appears similar to AVNRE, although QRS alternating amplitude at >200 bpm WPW apparent from δ- waves in SR trace
- Mechanism: Depolarisation spreads downwards via AVN, and upwards via accessory pathway (orthodromic)

Rx:

- Underlying cause
- 1st-line (assists diagnosis):
  - Carotid sinus massage
  - Adenosine
- 2nd-line:
  - Digoxin
  - Verapamil
  - Beta-blocker, esp. sotalol
  - Amiodarone
- DC 25–50 J + overdrive pace
- RF ablation

Broad-complex = ventricular or supraventricular tachycardia with bundle branch block

Ventricular

- Tachycardia

Causes (p. 20)

Independent P wave activity

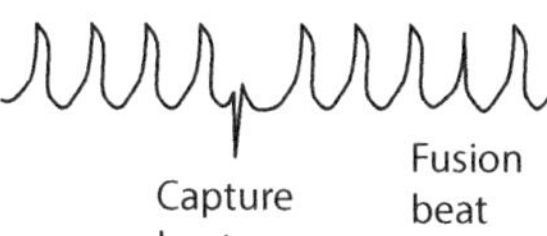

Rx:

- IV K^+, $MgSO_4$
- Lidocaine amiodarone
- DC 100 J

Ventricular tachycardia: R-R rate: 100–250, usually regular
Accelerated idioventricular rhythm: R-R rate: 50–100; Cause = MI, post-thrombolysis

- Torsades de pointes (polymorphic VT)

Causes:

QT interval >500 ms

Frontal axis slowly rotates

Rx:

- IV $MgSO_4$
- Isoprenaline beta-blocker (if congenital)
- Pacing

- Fibrillation

Causes:

VT
QT interval >500 ms

Rx:

- CPR!
- Epinephrine
- DC 100–360 J

SVT with BBB

- Intraventricular block (R BBB or L BBB) including K^+ ↑, subarachnoid haemorrhage

Rx:

As for SVT

- Pre-excitation (e.g. Wolff–Parkinson–White syn.)
  These SVTs are less commonly associated with WPW, but potentially more dangerous due to ↑ risk of R-on-T, and VF

Pre-excited AF (20%):
R-R rate 100, irregular

Pre-excited AFlutter (3%):
R-R rate 250, regular

Antidromic AVRE (2%):
R-R rate 200, regular

Rx:

- Drugs:
  - Fleicanide
  - Disopyramide
  - Propranolol
- DC 100J

NB: Avoid verapamil and digoxin as blockage of AVN ↑ anterograde conduction down bundle of Kent!

ATRIAL FIBRILLATION

Causes

A.T.R.I.A⁴.L. S.W.I.T.C.H.

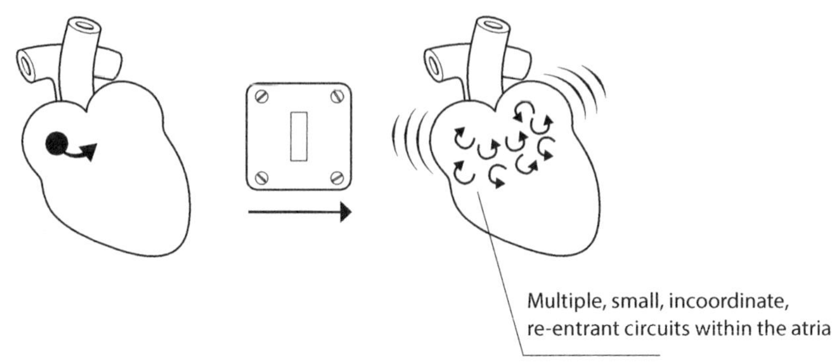

Acute: PE, MI, infection, post-surgery
Thyrotoxicosis
Rheumatic heart disease
Ischaemic heart disease – COMMONEST CAUSE
Arterial hypertension/**A**lcohol/**A**SD/**A**ortic regurgitation
Lung: Bronchial carcinoma, PE

Sick sinus syndrome
Wolff–Parkinson–White syndrome
Inflammation: Pericarditis (± effusion), myocarditis, endocarditis
Toxin: Digoxin toxicity
Cardiomyopathy esp. infiltrative disease, e.g. sarcoid
Hypokalaemia

PATH: AF arises because parts of the atria lose their refractoriness before the end of atrial systole, enabling recurrent but uncoordinated atrial activation. This may be due to:

- Atrial enlargement, e.g. CCF, rheumatic heart disease
- Conduction velocity ↓, e.g. inflammation, ischaemia, fibrosis
- Refractory period ↓, e.g. ischaemia, T4, sympathetic tone ↑

Management

Management is guided by 4 principles:

1. **Underlying cause**

   e .g. anti-hypertensives, thyroid medication, replace electrolytes

2. **Rate control**

- Beta-blockers (careful in asthmatics)
- Non-dihydropyridine calcium channel blockers (e.g. diltiazem, verapamil)
- Digoxin

3. **Rhythm control *aka* cardioversion**

- Chemical cardioversion: Amiodarone, flecainide
- Electrical: DC cardioversion with 100–200 J
  - If AF present for >48 h, must first anti-coagulate for 4 weeks
- Maintenance of sinus rhythm:
  - Antiarrhythmic:
    - Type III – amiodarone/sotalol
    - Type Ic – propafenone/fleicanide
    - Type Ia – quinidine
  - Radiofrequency ablation of left atrium to prevent AF recurring
- Indications: There is no difference in mortality rate between rate control and rhythm control, but the following groups are selected for cardioversion:
  - Acute – for cardiovascular compromise, e.g. hypotension
  - Elective – good chance of cardioverting, e.g. young, normal heart size, first episode

4. **Anti-coagulation**

- Mandatory in AF if **CHADSVASC** score >0 (or >1 in women) to prevent stroke:
  - **C**ongestive heart failure = 1
  - **H**ypertension = 1
  - **A**ge >75 = 2
  - **D**iabetes mellitus = 1
  - **S**troke/TIA = 2
  - **V**ascular disease = 1
  - **A**ge > 65 = 1
  - **S**ex **C**haracteristic (female) = 1

VENTRICULAR TACHYCARDIA

Appearance

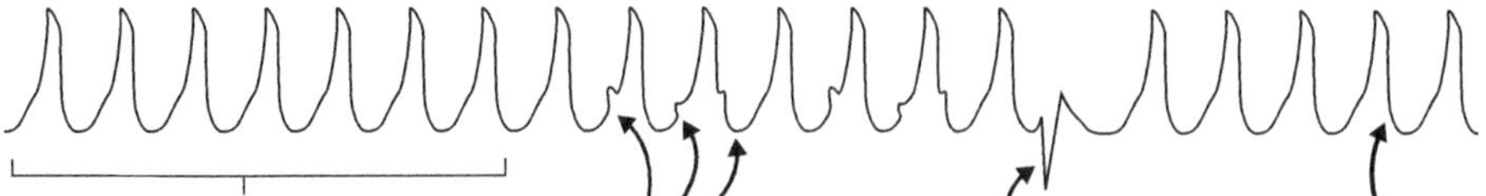

Broad-complex tachycardia: usually regular and monomorphic

Independent P wave activity

Capture beat: Normal QRS complex occurring earlier than expected ventricular beat

Fusion beat: Ventricle activated from 2 different foci, one of which is ventricular

Rate and duration

Ventricular tachycardia:	R-R rate: 100–250
• Ventricular ectopics, ventricular bigeminy	1–2 beats
Non-sustained VT	3 beats–30 s
Sustained VT	>30 s

Distinguishing features from SVT with BBB

Atrio-ventricular dissociation:
Independent P waves/retrogradely conducted P waves
On exam: Cannon waves; variable S1

Bundle branch block:

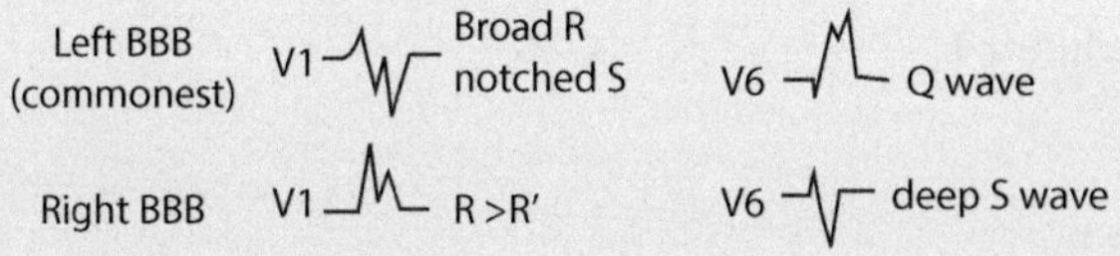

Left BBB (commonest)	V1	Broad R notched S	V6	Q wave
Right BBB	V1	R >R′	V6	deep S wave

Concordance in precordial leads

Duration of QRS complex: >140 ms (>160 ms if LBBB)

Extreme **LE**ft axis deviation with LBBB
or **LE**ft axis deviation with RBBB

Fusion or capture beats

History of ischaemic heart disease

Intervention: Carotid sinus massage and adenosine do NOT terminate
(Verapamil may induce VF if actually in VT!!)

Causes

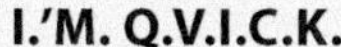

I.'M. Q.V.I.C.K.

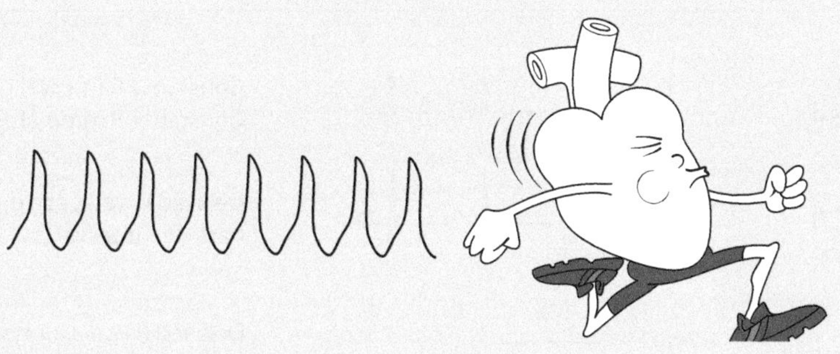

Infarction (esp. with ventricular aneurysm); ischaemia
Myocarditis

QT interval ↑
Valve abnormality: Mitral valve prolapse, aortic stenosis
Iatrogenic, e.g. digoxin, antiarrrhythmics, surgery
Cardiomyopathy, esp. dilated
K$^+$ ↓, Mg^{2+} ↓, O_2 ↓, acidosis

Management

Acute, unstable (hypotensive):

- Precordial thump (if witnessed and no defibrillation kit available)
- Synchronized DC shock 150 J

Acute, stable:

- IV K^+ to keep levels between 4.5 and 5.5 mmol/l
  IV Mg^{2+} 8 mmol bolus over 5 min → 60 mmol in 50 ml 5% dextrose over 24 h
- Chemical cardioversion: Amiodarone IV 300 mg/1 h, followed by 900 mg /23 h via CVP line
- Synchronized DC shock 100 J → 150 J → 200 J

BRADYCARDIA

Sinus or junctional rhythm

Sinus:

- Bradycardia

Constant PR interval of <200 ms
Constant PP interval

- Sino-atrial exit block

Delayed P wave, at a multiple of the basic P-P interval

- Sinus pause

Delayed P wave, out of phase

Junctional escape

No P wave, or
P wave immediately before, during or after QRS complex

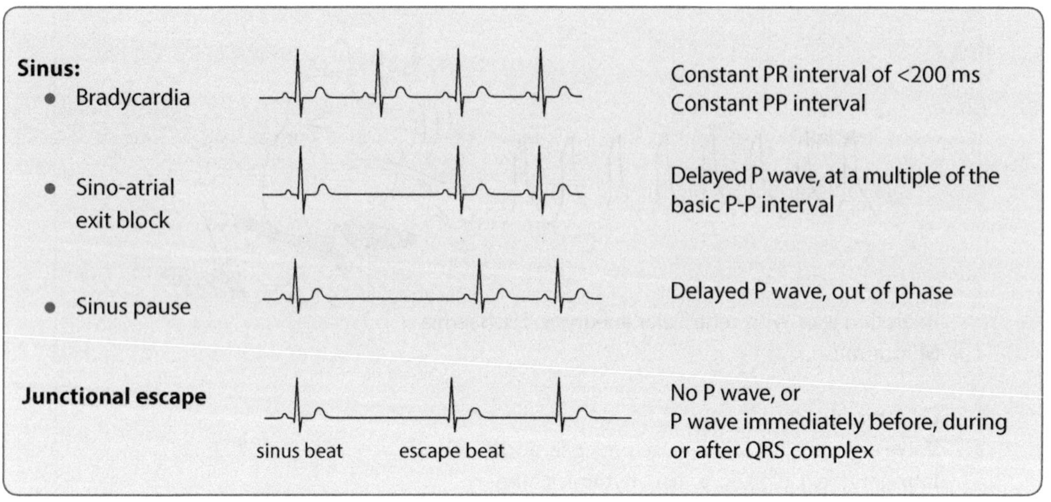

Heart block = AV conduction defect

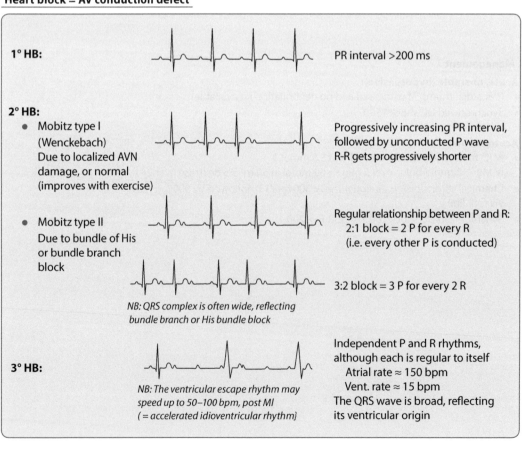

1° HB:

PR interval >200 ms

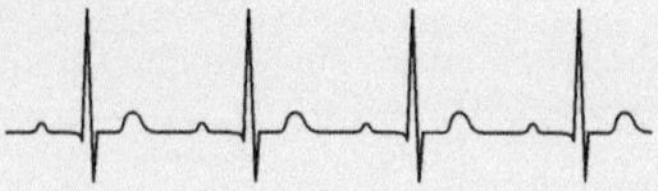

2° HB:

- Mobitz type I (Wenckebach)
  Due to localized AVN damage, or normal (improves with exercise)

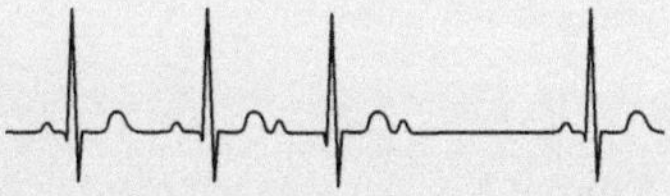

Progressively increasing PR interval, followed by unconducted P wave
R-R gets progressively shorter

- Mobitz type II
  Due to bundle of His or bundle branch block

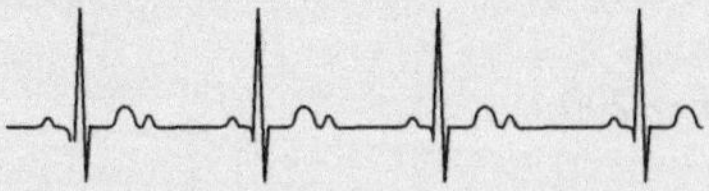

Regular relationship between P and R:
2:1 block = 2 P for every R
(i.e. every other P is conducted)

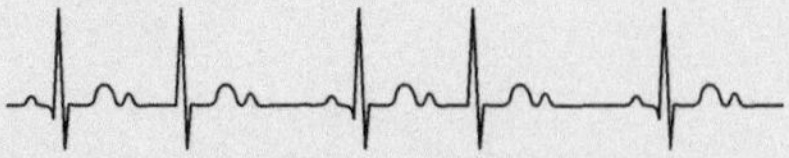

3:2 block = 3 P for every 2 R

NB: QRS complex is often wide, reflecting bundle branch or His bundle block

3° HB:

NB: The ventricular escape rhythm may speed up to 50–100 bpm, post MI (= accelerated idioventricular rhythm)

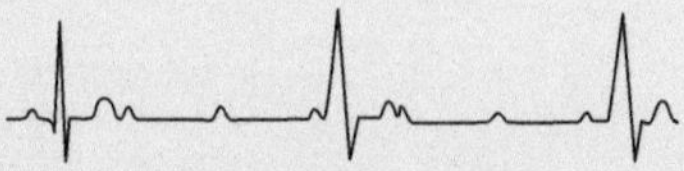

Independent P and R rhythms, although each is regular to itself
Atrial rate ≈ 150 bpm
Vent. rate ≈ 15 bpm
The QRS wave is broad, reflecting its ventricular origin

Causes

The rates are **D.I.V.I.S.I.O³.N.S**. of the usual sinus rhythm:

Drugs:
- Anti-arrhythmics (type Ia, amiodarone)
- Beta-blockers
- Ca^{2+} antagonists
- Digoxin

Ischaemia/infarction:
- Inferior (right coronary artery), or anteroseptal MI (if large)

Vagus hypertonia:
- Athletes, vasovagal syncope, hypersensitive carotid sinus syndrome

Infection:
- Typhoid, brucella (sinus bradycardia)
- Rheumatic fever
- Endocarditis, esp. involving aortic root
- Myocarditis (heart block)

Sick sinus syndrome = Tachy–Brady syndrome

PATH: Majority are due to senile amyloid or fibrosis of SAN, AVN and conducting tissue. May also be due to other structural causes of bradycardia, e.g. ischaemia, infiltration

PC: Comprises combinations of the following brady-tachyarrhythmias:
- Any of the bradycardias shown opposite, esp. sinus pauses, sinoatrial or AV block
- SVT, esp. AF with slow ventricular response; VT or torsades de pointes

Infiltration: Restrictive or dilated cardiomyopathy, esp. autoimmune, sarcoid, haemochromatosis, amyloid, muscular dystrophy

O: hyp**O**thyroidism, hyp**O**kalaemia (or hyperkalaemia), hyp**O**thermia

Neuro: Raised intracranial pressure

Septal defect: ASD, surgery or catheterisation (near AVN)

Management of bradycardia

Urgent
- Underlying cause
- Medical:
  - Atropine IV 0.6–3 mg
  - Isoprenaline
- Pacing:
  - External transcutaneous (using defibrillator machine)
  - Transvenous via a pacing wire

Elective
- Permanent pacemaker insertion
- Amiodarone when controlling sick sinus syndrome

ACUTE CORONARY SYNDROMES

Def

Acute coronary ischaemia, with or without myocardial infarction, due to unstable atheromatous plaque

Types

- Unstable angina
- NSTEMI
- STEMI

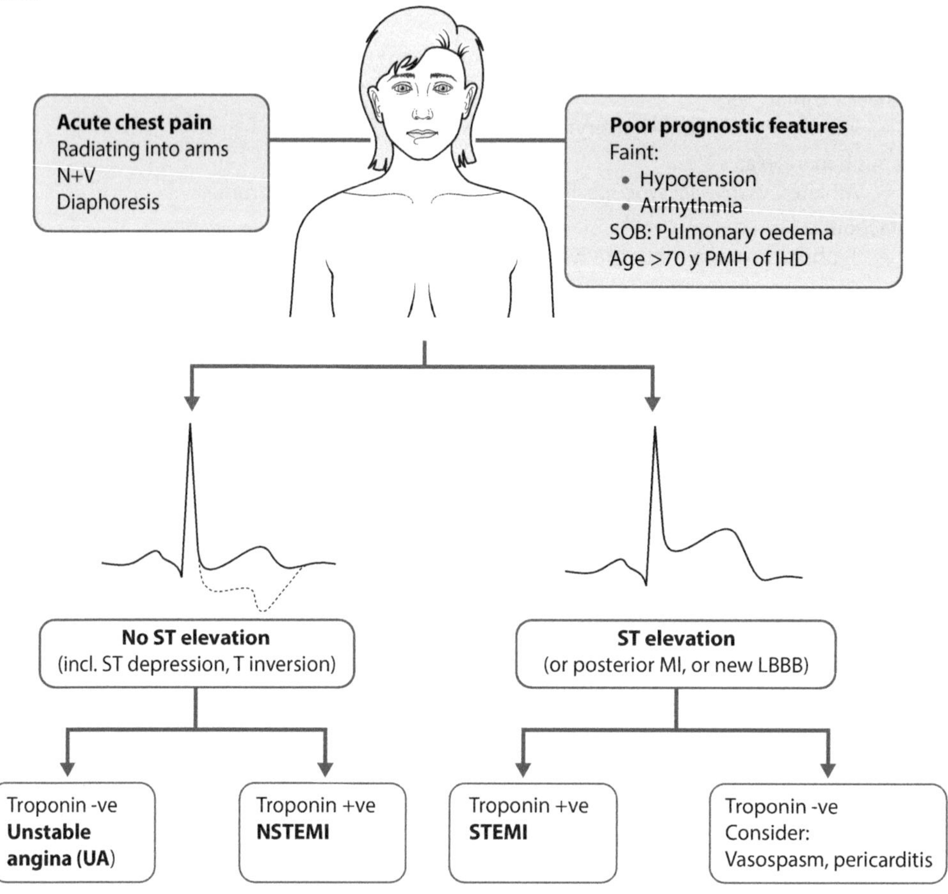

MYOCARDIAL INFARCTION – COMPLICATIONS

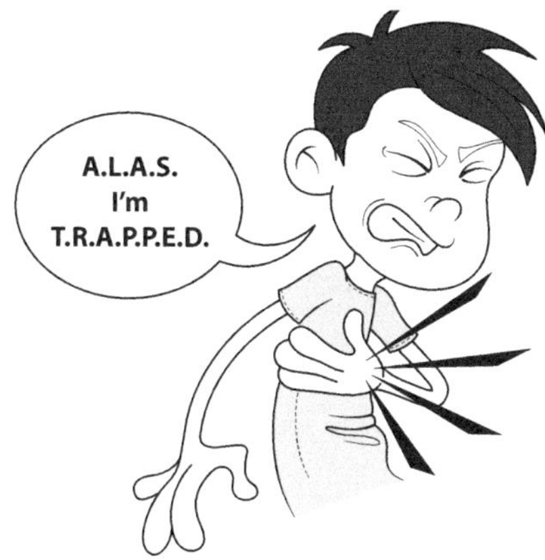

Arrhythmias (VT, VF, AF, heart block, esp. in inferior MI)
LVF or RVF failure
Arterial hypertension
Shock (cardiogenic)

Thrombus: mural/DVT
Ruptured:
- Septum (VSD)
- Papillary muscle/chordae tendinae (acute MR)
- Ventricular wall (cardiac tamponade)

Aneurysm, ventricular
Pericarditis: Early (<1 week) – infarction
Pericarditis: Late (2–12 weeks) – Dressler syndrome
Extension of Infarction
Death (e.g. due to VF, LVF, CVA)

Arrhythmias/heart block
Tachycardias

- SVT:
  - Sinus tachycardia – poor prognosis, if persists despite control of pain and heart failure. Treat with beta-blockers
  - AF or AFlutter – assoc. with LVF
  - Accelerated junctional rhythm, esp. inferior MI
- Ventricular:
  - Ventricular ectopics:
    - Frequent VPBs (>10/h) are seen in 70% of patients, in the first 3 days
    - Rx: Do not treat, unless they become sustained. Maintain K^+ >4.5, Mg^{2+} >2.0 mmol/l
  - VT, VF:
    - 1° VF (i.e. within hours), due to reperfusion; carries a good prognosis if corrected
    - 2° VF (i.e. after days or weeks), due to extensive heart damage, carries a poor prognosis

Myocardial Infarction – Complications continued →

Myocardial Infarction – Complications continued

Bradycardias
- Sinus bradycardia, esp. inferior infarction, due to diaphragmatic/vagus stimulation
- Ventricular bradycardia/idioventricular rhythm: SAN, AVN damage
- Heart block:
  - 1°, 2° (Mobitz Type I), 3° – associated with inferior MI (right coronary artery)
  - 2° (Mobitz Type II) – associated with anterior MI (left coronary artery)

Left- or right-sided heart failure
- LVF = anterior MI; RVF = inferior MI
  Treat with oxygen and diuretics

ABP ↑ : Hypertension
e.g. due to heart failure, tachycardia, pain, catecholamine response

Shock (SBP <100 mmHg)
Causes:
- Myocyte loss (>30%)
- Arrhythmia
- Pain
- Diamorphine, nitrate, beta-blockers

Thrombus
- Mural thrombi typically occur in a dyskinetic area of heart wall, or in AF → CVA/ARF/PVD
- DVT may occur in any bed-bound patient

Rupture of septum, papillary muscle, wall
- These typically occur after several days
- Both VSD and MR give a pan-systolic murmur

Aneurysm, ventricular
- A true aneurysm is a dyskinetic area of wall that becomes thin
- A false aneurysm is a cardiac rupture with adherent blood clot

Pericarditis
- Early pericarditis represents infarction of the pericardium
- Dressler syndrome is due to autoantibodies against sarcolemma + subsarcolemma of myocytes

MANAGEMENT OF ACS

ABCDE assessment

5 Ps

Pain: IV morphine and IV GTN infusion
Platelets: Give 300 mg aspirin and 300 mg clopidogrel
Pressure: Morphine and GTN often cause hypotension. Check patient not in shock
Vene**P**uncture: Check troponin, full blood count, clotting and electrolytes
Pulse: Give beta-blocker if HR >100 bpm

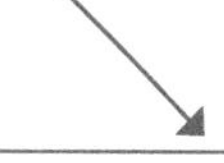

STEMI
Refer for emergency PPCI (primary percutaneous coronary intervention)

NSTEMI AND UA
Aspirin and clopidogrel 75 mg daily
LMWH (e.g. enoxaparin) bd for 3 days
Coronary angiogram before discharge

Secondary prevention

ACE inhibitors
Beta-blocker
Cholesterol (statin therapy)
Diabetic control (if appropriate)
Exercise (as part of cardiac rehabilitation)
Follow-up
Give up smoking!

SHOCK

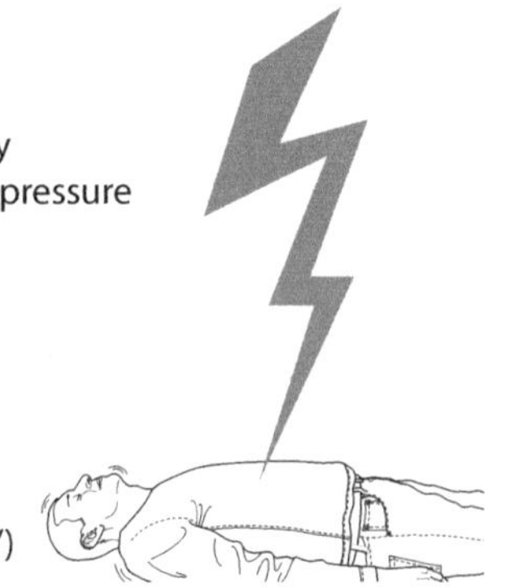

Def

Hypotension resulting in critical organ hypoperfusion. Incipient shock may occur with normal blood pressure, but with tachycardia and narrow pulse pressure (esp. in young people).

Remember:

BP = CO x TPR

and CO = SV x HR

and SV depends on good ventricular diastolic filling (= 'pre-load')

Causes

Cardiogenic

- Acute pump failure, e.g. acute anterior MI
- Arrhythmias

DESPITE INCREASING HR, CO DROPS DUE TO BIG DROP IN SV

TACHYCARDIA: RAPID HR LEADS TO DROP IN SV → CO FALLS

Hypovolaemic

Due to loss of either:

- Fluid – dehydration
- Blood – 'haemorrhagic shock'

DROP IN TPR AND SV LEADS TO HYPOTENSION

Distributive

Due to profound vasodilation:

- Septic shock
- Anaphylactic shock
- Neurogenic shock (loss of sympathetic tone)

VASODILATION CAUSES MASSIVE DROP IN TPR

Obstructive

LV unable to eject blood due to obstruction:

- Cardiac tamponade
- Massive PE
- Severe AS

HIGH AFTERLOAD AND LOW SV → DROP IN CO

PC

Non-localising: Dizzy, weak, light-headed or syncope

Localising, e.g.

- Chest pain: MI, PE, aortic dissection, gastric perforation, anaphylaxis
- Abdominal pain: Bowel perforation, ectopic pregnancy, DKA
- Back pain: Aortic aneurysm, pyelonephritis → urosepsis

O/E

General
Pale, grey (hypovolaemia)
Fever, sweaty (sepsis)
Red face + eyes, urticaria, stridor (anaphylaxis)

JVP
↓ : Hypovolaemia, septic
↑ : Cardiogenic

ABP
Systolic
Pulse pressure
Differential R-L arm pressure (aortic dissection)

Pulse
Fast (except if bradycardia is cause of shock)
Small, thready (hypovolaemia)
Bounding (sepsis)

Hand
Poor capillary refill (hypovolaemia)
Erythema (sepsis, anaphylaxis)

Auscultation
New murmur
Chest: Pulmonary oedema, pneumonia

Abdominal
Tender, guarding
PR: Melaena
PV: Tenderness, gravid uterus

Ix

Bloods: U&E (pre-renal failure); WCC and CRP (sepsis); LFT (liver failure); amylase (pancreatitis); troponin-I (MI); TFT; Hb (haemorrhage); FBC (anaemia – not acute blood volume loss); clotting; Group & Save
Urine: Volume (anuric, polyuric); glucose; ketones (DKA); β-HCG (pregnant, incl. ectopic)
Micro: Blood cultures
Monitor: BP; temperature; fluid-balance chart
ECG (arrhythmia. MI); ECHO (MI, endocarditis)
Radiol:
- CXR – pneumonia, pulmonary oedema, GIT perforation (erect CXR)
- CT–pulmonary angiogram – PE
- Abdo. USS – aorta, pregnancy

Special, e.g. OGD endoscopy

Rx

Septic: **'SEPSIS 6' B.U.F.f.A.L.O.**
Blood cultures
Urine output measurement
Fluid resuscitation
Antibiotics
Lactate measurement
Oxygen

Hypovolaemia: Haemorrhage: Red blood cells, fresh frozen plasma, platelets, stop the bleeding
Fluid depletion: IV fluid resuscitation

Cardiogenic: IV inotropes, high flow O_2, diuretics for pulmonary oedema, cardioversion if in unstable tachyarrhythmia

Anaphylaxis: **S.A.U.N.A. FLUIDS**
Steroid – IV hydrocortisone 100 mg
Adrenaline – IM adrenaline 1:1000 0.5 mg
Urgent anaesthetic review for airway oedema
Nebulized salbutamol 2.5 mg
Anti-histamine – IV chlorpheniramine 10 mg
FLUIDS High volume of fluid resuscitation

> **Septic shock** mandates transfer to critical care for vasopressors via a central line, e.g. noradrenaline

HYPERTENSION

P.R.E.D.I.C.T.I.O.N. *of arteriopathy*

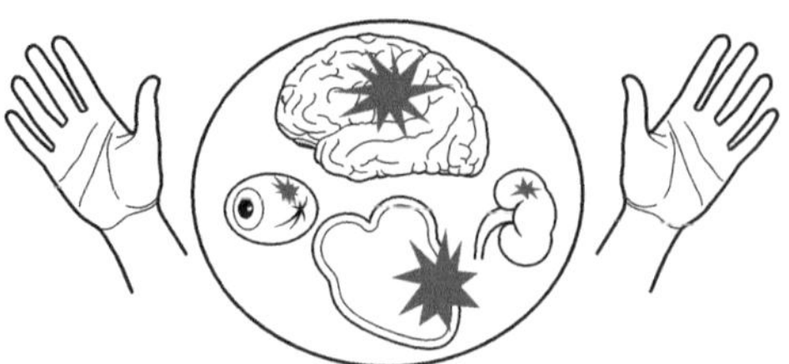

Causes

Primary

Essential: Risk factors

- Irreversible: Age, genetic
- Reversible: Exercise, diet (salt, alcohol, weight), smoking

Isolated systolic:

- Arteriosclerosis (elderly)
- Hyperdynamic circulation, e.g. anxiety, pain

Renal

- Vascular (e.g. renal artery stenosis, scleroderma, SLE)
- Glomerulonephritis, or tubulointerstitial nephritis
- Structural – APKD, tumour (e.g. Wilms, periangiocytoma)

Endocrine

- Hypercortisolism, e.g. Cushing disease
- Hyperaldosteronism, e.g. Conn syndrome
- Hyperadrenalism, e.g. phaeochromocytoma
- Hyperthyroidism, e.g. Graves disease
- Hyperparathyroidism
- Excess growth hormone, e.g. acromegaly

Drugs

- Drugs of abuse: Alcohol, cocaine, amphetamines (incl. adrenaline)
- Anti-inflammatory: NSAIDs (renovascular dysfunction), steroids, cyclosporin

Inborn errors of metabolism (porphyria)

Coarctation of aorta

Toxaemia of pregnancy = pre-eclampsia

Increased viscosity: Polycythaemia

Overloaded with fluid (iatrogenic)

Neurogenic: Autonomic neuropathy, diffuse brain injury, spinal section, thalamic stroke

O/E

ABP
Definition
- 3 measurements over 3 months (or 1 week if DBP >110)
- Cuff size >2/3 arm circumference
- 4th Korotkoff sound (i.e. muffling of pulse)

Factors
- Position: Measure semi-recumbent
- Time of day/temperature
- Activity/anxiety

Pulse
1. Rate: Thyrotoxicosis/phaeochromo, heart failure
2. Rhythm: AF (complication of ABP ↑)
3. Volume: Bounding (arteriosclerotic)
4. Peripheral pulses: Atherosclerosis
5. RF-Delay: Coarctation

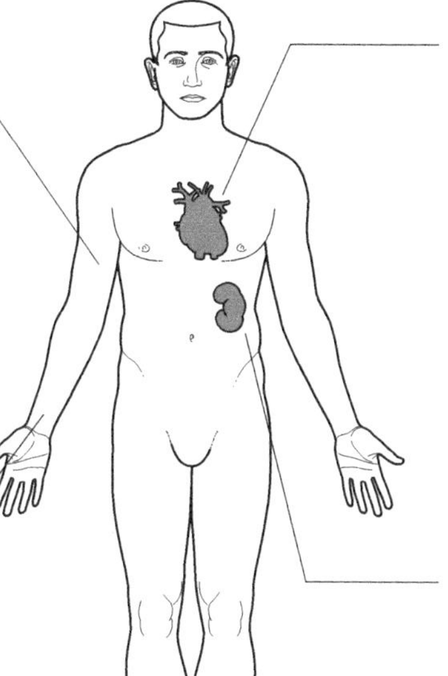

Precordium
Apex beat:
Heaving, sustained, non-displaced (pressure overload)
Heart sounds:
- Loud A2, reverse splitting
- 4th (later 3rd) ejection click

Murmurs:
- Ejection-systolic
- Aortic regurgitation

Lung bases:
Pulmonary oedema

Kidneys
- Renal bruit
- Palpable: APKD

End-organ damage – **C.A.R.N.A.G.E.**

Cardiac
- IHD, incl. MI
- lVH → later, CCF → pulmonary oedema
- AR, MR

Aortic
- Aneurysm
- Dissection

Renal
- Proteinuria
- Chronic renal failure

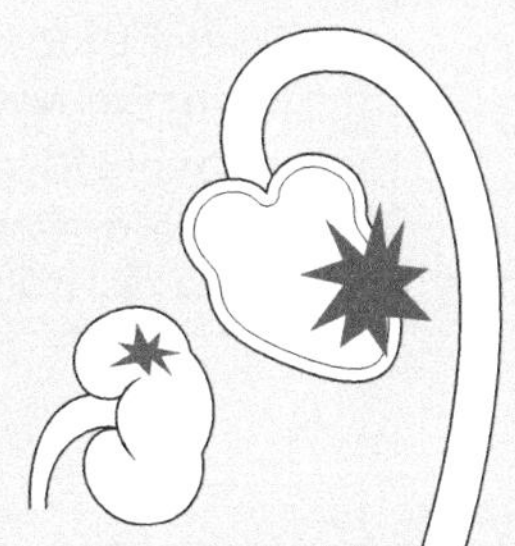

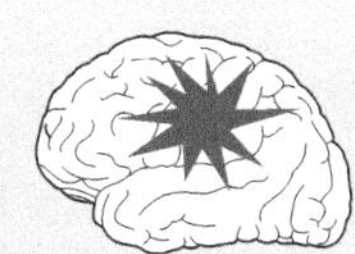

Neurological
- Ischaemic CVA
- Haemorrhagic CVA: Intracerebral, subarachnoid (berry aneurysm)
- Lacunar state: Dementia, parkinsonism
- Encephalopathy: Headache, dizzy, syncope, fits (posterior cortical oedema)

Anaemia: Microscopic angiopathic haemolytic anaemia (accelerated hypertension)

GIT: N+V

Eyes
Retinopathy grade:
- Silver wiring, tortuosity, irregular calibre
- AV-nipping
- Flame haemorrhages; hard exudates, cotton-wool spots
- Papilloedema
+ retinal detachment, retinal vein thrombosis

HEART FAILURE

Def

Inability of heart to pump blood at a rate commensurate to the metabolic demands of peripheral tissue, in the presence of normal filling pressures (cf. shock)

Epi

Prevalence: 2% at 50 years → 10% at 80 years. Mortality rate: 50% at 5 years

Causes

D.I.V.A. C.O.P

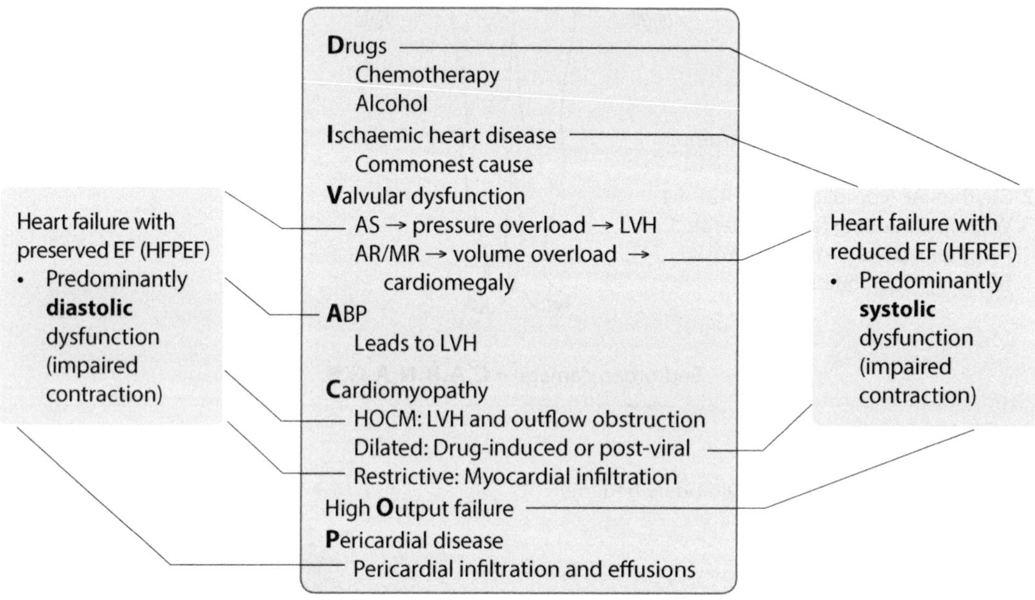

Drugs
Chemotherapy
Alcohol
Ischaemic heart disease
Commonest cause
Valvular dysfunction
AS → pressure overload → LVH
AR/MR → volume overload → cardiomegaly
ABP
Leads to LVH
Cardiomyopathy
HOCM: LVH and outflow obstruction
Dilated: Drug-induced or post-viral
Restrictive: Myocardial infiltration
High **O**utput failure
Pericardial disease
Pericardial infiltration and effusions
Heart failure with preserved EF (HFPEF)
• Predominantly **diastolic** dysfunction (impaired contraction)
Heart failure with reduced EF (HFREF)
• Predominantly **systolic** dysfunction (impaired contraction)

NB: High output failure - *Hyperdynamic circulation – i.e. uses up a lot of* $\mathbf{A^4.T^3.P^2.}$ *molecule***S**:

Anaemia, **A**lcohol (beri-beri), **A**VM (e.g. Paget), **A**ortic regurgitation
Thyrotoxicosis, **T**emperature, **T**oxins (e.g. salbutamol, diuretics)
Pregnancy (+ infants); **P**roliferative: Leukaemia, psoriasis; severe obesity
Systemic: CO_2 retention, cirrhosis

Pathogenesis of heart failure

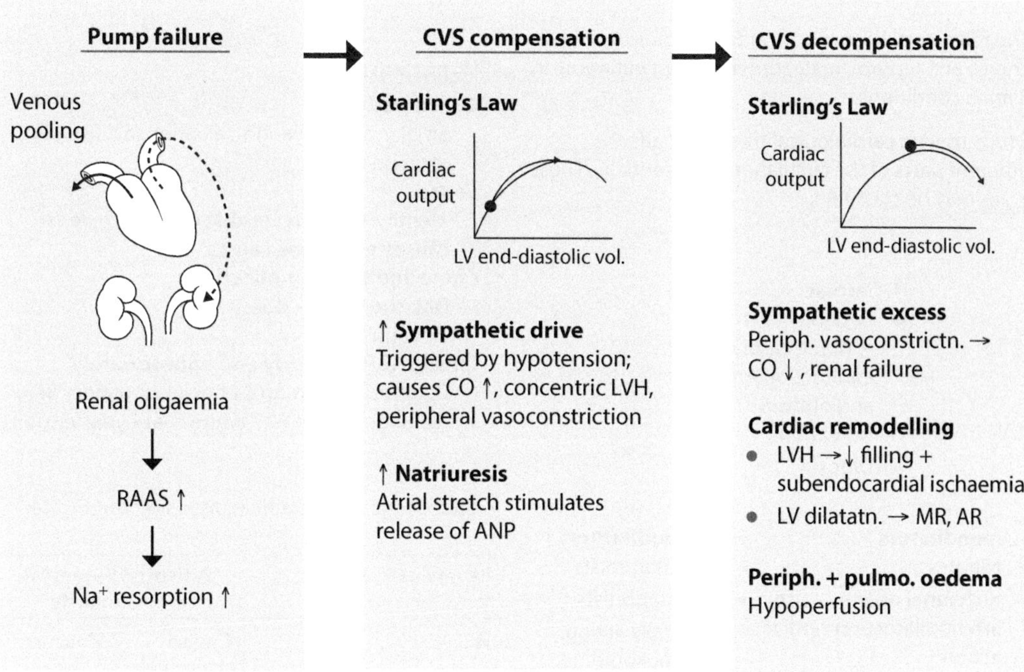
Pump failure
Venous pooling
Renal oligaemia
RAAS ↑
Na⁺ resorption ↑
CVS compensation
Starling's Law
Cardiac output
LV end-diastolic vol.
↑ Sympathetic drive
Triggered by hypotension; causes CO ↑, concentric LVH, peripheral vasoconstriction
↑ Natriuresis
Atrial stretch stimulates release of ANP
CVS decompensation
Starling's Law
Cardiac output
LV end-diastolic vol.
Sympathetic excess
Periph. vasoconstrictn. → CO ↓, renal failure
Cardiac remodelling
LVH → ↓ filling + subendocardial ischaemia
LV dilatatn. → MR, AR
Periph. + pulmo. oedema
Hypoperfusion

CARDIOLOGY TREATMENTS

The following diagrams are aides-memoires for the choice and (approximate) order of drug initiation, in 3 main conditions.

Drugs used in cardiological treatment affect different parts of the circulation preferentially. These areas may be classified:

1. **Cardiac**
   - Beta-blockers – inhibit cardiac contraction AND angiotensin formation
   - Digoxin

5. **Venodilators**
   - Nitrates
   - K-channel opener – also arteriodilator and cardiac action

2. **Arteriodilators**
   - Ca antagonists
   - α_1 antagonists
   - Centrally acting, e.g. moxonidine, methylDOPA

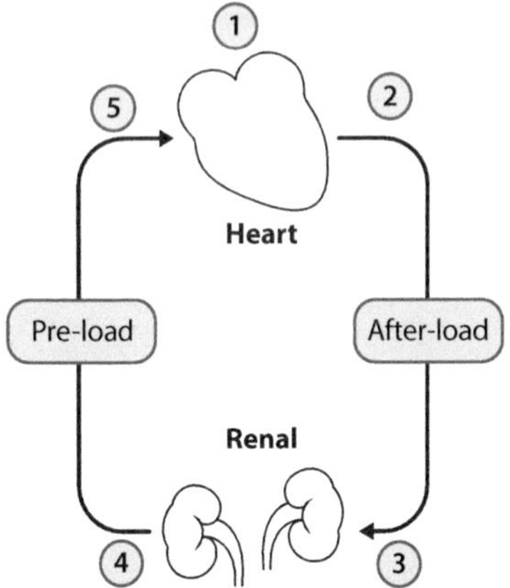

4. **Venodilators + renal**
   - Diuretics

3. **Arteriodilators + renal**
   - ACE inhibitors
   - Angiotensin-II receptor-1 inhibitors

Hypertension

Conservative
Smoking; diet (weight, alcohol, salt, fish oil), exercise

Cause
Identify + treat reversible causes, e.g. renal causes, endocrine causes

Comorbidity + complications
DM, cholesterol, obesity
TIA, angina

Check: ABP regularly and appropriately
Diagnosis based on 24 hour ambulatory BP readings (eliminates 'white coat hypertension')

Choose the right medications using ABCD rule:

Patient <55 years		**Patient >55 years OR black ethnicity**	
ACEI	**B**eta-blocker	**C**alcium channel blockers	**D**iuretics
10% develop cough and need to switch to ARB	Largely disappeared from managing hypertension	Dihydro-pyridines only, e.g. amlodipine	Thiazide diuretics, e.g. indapamide
Monitor renal function		Peripheral oedema is common side-effect	May cause hypo-natraemia

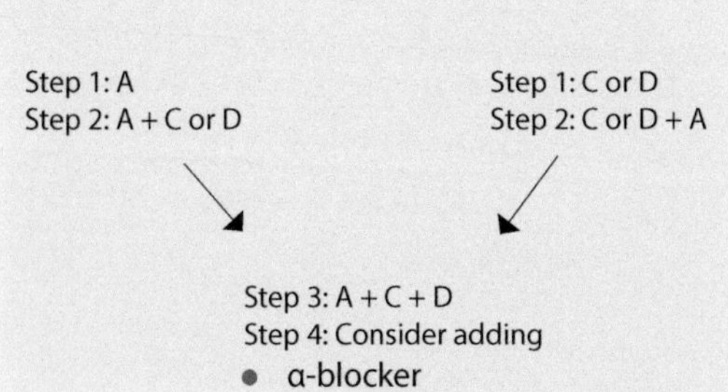

Heart failure

Conservative
- Smoking
- Low salt diet
- Cardiac rehabilitation (graded exercise)

Cause
- Identify + treat reversible causes, e.g. high output states, ischaemic heart disease

Comorbidity + complications
- Close glycaemic control in DM
- Tight BP control

Choose the right medications using **A.B.C.D.**
- **A**CEI
- **B**eta-blocker
- **C**holesterol control (statin)
- **D**iuretics – loop diuretic (furosemide) improve symptoms only

ACEI, Beta-blocker → **PREVENT CARDIAC REMODELLING AND IMPROVES MORTALITY**

Angina

Conservative
- Smoking
- Exercise
- Weight loss

Cause
- Identify + treat reversible causes, e.g. aortic stenosis, HOCM

Comorbidity + complications
- Close glycaemic control in DM
- Tight BP control

Choose the right medications to treat angina (GTN spray)

Choose the right medications to prevent angina

1st line **A.B.C.**
- **A**spirin (secondary prevention of coronary disease)
- **B**eta-blocker
- **C**alcium channel blockers (non-dihydropyridines, e.g. diltiazem) if beta-blocker contraindicated

2nd line **N.I.N.A.**
- **N**itrates (long acting, e.g. ISMN)
- **I**vabradine
- **N**icorandil
- **A**ngiogram and possible stenting

RHEUMATIC FEVER

Def

Autoimmune response to Group A beta-haemolytic streptococcus infection (– haemolytic streptococcus), occurring typically 2–3 weeks after streptococcal pharyngitis.

Epi

Inc: Rare in West; common in resource-poor countries
Only 3% of population are susceptible
Half of previous sufferers will develop recurrences after streptoccocal outbreaks

Age: 3–30 (esp. 5–15 y)
Children more likely to develop **C**arditis + **C**horea + **C**utaneous rash; **A**dolescents + **A**dults develop **A**rthritis

Sex: M:F = 1:1

PC

Diagnosis made by Revised Jones Criteria:

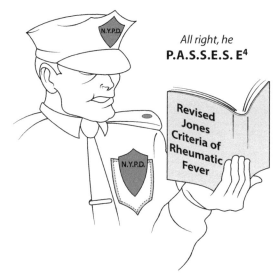

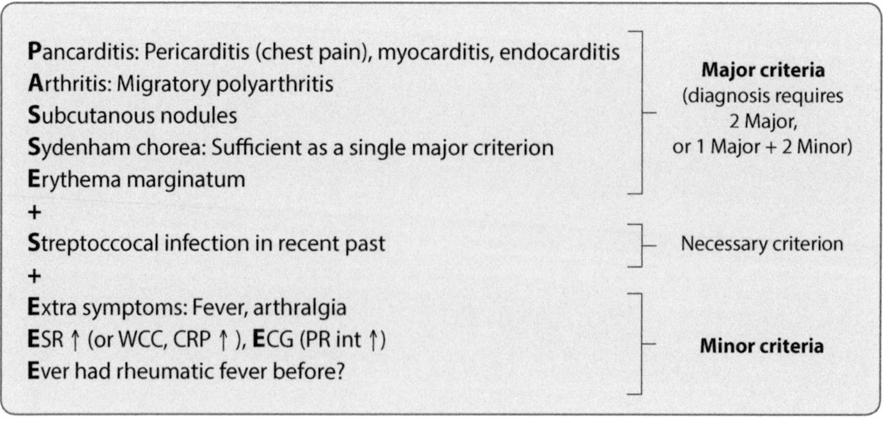

Pancarditis: Pericarditis (chest pain), myocarditis, endocarditis
Arthritis: Migratory polyarthritis
Subcutanous nodules
Sydenham chorea: Sufficient as a single major criterion
Erythema marginatum

— **Major criteria** (diagnosis requires 2 Major, or 1 Major + 2 Minor)

\+
Streptoccocal infection in recent past — Necessary criterion

\+
Extra symptoms: Fever, arthralgia
ESR ↑ (or WCC, CRP ↑), **E**CG (PR int ↑)
Ever had rheumatic fever before?

— **Minor criteria**

PC

Major criteria – explanations:

Pancarditis (60%)
- Pericarditis:
  - Chest pain
  - Friction rub
- Myocarditis:
  - PATH: Aschoff nodules = granulomas
  - Sinus tachycardia (nocturnal) or AV conduction block
  - Cardiac failure
  - CK↑, T inversion
- Endocarditis:
  - Acute:
    - Changing murmur
    - Mitral valvulitis (Carey Coombs' murmur = mid-diastolic murmur)
  - Chronic: Valve disease may present up to 50 years after rheumatic fever; 90% cases involve mitral valve

Arthritis (75%): Migratory polyarthritis
- Flits but persists symmetrically, esp. knees
- Effusions: Painful, red, hot joints
- Jaccoud arthropathy (non-deformative subluxations)

Subcutanous nodules (10%), esp. on elbows

Sydenham chorea:
- Grimacing, clumsy, hypotonia – stops during sleep
- Chronic: Tourrette syn; ADHD, parkinsonism (post-encephalitic lethargicum)

Erythema marginatum:
- Macules that extend centrifugally on trunk, thighs, arms (not face)

Streptoccocal infection in recent past:
- Scarlet fever
- Throat swab: Culture +ve
- Serology: ASO or anti-DNase B titre – ↑ by 200 U/ml

Rx

Medical

Penicillin: IM benzylpenicillin stat + PO penicillin V for 5 years, due to risk of recurrence (or erythromycin) + pre-procedure antibiotics if permanent cardiac valve damage as endocarditis prophylaxis
Steroids if severe

Symptomatic

Arthritis – high-dose aspirin, physiotherapy; pericarditis – aspirin; chorea – haloperidol

INFECTIVE ENDOCARDITIS

Def

Cardiac valves develop surface vegetations, that comprise bacteria and a platelet–fibrin thrombus

Types

Infective
Culture +ve

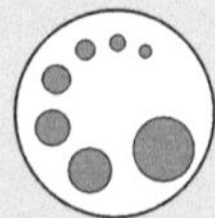

Streptococci
S. viridans: Oropharynx
S. bovis, faecalis: Bowel
S. pneumoniae
Staphylococci
S. aureus: IVDU, distant abscess
S. epidermidis: Prosthesis
NB: Poor prognosis
Gram negatives
Pseudomonas

Infective
Culture −ve

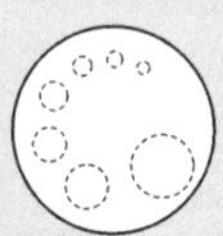

Pre-treatment with antibiotics
Fastidious bacteria
Nutritionally-dependent strep:
S. defectivus or *adjacens*
CO_2-dependent HACEK orgs.
Haemophilus, Actinobacillus
Brucella
Atypical bacteria/fungi
TB
Chlamydia
Coxiella
Candida

Non-infective
(Marantic)

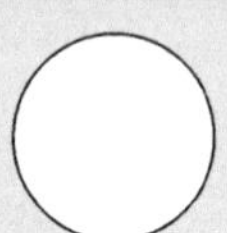

Autoimmune
SLE (Libman–Sacks)
Anti-phospholipid syn.
Rheumatoid arthritis
Rheumatic fever
Neoplasia
Adenocarcinoma
Atrial myxoma
Other
Thrombus on valve
Stitch on prosthetic valve

Predisposing

Pre-existing cardiac disease

Usually subacute

Congenital
VSD, PDA, MV prolapse, HOCM
Adolescent
Rheumatic heart disease
Elderly
Degenerative valvulopathy
Prosthetic heart valves
Early (<1 y): *Staph. epidermidis, Candida*
NB: Poor prognosis
Late: (>1 y): *Strep. viridans*

Haematogenous spread

Usually acute

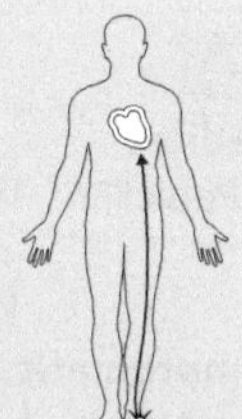

Infection elsewhere
- Dental caries
- Diverticulae, colon carcinoma (*S. bovis*)
- Pneumonia, UTI

Iatrogenic
- Dental, ENT procedure, GIT or GU endoscopy
- IV cannula, acupuncture
- IUCD insertion, labour

IVDU: *S. aureus* or *Candida*: Rt-sided endocarditis
Immunocompromised: DM tend to get *S. aureus*

PC

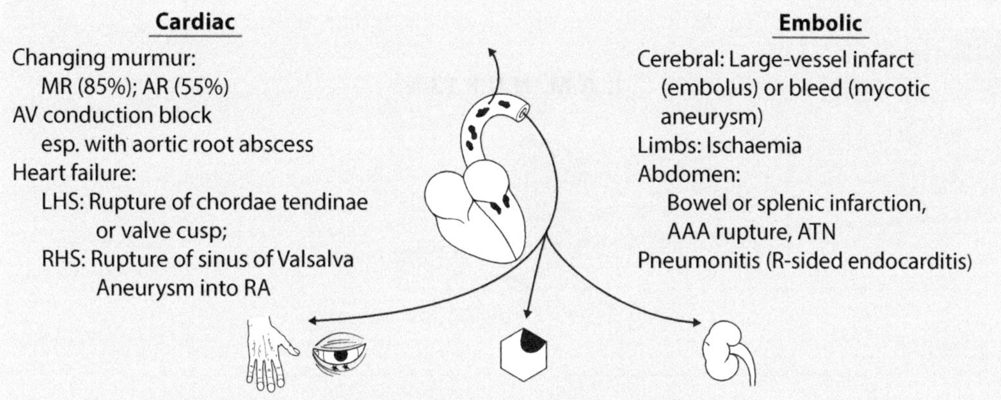

Cardiac

Changing murmur:
MR (85%); AR (55%)
AV conduction block
esp. with aortic root abscess
Heart failure:
LHS: Rupture of chordae tendinae or valve cusp;
RHS: Rupture of sinus of Valsalva Aneurysm into RA

Embolic

Cerebral: Large-vessel infarct (embolus) or bleed (mycotic aneurysm)
Limbs: Ischaemia
Abdomen:
Bowel or splenic infarction, AAA rupture, ATN
Pneumonitis (R-sided endocarditis)

Peripheral

Hands:
- Splinter haemorrhages
- Osler nodes:
  - Painful, purple papules on finger pulp
- Janeway lesions: Palmar macules
- Clubbing

Eyes:
- Conjunctival haemorrhages
- Roth spots = retinal infarct + bleed

Constitutional

Fever
Splenomegaly
Weight loss
Arthralgia, myalgia, arthritis

Renal

Microscopic haematuria:
- Due to proliferative glomerulonephritis
- Also proteinuria, reversible renal failure

Murmur, fever, splenomegaly, haematuria = most reliable signs

Ix

Bloods: N. chromic N. cytic anaemia; ESR ↑, CRP ↑
Urine: Microscopic haematuria, RBC casts
Micro: Blood cultures × 3 serology for atypical organisms
Monitor: Temperature, murmur
ECG: Heart block
ECHO: Trans-thoracic or TOE – detects vegetations >3 mm
Radiol: CXR – cardiomegaly, pulmonary oedema

Rx

Medical:

Antibiotics for 6 weeks:
- Blind or streptococci: Benzylpenicillin + gentamicin (IV for 2 weeks)
- Staphylococci suspected: Flucloxacillin + gentamicin (and/or vancomycin, rifampicin)

Surgical:

IND: Acute heart failure, emboli, prosthetic valve

PERICARDIAL DISEASE

Causes

I. A.M. H.U.R.T.I.N.'

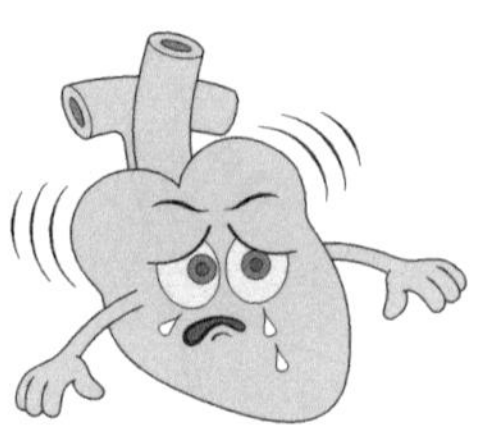

Infection:
- Viruses, esp. coxsackie, echo, EBV, influenza, HIV
- Bacteria: *Strep. pneumoniae*, mycoplasma, TB, rheumatic fever
- Other: Fungal (candida, aspergillosis), protozoal (toxoplasmosis)

Autoimmune: Rheumatoid arthritis, SLE, scleroderma, PAN

Myocardial Infarction:
- Early: Self-limiting
- Late (2–12 weeks): 'Dressler syn.' – anti-myocardial Abs

Haemorrhage:
- Aortic dissection
- Rupture: Trauma, MI, catheterisation, cardiac surgery

Uraemia

Radiotherapy: Acute or chronic pericarditis

Thyroid ↓/cholesterol ↑

Iatrogenic: Procainamide, hydralazine

Neoplasia:
- Local: Lung cancer, thymoma
- Systemic: Metastases, leukaemia, lymphoma
- Amyloid

Rx

Conservative: Bed-rest, avoid anti-coagulants

Symptomatic: NSAIDS (aspirin, naproxen)
Colchicine
Prednisolone

Pericardiectomy for multiple, recurrent episodes of pericarditis

PC

Pericarditis

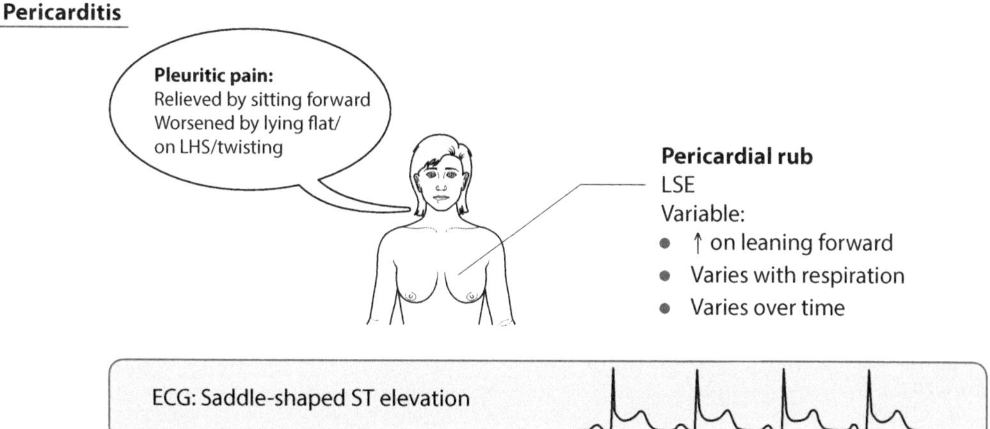

Pericardial effusion → cardiac tamponade

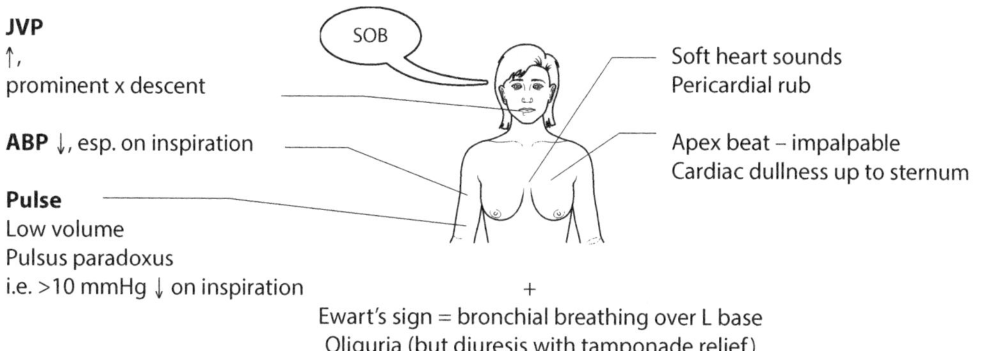

+

Ewart's sign = bronchial breathing over L base

Oliguria (but diuresis with tamponade relief)

NB: Sx most prominent in tamponade

CXR Symmetric, globular heart
ECG Low voltage or 'electrical alternans' (alternating QRS amplitude)

Constrictive pericarditis

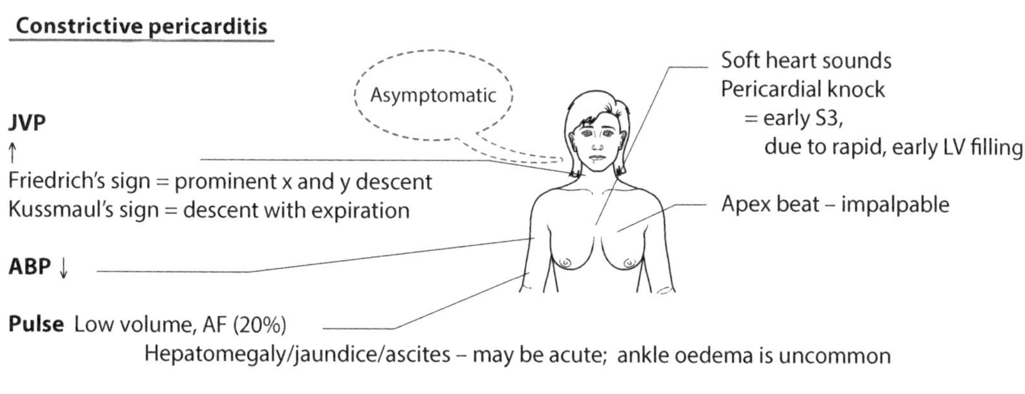

Hepatomegaly/jaundice/ascites – may be acute; ankle oedema is uncommon

CXR Calcification of posterior border (lateral CXR) = TB
ECG Low voltage and T inversion

MYOCARDITIS

Causes

Infection
Viral:
- Enterovirus, esp. coxsackie B
- HIV

Bacteria:
- *S. aureus* (complication of staphylococcal endocarditis – abscess of valve ring or septum)
- Diphtheria toxin
- Lyme disease: Often requires a temporary pacemaker

Protozoa:
- Chagas
- Toxoplasmosis

Autoimmune: Giant cell myocarditis – assoc. with SLE, thymoma, thyrotoxicosis
Iatrogenic: Toxins, radiation, trauma

PC

Viral myocarditis
- Prodromal flu-like symptoms, e.g. fever, sore throat, myalgia (may co-exist with Bornholm disease)
- Chest pain
- Contact with other cases (epidemic)
- Arrhythmias, ↑ by exertion
- Heart failure: Acute, or dilated cardiomyopathy (10%)

O/E

Pyrexia

JVP May be ↑

ABP May be ↓

Pulse
Rapid + feeble
AF

Heart sounds
Muffled S1
S3
Pan-systolic murmur (MR)
Pericardial rub
(if coexisting pericarditis)

Apex Palpable

± Pulmonary oedema

Ix

Bloods: Massive rise in troponin
Micro: Throat swab + stool sample virology cultures
ECG: Widespread ST depression; T inversion

Rx

Symptomatic only

MYXOMA

Epi

Inc: Commonest 1° cardiac tumour
Age: 50–60s (except familial syndromes – present <30 y)
Sex: Females 70%
Assoc: Familial (AD) in 7%: The Carney Complex of Syndromes:

- **NAME syn.**: **N**aevi, **A**trial myxoma, **M**yxoid neurofibromas, **E**phelides (facial freckles)
- **LAMB syn.**: **L**entigines, **A**trial **M**yxoma, **B**lue naevi
- Multiple tumours

PATH: Location: L atrium, in fossa ovalis – 90%
Solitary
Gelatinous, friable, attached by pedicle to fossa ovalis

PC

F.L.E.C.K.S. *fall off*

Failure, cardiac: LHS or RV failure, depending on site of tumour
LOC or sudden death: Due to prolapse via mitral valve/AF
Emboli:

- CVA
- PVD, incl. aortic saddle embolus/Raynaud
- MI

Clubbing
Koagulation (prothrombotic): + polycythaemia, thrombocytosis → DVT, PE
Systemic: Fever, LOW, myalgia

O/E

- LA tumour: Signs are similar to mitral stenosis:

Similarities	**Differences**
• Loud S1	• Sinus rhythm
• Mid-diastolic murmur	• Postural changes affect murmur
• Pre-systolic accentuation	• Early diastolic plop: Tumour prolapses via valve in place of opening snap

- RA tumour – RV failure

Ix

Bloods: ESR ↑↑, Ig ↑;
Albumin ↓;
WCC ↑, Plts ↓ or ↑ Hb ↓ (chronic disease or haemolytic)
ECHO: Diagnosed on ECHO
Radiol:
CXR:

- Small heart with LA appendage enlargement (± pulmonary oedema)
- Calcification of tumour (not MV)

Special: Histology

Rx

Surgical: Cardiopulmonary bypass ± atrial septectomy/interatrial patch
RECURRENCE IS VERY RARE!

CARDIOMYOPATHY

Def

Structural pump failure due to primary myocardial damage

Hypertrophic – HOCM

Autosomal dominant (AD) or spontaneous mutation

Features

Hypertrophy: Either **ASH** =**A**symmetric **S**eptal **H**ypertrophy, or concentric **LVH**
Obstruction: **SAM** = systolic anterior motion of anterior leaflet of mitral valve that obliterates LV outflow tract in systole
Cardiac death: Commonest cause of sudden cardiac death in young people
Myosin: ß-myosin heavy chain is commonest mutation (AD)

PC

Angina
Arrhythmias, esp. AF, WPW, VT

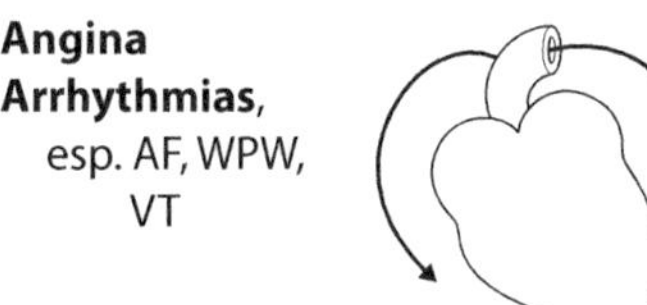

Exertional syncope, or sudden death, due to:

- Peripheral vasodilation
- Catecholamine-induced outflow obstruction
- Vagal-bradycardia/WPW/VT-VF

Diastolic heart failure , i.e. ↑ LVEDP

O/E

General Friedrich ataxia

JVP Large a wave

ABP ↓ on exercise

Pulse
Jerky
Small, collapsing
AF

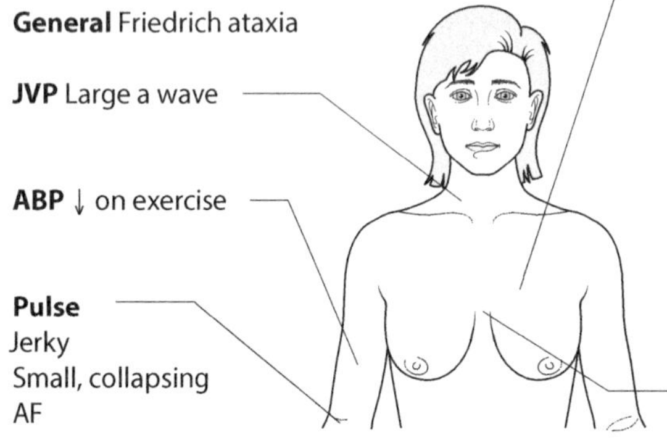

Auscultation
HS: 4th HS; single/reversed S2 splitting
Mid-late ejection systolic murmur over LSE
Mitral regurgitation or stenosis-like murmurs

Manoeuvres that ↑ murmur + ↑ outflow obstruction =

↓PRE-LOAD	↓AFTER-LOAD	↓CONTRACTILITY
Valsalva	Standing	Exercise
Nitrate/diuretic	Nifedipine/ACEI	Digoxin

Palpation Pressure overloaded APB
Double/triple impulse/LV lift
Systolic thrill

Ix

ECG:
- LVH/LAD/L-sided strain
- Widespread Q waves
- Pre-excitation

ECHO: ASH – ground-glass appearance

Radiol:
- Normal or RA or LA dilation on CXR
- SAM
- Hypertrophied, dilated atria due to LVEDP ↑
- Intra-cavity pressure gradient within the LV

Special: Cardiac catheterisation – large intra-cavity pressure gradient

Rx

Medical: –ve inotropes ↓ obstruction/diastolic failure: ß-blockers, verapamil (AVOID nitrates, ACEI , diuretics, nifedipine)

Surgical:

- Pacemaker DDD: Delays septal depolarisation and ↓ obstruction
- Myomectomy/ MVR/ alcohol ablation

Dilated

Causes

D.I.L.A.T.E.D.

Dystrophy: Primary; muscular dystrophy, myotonic dystrophy, glycogen storage disease
Infection: Sequela of myocarditis, esp. enterovirus
Late pregnancy: 3rd trimester – 6 months post-partum
Autoimmune: SLE
Toxin:
- Alcohol (thiamine deficiency), cocaine
- Doxorubicin, cyclophosphamide (and radiotherapy)

Endocrine: Dysthyroidism; acromegaly; Addison; diabetes
DNA: Either autosomal dominant or recessive

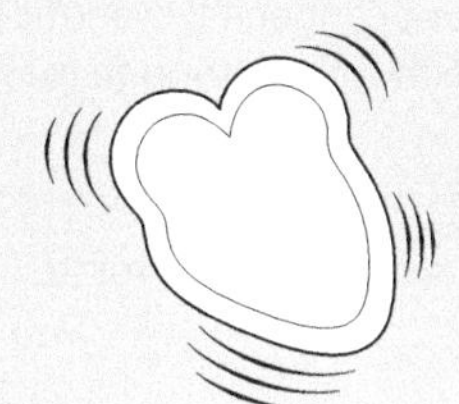

PC

LVF
- Pulmonary oedema
- Pleural effusion
- Renal failure

RVF
- Peripheral oedema
- Liver failure, ascites

Arrhythmias

O/E

JVP ↑↑cv wave (TR)

ABP ↓ pulse pressure

Pulse
Fast, thready; pulsus alternans

Auscultation
HS: 3rd + 4th gallop
MR, TR

Apex
Displaced, diffuse

Ix

ECG: T inversion, poor R wave progression, AF, VT
ECHO: LVEDV ↑; LV ejection fraction ↓; LV thrombus
Radiol: CXR: Dilated RV + LV
Catheter + Bx: Myocardial fibre disarray

Rx

Medical:
- Diuretics, ACEI, beta-blockers
- Anticoagulation if cardiac thrombus or AF

Surgical: LV assist device/transplant

Restrictive

Causes

S.I.N.E.

Storage diseases
Fabry
Gaucher
Haemochromatosis (the only reversible cause)
Glycogen storage diseases
Infiltrative diseases
Sarcoid
Amyloid
Non-infiltrative
Idiopathic
Scleroderma
Pseudoxanthoma elasticum
Endocardial
Hypereosinophilia
Radiotherapy
Carcinoid

PC

Heart failure with preserved systolic function, i.e. primarily diastolic dysfunction

O/E

Similarities to Constrictive pericarditis:
- JVP + prominent x, y descents, Kussmaul Sx.
- Peripheral oedema, hepatomegaly, ascites

Differences:
- Palpable apex beat
- MR/TR (sarcoid, amyloid)

Ix

Catheter: Difference in LVEDP and RVEDP >7 mmHg at end-expiration (cf. constriction)
Biopsy
Amyloid screen Ix, e.g. BJP, SEP, SAP-scan

CONGENITAL HEART DISEASE – CYANOTIC

Fallot tetralogy

EPI

Commonest congenital cyanotic heart disease presenting after 1 year
Age: >3–6 months, although most are cyanosed at birth

PATH

Failure of bulbis cordis to rotate:

You can see Fallot tetralogy with the **R**ight **P.O.V.**

Right ventricular hypertrophy
→ Right left shunting: cyanosis
Pulmonary stenosis
Over-riding aorta with wide aortic ring
(aorta displaced anteriorly and rightwards)
VSD: Infundibular-subaortic

O/E

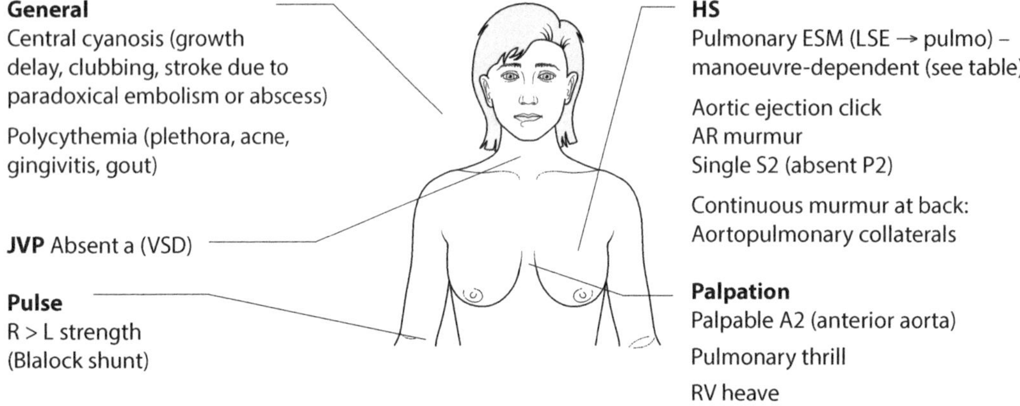

Murmur/cyanosis variability
The murmur reflects flow through the pulmonary artery, so that the **louder** the murmur, the **less** the cyanosis!

Mechanism	Murmur	Cause		
Shunting ↓ no cyanosis	Intensity ↑	After-load ↑: Squatting	Pre-load ↑: Leg elevation	Cardiac contractility ↓: Beta-blockers
Shunting ↑ cyanosis	Intensity ↓	After-load ↓: Exercise, sepsis	Pre-load ↓: Nitrates, ACEI	Cardiac contractility ↑: Digoxin

ECG:
- RAD
- R BBB
- VEs, paroxysmal VT

Radiol: CXR
- Coeur en sabot
- Pulmonary oligaemia/absent L pulmonary artery
- Large aortic knuckle

Special: Heart catheter

Rx

Surgical:
Shunt:
- Blalock Taussig: L saubclavian artery → pulmonary artery
- Pulmonary valvuloplasty/infundibular resection

Eisenmenger syndrome

PATH

Reversal of shunt flow in ASD/VSD/PDA

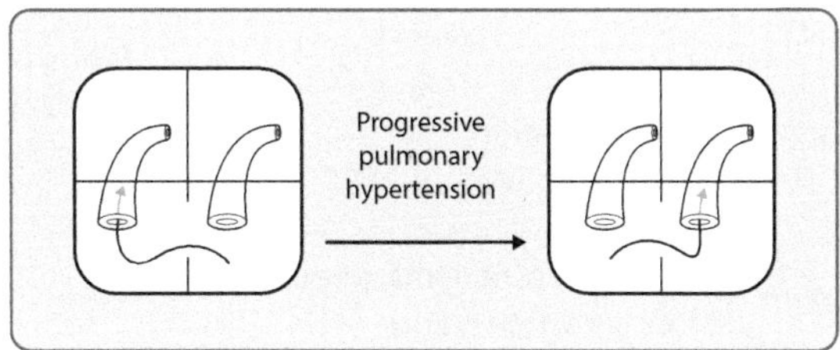

Rarities (4Ts)

TGA + essential shunt: Hyperdynamic circulation
TGA – congenitally correct
TAPVD
Tricuspid atresia/Ebstein's anomaly

CONGENITAL HEART DISEASE – NON-CYANOTIC

Epi

Congenital heart defects occur in <1% live births, or 4% if mother had congenital heart disease. Of these, 50% require medical/surgical intervention in infancy, and a further 30% in later life

Atrial septal defect (ASD) (30%)

1°: Primum

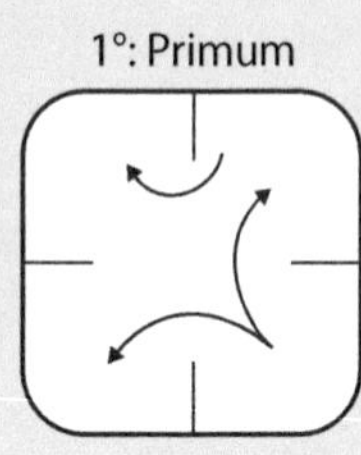

AV-canal defect: Associated MR and VSD

☠

Mitral reurgitation: LVH/LSH failure

Pulmonary hypertension

SBE: Due to low atrial pressure

2°: Secundum (70%)

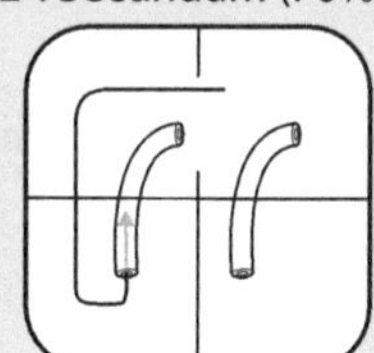

Fossa ovalis defect

☠

Atrial dilation:
- AF or SVT
- TR
- PE

Pulmonary hypertension:
- Pulmo. oedema, pneumonia
- RVH/RSH failure
- Eisenmenger (cyanosis)

Other:

Patent foramen ovale

Asymptomatic finding in 25% population

No shunting occurs ∴ strictly not ASD!

Associated with CVA (paradoxical embolism during Valsalva)

Sinus venosus defect

Upper atrial defect

Associated anomalous R pulmonary venous drainage → RA

O/E

General
M:F = 3:1
Holt–Oram syn. – 2° (clavicle, thumb defects)
Down, Turner syn. –1°

JVP
Large a (PHT)/cv waves (TR)
Raised level (RSH failure) – esp. 2°

ABP ↑ if coarctation (assoc. with 1°)

Pulse AF/SVT – esp. 2°

HS
Fixed split S2, because inspiration ↑ RA filling but ↓ L → R shunt

Wide split S1

Pulmonary ejection systolic murmur
Tricuspid mid-diastolic flow murmur

NB:
Eisenmenger – Flow murmurs disappear; loud P2, ejection click, PR
Assoc. MVP (2°), MR (1°)

Palpation
APB: Undisplaced (2°); volume-overload (1°)
Parasternal heave; palpable S2 (PHT)

Ix

ECG: Long PR, R BBB, RAD (2°), LAD (1°)
ECHO: (+ bubble injection)
Radiol: CXR Pulmonary plethora, prominent pulmonary arteries

Rx

Rarely close spontaneously

Surgical: Closure via catheter-inserted device or surgical
IND = P:S flow ratio >1.5
CI = Eisenmenger (P:SVR >0.7)

Ventricular septal defect (VSD) (70%) = Maladie de Roger

Types

Membranous: Commonest – closes spontaneously due to adjacent papillary muscle

Muscular: Post-MI, multiple – closes spontaneously

Infundibular: Assoc. AR, Fallot

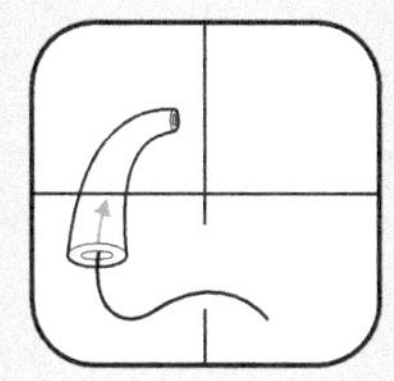

☠

LVH/LSH failure

PHT (as for ASD 2°)

SBE, R-sided → pneumonia/pleurisy

O/E

General Scars:

- CABG scar
- Childhood correction

JVP Large a (PHT)

ABP ↑ if coarctation –1°

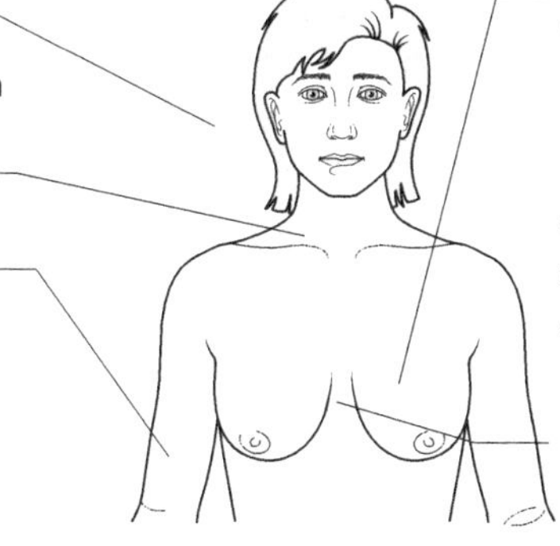

HS

Wide, but variable S2

PSM at LSE → apex

Mitral mid-diastolic flow murmur

Eisenmenger:

- Single S2 (equal ventric. pressures)
- Soft ESM at LSE, or no murmur
- Loud P2 + ejection click + PR

Palpation

APB: Volume overload

Parasternal heave

LSE thrill

Rx

Often close spontaneously (50% by 10 y)

Surgical: Double clamshell device

Patent ductus arteriosus (PDA) (10%)

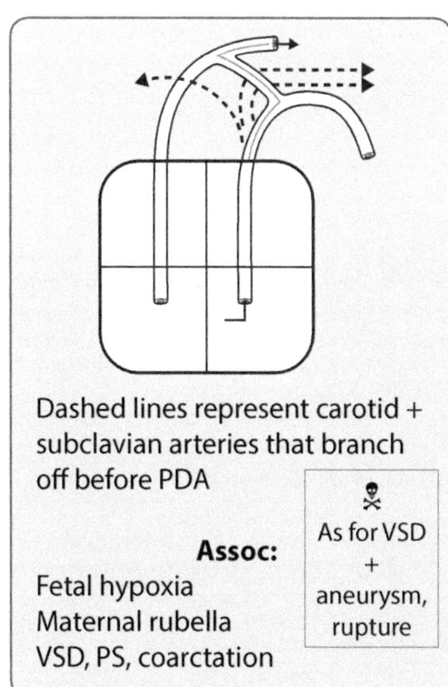

Dashed lines represent carotid + subclavian arteries that branch off before PDA

Assoc:

Fetal hypoxia

Maternal rubella

VSD, PS, coarctation

☠

As for VSD + aneurysm, rupture

O/E

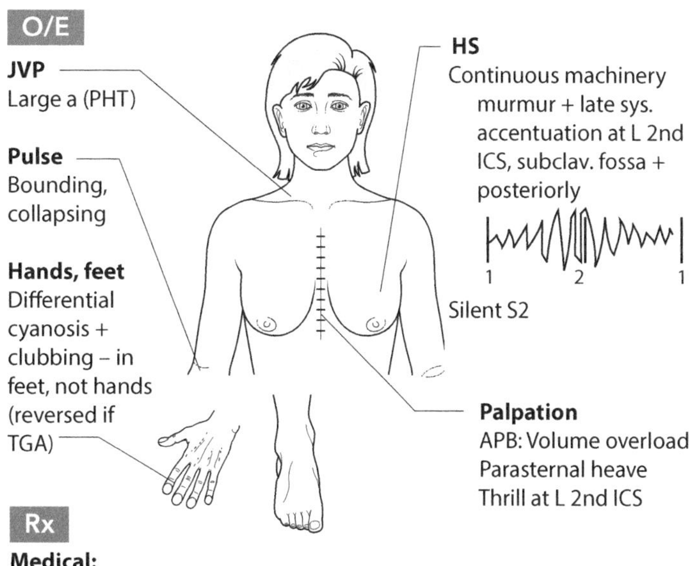

JVP

Large a (PHT)

Pulse

Bounding, collapsing

Hands, feet

Differential cyanosis + clubbing – in feet, not hands (reversed if TGA)

HS

Continuous machinery murmur + late sys. accentuation at L 2nd ICS, subclav. fossa + posteriorly

Silent S2

Palpation

APB: Volume overload

Parasternal heave

Thrill at L 2nd ICS

Rx

Medical:

Indomethacin in neonatal period

Surgical:

Closure – ligation, catheter-placed device

Respiratory Medicine

RESPIRATORY EXAMINATION

1. Hands

Clubbing (ca., bronchiectasis)
Nicotine staining (actually due to tar)
Hand wasting: T1 wasting (Pancoast tumour)
Arthritis, sclerodactyly {fibrosis)
Hand flap: CO_2 retention

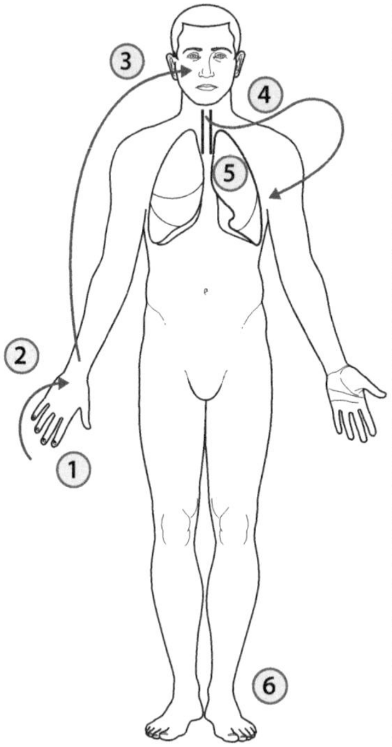

2. Pulse, ABP, RR

Pulse: ↑ in PE, infection, severe asthma
ABP:
- ↓ in PE, infection, severe asthma
- Pulsus paradoxus: >10 mmHg ↓ on inspiration (severe asthma)

RR: Rate and pattern (periodic?)
Measure surreptitiously, while appearing to take pulse, so as not to make patient self-conscious

3. Face – General

Eyes:
- Conjunctivae: Pallor (anaemia)
- Sclera: Jaundice (cor pulmonale, cystic fibrosis)
- Horner syn. (Pancoast tumour)

Mouth:
- Central cyanosis

Cheeks, nose:
- Flushed (polycythaemia, SVCO, mitral stenosis)
- Rash (SLE, scleroderma, sarcoid, carcinoid)

General habitus:
- Obese (Pickwickian syn.)
- Cachexia (TB, ca., bronchiectasis)
- Marfanoid (pneumothorax)

4. Neck

Accessory muscles of respiration:
Sternocleidomastoid, arm support, alae flaring
JVP: ↑ in:
- Pulmonary hypertension
- SVCO (non-pulsatile), due to bronchial ca. (90%), lymphoma, Hodgkin (8%)

5. Chest

Inspection:
- Barrel chest, pectus carinatum
- Kyphosis: Ankylosing spondylitis thoracic vertebral fracture (TB)
- Concavity: Lobe- or pneumonectomy
- Scars: Chest drain, thoracotomy, radiation marks

Palpation:
- Front: Trachea + apex beat (mediastinal shift, LVF) parasternal heave
- Back: Lymphadenopathy

Expansion: ↓ with most pathologies
Percussion: Include clavicle + axillary areas
Auscultation:
- Air entry: Intensity, quality
- Added sounds: Creps, wheeze

Manoeuvres:
- Tactile vocal fremitus (TVF)
- Vocal resonance
- Whispering pectoriloqy

(For all: Transmission loud with consolidation, soft with effusion, collapse)

Order

1. *Recline patient at 45°*
2. *Stand back and get pt. to take 2 deep breaths in and out, while inspecting*
3. *Examine front; palpation, expansion ...*
4. *Sit patient forward, inspect and palpate for cervical + axillary lymph nodes; then repeat palpation, etc.*

6. Elsewhere

Ankle oedema (cor pulmonale)
Ascites, liver edge

7. And finally ...

Talking in sentences?
- Indicates severity of respiratory distress

PEFR; temperature charts
Surrounds: Sputum pot

Patterns

1. **Consolidation**
   Palpation: Lymphadenopathy in TB, HIV
   Expansion ↓
   Percussion note dull
   Auscultation: • Air entry ↓, bronchial breathing
   • Added: Coarse creps
   Tactile vocal fremitus or vocal resonance ↑, whispering pectoriloquy (whispering sounds loud + harsh)

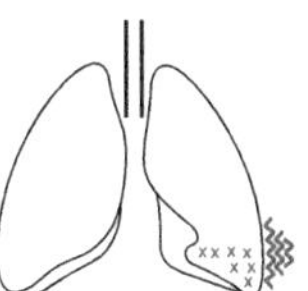

2. **Pleural effusion**
   Palpation: Mediastinum shifts away
   Expansion ↓
   Percussion note stony dull
   Auscultation: • Air entry – absent
   • Bronchial breathing just above effusion
   Tactile vocal fremitus or vocal resonance ↓, egophony (patient's voice sounds like bleating sheep just above effusion)

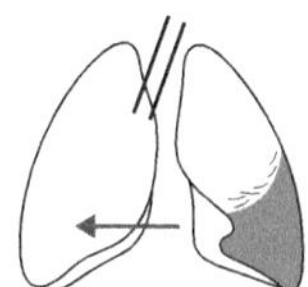

3. **Collapse (or lobectomy, or pneumonectomy or thoracoplasty)**
   Palpation: Mediastinum shifts towards
   Expansion ↓
   Percussion note: • Dull (collapse)
   • Stony dull (pneumonectomy, due to fluid replacement)
   Auscultation: Air entry ↓
   Tactile vocal fremitus or vocal resonance ↓

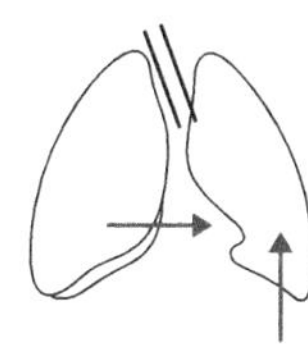

4. **Fibrosis**
   Palpation: Mediastinum shifts towards
   Expansion ↓
   Percussion note dull
   Auscultation: • Air entry ↓, bronchial breathing
   • Added: End-inspiratory fine or coarse creps, don't shift with coughing

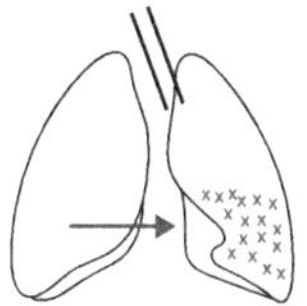

5. **Pneumothorax**
   Palpation: Mediastinum shifts away (with large or tension pneumothorax)
   Expansion ↓
   Percussion note hyper-resonant
   Auscultation: Air entry ↓
   Tactile vocal fremitus or vocal resonance ↓
   + Hamman's sign: Systolic click, heard in time with heart (left-side pn.tx.)
   + Coin sign (tap on coin placed on chest → ringing sound heard)

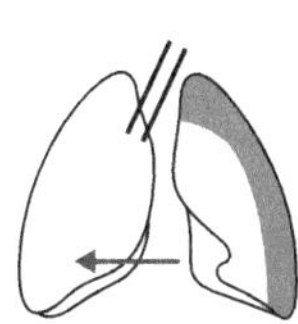

6. **Bronchiectasis**
   Clubbing, cyanosis
   Coarse crepitations
   Extra: Fever, copious green sputum in pot

7. **Pulmonary fibrosis**
   Clubbing, cyanosis
   Fine crepitations

8. **Cavity**
   Amphoric breathing (like blowing over a bottle top)

CLUBBING

O/E

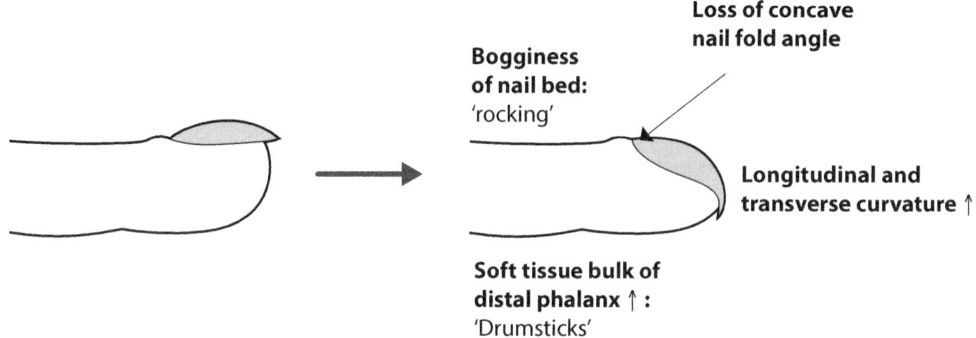

Causes

All the **Cs**

Respiratory

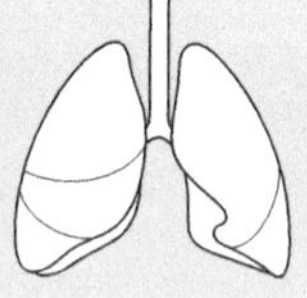

Cancer:

- Bronchial, esp. squamous cell carcinoma – assoc. hypertrophic pulmonary osteoarthropathy (HPOA)
- Mesothelioma (or asbestosis)

Cystic fibrosis + other **C**hronic suppurative disease:

- Lung abscess/bronchiectasis
- Empyema – may occur within a few weeks
- TB – uncommonly associated

Idiopathic pulmonary fibrosis (formally **C**ryptogenic fibrosing alveolitis)

Cardiac

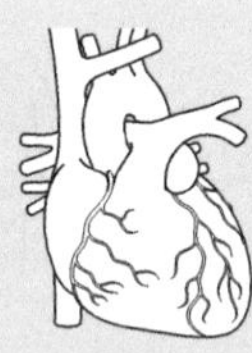

Congenital cyanotic heart disease
Infective endo**C**arditis
Cancer: Myxoma

GIT

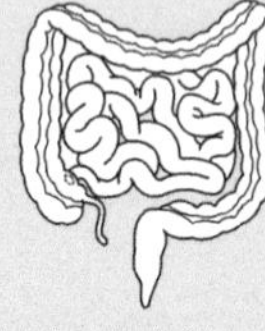

Cirrhosis
Crohn
Coeliac
Cancer: GI lymphoma

Other

Congenital
a**C**ropachy

CYANOSIS

Def

Blue discolouration of mucosal membranes/skin, caused by hypoxaemia

Types: 1. Peripheral: Cold, blue peripheries, e.g. nail beds
2. Central: Blue tongue, lips; warm peripheries; digital pulses present

Causes

Think of the path of O_2 from air to red blood cells:

Atmosphere

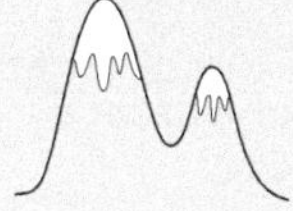

High-altitude acclimatisation:

- ↑ bicarbonate excretion: Counters hypoxia-driven hyperventilation and respiratory alkalosis
- ↑ Hb 2,3-DPG → ↓ affinity for O_2
- Polycythaemia

Nitrite-contaminated water

Cold exposure (peripheral cyanosis)

Respiratory

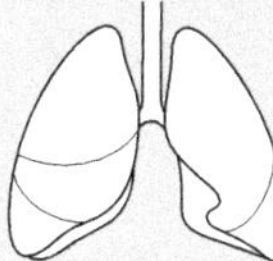

Ventilation ↓: COPD, ventilatory muscle weakness

O_2 diffusion ↓: Pulmo. oedema, pneumonia, fibrosis, alveolar haemorhage, aspiration

Pulmonary blood perfusion ↓: PE

Cardiac

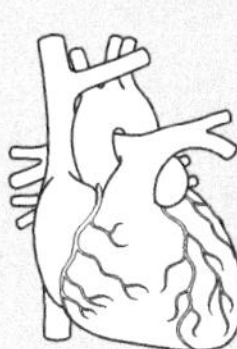

Congenital:

- R→L shunt: Eisenmenger (ASD, VSD, PDA), Fallot
- R+L mixing: Transposition of great arteries
- Pulmonary blood flow ↓: Pulmonary atresia

Cardiac output ↓:

- Mitral stenosis
- Severe heart failure

Vascular (peripheral cyanosis):

- Arterial obstruction: Raynaud, thromboembolic disease
- Venous obstruction: DVT, constrictive pericarditis
- Shock: Sympathetic redistribution

Red-**blood** cells

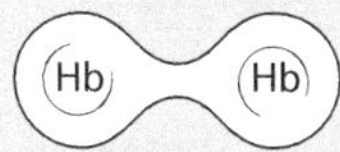

Hereditary low-affinity **Hb**:

- **Hb** Kansas
- Methaemaglobinaemia = Cyt B5 reductase deficiency

Acquired low-affinity **Hb**:

- Met**Hb**aemia
- Sulp**Hb**aemia
- Carboxy**Hb**aemia: (CO poisoning): Pt. appears cherry red

Polycythemia (peripheral cyanosis): Due to sluggish circulation

RESPIRATORY FAILURE

Def

Type 1 failure hypoxaemia – failure of oxygenation
Type 2 failure hypoxaemia and hypercapnia – failure of oxygenation and ventilation

Causes

Alveolar ventilation failure

PaO_2 ↓ $PaCO_2$ ↑ pH ↓
Alveolar–arterial grad. normal

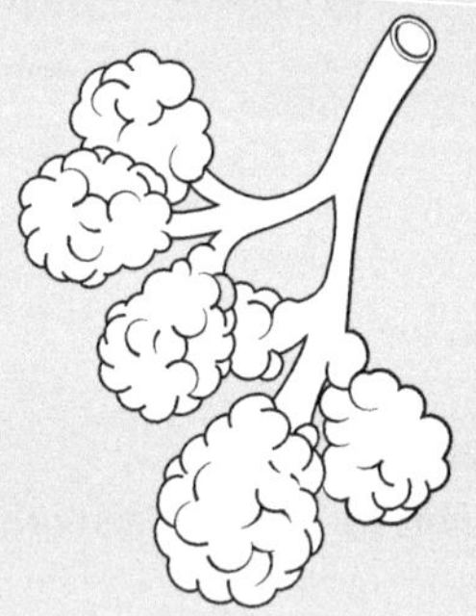

Obstructive

Small airway:
- COPD
- Asthma – severe
- Bronchiectasis
- Bronchiolitis

Large airway:
- Intra-thoracic:
  - Ca., LN, FB
- Extra-thoracic:
  - Ca., OSA, epiglottitis

Restrictive

Extraparenchymal:
- Neuromuscular:
  - CNS Δ, sedatives
  - High – cervical cord Δ
  - Lower-motor neurone: MND, GBS, myasthenia
- Structural:
  - Ankylosing spondylitis + other skeletal Δ
  - Pleural disease
  - Obesity

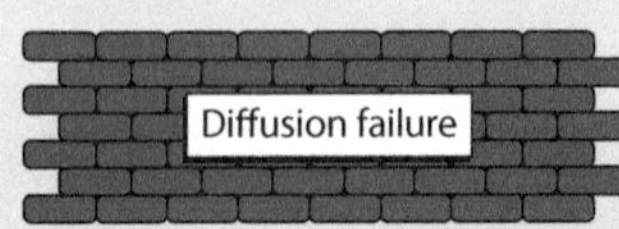

Fluid

Pulmonary oedema
Pneumonia
Infarction
Blood

Fibrosis

Both also cause V/Q mismatch + alveolar ventilation failure, due to lung compliance ↓
=> work of breathing ↑

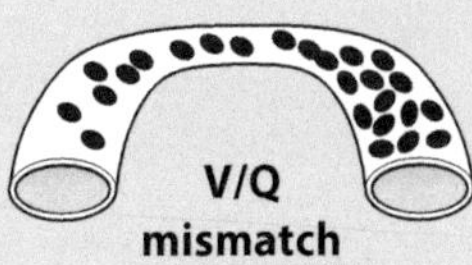

mismatch

PaO_2 ↓ $PaCO_2$ ↓ pH ↑
Alveolar–arterial grad. ↑

Vascular

PE
PHT
Pulmonary shunt

Asthma – early

Atelectasis

Pneumothorax

PC

	$PaO_2\downarrow$	$PaCO_2\uparrow$ or pH$\downarrow$
Acute	Cyanosis (deoxyHb ≥5 g/dl) Cardiac: • Angina, MI • Arrhythmias, esp. VT Cerebral: Encephalopathy	Tachypnoea Cardiac: • Peripheral vasodilation (warm), pulse volume ↑ • Arrhythmia, esp. sinus tachycardia, SVT Cerebral: Encephalopathy, incl.: asterixis, papilloedema, miosis, reflexes ↓
Chronic	Polycythaemia Pulmonary hypertension/cor pulmonale Renal: ATN (vasoconstriction)	Renal compensation: HCO_3^- ↑ Cl^- ↓

Ix

ABG:

pH/HCO_3: Determines chronicity and whether renal compensation has occurred:

Alveolar–arterial gradient (PAO_2 – PaO_2)

PAO_2 (Alveolar O_2) = 20 –($PaCO_2$ × 1.25)

Normal A–a gradient = 2 kPa (50-y-old, at sea-level, room air)

Raised A–a gradient indicates diffusion failure or V/Q mismatch

PEFR, spirometry, transfer factor

Rx

Underlying cause, e.g. opiates – naloxone

Oxygenation failure (PaO_2 <8.0 kPa):

- Low/high-flow O_2, e.g. nasal cannulae, Venturi face-mask, reservoir bag
  ☠: Chronic ventilatory failure: Ventilation depends on hypoxaemic drive!
- Continuous positive airway pressure (CPAP) – tight-fitting mask (non-invasive)
- Alternative to CPAP is high-flow nasal oxygen
- Mechanical ventilation via intubation or tracheostomy

Ventilatory failure ($PaCO_2$ >6.5 kPa)

- BiPAP
- Mechanical ventilation

RESPIRATORY FUNCTION TESTS – SPIROMETRY

FEV_1: Forced expiratory volume in 1 s
FVC: Forced vital capacity
KCO: Transfer factor (diffusion rate)
PEFR: Peak expiratory flow rate
RV: Residual volume
TLC: Total lung capacity

Obstructive

FVC slightly ↓
FEV_1: Dramatically ↓ (determines severity)
FEV_1/FVC = <0.7
TLC ↑, RV ↑
KCO ↓ emphysema

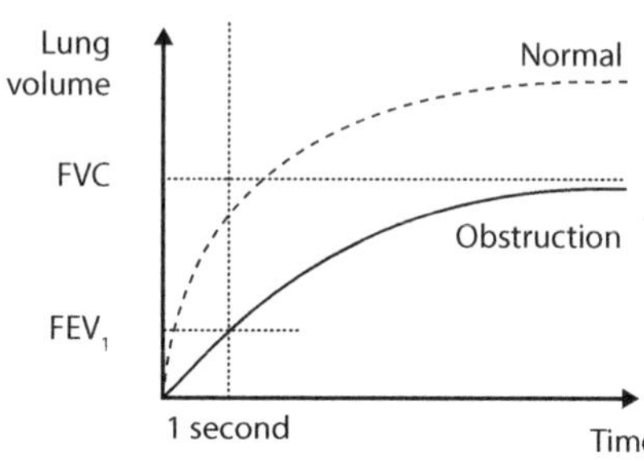

Causes

C.A.B.B.I.E.

Small airways
COPD, irreversible
Asthma
Bronchiectasis
Bronchiolitis

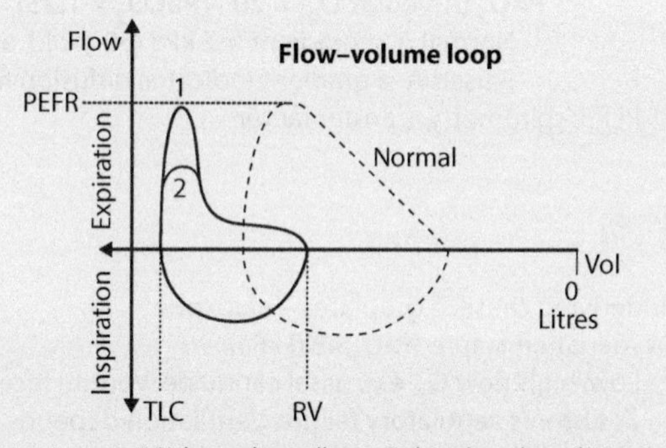

1. Volume-dep. collapse: Early asthma, bronchitis
2. Pressure-dep. collapse: Emphysema, bronchiolitis

Large airways
Intra-thoracic – fixed obstruction

- Bronchial carcinoma, lymph node, foreign body
- Relapsing polychondritis: Intermittent bronchial collapse

Extra-thoracic – collapse on inspiration only

- Laryngeal carcinoma, epiglottitis, tracheal stenosis
- Foreign body in throat
- Goitre, cervical lymph nodes

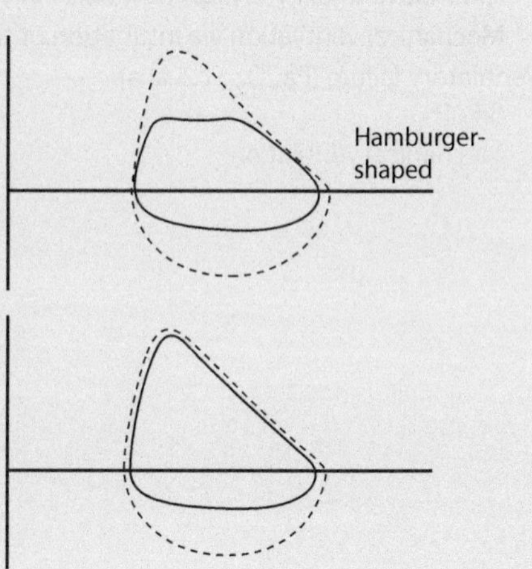

Restrictive

Intra-parenchymal
FVC↓ ↓
TLC↓, RV↓
KCO↓

Extra-parenchymal
FVC↓ ↓
TLC↓, RV↓
KCO normal

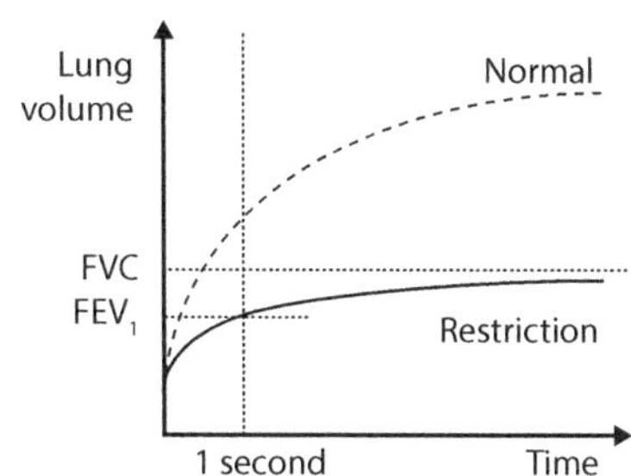

Causes

Intra-parenchymal
Pulmonary fibrosis
Pulmonary oedema, severe
Pulmonary hypertension

Flow–volume loop

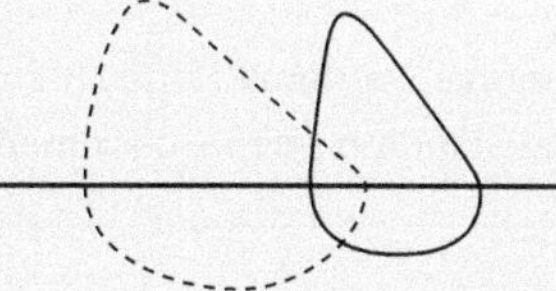

Extra-parenchymal
= expiratory and inspiratory weakness
Neuromuscular:
- High spinal cord injury,
- Guillain–Barré syndrome, motor neurone disease

Pleura:
- Mesothelioma

Chest wall:
- Ankylosing spondylitis, severe kyphosis

Severe obesity

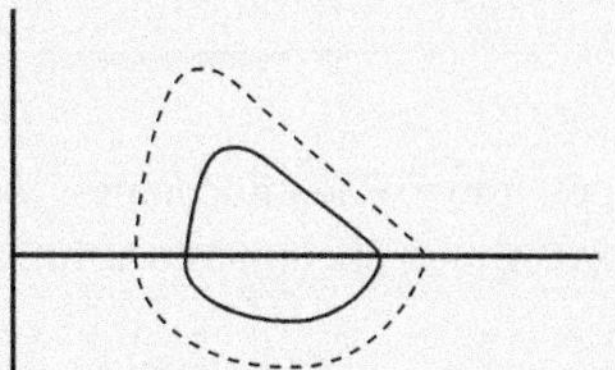

CHEST X-RAY PATTERNS

Reticulo-nodular shadowing

F.I.N.E. *shadows*

Fibrosis:
- Upper zones: Pneumoconioses, extrinsic allergic alveolitis seronegative arthropathies, TB, aspergillosis
- Mid zones: Sarcoid
- Lower zones: SLE, CFA, asbestosis, radiotherapy, drugs

Infection:
- Atypical pneumonia: Psittacosis, Q-fever
- Viral, VZV pneumonitis (nodular)

Neoplasia:
- Lymphangitis carcinomatosis (reticular)
- Thyroid carcinoma (follicular) ('snowstorm' appearance)
- Other: Renal cell, melanoma, lymphoma (nodular)

O**E**dema:
- Pulmonary oedema: Kerley B-lines (horizontal, peripheral)
- Long-standing pulmo. oedema/haemosiderosis (nodular)

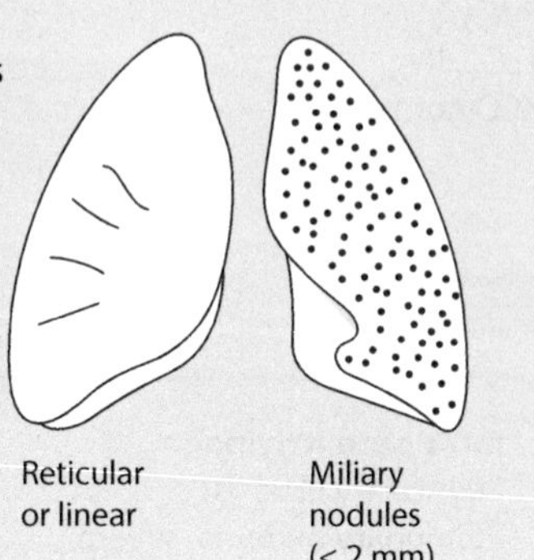

Coin lesions, cavities

F.A.N.G.S.

Fibrosis:
- Upper zones: Pneumoconioses (progressive massive fibrosis)
- Lower zones: Rheumatoid arthritis

Abscess:
- Bacterial: Staphylococci, TB, *Klebsiella*
- Mycetoma, *Aspergillus*
- Hydatid cyst; amoebic cyst

Neoplasia:
- 1°, 2°
- Benign: Hamartoma, bronchial cyst

Granulomatous: Rheumatoid arthritis, granulomatosis with polyangiitis

Structural:
- AVM
- Pulmonary infarction
- Traumatic haematoma

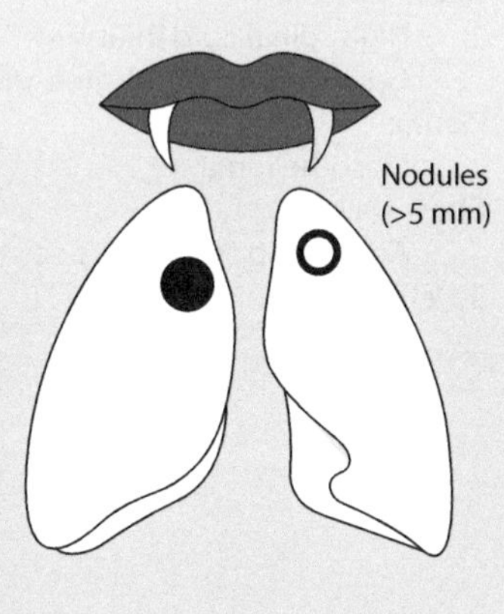

Opacification

- Consolidation: Air-space infiltration

Confluent shadowing
Air bronchogram

Fluid: Oedema 2° to LVF or ARDS
Alveolar proteinosis

Cells: Neutrophils:
- Pneumonia: Bacterial, viral, TB, PCP
- Infarction 2° to PE

Eosinophils:
- Pulmonary eosinophilia, ABPA

Red blood cells (pulmonary haemorrhage):
- Goodpasture, granulomatosis with polyangiitis
- Mitral stenosis, L → R shunt, e.g. VSD
- Idiopathic pulmonary haemosiderosis

Tumour:
- Bronchioalveolar cell carcinoma, Kaposi's sarcoma

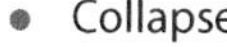

- Collapse

Lobar
Segmental atelectasis
Surgery: Pneumonectomy, thoracoplasty (for TB)

Patterns observed with lobar collapse:

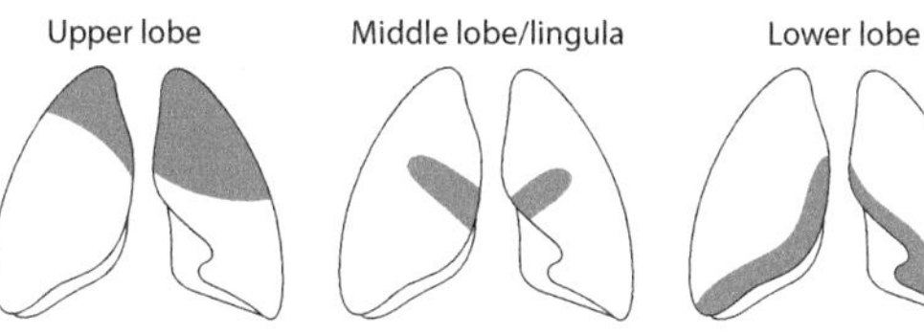

- Pleural disease

Effusion
Plaques – holly-leaf plaques or linear shadows
Asbestos exposure/mesothelioma (but not asbestosis)
TB
Old haemothorax

Mediastinal mass

Thyroid (retrosternal goitre)
Thymoma
Teratoma
TB (or sarcoid) lymph nodes
Terrible diagnoses!!!: Lymphoma or aneurysm/dissection!!!

PNEUMONIA – CLINICAL FEATURES

PC

Specific: Pleuritic pain, cough productive of rusty sputum, SOB
Constitutional: Fever, rigors, malaise, myalgia,
D+V (esp. *Legionella*), headaches (esp. *Mycoplasma*) confusion, falls
Other history: PMH – pulmonary disease or immunocompromised
PH: Smoking, pets (psittacosis),
travel (Legionnaire, typhoid, TB)
SH: Job, contacts

O/E

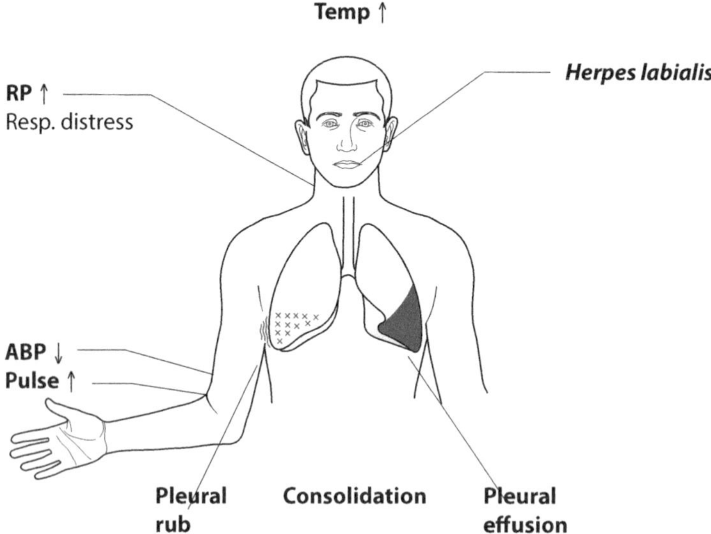

Poor prognostic features

H^2.A.R.M.F.U.L^2.

History: Age >50, comorbidity (e.g. IHD, ca.)
Hypoxia: Sats <92%, PaO_2 <8 kPa on room air
ABP: SBP <90 mmHg, or DBP <60 mmHg
RR: >30/min
Mental confusion
Fluid: Pleural effusion
Urea: >7 mmol/l
Leucocytosis: WCC <4 or >20 x10^9/l
Lobar, multi-, appearance of CXR

Ix and Rx

WARN ITU
if still hypoxic or $PaCo_2$
>6 kPa

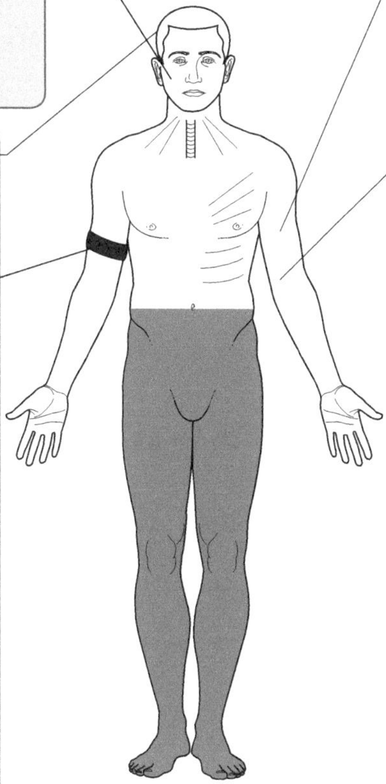

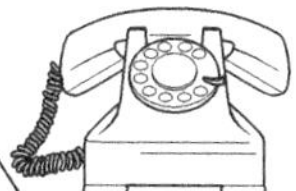

B. Ventilatory support
Sit patient up (aids respiration)
Oxygen: 35–100% OPD
± rebreath bag
Nebulizers if COAD or wheeze
CPAP or intubate

A. Assessment
A.B.C.D.

C.O.A.T.

Cardiac monitor,
O_2 stats, **A**BP, **T**PR

Investigations

Bloods:
- ABGs:
  - PaO_2 – index of severity
  - $PaCO_2$ – should be low; if normal or high, suggests fatigue and need for ventilatn
- U&E: Fluid depletion, *Legionella*
- LFT: *Mycoplasma, Legionella*
- FBC: Neutrophilia (not *Mycoplasma*)
- ESR, CRP – allows monitoring
- Clotting, FDP: DIC is complication
- Igs: Is patient immunodeficient?

Urine:
- Glucose; *Legionella* antigen serology

Micro:
- Blood cultures
- Serology: *Mycoplasma, Legionella, Chlamydia, Coxiella* (4× ↑ over 10 days)
- HIV
- Sputum: Gram, silver, AAFB stains; ELISA

Monitor: PEFR, O_2

ECG: AF may occur

Radiol: CXR

Special:
- Bronchoscopy – if PCP or carcinoma possible
- Pleural aspirate or biopsy
- Lung biopsy

C. Hydration
e.g. N. saline IVI, unless possibility of pulmonary oedema

D. Medication
Antibiotics:
selected according to likely organism:

C.R.A.N.E.

Community-acquired:
S. pneumoniae, H. influenzae, Mycoplasma, Legionella
amoxicillin + erythromycin

Recent- flu:
Staphylococcus
above + flucloxacillin

Aspiration possible, e.g. alcoholic:
Anaerobes, Gram –ves
cefuroxime + metronidazole

Nosocomial:
Gram –ves, MRSA
cefotaxime ±
vancomycin (if MRSA possible)

Extra:
HIV (consider PCP)
add co-trimoxazole
TB: Consider R.I.P.E.

Optional
- Analgesics, e.g. NSAID OPD if not asthmatic
- Glucocorticoids if COAD

E. Other
Physiotherapy:
Clear pooled secretions

On discharge
Follow-up
1. Advice on smoking, pets, job
2. Isolate TB until smear –ve
3. Vaccine: *Pneumococcus*, flu – in immunocompromised

ASTHMA – CHRONIC

Def

Episodic, reversible small airways obstruction, due to bronchial hyper-reactivity to various stimuli

Epi

Inc: Children 5%; adults 2%
Age: Peaks at 5 years; most outgrow in adolescence
Sex: M:F =1:1, except under 5, when boys predominate (3:2)
Geo: Western world
Aet: Acute phase (30 min): Mast cell–Ag interaction → histamine → local axon + central reflexes
Late phase (12 h): TH2 cell → interleukins-3,4,5 → mast cells, eosinophils, B cells
Micro: Sputum contains mucus casts, eosinophils, Curschmann spirals, Charcot–Leyden crystals

Causes

All the **As**

Atopy – presents in childhood, hay fever, eczema, asthma, tendency to type 1 reactions
Auto-immune – eosinophilic granulomatosis with polyangiitis (formerly Churg–Strauss)
At the workplace – occupational asthma
Adult onset – unknown pathogenesis, seems to follow respiratory tract infection

PC

Cough: Often at night, tenacious yellow sputum
Wheeze: Often post-exercise, early morning; relieved by empirical salbutamol Rx
SOB, or 'chest tightness'
+ failure to thrive children

O/E

General: Underweight (hypermetabolic)

Inspection:
Hyperexpanded
Harrison sulci: Indraw subcostal margins

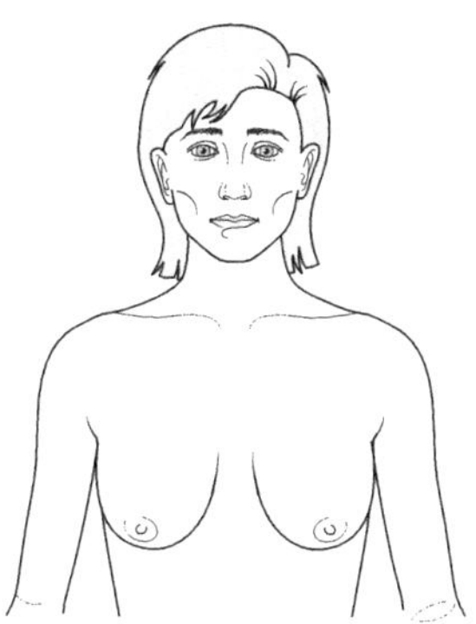

Auscultation:
Widespread, polyphonic high-pitched wheeze (small-airways obstruction)
Often normal – as characteristically episodic

Ix

Bloods: FBC – eosinophilia; ANCA
Urine: Glucose (if on chronic steroids)
Micro: Sputum – microscopy; serology: *Aspergillus*, *Ascaris*, *Strongyloides*
Monitor: PEFR – varies according to sex, age, height (normal = 300–600 l/min); characteristic daily pattern

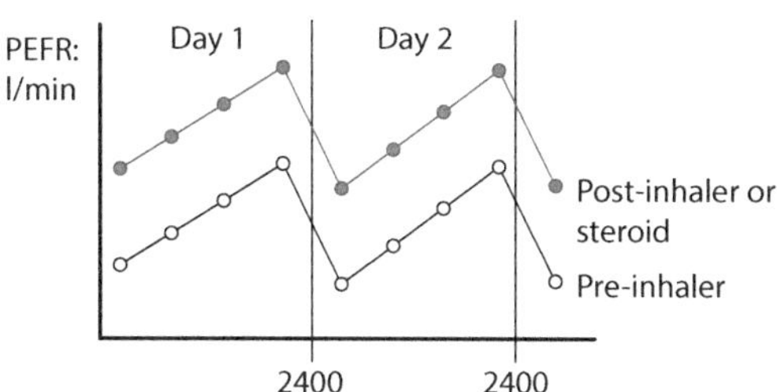

- Early morning dips; may be fatal despite normal daytime values
- β2-agonist improves
- 3 weeks prednisolone 30 mg od: Improvement suggests COPD reversibility, and hence utility of steroids

Radiol: CXR – hyperexpanded
Special: Spirometry:

- FEV_1/FVC ↓ (20–40%, cf. 70–80%)
- RV, and TLC↑
- Flow–volume loop – peak flow depressed most at lower lung volumes

ASTHMA MANAGEMENT – GENERAL

Remember to **T.A.M.E.** *your patient . . .*

Technique for inhaler use

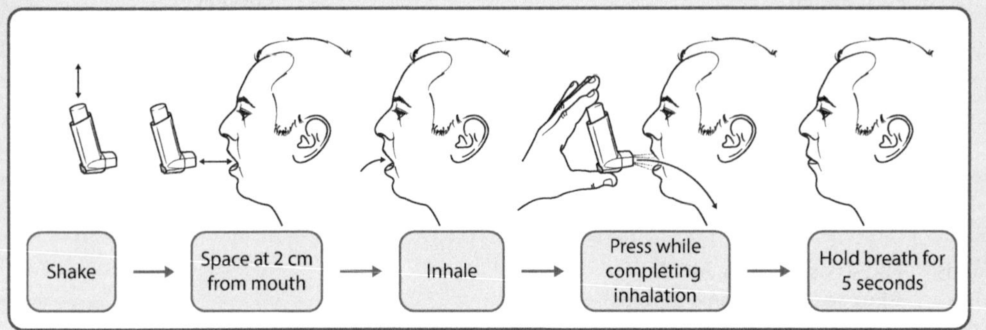
Shake
Space at 2 cm from mouth
Inhale
Press while completing inhalation
Hold breath for 5 seconds

Avoidance:

- Allergens: Smoke, carpets, grass in summer
- Prophylactic measures: Dust covers, synthetic pillows

Monitor:

- Peak flow monitor (2–4×/day) on chart → adjust drugs accordingly

Educate:

- Liaise with specialist respiratory nurse and/or district nurse
- Pt. to be able to assess severity based on symptoms and PEFR
- Reinforce need for compliance with Rx

Methods of drug delivery

Inhaler:

- **Metered-dose inhaler (MDI)**: Needs correct technique
- **Spacer + MDI**: Spacer acts as a short-term reservoir for aerosol, and creates smaller particles for inhalation
  Advantage – better for children or elderly who cannot coordinate technique, and may be administered by carer
- **Breath-activated** depends on pt.'s. effort

Nebulizer:

Mechanism: Finer particle size (3–10 μm) allows tracheobronchial deposition
Advantage: Allows high-dose drug to be administered; coordination not required
Disadvantage:

- Higher doses causes systemic effects
- Expensive + bulky

Drug ladder

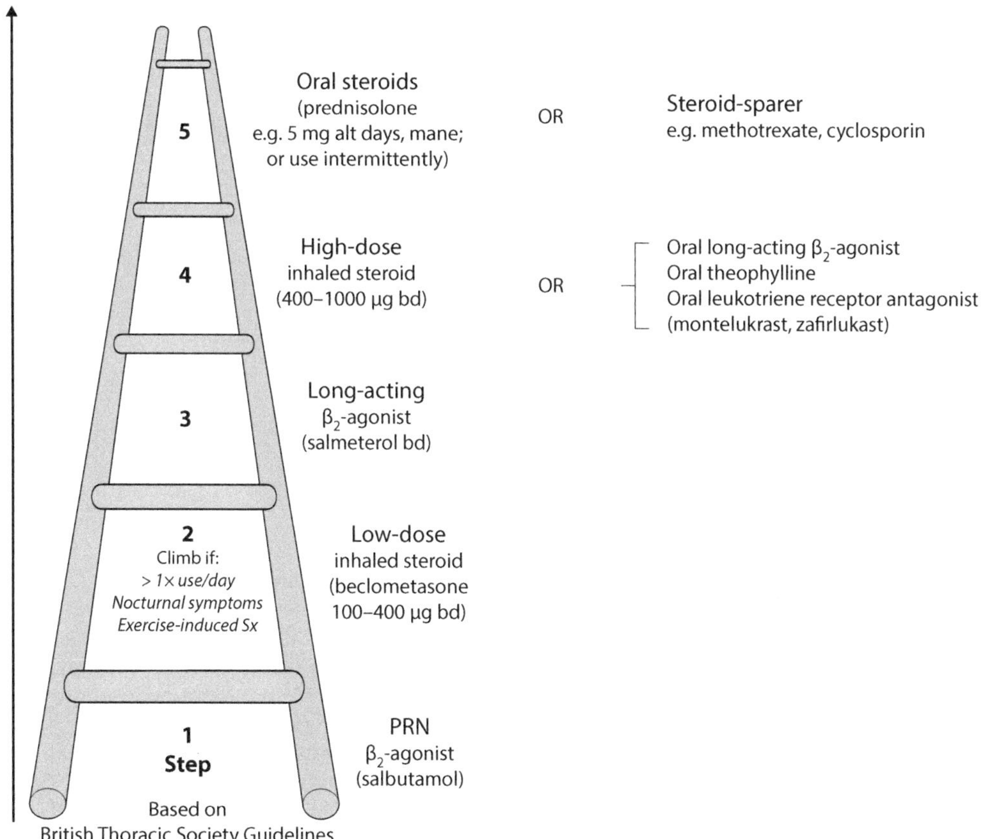

Rules

1. Start on step commensurate with present severity
2. Move up and down 1 step at a time
3. Take each lower step medication in addition to medication of new step

ASTHMA MANAGEMENT – DRUGS

Pharmacology

Drugs can be classified depending on when they act:

Early phase:	Bronchodilators	Immediate onset (min)
Early AND late phases:	Prophylactic	Delayed onset (hours – days – weeks)

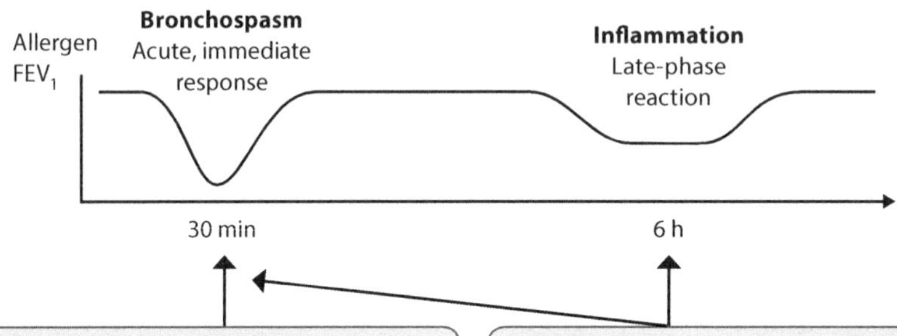

ß$_2$-Agonists

Short-acting: Salbutamol (inhaler, nebulizer, IV)
Long-acting: Salmeterol (inhaler, PO – bd)

Action: cAMP ↑ + cGMP ↓

Reduces **S.E.E.PA.G.e.**

Smooth muscle: Bronchospasm ↓
Epithelium: Mucociliary clearance ↑
Endothelium: Permeability ↓
PArasympathetic ganglia: Vagal tone ↓
De**G**ranulation of mast cells ↓

Onset = 3, Offset = 5 h

Muscarinic antagonists

Ipratropium bromide (inhaler, nebulizer)

Action: non-selective, but M3 receptor mediates:

Smooth muscle: Bronchospasm ↓
Epithelium: Submucosal gland secretion ↓
Endothelium: Permeability ↓

More effective in COAD than in asthma
Onset = 30 min Offset = 6 h

Steroids/steroid sparers

Inhaled: Beclomethasone (activated in lungs), budesonide, fluticasone
Systemic: Prednisolone PO, hydrocortisone IV
Steroid sparers: Methotrexate, cyclosporin

Action: Blocks early + late phases:

- Early: Histamine, leukotrienes, prostaglandins, PAF (platelet activating factor)
- Late: Interleukins-3,4,5
  Upregulation of ß$_2$-receptors

Onset: 3–7 days

Mast cell stabilizers

Na cromoglycate, Na nedocromil

Action:

- Mast cell stabilizer (not main effect) ⇒ release of preformed cytokines ↓
- Neuronal reflexes (central + axonal) ↓
- Substance P + PAF antagonist

Leukotriene receptor antagonists

Montelukast, zafirlukast

Action:

- Competitive antagonists at cysteinyl-leukotriene receptor (LTC4, D4, E4)
- Effective for NSAID, allergen or exercise-induced asthma

Side-effects

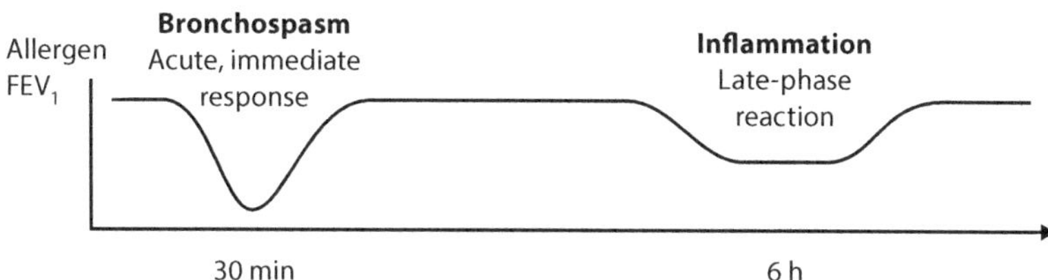

β_2-Agonists

Local:

- Rebound hyper-reactivity
- Tolerance (↓ by steroids)
- Paradoxical bronchospasm
- V/Q mismatch ↑ due to pulmonary vasodilation
- Long-term worsening ↑ (due to ↓ mast cell release of heparin that ↓ late-phase reaction)

Systemic:

- Fine tremor, muscle cramps, anxiety
- Dysrhythmias
- Periph. vasodilation – headache, flushing
- K^+ ↓ (↑ uptake of K^+ into skeletal muscle)

Muscarinic antagonists

Local:

- Glaucoma, diplopia (with face-mask)
- Dry mouth
- Paradoxical bronchospasm

Systemic: Rare, as 4° NH_4^+ compounds, e.g. urinary retention

Steroids

Local:

- Oral candidiasis
- Dysphonia (vocal cord myopathy)

Systemic (high-dose inhaled or oral):

- Osteoporotic-bone change/skin-thinning, bruising
- Growth suppression in children (>400 µg/day)
- Adrenal suppression

Minimize by:

- Titrating dose upwards
- Using inhalers with high 1st-pass metabolism, e.g. budesonide (90%) or fluticasone (99%), esp. in children
- Steroid-sparing agents

Mast cell stabilizers

- Transient bronchospasm – give salbutamol 1st!
- Minor URT irritation/cough
- Hypersensitivity

Leukotriene receptor antagonists

- Dry mouth
- URTI/flu-like symptoms

ACUTE SEVERE ASTHMA

Epi

75% hospitalisations could be avoided in that effective Rx should have begun 48 hours earlier

At-risk groups

R.A.M^3.P^5.

Recent deterioration: Noctural symptoms, diurnal lability, ↓ PEFR
Allergen exposure: Pollen (e.g. summer, holiday), storm, evening
Misjudged perception of severity; **M**eter use inadequate (PEFR); **M**iserly use of systemic steroids
Personal characteristics: **P**revious recent attacks, **P**sychiatric, **P**oor, **P**uberty

PC

- Respiratory distress

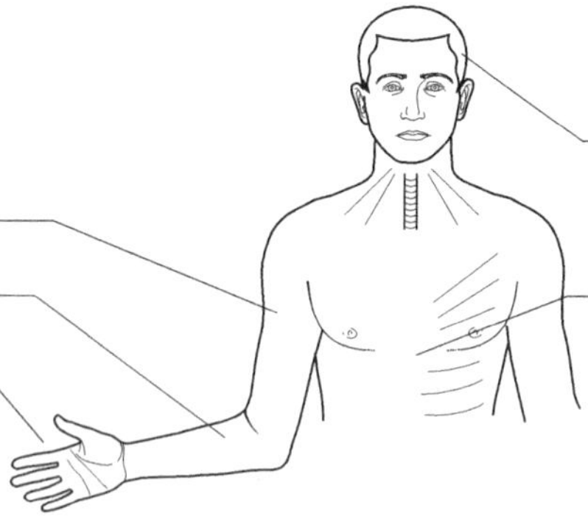

Central cyanosis

ABP: Pulsus paradoxus
SBP ↓ by >10 mmHg on inspiration

Pulse: Bounding

Hands: Warm, flap

Encephalopathic:
Headache, confused, papilloedema

Breathing:
Accessory muscles/alae flaring
Tracheal descent
Intercostal recession/subcostal (Harrison sulcus)

- Specific markers of severity

	Severe	Life-threatening
Airway	PEFR <50%	PEFR <33%
Breathing	RR ≥25	Resp. effort ↓, silent chest, central cyanosis
Circulation	Pulse >110	Pulse <60, hypotension
Disability	Can't complete sentence in 1 breath	Exhaustion/confusion/coma
Exchange, gas		$PaCO_2$ normal or ↑ (>5.0 kPa) PaO_2 ↓(<8.0 kPa) pH ↓ (<7.36)

- Complications

Lung:
- Collapse: Segmental/lobar
- Pneumothorax/pneumomediastinum
- Pulmonary oedema

Heart:
- Dysrhythmia (esp. due to O_2 ↓ and K^+, exacerbated by salbutamol)
- Myocardial infarction

Ix and Rx

WARN ITU
if any life-threatening
features

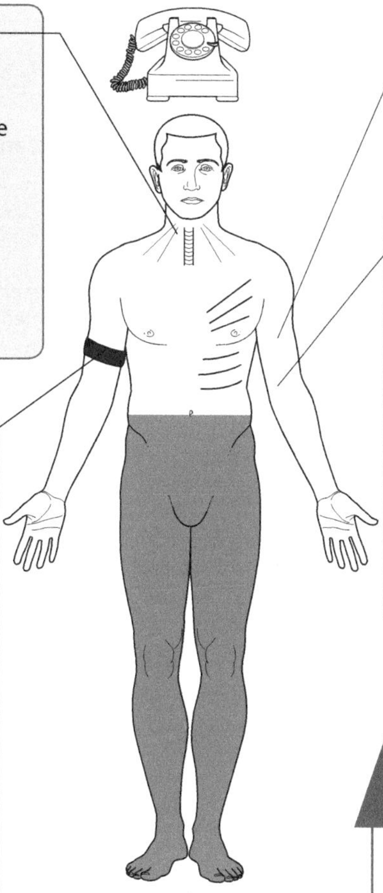

B. Ventilatory support

Sit patient up (aids respiration)
Oxygen: 60%,
unless Type II respiratory failure
Nebulizers:
Salbutamol (5–10 mg) +
Ipratropium bromide (0.5 mg):
every 4 hours, or every
15–30 min if Sx persist
CPAP, nasal IPPV,
intubate/IPPV → ITU

C. Hydration

e.g. N. saline IVI, unless
possibility of pulmonary
oedema

A. Assessment

A.B.C.D.

C.O.A.T.
- **C**ardiac monitor
- **O_2**
- **A**BP
- **T**PR

Investigations
- **B**loods:
  - U&E: K^+ ↓
  - FBC: WBC, Hb
  - ABGs:
    - $PaCO_2$ ↓ : Early
    - Normal or ↑ : Late
- **U**rine:
  - Glucose
- **M**icro:
  - Blood cultures; serology
- **M**onitor:
  - PEFR
- **E**CG
- **R**adiol:
  - CXR

D. Medication

Glucocorticoid:
IV hydrocortisone,
PO prednisolone
30–60 mg/day
IV magnesium
if not responding to nebs
Consider IV salbutamol

Optional
Antibiotics, e.g. augmentin,
erythromycin

DISCHARGE when:
- No nocturnal Sx
- Morning PEFR >75% expected
- Diurnal variation <25%

Other

Physiotherapy
Education via respiratory nurse:
- Inhaler technique
- PEFR monitor
- Compliance, esp. to steroid inhaler

COPD

Def

Chronic and irreversible small away obstruction with:

Mucus production and inflammation (chronic bronchitis)

+

Permanent enlargement of air spaces distal to terminal bronchiole, and alveolar wall destruction (emphysema)

Aet:

Chronic bronchitis

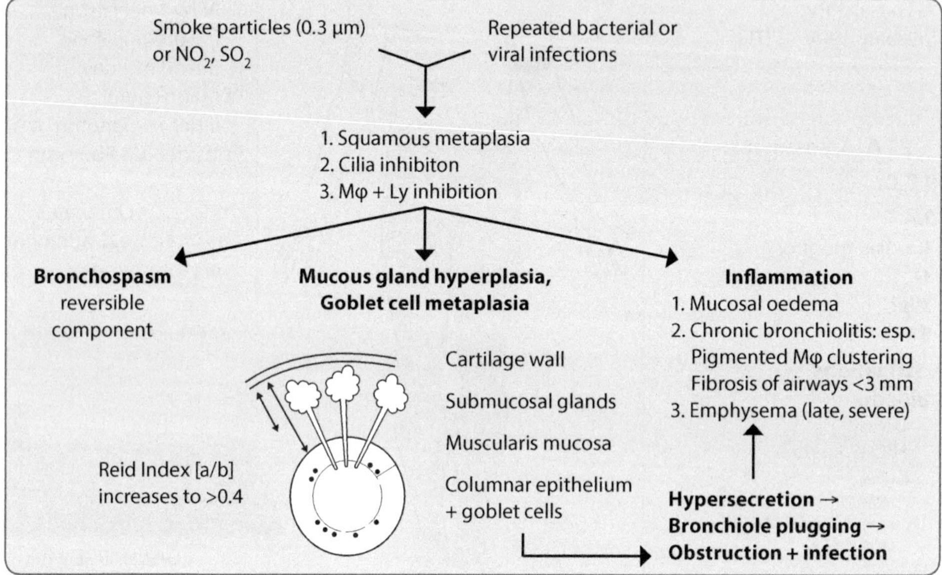

Emphysema

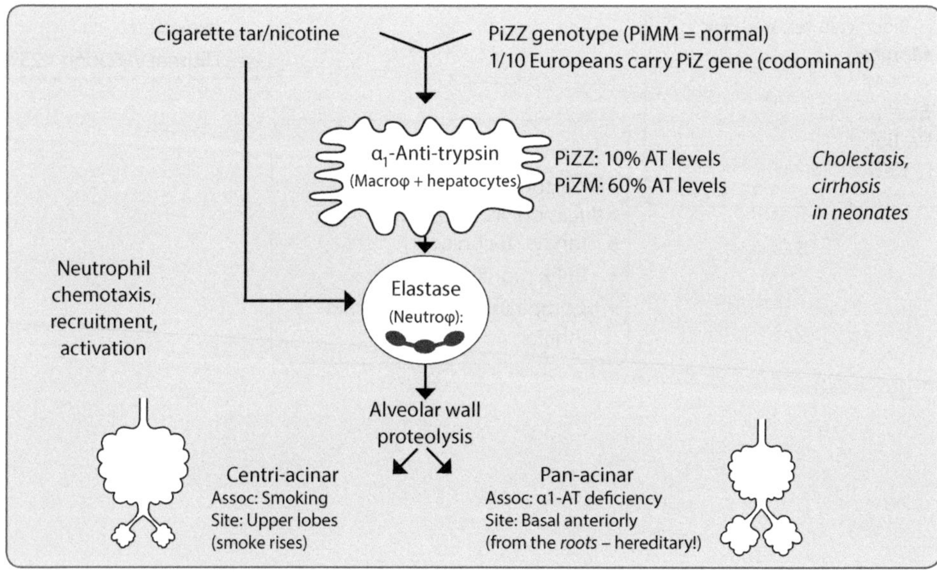

PC

Chronic cough
Exertional dyspnoea
Wheeze
Regular chest infections
Regular sputum production

Ix

Radiol:
  CXR: Hyperexpanded lungs
  HRCT: Bullous disease (emphysema)
Special:
  Spirometry: Obstructive defect (FEV1/FVC < 0.7)
  FEV1 correlates with severity

Rx

STOP SMOKING!

Regular influenza and pneumococcal vaccination
Pulmonary rehabilitation
Surgical: Lung volume reduction
lung transplant

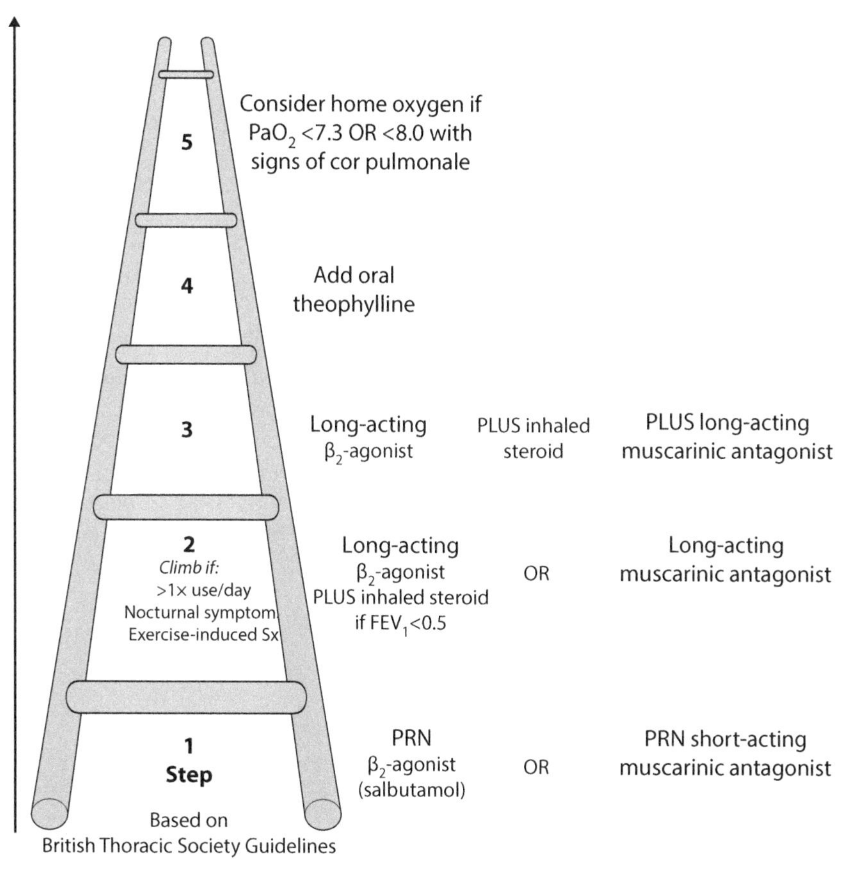

PULMONARY FIBROSIS

Causes

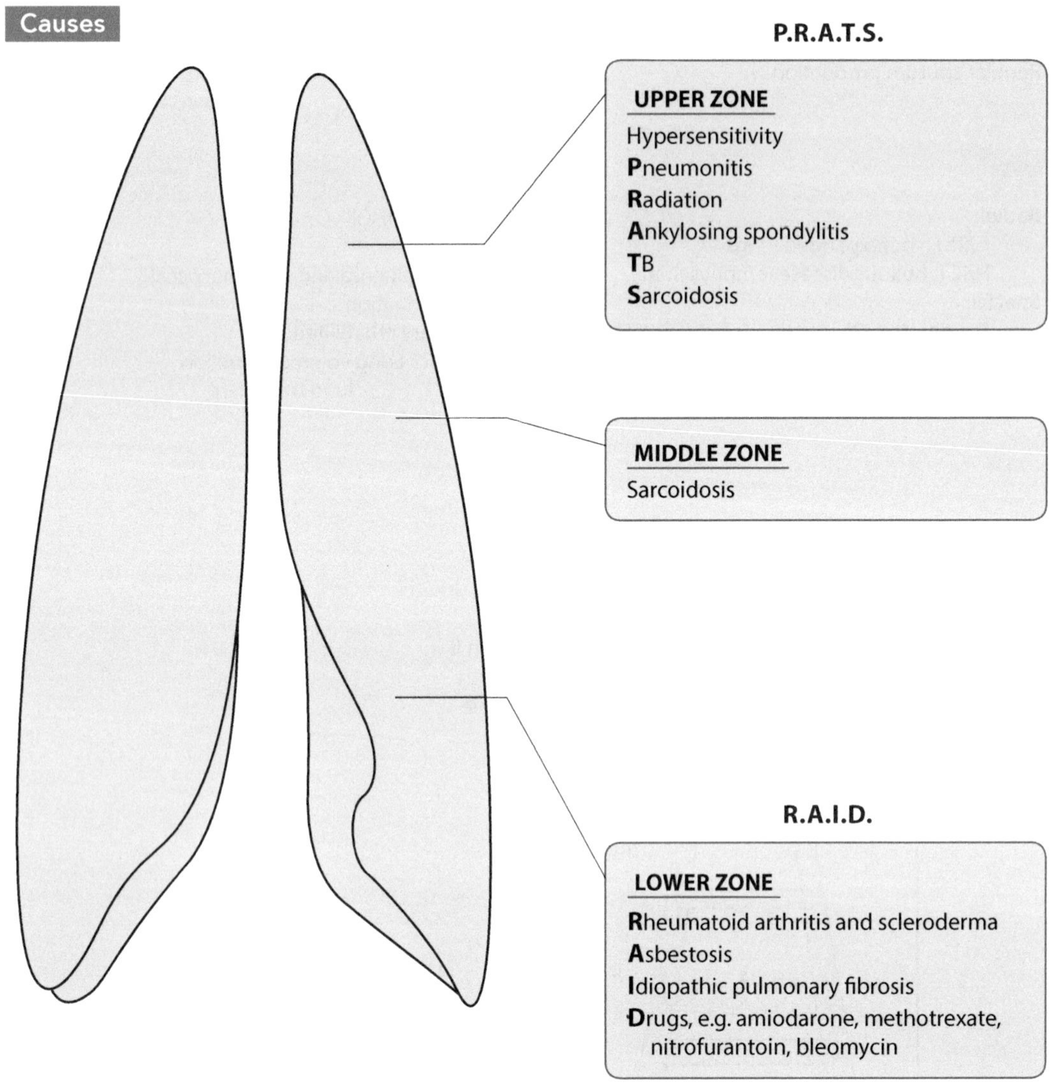

P.R.A.T.S.
UPPER ZONE
Hypersensitivity
Pneumonitis
Radiation
Ankylosing spondylitis
TB
Sarcoidosis
MIDDLE ZONE
Sarcoidosis
R.A.I.D.
LOWER ZONE
Rheumatoid arthritis and scleroderma
Asbestosis
Idiopathic pulmonary fibrosis
Drugs, e.g. amiodarone, methotrexate, nitrofurantoin, bleomycin

IDIOPATHIC PULMONARY FIBROSIS

= Usual interstitial pneumonitis (UIP)

PATH

Leaky alveolar-capillary membrane → macrophage and neutrophil infiltrate
Antibodies to unknown antigen, e.g. viral
Macrophage–T-cell interaction → IL-8, LT-B4, TNF → fibrosis and lung destruction

Epi

Age: Middle age
Sex: M:F = 2:1
Assoc.: Autoimmune disease in 1/3

HPC

PC

Constitutional: Malaise/weight loss/ arthralgia
Cough (dry)/Progressive SOBOE (acute form = Hamman–Rich syndrome)

O/E

Cyanosed
Clubbed
Creps: Basal, fine end-inspiratory; best heard in axillae, patient lying on side

COMPS

Carcinoma, lung: 15%

Ix

Bloods: ESR, immunoglobulins ↑
AutoAbs, e.g. ANA, RhF in 35%
ABG: ↓ O2, ↓ CO_2
Radiol: CXR: Bilateral basal; diffuse reticulonodular shadowing: 'honeycombing'
High-resolution CT: Cystic spaces
Special: Spirometry: Restrictive picture with ↓ KCO
BAL: Neutrophils + eosinophils (if lymphocytes, then suggests Rx-responsive)

Rx

Perfenidone
Nintedanib
Lung transplant

(Perfenidone, Nintedanib, Lung transplant: MAY SLOW DISEASE PROGRESSION ONLY)

Prog

5-year SR = 50%; highly variable: 65% if steroid-responsive (1/3); 25% if steroid-unresponsive (2/3)
Life expectancy: 1–20 years

OCCUPATIONAL LUNG DISEASES

Pneumoconioses

PATH

Inhaled inorganic dust is phagocytosed by alveolar macrophages, resulting in:

- Disruption of lysosomal membranes and release of proteolytic enzymes, e.g. elastase
- Impaired immunity (also caused by defective ciliary flow)

Epi

Coal worker's pneumoconiosis (dust = coal + kaolin + mica + silica; anthracite mine dust is more antigenic): 2% miners in resource-poor countries (rare where precautions heeded)

Silicosis: Seen in other types of miners, quarryworkers, sandblasters, pottery man

Asbestosis: Shipworkers; demolition or boilers; pipe-laggers; sputum reveals 'asbestos bodies' in macrophages

HPC

Acute (uncommon – usually silicosis or talcosis):

- Rapidly progressive SOB
- Respiratory failure
- Fever

Chronic (common):

- Slowly progressive SOB
- Cough (haem- or melanoptysis)
- Cyanosis, Clubbing, Crepitations

CXR

Coal worker's pneumoconiosis

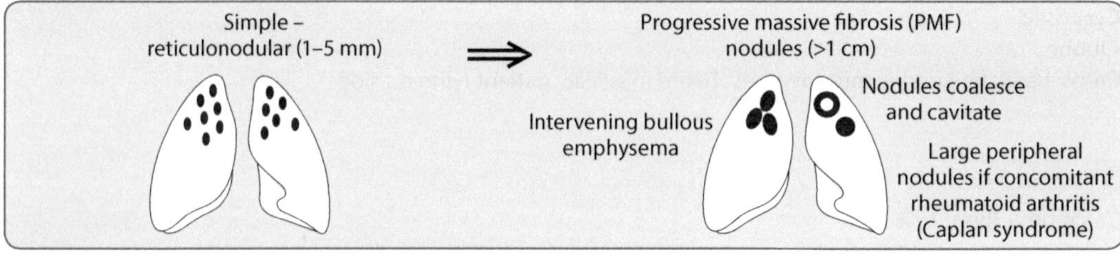

Silicosis

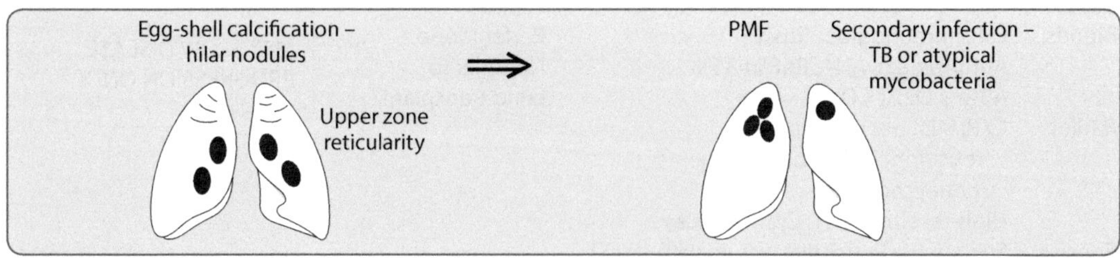

Asbestos exposure

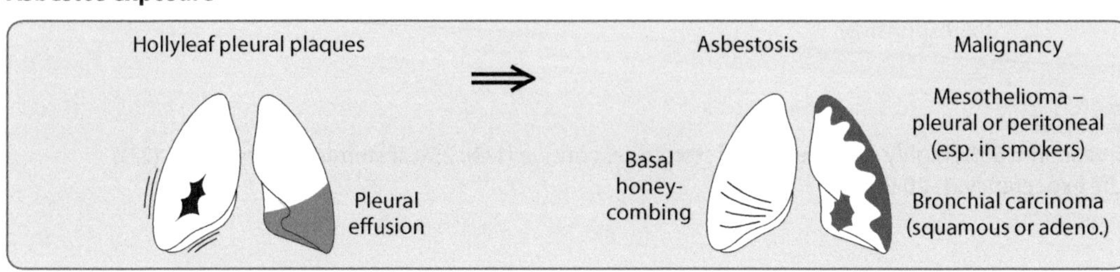

Hypersensitivity pneumonitis

PATH

Inhaled organic dusts result in acute or chronic alveolar sensitisation to particular antigen:

- Acute: Type III hypersensitivity reaction (starts 4–8 hours post-exposure; lasts 1–2 days)
- Chronic: Type IV hypersensitivity reaction, with granulomas (starts after 5–20 years)

Epi

Farmer's lung: Antigen = *Actinomycetes* spores (thermophilic filamentous bacteria), found in moist hay; worsens in winter (hay is moved); improves with smoking!

Bird fancier's lung: Antigen = serum proteins in bird droppings or feathers

Byssiniosis: Antigen = cotton dust, flax, hemp; worst on 1st day of week, and improves as week progresses; worsens with smoking

Other: Baggasosis (sugar); mushroom-worker's; grain-worker's; ventilator's lung

HPC

Acute:

- Flu-like (fever, myalgia)
- Cough (dry)
- SOB

Chronic:

- Constitutional (malaise, LOW)
- Cough (dry)
- SOB
- Fine creps or squeaks (NB: No wheeze!)

Ix

Bloods: Neutrophilia (NB: Eosinophils normal)
ESR ↑

Micro: Serum precipitins farmer's lung (ELISA): 80% sensitivity + 80% specificity

Radiol: CXR:

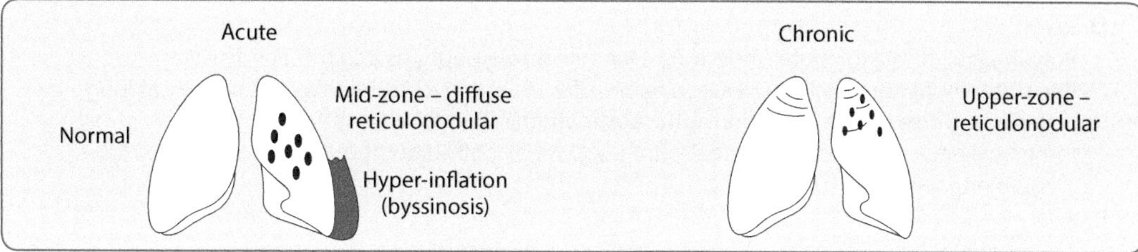

Special: Spirometry: Restrictive/obstructive picture, ↓ KCO
BAL: Lymphocytes + mast cells
Intradermal skin test (6 hours)

Rx

Avoidance
Prednisolone – acutely/long-term
Lung transplant

SARCOIDOSIS

PC

Characterized by **G.R.A.N.U.L.O.M.A.S.**

General
- Fever (Löfgren syndrome = acute fever + arthralgia + cough + erythema nodosum)
- Anorexia: Weight loss, fatigue
- Lymphadenopathy, hepatosplenomegaly

Respiratory
- Upper tract: Otitis, sinusitis, rhinitis, laryngitis
- Lower tract:
  - Bihilar lymphadenopathy (BHL): CXR = egg-shell calcification (stage 1)
  - Parenchymal infiltration: Diffuse, miliary nodules (stage 2)
  - Fibrosis: Apical and perihilar linear streaks (stage 3)
  - Complications: Cavitation ± mycetoma; collapse 2° to bronchial obstruction

Arthralgia
- Painful joints more common than arthritis
- Dactylitis, bony cysts, tufting + sclerosis of terminal phalanges
- Soft tissue calcinosis

Neurological
- Brain:
  - Diffuse, meningeal thickening: Dementia, meningo-encephalitis
  - Focal granulomas: Seizures, focal signs, hydrocephalus
- Cord: Transverse myelitis
- Peripheral and cranial neuropathy, e.g. bilateral VII cranial nerve palsy
- Myopathy

Urine
- Polyuria, polydipsia (diabetes insipidus): Due to neurohypophysis and tubular disease
- Renal stones, nephrocalcinosis: Due to hypercalcaemia: due to 1α-hydroxylase activity in lung lesions; worse in summer when light causes vitamin D synthesis
- Interstitial nephritis: Due to hypercalcaemia and renal infiltration (tubulointerstitial nephritis + glomerulonephritis)

Liver
- Causes cholestatic LFTs, but only rarely liver failure or cirrhosis

Ophthalmological
- Lacrimal: Xerophthalmia, Mikulicz syndrome – enlarged lacrimal + 3 salivary glands; 'uveoparotid fever' (Heerfordt syn.)= acute fever + Mikuliczs syn. + uveitis + Bell's palsy
- Anterior: Conjunctivitis (incl. due to sicca), band keratopathy, cataract, anterior uveitis, glaucoma
- Posterior: Posterior uveitis – perivascular cuffing of equatorial veins, optic atrophy

Myocardial
- Restrictive cardiomyopathy, 2° to myocardial granulomas + fibrosis → 3° heart block/VT
- Pericardial effusion

Amenorrhoea etc: Hypopituitarism

Skin
- Lupus pernio: Raised, dusky-purple plaque on nose, cheeks, fingers
- Boeck sarcoid: Purple-red nodules on face, back, extensor surfaces
- Scar infiltration
- Erythema nodosum: Painful, erythematous nodules on legs, forearms

Epi

Inc: 10/100,000 pa
Age: Peaks in 20s–30s, but can occur at any age
Sex: F>M
Geo: Afro-Caribbeans have 10× higher incidence, and have more severe disease
Chinese: Rarely occurs
Aet: Immune:
- T-cell function impaired, although CD4 T cells, activated macrophages and soluble IL-2R levels ↑
- B-cell function ↑: Hypergammaglobulinaemia

Infection: Unidentified mycobacteria? since similar immune response (granulomas, ↑ T cells) and PCR +ve in some cases

Ix

Bloods: Serum ACE↑ (+ve in 75%; false +ves = atypical mycobacteria; leprosy; Gaucher)
Other: Ig ↑, ESR ↑, Ca^{2+}↑
Urine: Ca^{2+}↑
Radiol: CXR: 'Bihilar lymphadenopathy, apical fibrosis'
Gallium scan:
- Taken up by activated macrophages in granuloma
- 'Panda appearance' due to uptake in salivary + lacrimal glands
- Can be used to monitor disease activity

Special: Tuberculin skin test: –ve in sarcoid (cf. TB = +ve)
Kveim test: Intradermal injection of sarcoid-spleen suspension → skin biopsy at 6 weeks shows granulomas
Lung function tests: KCO ↓ (1st sign of parenchymal disease); restrictive picture (FVC ↓, FEV_1/FVC norm or ↑)

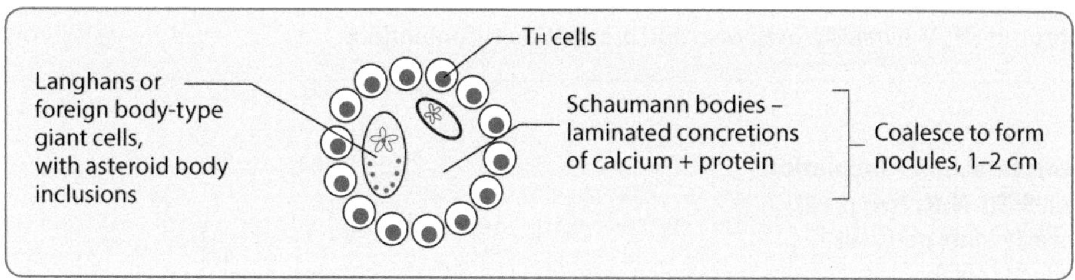

Rx

Serum **A.C.E.**
Steroids: Prednisolone, 3 month course
Indications: Respiratory, cardiac, ophthalmic, neurological, renal disease, hypercalcaemia
Azathioprine/methotrexate/hydroxychloroquine: Act as steroid sparers/maintenance therapy
- Need to check FBC (Aza, MTX) + LFT (MTX)
- Need to check central visual field (Amsler eye test)

Calcium reduction: see p. 389
Eye drops: Cyclopentolate: mAch receptor inhibitor
Fluorometholone: Steroid with least tendency to ↑ intraocular pressure

Prog

70% recover within 1–2 years, esp. acute presentation, e.g. Lofgren syndrome, young, Caucasian
25% relapses or chronic disease: More likely if insidious onset, e.g. lupus pernio, chronic uveitis, middle aged, black ethnicity
5% death due to complications

BRONCHIECTASIS

Causes

B.R.O.N.C.H.I.E.C.T.A.T.I.C.

Bronchial asthma
Rheumatoid arthritis
Obstruction of airways, due to inhaled foreign body or bronchial tumour
Yellow **N**ail syndrome: Rare disease comprising bronchiectasis, lymphoedema, pleural effusions and yellow nail dystrophy
Cystic fibrosis
Hypogammaglobulinaemia and other congenital immunodeficiency disorders (recurrent childhood lung infections)
Idiopathic
Eponymous syndromes
- Kartagener syndrome: Primary ciliary dysmotility, autosomal recessive
- William Campbell syndrome: Congenital bronchiomalacia
- Young syndrome: Viscous sputum, bronchiectasis, sinusitis and subfertility

Chronic gastric reflux
TB
Allergic broncho-pulmonary aspergillosis (ABPA): Hypersensitivity inflammatory response to inhaled aspergillus, most common in patients with asthma or CF
Traction bronchiectasis: Distortion of lung architecture due to severe COPD or fibrosis
Infections, repeated
Crohn and UC: Mechanism unknown and association is contentious

1. Chronic infection – Inhalation
Bacterial: **S.T.I.N.K.** (see p. 82)
Viral (measles, flu); pertussis
Aspergillosis (ABPA)
Toxic gas inhalation

2. Bronchial obstruction
Foreign body
Tumour (esp. carcinoid); lymph node, e.g. sarcoid
Congenital, e.g. pulmonary sequestration

3. Host defences ↓
Secretions:
- Cystic fibrosis: ↑ viscosity → bronchial clogging
- Yellow nail syndrome: ↓ lymphatic drainage

Structural:
- Kartagener syndrome: Ciliary dyskinesia
  PC: Sinusitis. male infertility, dextrocardia
- Marfan syndrome: ↓ bronchial elasticity

Immune:
- Hypogammaglobulinaemia, HIV

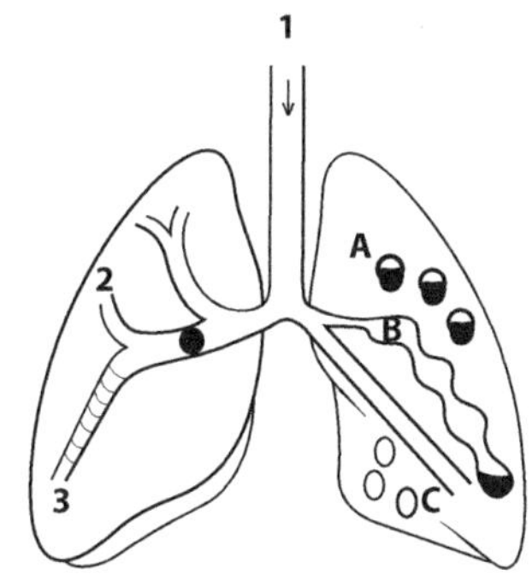

Pathology
A. Cystic: Blind-ending saccules with fluid levels
B. Varicose: Irregular beading
C. Cylindrical: 'Tram-tracks'

Complications
- Abscess
- Emphysema – fibrosis
- Amyloidosis

PC

Cough: Haemoptysis
Chest pain: Pleuritic
Systemic: Fever, weight loss

O/E

Inspection: Cyanosed, clubbed, cachectic
Auscultation: Creps – coarse, clicks – inspiratory, Wheeze
Sputum: Copious, purulent, bloody (cf. IPF – dry)

Ix

Bloods: Inflammatory markers, CF genetic testing, rheumatoid factor/CCP
Micro: Sputum culture including for TB
Radiol: CXR: 'Tram-tracks', cystic cavities
CT: 'Signet-ring sign' = large bronchiole + paired vascular bundle
Special: Bronchoalveolar lavage for culture

Rx

Physiotherapy: Chest wall percussion with head-down postural drainage
O_2, long-term – to prevent cor pulmonale

Medical:

- Bronchodilators
- Mucolytics (DNase) – degrade DNA released from neutrophils
- Daily prophylactic antibiotics, e.g. azithromycin 3 times/week or daily colomycin nebs

Surgical:

- Resection
- Artery embolisation (for hemoptysis)
- Lung transplant

LUNG ABSCESS

Causes

Sputum tends to **S.T.I.N.K.** *(due to anaerobes)*

1. Infection

S*taphylococcus aureus*

Risk:

- Post-pneumonia, e.g. post-influenza
- Haematogenous, e.g. IVDU, CVP line

TB

Upper zone ± 2ndary *Aspergillus* infection

Intestinal bacteria

Organisms:

- Anaerobes: *Bacteroides, Actinomyces*
- Coliforms
- *Enterococcus*

Risk:

- Dental caries, pharyngeal abscess
- Aspiration pneumonia
- Liver abscess via diaphragm:

Strep. ml7/eri (anaerobic), *Entamoeba*

N*ocardia*

K*lebsiella*

2. Bronchial obstruction

Due to FB, tumour, lymph node – mixed organisms

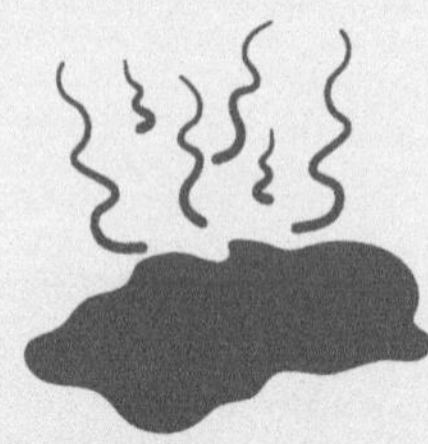

3. Host defences ↓

AIDS, leukaemia, chronic granulomatous disease

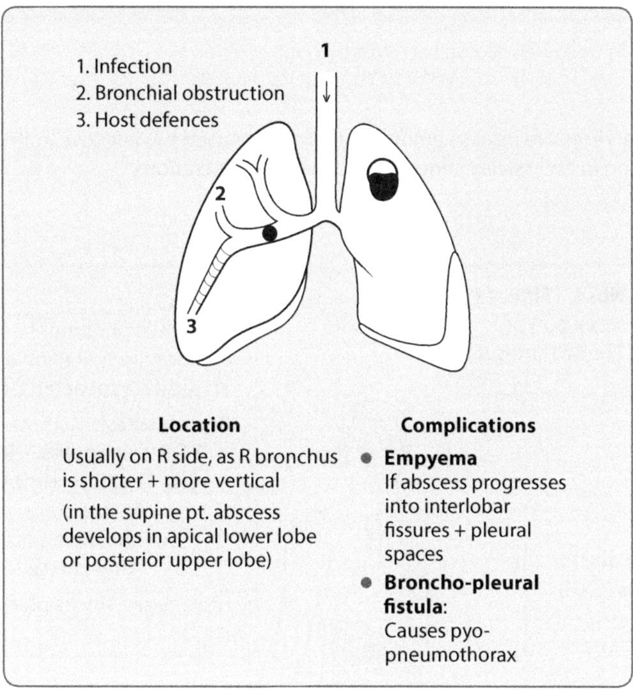

Location

Usually on R side, as R bronchus is shorter + more vertical

(in the supine pt. abscess develops in apical lower lobe or posterior upper lobe)

Complications

- **Empyema**
  If abscess progresses into interlobar fissures + pleural spaces
- **Broncho-pleural fistula**:
  Causes pyo-pneumothorax

PC

As for bronchiectasis

O/E

As for bronchiectasis +
Amphoric breathing = breath sound, like blowing over a jar, suggests air–fluid level

Ix

Micro: Culture – sputum, blood, bronchoalveolar lavage

Radiol: CXR (AP & lateral): cavity ± fluid-level
CT

Rx

Physiotherapy

Medical: IV antibiotics

Surgical:

- Bronchoscopy: Repeated bronchoalveolar lavage
- Resection

CYSTIC FIBROSIS

Def

Commonest autosomal recessive disease among Caucasians, caused by defective epithelial chloride channel (CFTR), resulting in excessively concentrated epithelial secretions

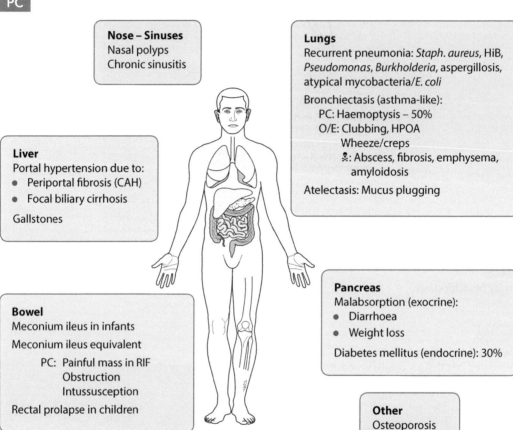

Nose – Sinuses
Nasal polyps
Chronic sinusitis

Lungs
Recurrent pneumonia: *Staph. aureus*, HiB, *Pseudomonas*, *Burkholderia*, aspergillosis, atypical mycobacteria/*E. coli*

Bronchiectasis (asthma-like):
- PC: Haemoptysis – 50%
- O/E: Clubbing, HPOA
  - Wheeze/creps
  - ☠: Abscess, fibrosis, emphysema, amyloidosis

Atelectasis: Mucus plugging

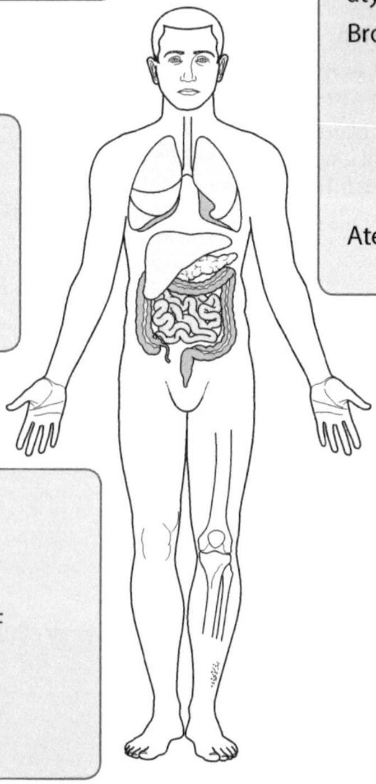

Liver
Portal hypertension due to:
- Periportal fibrosis (CAH)
- Focal biliary cirrhosis

Gallstones

Pancreas
Malabsorption (exocrine):
- Diarrhoea
- Weight loss

Diabetes mellitus (endocrine): 30%

Bowel
Meconium ileus in infants

Meconium ileus equivalent
- PC: Painful mass in RIF
  - Obstruction
  - Intussusception

Rectal prolapse in children

Other
Osteoporosis
Arthropathy
Rash, vasculitic

Sexual organs
Male infertility:
- Hypogonadism
- Azoospermia
- Vas deferens maldevelopment

Female infertility: Cervical mucus thickening

Hazardous pregnancy

Epi

Inc: Carrier = 1/25; disease = 1/2500 (in Caucasians)

Age: Neonatal presentation: Meconium ileus; Guthrie heel-prick (serum trypsin ↑
Childhood presentation: Failure to thrive; asthma; diarrhoea

Sex: M:F =1:1

Geo: Caucasians predominantly

Aet: Law of **7s**:
- Chromosome **7p**
- **70%**: ΔF508 = Phenylalanine substitution or deletion
- >**70** mmol/l: NaCl concentration in sweat test

Micro:

Normal epithelial lumen, e.g. pancreas, bronchus

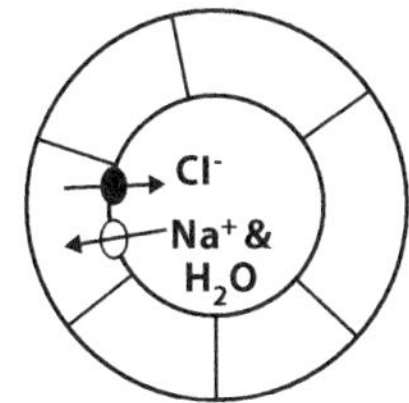

Cystic fibrosis

Cl^- channel (CFTR) fails due to:
- Intracellular trafficking defect
- Abnormal functioning

X
Na^+ & H_2O

Also:
Cl^- influx ↓
⇒
$NaHCO_3$ and trypsin secretn ↓

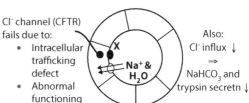

Ix

Sweat test: NaCl >70 mmol/l (adults >90); fludrocortisone ↑ sensitivity
Nasal transepithelial potential difference more negative than normal
Faecal elastase ↑

Rx

Lungs

Conservative: Physiotherapy (postural drainage), O_2, vaccinate

Medical:
- Mucolytic: DNase
- Bronchodilators, incl. aminophylline; steroids for COPD
- Antibiotics, e.g. flucloxacillin, piperacillin, gentamicin, ceftazidime, ciprofloxacin

Surgical: Lung transplantation

Liver
- Ursodeoxycholic acid
- Injection sclerotherapy
- Liver transplant

Bowel: Surgery

Pancreas
- Oral pancreatin
- Insulin

Other
- Genetic counselling (screen family with gene probes)
- Chorionic villous sampling for prenatal Dx, at 9–12 weeks
- DEXA scan for osteoporosis; Rx with bisphosphonates

PNEUMOTHORAX

Def

Accumulation of air in pleural space, with secondary partial collapse of lung

Types

Primary – in a normal lung
Secondary – due to lung pathology, e.g. COPD, asthma

Either type may be under **tension** = air moves in, but not out, due to fistula or defect acting as one-way valve

Causes

S.T.R.I.P.

Spontaneous, associated with
Smoking
Structural:
- Congenital, apical bleb ruptures
- Young, thin men (M:F=6:1), esp. Marfan syndrome; recurrence common (unilateral): 25% if had one; 50% if had two

Trauma: Blunt (e.g. CPR) or penetrating (e.g. stab wound)
Ruptured oesophagus: Boerhaave syndrome (severe vomiting causing rupture) → hydropneumothorax
Iatrogenic: CVP line, esp. subclavian; positive-pressure ventilation; bronchoscopy, esp. with biopsy
Pulmonary disease
Diffuse:
- Obstructive: Asthma, emphysema, bronchiectasis
- Restrictive: Pulmonary fibrosis, sarcoid, rheumatoid arthritis

Focal: Infection, tumour, esp. metastases, congenital

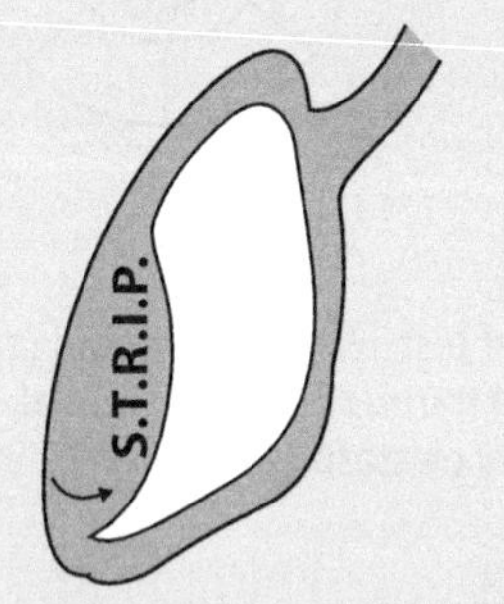

Simple: Pain (sudden, pleuritic, radiates to shoulder); dry cough; SOB
Tension: Acute respiratory distress; collapse; cardiac arrest

O/E

Chest exam
Ipsilateral chest movement ↓
Hyper-resonance
Auscultation: AE ↓
Subcutaneous emphysema

If tension:
Obstructive shock
Elevated JVP
Tracheal deviation away from affected side

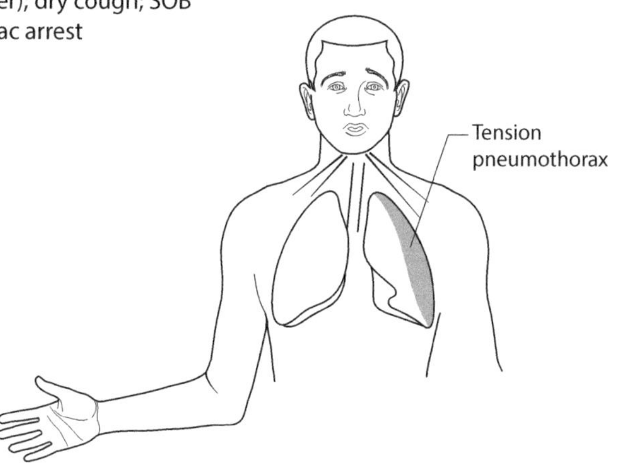

Ix

Radiol: CXR:

- Translucency + collapse visible rim between lung and chest-wall >2 cm = >50% lung volume loss
- Mediastinal shift
- Pneumomediastinum or surgical emphysema – air in local tissues
- Underlying lung disease

CT: Distinguishes loculated pneumothorax from bullae

Rx

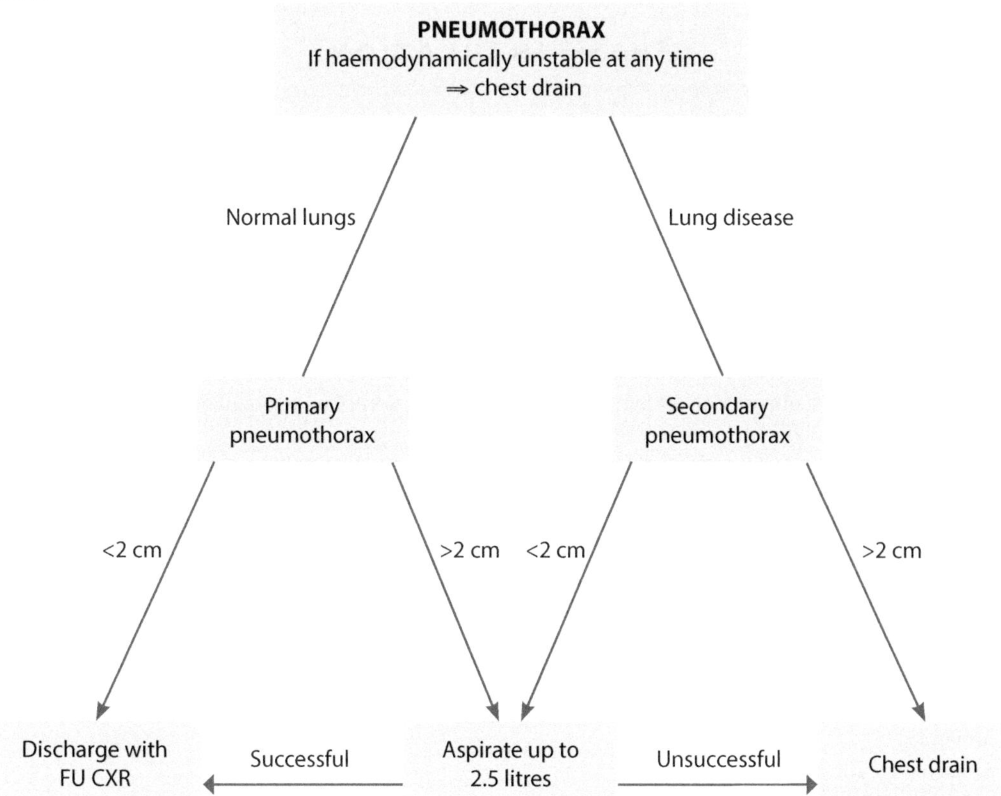

Refractory or recurrent

Lateral thoracotomy or thoracoscopy:

IND: Required if no improvement with intercostal drain after 1 week, or if recurrent pneumothorax

Method: Pleurodesis, e.g. tetracycline, bleomycin, talc injection
Pleural abrasion or pleurectomy
Bulla stapling or lasering

Tension pneumothorax:

Immediate insertion of wide-bore cannula into 2nd I/C sp., mid clavicular line (don't wait for CXR)
Rapid insertion of chest drain

PLEURAL EFFUSION

Causes

Categorized according to protein or LDH (lactate dehydrogenase) content of pleural fluid:

Transudate: Redistribution of Starling forces across microcirculation (as for pulmo. oedema – p. 90) protein <35 g/l or pleural/serum LDH < 2/3

Exudate: Capillary permeability increases or lymph drainage decreases, protein >35 g/l or pleural/serum LDH > 2/3

C^2.H.E.S^2.T. I.N.S.U.L.A.T.I.O.N.

Transudate

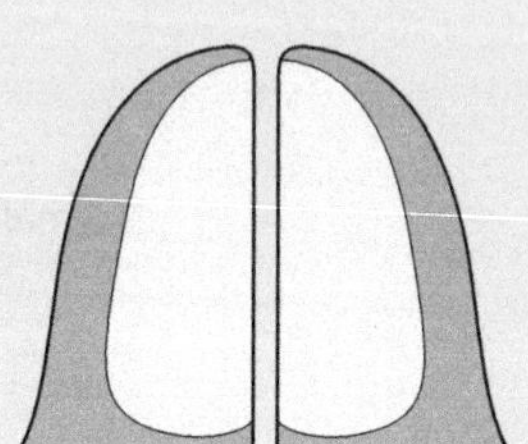

Cardiac failure: LVF, RVF, pericardial effusion or constriction: due to pulmonary (LVF) or bronchial (RVF) capillary hydrostatic pressure ↑

Cirrhosis, nephrosis, malnutrition, malabsorption, protein-losing enteropathy (e.g. intestinal lymphangectasia) – often R-sided effusion and concomitant ascites

Hypoalbuminaemia – plasma oncotic pressure ↓

Embolism, pulmonary: Due to hydrostatic pressure redistribution

Superior vena cava obstruction (or inferior vena cava obstruction): Due to drainage of bronchial veins into SVC/IVC

Subclavian or jugular vein catheter misplacement with infusion of crystalloid, or peritoneal dialysis in presence of congenital pleuro-peritoneal communication

Thyroid ↓: Due to myxoedema

Exudate

Infection: *Strep. pneumoniae, Mycoplasma,* TB, viruses (EBV, coxsackie), rheumatic fever: may cause either a parapneumonic effusion or empyema (i.e. bacterial infection of pleural fluid)

Neoplasia: Bronchial carcinoma, pleural mesothelioma or fibroma, breast, ovarian, lymphoma

Surgery or trauma: CABG, mastectomy, radiotherapy, lung contusion

Uraemia

Liver, pancreatic, ovarian disease:
- Subphrenic or hepatic abscess
- Pancreatitis or pancreatic pseudocyst or carcinoma; pleural fluid amylase ↑
- Ovarian fibroma (Meigs syndrome); ovarian hyperstimulation; pleural endometriosis

Autoimmune: SLE, rheumatoid arthritis, scleroderma, polyarteritis nodosa

Toxins: **B.A.N. M.E.** – **B**romocriptine, **A**miodarone, **N**itrofurantoin; **M**ethysergide, **E**nvironmental – asbestosis

Infarction: Pulmonary (due to multiple PEs), myocardial (Dressler syndrome)

Oesophageal rupture: Pleural fluid amylase ↑

Nail syndrome, yellow: Due to lymphatic hypoplasia, and also associated with pitting oedema and sinusitis + familial Mediterranean fever: periodic fever + pains in pleura, peritoneum and joints, due to pyrin mutation

PC

SOB, progressively worsening
Chest pain

O/E

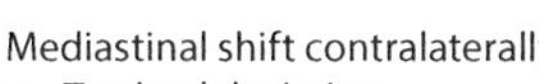

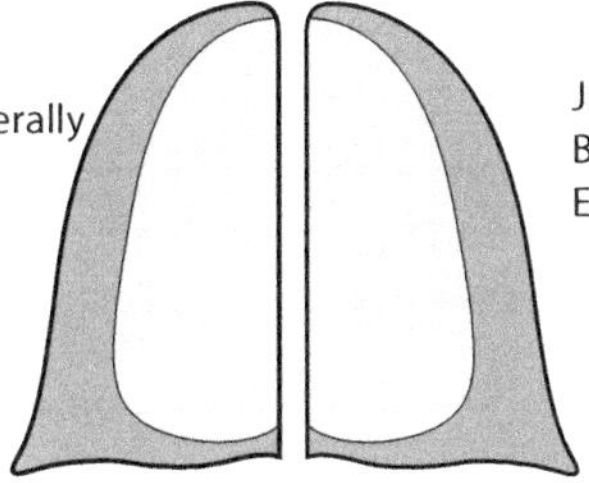

Ix

Radiol: CXR: Meniscus-shaped, rises towards axilla; repeat after drainage to look for tumour/lymph nodes
USS: Localizes small effusions, and allows their tapping
CT: Allows underlying lung and mediastinum to be visualized

Special: Pleural fluid aspiration

Appearance:

- Clear, straw-coloured suggests transudate
- Turbid, green indicates exudate (pus cells) or empyema (i.e. actual bacterial infection)
- Bloody (i.e. haemothorax): Tumour; pulmonary embolism; acute pancreatitis, trauma
- White (i.e. chylothorax = lymph): Blocked thoracic duct, usually due to tumour

Analysis:

- Protein and LDH: Determine whether transudate or exudate; glucose ↓ in most exudates
- Amylase ↑ in pancreatitis, tumour, oesophageal rupture
- Microbiology, incl. AAFB staining and cultures
- Cytology

Rx

Underlying cause

Specific:

Transudate: Diuretics can result in rapid resolution
Exudate:

- Repeated drainage (thoracocentesis): Limit drainage rate to <2/24 h
- Intrathoracic streptokinase via chest drain: Lyses fibrinous adhesions
- Pleural adhesion: Tetracycline, bleomycin, talc
- Decortication surgery

PULMONARY OEDEMA

Causes

May be classified in accordance with Starling forces:

C.O.I.L.ED.

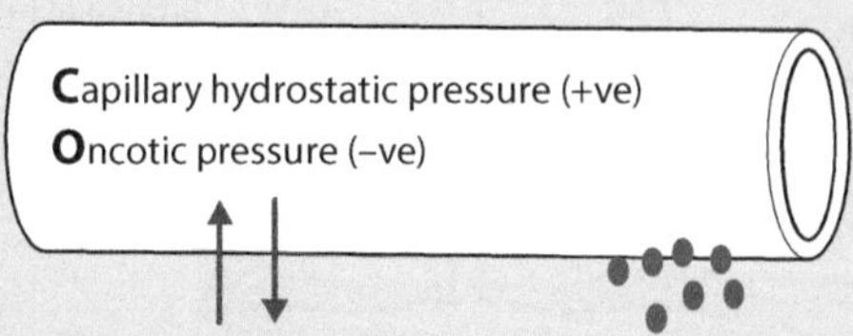

Interstitial hydrostatic pressure (–ve)
contributed to by alveolar air pressure

Exu**D**ate – capillary permeability ↑

Lymph drainage (–ve)

Transudate

Capillary hydrostatic pressure ↑
- LVF
- PE
- Overhydration, e.g. with normal saline

Oncotic pressure ↓
- Malnutrition, malabsorption, protein-losing enteropathy
- Cirrhosis
- Nephrosis

Interstitial negative hydrostatic pressure ↑
- Asthma: Acute airway obstruction with high end-expiratory volume (more –ve pleural pressure required)
- Aspiration of pneumothorax or pleural effusion – if too rapid
- Altitude – unacclimatized athletes

Lymphatic drainage ↓
- Lymphangitis carcinomatosis
- Fibrosis, esp. secondary to silicosis
- Lung transplant

Exu**D**ate

Capillary permeability ↑ = ARDS (see opposite)

PATH: Diffuse endothelial + alveolar epithelial damage
Acute inflammatory exudate: Fibrin forms in airspaces ('hyaline membrane')
Pulmonary thromboemboli

Adult respiratory distress syndrome

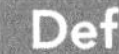

ARDS is a common inflammatory response to various lung insults, resulting in:

T.O.X.I.C.

Tachypnoea
Oxygen ↓: Progressive respiratory failure
X-ray: Bilateral pulmonary infiltrates
Interstitial fluid ↑
- Lung compliance (volume/pressure) ↓, so ↑ positive end-expiratory pressure (PEEP) required
- V/Q mismatch: Due to alveolar flooding + microvascular occlusion with platelets and neutrophils
- Fibrosis: >4 weeks

Cardiac function is normal (i.e. normal left atrial pressure or PAWP)

Causes

Lungs get **T.I.G.H.T.** *due to poor compliance*

Toxins:
- Aspirated
- Inhalation: Smoke, paraquat, O_2
- Systemic: Opiates, barbiturates, anaesthesia, aspirin, heparin

Infection:
- Pneumonia: Bacterial, viral, PCP
- Septicaemia, esp. acute pancreatitis

Gynaecological: Eclampsia, amniotic fluid embolism
Hypotension (shock): Hypovolaemic, anaphylaxis, anaesthesia/massive transfusion, cardiopulmonary bypass, cardioversion neurogenic: ICP ↑, e.g. SAH/status
Trauma: Lung contusion, DIC, fat embolism

Underlying cause, e.g. antibiotics, pleural drainage
Ventilation

Aims: High PEEP to recruit unused alveoli
Low tidal volume to avoid pneumothorax
Low FiO_2, e.g. 0.6 to avoid O_2 toxicity + permissive hypercapnia

☠: Pneumothorax: Due to high PEEP, high tidal volume, fibrosis; more apparent in lungs with near-normal compliance
Nosocomial infection: Ventilator-assoc. pneumonia; IV lines; catheters
Organ failure:
- Cardiac, renal, neuro: Avoid by keeping tight fluid control
- GIT: Enteral nutrition; H_2-antagonists, sucralfate

Medical: Adjuvants
- Prone positioning: Aerates better perfused dorsal lung segments
- Nitric oxide ± nebulized prostacyclin: Vasodilate in vicinity of ventilated alveoli
- Corticosteroids: Decrease fibrosis

LUNG CARCINOMA

PC + O/E

Lung carcinoma may present at 5 different levels:

1. Lung

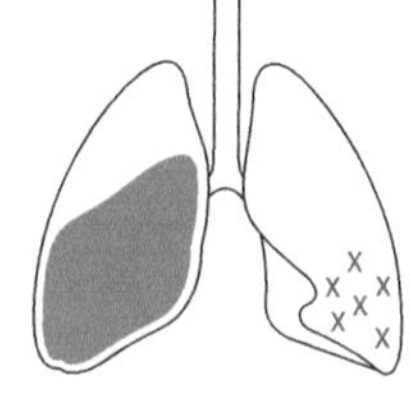

PC: SOB/cough (esp. haemoptysis)/chest pain
Recurrent pneumonia

O/E: Quiet breath sounds:

- Tumour; lobar collapse; pleural effusion
- Elevatated hemidiaphragm (phrenic N. palsy)

Crepitations: Consolidation; bronchiectasis; (radiotherapy: fibrosis)
Pneumothorax esp. pulmonary mets, e.g. osteosarcoma, Wilms

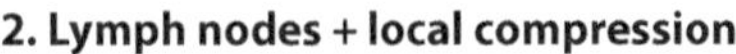

2. Lymph nodes + local compression

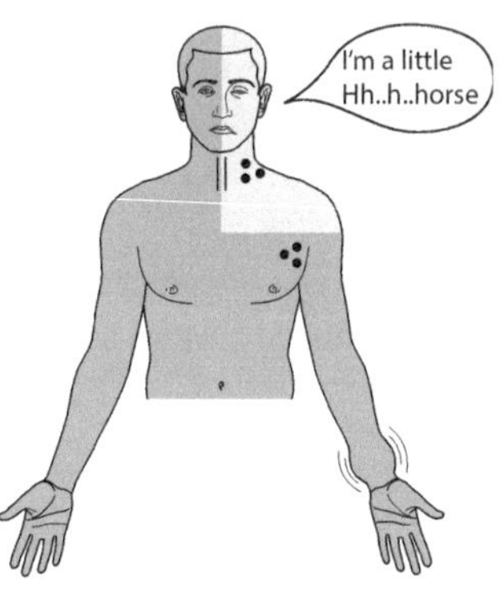

PC: Hoarseness: Due to L recurrent laryngeal N. palsy
Dysphagia, stridor

O/E: Lymphadenopathy: Supraclavicular, axillary
Neuro: Pancoast tumour infiltrates T1 stellate ganglion → Horner syn; wasting of intrinsic hand muscles; shoulder pain
Hands: Clubbing; tender wrists = hypertrophic pulmonary osteoarthropathy; hyperhidrosis; tar staining fingers (smoker)

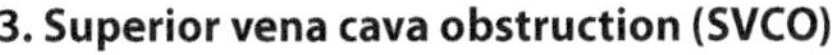

3. Superior vena cava obstruction (SVCO)

PC: Headache, SOB

O/E: Conjunctival oedema, plethora, vein dilatation

Pericardial tamponade: JVP ↑, ABP ↓, quiet HS

4. Metastases

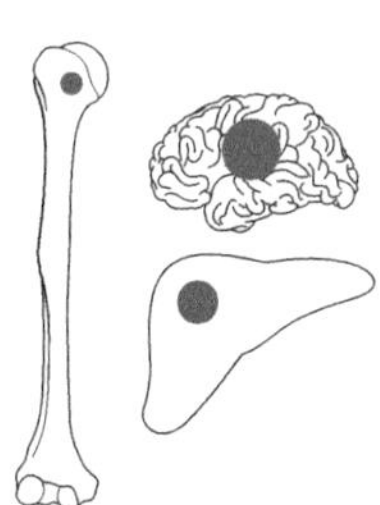

B.L.O.B.S.

Bone pain
Liver, adrenal (Addison)
Other: Lung, pleura, thoracic cage
Brain (stroke); spinal cord
Skin: Slightly blue umbilicated lesions

5. Constitutional + paraneoplastic

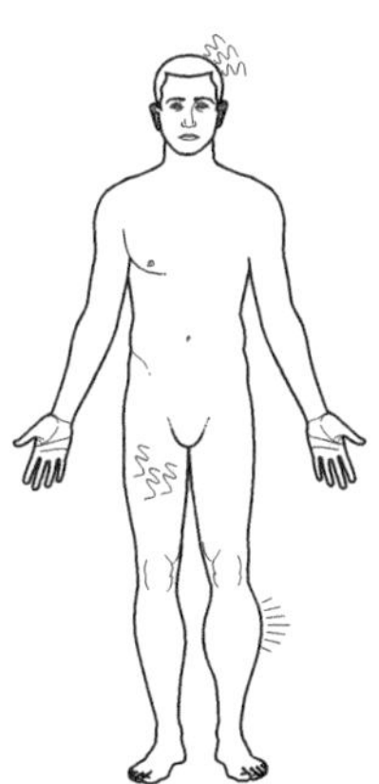

Constitutional: Cachexia; leucoerythroblastic anaemia; immunocompromise, e.g. shingles

Neurological (assoc. with small-cell carcinoma): Cerebellar degeneration; limbic encephalitis; peripheral neuropathy; dermatomyositis; Lambert–Eaton myasthenic syndrome

Endocrine: Ectopic secretions (mostly assoc. with small-cell ca.)
ACTH: Cushing; SIADH: confusion; β-HCG: gynaecomastia, body hair loss
PTHrp: Hypercalcaemia (esp. squamous cell carcinoma)

Skin: Dermatomyositis: Acanthosis nigricans; erythema gyratum repens; pruritus (also radiotherapy marks; burns)
Hypercoagulable state (assoc. with adenocarcinoma)
DVT, thrombophlebitis migrans, marantic endocarditis

Types of lung neoplasia

PRIMARY

Squamous cell carcinoma

Epi: 30% of all primary lung tumours, but decreasing incidence
Prog: Relatively good prognosis if localized (5-y survival ≈ 50%) – metastases occur late
Histo: Squamous metaplasia; keratin whorls
Characteristics: **C**entral location, **C**avitates, **C**lubbing (+ HPOA); **C**alcium ↑ (PTH-rp secretion)

Adenocarcinoma

Epi: 30%; increasing incidence, esp. women, less association with smoking
Prog: Poor (1 y median survival) – metastases occur early
Histo: Gland-like, mucin-secreting
Characteristics: Peripheral location; pleural effusions; hypercoagulable state

Small-cell carcinoma

Epi: 20%; strongest association with smoking
Prog: Poor (1 y median survival) – metastases occur early
Histo: Small APUD cells with neurosecretory granules; dark, oval nuclei, little cysts
Characteristics: Central location; paraneoplastic syndromes common

Large-cell carcinoma

Epi: 10%
Prog: Poor – metastases occur early
Histo: Giant cells; clear cells; anaplastic
Characteristics: Local invasion into mediastinum

RARE

Bronchoalveolar cell carcinoma:

- Variant of adenocarcinoma that is associated with chronic lung inflammation, rather than smoking. Prognosis relatively good
- Characteristics: Copious, clear mucoid sputum; SOB; recurrent bilateral pneumonia (cells carried in sputum)

Adenoma:

- Majority are carcinoid tumours (APUDomas) that occur in young people and have good prognosis
- Characteristics: Haemoptysis, lobar collapse, wheeze; 2% develop carcinoid syndrome or acromegaly; tumours occupy a central location, so often not visible

Hamartoma: Benign tumour of older men, seen on CXR as a peripheral calcified mass, and consisting of disordered but differentiated smooth muscle and cartilage

SECONDARY

B.O.M.B.E.R.S.

Breast
Oesophago/gastric/head–neck (+ colon if liver mets.)
Melanoma
Bone, sarcomas
Endocrine: Thyroid
Renal, prostate
Sex: Ovary, choriocarcinoma, testes

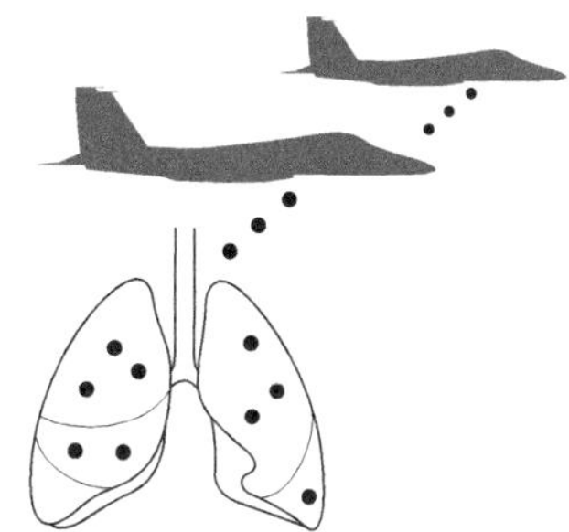

Non-small cell: Surgical resection possible in 1/3; adjuvant chemo/radiotherapy
Small cell: Radiotherapy + chemotherapy; 90% show limited regression

OBSTRUCTIVE SLEEP APNOEA

Def

Obstruction: Obstruction of upper airway occurs at night with loss of muscle tone in sleep
Sleep: Sleep disruption, snoring, sleepiness during day
Apnoea: Apnoeic spells: O_2 ↓, patient awakes from sleep

Causes

O.S³.A².

Obesity, central
The strongest risk factor for OSA is central obesity
This is measured as neck circumference (rather than Body Mass Index)
PATH: Fat deposition around upper airway → airway narrowing and resistance ↑
Abdominal fat ↑ elevates diaphragm

Structural features of upper airway

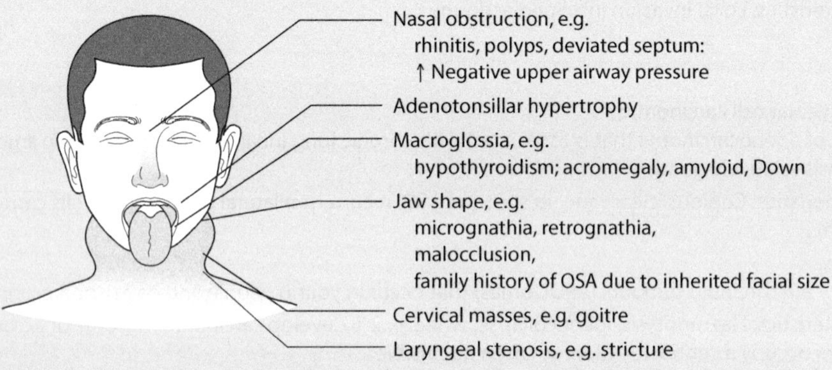

Smoking: Exacerbates hypoxia
Sex: Male
Atony:
Neuromuscular: Motor neurone disease, myopathy, myotonic dystrophy
CNS: CVA, multiple systems atrophy, encephalitis
Connective tissue laxity: Marfan syndrome (also because of high-arched palate)
Alcohol: Acts as a sedative thereby reducing upper airway tone (same for anaesthetics, benzodiazepines)

PC

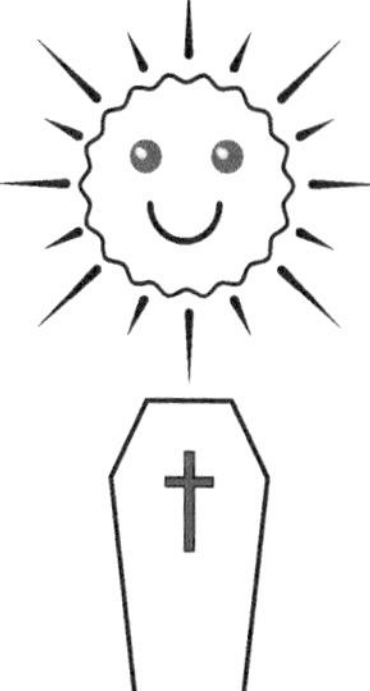

Nocturnal Sx
Obstruction and apnoea:
- Snoring, choking, gasping
- Awakening with nocturia

Gastro-oesophageal reflux

Daytime Sx:
Morning headache
Daytime somnolence
Memory + attention ↓, → accident risk!
Irritability, depression

Complications
Cyanosis → polycythaemia
Systemic hypertension (loss of normal nocturnal dipping)
Pulmonary hypertension – late (2° to chronic hypoxia) → cor pulmonale

Bloods: Causes: TFTs: hypothyroidism; LFTs: alcoholism
Effects: Hb ↑; ABG: CO_2 ↑
Urine: Glucose (Type II DM assoc. with obesity)
Monitor: Overnight oximetry
ECG: R-sided strain
Radiol: CXR: Cardiomegaly
Special: Polysomnography (overnight sleep study):
- Apnoea–hypopnea Index: >5/h abnormal (except elderly)
- 02 dipping: Titrate nasal CPAP to ↑ O_2
- EEG: Categorizes apnoea as REM or NREM sleep predominant

Conservative:
Weight loss
Avoid smoking, alcohol, sedatives
Sleep: Avoid supine position and sleep deprivation

CPAP (continuous positive airway pressure)
Method: 4–20 cm H_2O for >4 h per night, via nasal mask, maintains upper airway patency
Benefits: Reverses daytime Sx. (incl. accidents); prevents complications; MR ↓
Side-effects: Poor compliance due to encumbrance; skin ulceration; rhinorrhoea, epistaxis; aerophagia

MAD (mandibular advancement device) – intra-oral device that ↑ A-P diameter of upper airway →, ↓ snoring + apnoea

Surgical:
Adenoidectomy (curative in children)
Uvulopalatopharyngoplasty (50% benefit)
Maxillomandibular osteotomy
Tracheostomy if CPAP-intolerant

PULMONARY EMBOLISM

PATH

Embolus originates from deep-vein thrombosis in proximal leg or iliac veins (peri-operative), renal vein or IVC (renal or pelvic tumour), or cerebral venous or SVC thrombosis.

Types

PE may be classified according to size, with different pathologies and presentations for each:

Small–Medium

PATH:
- Infarction
- Haemorrhage

PC:
- Pleuritic pain
- Haemoptysis
- Acute SOB

O/E:
- Fever, low-grade
- Tachycardia (incl. AF)
- Pleural rub, wheeze

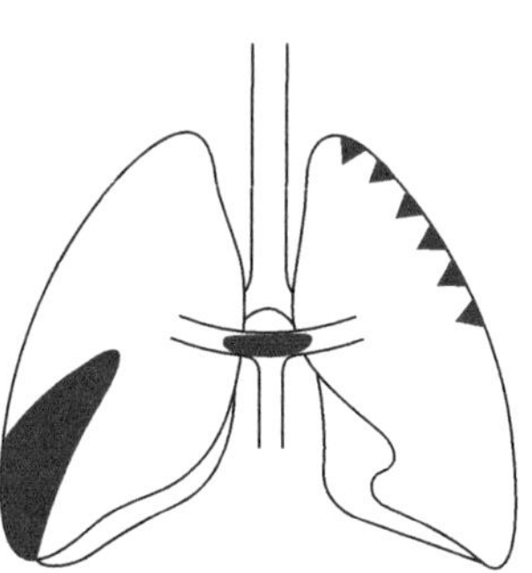

Multiple

PATH:
- Widespread infarction
- Pulmonary hypertension

PC:
- Cough, wheeze
- Progressive SOB, due to subacute right-sided heart failure

O/E:
- Respiratory distress, cyanosis
- Pulmonary hypertension: JVP ↑, gallop rhythm (S3), loud P2

Large

PATH: Pulmonary insufficiency due to occlusion of pulmonary trunk or main artery
PC: Acute right-sided heart failure; collapse, EMD, sudden death

Ix

Bloods: ABGs: O_2 ↓, CO_2 ↓
D-Dimers: Very sensitive, but poor specificity (false +ves)

ECG: Sinus tachycardia, AF
SI-QIII-TIII (R axis deviation)
R-sided strain; R bundle branch block

Radiol: CXR:
- Normal
- Decreased vascular markings or focal oligaemia
- Wedge-shaped infarct
- Linear atelectasis
- Small pleural effusion

V/Q isotope scan
CT pulmonary angiogram

Special:
Establish underlying cause: Doppler USS thigh, pelvis (+ve in 40%); thrombophilia screen
ECHO: Look for right heart strain

Rx

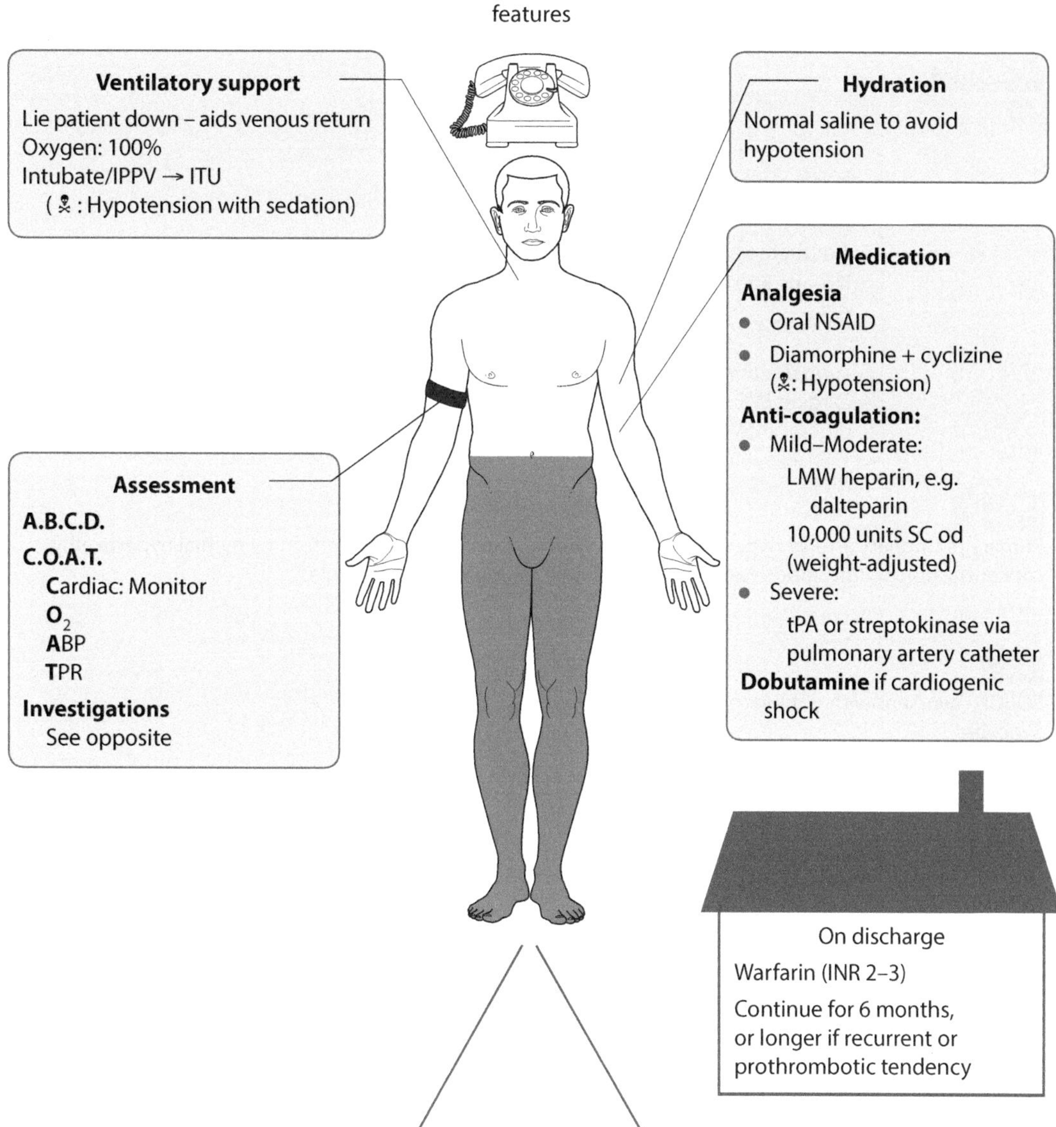

WARN ITU
if any life-threatening
features
Ventilatory support
Lie patient down – aids venous return
Oxygen: 100%
Intubate/IPPV → ITU
(☠: Hypotension with sedation)
Hydration
Normal saline to avoid
hypotension
Medication
Analgesia
Oral NSAID
Diamorphine + cyclizine
(☠: Hypotension)
Anti-coagulation:
Mild–Moderate:
LMW heparin, e.g.
dalteparin
10,000 units SC od
(weight-adjusted)
Severe:
tPA or streptokinase via
pulmonary artery catheter
Dobutamine if cardiogenic
shock
Assessment
A.B.C.D.
C.O.A.T.
Cardiac: Monitor
O2
ABP
TPR
Investigations
See opposite
On discharge
Warfarin (INR 2–3)
Continue for 6 months,
or longer if recurrent or
prothrombotic tendency

Surgery

Thrombendarterectomy if life-threatening

Radiology

Inferior vena cava filter

IND: Recurrent or chronic PE

☠ Recurrent PE

IVC occlusion; leg + genital oedema

PULMONARY HYPERTENSION

Causes

It can **C.H.A.N.GE.** *you…*

Connective tissue diseases, e.g. RA, SLE
HIV
Amphetamines
No-one knows (idiopathic)
GEnetic

Lung disease: Cor pulmonale due to COPD, ILD, bronchiectasis, OSA
Cardiac: LVF, MS, right-to-left shunt
Chronic PEs

PATH

Primary pulmonary arterial hypertension and systemic causes are characterized by medial hypertrophy, concentric fibrosis, thrombosis and vasoconstriction of arterioles and venules

PC

SOBOE – worsens with right ventricular failure
Syncope
Angina or myocardial infarction (right ventricle)

O/E

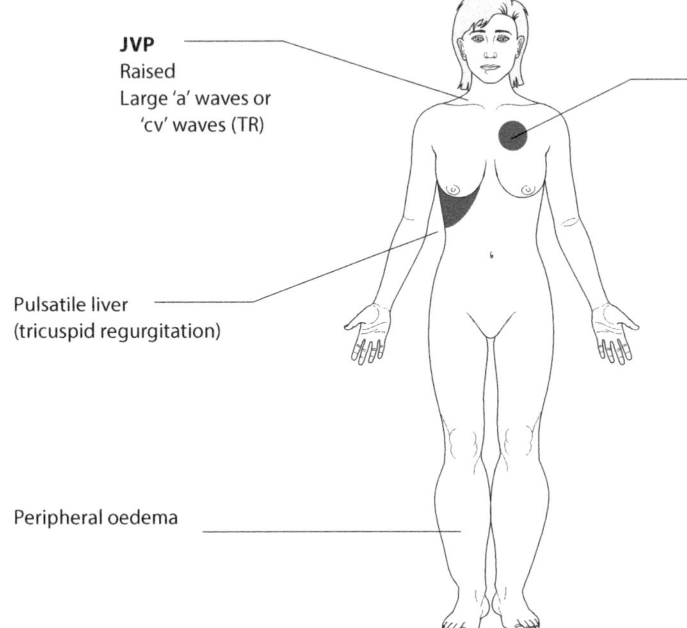

Ix

Bloods: ABG: O_2 ↓ CO_2 ↓; respiratory alkalosis
ECG: Sinus tachycardia, AF
SI-QIII-TIII (R axis deviation)
R-sided strain; R bundle-branch block
Radiol: CXR: Large pulmonary arteries; clear lung fields
V/Q isotope scan: Diffuse patchy filling defects (non-segmental, cf. PE = segmental)
Angio: Risk of bradycardia (give atropine)
Special: Lung function tests: Mild restrictive picture; KCO ↓

Rx

Conservative: Avoid exercise
Medical:
Diuretics
Warfarin (INR 1.5–2.5)
Vasodilators:

- Bosentan (endothelial receptor antagonist)
- Sildenafil, tadalafil (phosphodiesterase type 5 inhibitors)
- IV prostacyclin via indwelling central venous catheter
- Calcium channel blockers if patient is vasoreactive (only 5%)

Bilateral lung (± heart) transplantation

Prog

Survival: 3 years from diagnosis if untreated; 6 months from symptomatic heart failure (grade IV)

Gastroenterology

ABDOMINAL PAIN

Causes

Abdominal pain has the **P^2.O^2.T.E.N.T.I.A.L.** *to be serious*

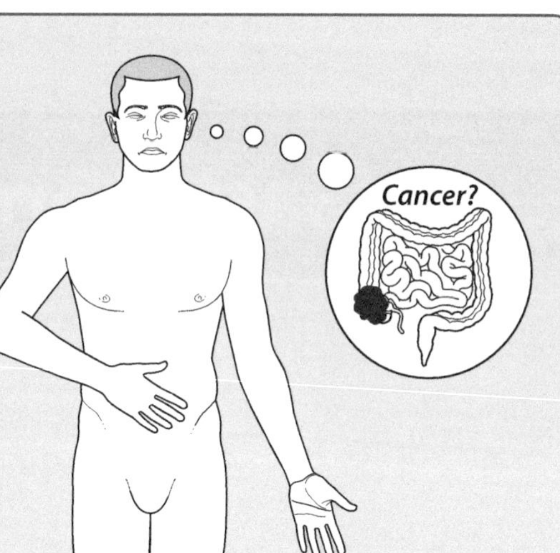

Peritonitis/**P**erforation (see opposite)
- PATH: Inflammation of viscus with extension to local peritoneum
- PC: Constant, worsened by movement, patient tends to lie down and shallow breathe

Obstruction/c**O**lic
- PATH: Colic suggests excessive contraction of viscus, e.g. due to obstruction or infection
- PC: Waxes and wanes, patient tends to writhe and move around

Toxins
- Food poisoning
- Drugs, e.g. opioid addiction, antibiotics, anticholinesterases; radiotherapy
- Poisons: Chronic lead poisoning; black widow spider bite

Endocrine crises
- Diabetic ketoacidosis
- Addison
- Hypermetabolic state: Thyrotoxicosis; phaeochromocytoma; carcinoid

Neuro-psychiatric
- Functional: Irritable bowel; anxiety; Munchausen syndrome
- Radiculopathy: Shingles; spondylosis. NB: Dermatomal pattern and hyperaesthesia
- Syphilis: 'Tabetic crisis'

Thoracic origin (referred pain)
- Basal pneumonia, pulmonary embolism; myocardial infarction; pericarditis; thoracic radiculitis

Inherited
- Acute porphyria: Colic
- C'1-esterase inhibitor deficiency: Hereditary angioedema
- Familial Mediterranean fever

Abdominal wall
- Rectus sheath haematoma (e.g. over-anticoagulation); myositis. NB: Worsened by lifting head off pillow

Labour or other gynaecological disorder
- Ovarian torsion
- Ectopic pregnancy
- PID

Peritonitis

PC

Localized peritonitis: Constant localized pain, worsened by movement, patient tends to lie down and shallow-breathe; e.g. appendicitis: umbilical → **RIF** pain

Sub-diaphragmatic: L shoulder-tip pain

Retroperitoneal origin: Vague localisation or back pain; patient tends to sit up or move around

O/E

Inspection In pain, shallow breathing pattern, pale, shocked
Palpation Abdominal rigidity; guarding (involuntary abdominal wall contraction); rebound (pain on release); Murphy's sign (tenderness in RUQ on inspiration); pain per rectum – retrocaecal appendicitis
Auscultation Absent bowel sounds (paralytic ileus)

Ix

Erect CXR (air under diaphragm with oesophageal – bowel rupture)
USS: Free fluid in peritoneum or bowel
CT: Localizes area of pathology and any free fluid

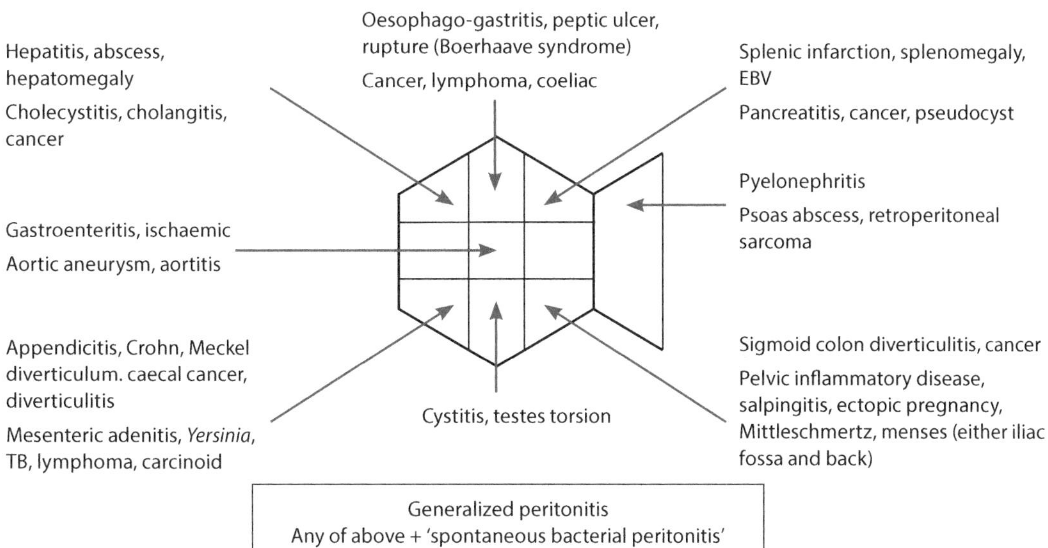

Generalized peritonitis
Any of above + 'spontaneous bacterial peritonitis'
(cirrhosis, nephrosis, e.g. from streptococcal pharyngitis)

Obstruction

Bowel

MECHANICAL

PC Colic:
- Umbilical: small bowel
- Lower half; lumbar: large bowel

Constipation + vomit
May progress to bowel infarction and/or perforation, with peritonitis

O/E
Abdominal distension
Tinkling bowel sounds
Hyperperistaltic movements

PARALYTIC

PC Constipation + vomit only
O/E Absent bowel sounds
Biliary: Cause – calculi
PC Colicky or constant; RUQ, worse after eating
Renal: Cause – calculi
PC Constant but migrates: loin → groin

V.A.N.I.S.H.I.N.G. P.O.o.
(i.e. constipated!)

Volvulus
Adhesions 2° to peritonitis, surgery
Neoplasia
Inflammation: Crohn, ischaemia, diverticulitis
Strangulated **H**ernia
Intussusception: Meckel diverticulum, polyp
Neonatal: Imperforate anus
Gallstone ileus; faecal bolus, FB, bezoar

Pseudo-**O**bstruction: Reflex atony – post-surgery; trauma; retroperitoneal haematoma

DIARRHOEA

Def

Reduction in stool consistency (essential)
>3× bowel opening per day, or >250 g stool per day – not essential

Causes

S.O.I.L.I.N.G.S².

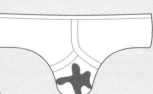

Secretory – diarrhoea persists with fasting

Infection

Food poisoning (toxin or organism pre-formed within food):

- Toxin-mediated: *Staph. aureus, Clostridium perfringens*
- Inflammation: *Salmonella, Camplylobacter*

Gastroenteritis (i.e. organism colonizes and multiplies within bowel):

- Toxin-mediated: Cholera, *E. coli* (enterotoxigenic – traveller's diarrhoea)
- Inflammation: *Shigella, E. coli* (enteroinvasive), *Clostridium difficile*, viral

Endocrine

APUDomas:

- Carcinoid
- Islet-cell tumour (VIPoma, somatostatinoma, glucagonoma, gastrinoma)
- Endocrine: Medullary carcinoma thyroid (via calcitonin), phaeochromocytoma

Systemic: Thyrotoxicosis, hypoadrenalism (Addison), hypopituitarism

Osmotic

Malabsorption – diarrhoea relieved by fasting

Causes: Intestinal wall disease; bile salt malabsorption; pancreatic disease (exocrine)

Haemorrhage into bowel

Inflammation or **I**schaemia

Inflammatory bowel disease: Ulcerative colitis, Crohn, microscopic colitis

Ischaemia, incl. vasculitis, mesenteric embolism

Laxatives or other drugs

Laxatives:

- Secretory: Phenolphthalein-containing, e.g. senna, bisacodyl
- Osmotic: Na, Mg or anion-containing

Antibiotics, esp. erythromycin; prokinetics

Radiation

Irritable bowel syndrome

Abdominal pain and bloating, relieved by defaecation

Altered stool passage

PR mucus

Neuropathy, autonomic, e.g. diabetes; MS

Gastrectomy + other surgery

Short-bowel syndrome: Extensive bowel resection; dumping syndrome – gastrectomy

Fistulae, e.g. jejuno-ileal bypass; anal sphincter disturbance

Structural

Rectal adenoma, neoplasia, diverticular disease

Special

Alcohol, dietary indiscretion

Overflow: Faecal impaction

CONSTIPATION

Def

Bowel opening <3× per week
Straining during defaecation >25%

Causes

O.P.E.N. I.T. W.I.D².E.

Obstruction
- Mechanical (colic) – see p. 103: Volvulus, adhesions, neoplasia, inflammation, strangulated hernia, intussusception, gallstone ileus
- Pseudo-obstruction (reflex atony), e.g. post-surgery

Pain
- Anal fissure; 3° piles

Endocrine/**E**lectrolytes
- Endocrine: T_4 ↓, DM (DKA, ↓ gastrocolic reflex)
- Electrolytes: Ca ↓, K ↓, uraemia

Neurological
- Brain: PD, CVA, MS
- Spine: Myelopathy, cauda equina, sacral plexopathy
- Neuropathy: Botulism, Hirschsprung disease, Chagas disease (*Trypanosoma cruzi* – S. America)

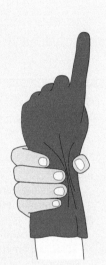

Inflammation or **I**schaemia
- IBD or diverticulitis, or ischaemia

Toxins
- Opioids, anticholinergics, nicotine (ganglion blocker), aluminium salt (antacid), iron

Gut **W**all disease
- Systemic sclerosis or visceral myopathy

Irritable bowel syndrome

Diet or **D**ehydration
- Inadequate roughage, diuretics, starvation

Elderly, pregnancy

Rx

Underlying cause
Laxatives:

B.O.S.S.E.S.

Bulking: Faecal mass ↑→ peristalsis ↑ – bran, ispaghula husk
Osmotic: Fluidity of faeces ↑ – lactulose, macrogol
Stimulant: GIT motility and secretion ↑ – senna, bisacodyl
Softeners: Sodium docusate
Enemas:
- Osmotic: PO_4, Na citrate
- Stimulant: Na picosulphate
- Softener: Arachis oil

Suppositories: Stimulant – glycerol

NAUSEA AND VOMITING

Causes

Too many **G.I.N. & T.O^2.N.I.C.S.**

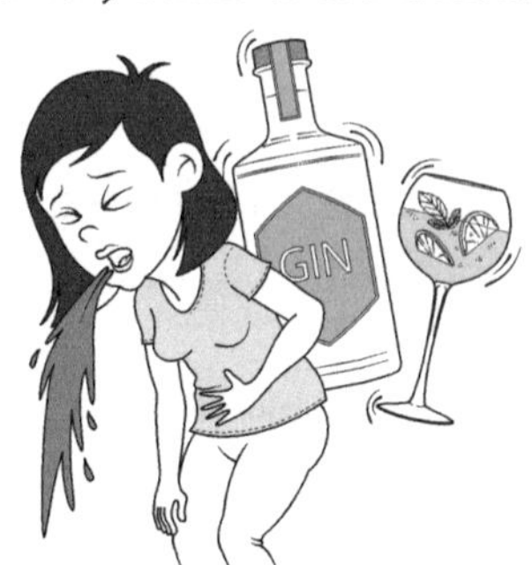

Gastrointestinal
- Gastro-oesophageal: Reflux; ulcer; pyloric stenosis
- Pancreatic, liver, gallbladder disease
- Obstruction
- Peritonitis

Infection
- GIT: Gastroenteritis; hepatitis; visceral abscess
- Systemic: RTI (esp. tonsillitis, otitis media); UTI; septicaemia

Neoplasia
- GIT: Oesophago–gastric–duodenal carcinoma; lymphoma; amyloid
- Other: Hypernephroma; hepatoma; ovarian
- Paraneoplastic

Toxins
- Chemotherapy, opioids
- Antibiotics, aminophylline, antiarrhythmics (esp. digoxin), L-DOPA
- Alcohol

Obstetric: Pregnancy

Ophthalmic: Acute closed-angle glaucoma

Neurology
- Labyrinthitis, Menière, brainstem-cerebellar disease, e.g. MS
- ICP ↑; meningo-encephalitis
- Migraine
- Vasovagal syncope
- Autonomic neuropathy/gastroparesis: Diabetes, acute intermittent porphyria
- Psychiatric: Bulimia or anorexia nervosa, psychogenic

Infarction: Myocardial, esp. posterior, transmural

Calcium ↑/endocrine dysfunction
- DKA gastroparesis
- Addison crisis
- Thyrotoxicosis

Systemic
- Respiratory failure: Acidosis
- Cardiac failure, esp. right-sided: Bowel oedema
- Renal or liver failure: Uraemia

Physiology

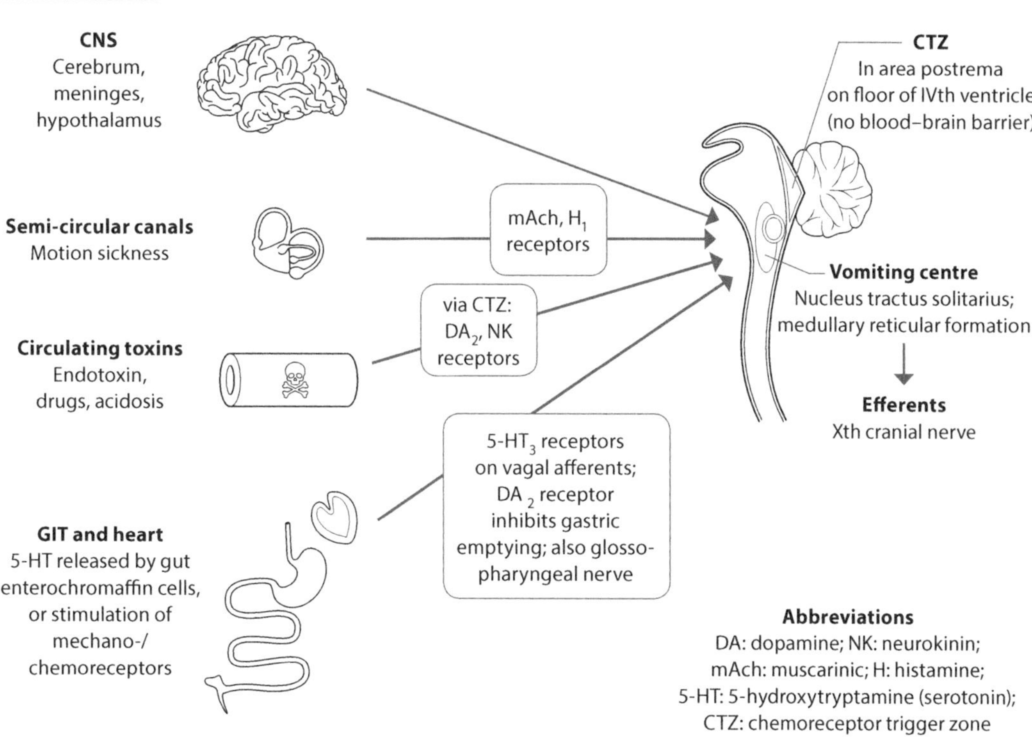

Abbreviations
DA: dopamine; NK: neurokinin;
mAch: muscarinic; H: histamine;
5-HT: 5-hydroxytryptamine (serotonin);
CTZ: chemoreceptor trigger zone

Rx

Underlying cause
Supportive: Hydration (PO/IV), NaCl replacement
Anti-emetics: Select according to receptor-type relevant to cause

A.1.2.3.

Muscarinic (**A**ch) receptor antagonist: Hyoscine
- Indication: Motion sickness, GIT causes
- ☠: Sedation, dry mouth

Histamine type **1** receptor antagonist: Cyclizine, cinnarizine, promethazine
- Indication: Motion sickness, GIT, cardiac causes
- ☠: Sedation, other anti-cholinergic side-effects

Dopamine type **2** receptor antagonist: Metoclopramide, domperidone
- Indication: Most causes, esp. gastro-oesophageal reflux (as pro-motility effect)
- ☠: Sedation, extrapyramidal reactions (less likely with domperidone), diarrrhoea

5-HT type **3** receptor antagonist: Ondansetron, granisetron
- Indication: Most causes, esp. chemotherapy, post-surgery, neoplasia, MS
- ☠: Headache, constipation

Others:
- Steroids for neoplasia
- Nabilone (cannibinoid, acts on opiate receptors) for chemotherapy, MS

SORE THROAT

Causes

I.N.T.E.R.N.A.L.S.

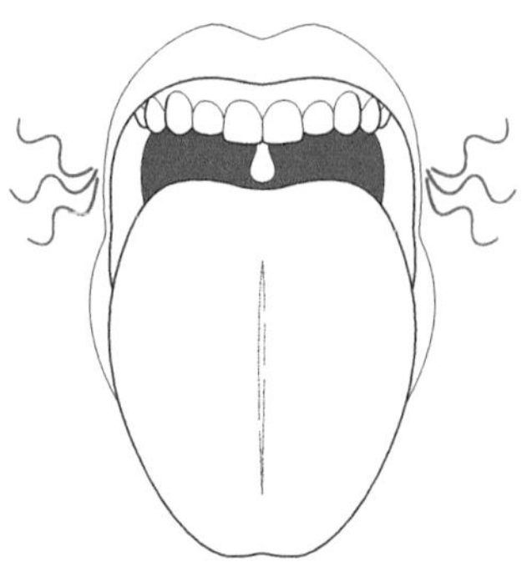

Infection

Viral:

- Influenza or coryza (coronavirus, adenovirus, rhinovirus, enteroviruses, coxsackie)
- Exanthems: Rubella, measles, hand, foot and mouth disease – coxsackie A16, enterovirus 71
- EBV: PC – pearly-white exudate + palatal petechiae
- Other: Parainfluenza, croup, haemorrhagic fever

Bacterial – localized

- *Streptococcus pyogenes* (β-haemolytic, Lancefield group A): Tonsillitis and quinsy (peritonsillar abscess) and rheumatic fever
- *Staphylococcus aureus*: Facial erysipelas
- *Haemophilus influenzae* type b: Epiglottitis
- Anaerobes: *Fusobacterium necrophorum* (necrobacillosis): Lemierre disease; also causes jugular thrombophlebitis; lung and brain abscesses

Bacterial – general:

- Pneumonia: *Streptococcus pneumoniae*, *Mycoplasma*, chlamydia, tularaemia, brucellosis
- GIT: Typhoid, leptospirosis
- STD: Gonorrhoea, 2° syphilis
- Neurological:
  - Diphtheria (bull neck, stridor, brassy cough, palatal weakness, myocarditis)
  - Meningococcus (Neisseria meningitidis), listeriosis (associated meningitis)

Fungal: Oral candidiasis

Neoplasia

Carcinoma of oral cavity or pharynx

Toxins

Smoking, alcohol, pollution, e.g. H_2S

Drugs: Carbimazole, clozapine, anti-epileptics (due to agranulocytosis)

Exogenous: Radiotherapy-induced mucositis

Reflux: Gastro-oesophageal

Nutritional: Vitamin B12, folate, iron deficiency: Mucositis, glossitis, cheilitis

Autoimmune: Sjögren syndrome – dry mouth

Long styloid process: Chronic sore throat in children

Sinusitis, chronic: Post-nasal drip

ORAL ULCERATION

Causes

I.N.T.E.R.N.A.L.

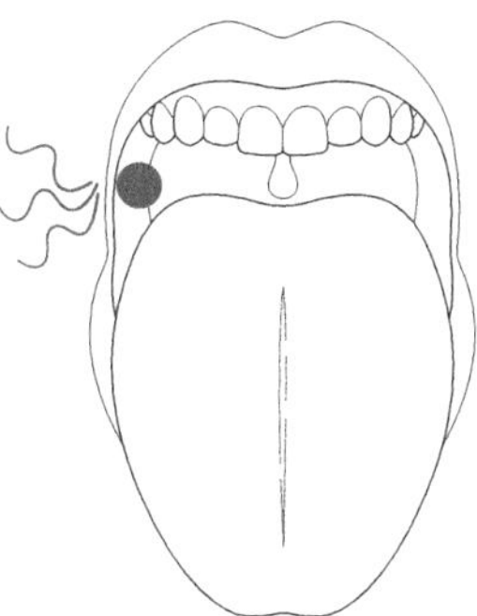

Infection

Viral:

- Herpangina: Enterovirus, coxsackie, echovirus – children
- Herpes: HSV-1 (acute gingivostomatitis or recurrent); VZV; EBV
- HIV: Acute gingivitis, ulceration; glandular fever-like illness

Bacterial:

- TB: Tip-of-tongue ulcers
- STD:
  - Gonorrhoea
  - Syphilis (1° – chancre; 2° – snail-track ulcer; tongue; 3° – gumma)
- Anaerobic:
  - Vincent angina = symbiosis of *Borrelia vincentii* + *Bacteroides* spp.
  - Actinomycoses: assoc. with tooth extraction or jaw fracture: inspection reveals yellow sulphur granules

Fungal: Histoplasmosis – ulcerative nodules, laryngitis, fever

Neoplasia: Carcinoma of oral cavity – raised edge

Toxins:

Sulphonamides, chloramphenicol, cytotoxics – neutropenia

Stevens–Johnson syndrome, erythema multiforme

Exogenous: Trauma/dentures

Recurrent aphthous ulceration

Epi: 20% lifetime incidence; assoc. with stress, menses

PC: Painful, single or cluster of ulcers with grey base and red surround

Types: Minor (1–5 mm); major (5–15 mm); herpetiform (200 × 1 mm)

Nutritional

Haematinics: Vitamin B, folate, iron deficiency

Vitamin C deficiency

Malabsorption, e.g. coeliac

Autoimmune: Most are aphthous ulcers (i.e. painful, grey base, red surround)

Behçet syndrome: Orogenital ulceration + anterior uveitis + arthritis

SLE

Seronegative arthropathies: IBD (esp. Crohn); Reiter syndrome

Pemphigus (ruptured bullae); pemphigoid (bullae); lichen planus (white striae)

Leukaemia, acute: esp, AML, 2° to neutropenia

DYSPHAGIA

Causes

Neuromuscular

Central (pseudobulbar palsy):

- CVA
- Parkinson, esp. progressive supranuclear palsy
- Motor neurone disease (MND)
- MS

Bulbar palsy (lower motor neurone):

- MND
- Syringobulbia
- Myaesthenia gravis
- Jugular foramen syndrome
- Guillain–Barré syndrome

Muscular/myenteric plexus

- Myopathy
- Ganglion/peristalsis dysfunction:
    - Scleroderma/CREST
    - Oesophageal spasm
    - Achalasia

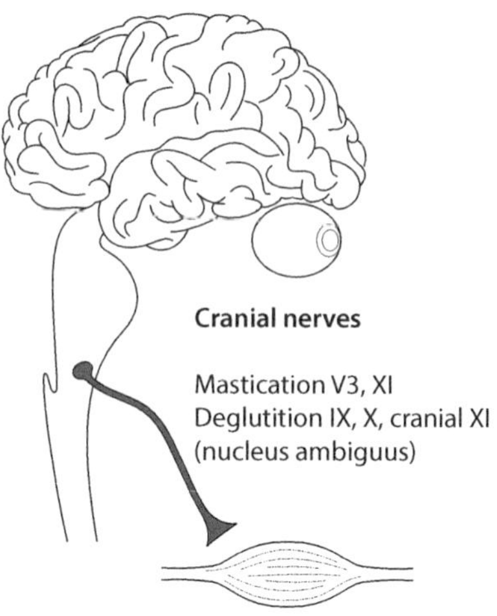

Oral

Pharyngitis and oral ulcers cause painful swallowing (odynophagia) with secondary dysphagia

Pharynx/oesophagus

Luminal: Foreign body, large bolus

Intrinsic:

- Upper:
    - Pharyngeal pouch
    - Post-cricoid web
- Middle:
    - Oesophagitis
    - Oesophageal stricture
    - Oesophageal carcinoma
- Lower:
    - Hiatus hernia
    - Schatzki ring

Extrinsic – **B.U^2.L.G.I.N.'**

Bone: Cervical spondylosis

U: Dysphagia L**U**soria – vascular compression:

Aberrant R subclavian artery, aortic aneurysm, mitral stenosis (enlarged left atrium)

Lymphadenopathy

Goitre

Infection: Retropharyngeal abscess

Neoplasia: Pancreatic cancer

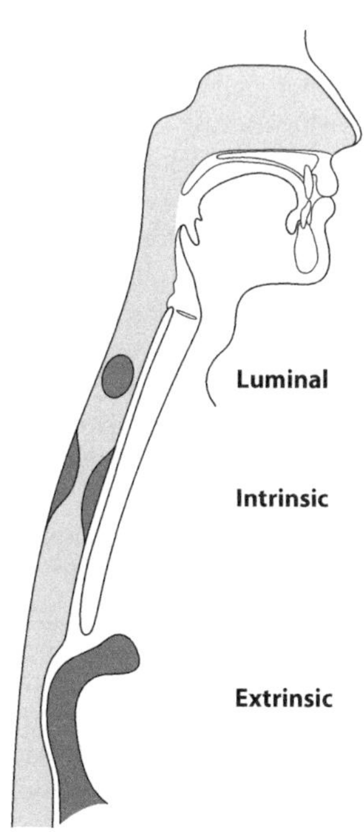

PC

Neuromuscular
Solids and liquid: Nasal regurgitation
Aspiration occurs while attempting to swallow
Other: Diplopia, ataxia

Oral
Odynophagia

Pharynx/oesophagus
Solids > liquids
Aspiration unrelated to swallowing
Other: Chest pain; dyspepsia, hiccups (lower oesophagus)

O/E

Neuromuscular
Other neurological deficits, e.g. ataxia, dysarthria, Horner syndrome

Oral
Erythema, aphthous ulcers, candida

Pharynx/oesophagus
Hoarse:

- Laryngitis (gastro-oesophageal reflux)
- Left recurrent laryngeal nerve palsy (carcinoma, lymph nodes)

Respiratory Sx:

- Right basal consolidation (aspiration pneumonia)
- Unilateral wheeze (main bronchus compression)

Ix

Neuromuscular
Videofluoroscopy: Identifies weakness or incoordination

Pharynx/oesophagus
Barium swallow
OGD
Oesophageal motility + manometry studies

Specific causes

Neuromuscular
Psychiatric 'globus pharyngis':

- Patient feels lump in the throat at level of cricoid
- Middle-aged female, depression

Achalasia: Chest pain

Pharynx/oesophagus
Pharyngeal pouch: Elderly
Post-cricoid web: Occurs as part of Plummer–Vinson or Paterson–Brown–Kelly syndrome, also characterized by iron-deficiency anaemia, koilonychia, glossitis, and risk of squamous cell carcinoma

HAEMATEMESIS

Causes

V.I.N.T.A.G.E.

Varices

Inflammation: Oesophago-gastroduodenitis or peptic ulcer; PC: coffee-grounds vomit

Neoplasia: Oesophageal or gastric (carcinoma, polyp, leiomyoma, Menetrier disease)

Trauma

Mallory–Weiss tear:

- Mucosal break <2 cm proximal to gastro-oesophageal junction
- Due to forceful vomiting, esp. males drinking alcohol

Surgery, ERCP (haemobilia), aorto-duodenal fistula, 2° aortic aneurysm/repair

Hypovolaemic shock: Ischaemic, stress ulcer in stomach

Angiodysplasia + other vascular anomalies

Angiodysplasia: Dilated vessel complexes in *clusters*

Hereditary haemorrhagic telangiectasia:

- Dilated vessels over entire bowel wall
- Autosomal dominant: Endoglin mutation (TGF-receptor on endothelium)
- PC: Haematemesis, haemoptysis (pulmonary AVM), cerebral abscess, epistaxis

Other:

- Dieulafoy lesion = protruding large submucosal vessel
- Watermelon stomach = gastric antral vascular ectasia
- Vasculitis, e.g. PAN

Generalized bleeding disorder

Connective tissue defects: Ehlers–Danlos syndrome, pseudoxanthoma elasticum

Coagulopathy, e.g. chronic renal failure, warfarin

Epistaxis or dental: Oropharynx; epistaxis or haemoptysis (swallowed blood)

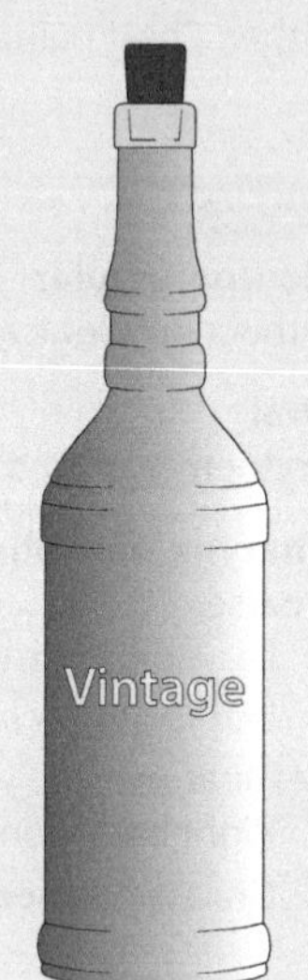

Ix for any GIT bleeding

Bloods: U&E: urea ↑↑ with upper GIT lesion; AKI
FBC: Chronic or acute
LFT: Liver disease
Coagulation screen + group and save + cross-match as appropriate

Radiol: CT angiogram

Special: Endoscopy
Laparotomy; investigative ileo-/colostomy

RECTAL BLEEDING

Causes

D.R.I.P.P.I.N.G. T.A^3.P^2.S.

Diverticulae
- Colonic: Diverticular disease
  - PC: Pellety stool, pain, PR bleeding + diarrhoea
- Ileal: Meckel diverticulum
  - PC: Childhood bleeding
- Jejunal:
  - PC: Usually present with malabsorption + vitamin B12 deficiency due to bacterial overgrowth

Rectal
- Piles
  - PC: Blood separated from stool; painless unless thrombosed
- Solitary rectal ulcer; proctitis, e.g. 2° to gonorrhoea

Infection
- Bacterial: *Salmonella*, *Campylobacter*, *E. coli*, *Shigella spp.*
- Other: HIV, CMV, *Candida*
- Parasite: Amoebic dysentery, hookworm (melaena)

Polyps – Benign
- Hyperplastic, esp. rectal
- Hamartomatous, e.g. Peutz–Jeghers syndrome
  - PC: Obstruction, intussusception → strawberry-jelly stool

Polyps – Neoplastic
- Adenoma → carcinoma

Inflammation
- Ulcerative colitis: Bloody diarrhoea
- Crohn: Ileal bleeding – uncommon

Neoplasia
- Carcinoma, lymphoma, Kaposi's sarcoma

Gastric–upper bowel bleeding
- PC: Melaena (black, tarry stool), or bloody, if rapid transit

Trauma
- Surgery, colonoscopy, e.g. polypectomy; radiation colitis

Arterial/**A**ngiodysplasia/**A**VM
- Ischaemic colitis
- Angiodysplasia
- AVMs, hereditary haemorrhagic telangiectasia

Pseudomembranous colitis/**P**arasites
- *see under Infection*

Systemic
- Coagulopathy
- Amyloid

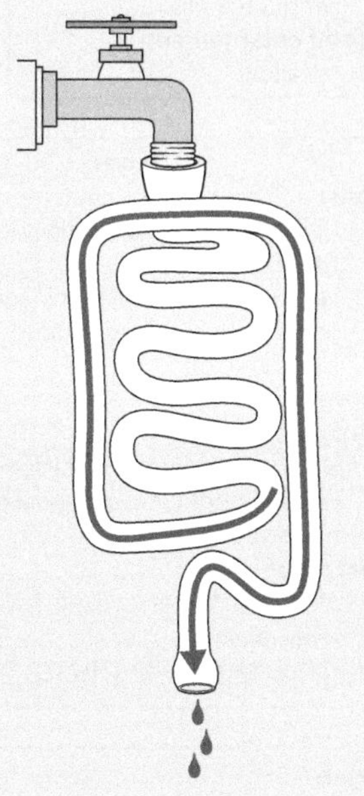

ABDOMINAL EXAMINATION

3. Neck

JVP ↑: A-sided cardiac failure as a cause of cirrhosis
Lymphadenopathy:
- Lymphoma, TB, HIV
- Gastric cancer: Supraclavicular LN = Troisier's sign

Goitre (dysphagia, T4-toxicosis causes diarrhoea)

2. Face

Eyes:
- Conjunctivae: Pallor - anaemia
- Cornea: Jaundice
- Xanthelasma: Lipids

Mouth:
- Pigmentation (Peutz-Jeghers syndrome Addison)
- Telangiectasia (HHT, scleroderma)
- Glossitis, cheilitis (vit B12 or Fe def.)
- Ulceration:
  - Crohn (also swollen lips),
  - Candida (white plaques – check genitalia)
  - Oral hairy leukoplakia (lymphoma, HIV)

Parotid enlargement:
Liver failure

1. Hands

Nails:
- Clubbing (cirrhosis, colitis, coeliac, lymphoma)
- Leuconychia (hypoalbuminaemia)
- Sclerodactyly, telangiectasia (scleroderma}

Palms:
- Asterixis (liver failure}
- Dupuytren contracture (alcoholism)
- Hyperkeratotic-oesophageal cancer (tylosis)

Forearms:
- AV-fistula thrill, excoriations: Chronic renal failure
- Tattoos: Hepatitis or HIV risk

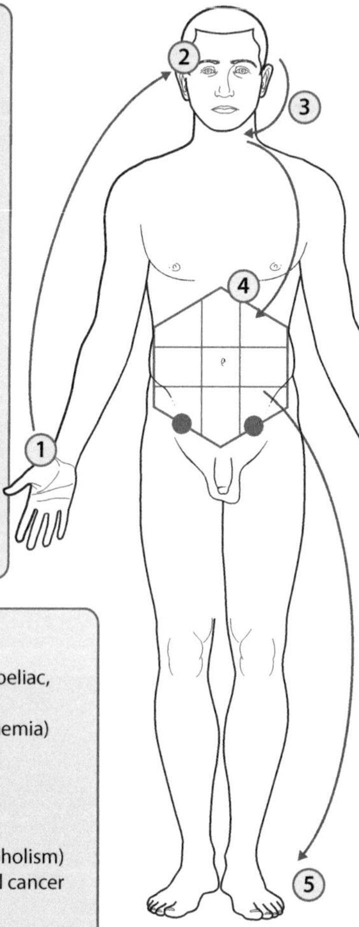

4. Abdomen

Inspection of trunk and back
- Skin of trunk and back:
  - Stigmata of chronic liver disease: Spider naevi, gynaecomastia, testis atrophy, sexual hair loss, caput medusa, dilated abdominal veins
  - Uraemic frost: Brown-yellow tinge
- Scars, stoma, sinuses, striae
- Masses, e.g.
  Sister Joseph nodule (umbilical 2°), hernia (on coughing and standing)
- Peristalsis: Obstruction

Palpation + percussion
- Peritonism – see page 103
- Masses, organomegaly
- Ascites: Shifting dullness, fluid thrill
- Pulsation: Expansile (aneurysm) transmitted (overlying mass) liver (tricuspid regurgitation}

Auscultation
- Bowel
  - Tinkling or succussion splash (obstruction}
  - Hyperactive
- Renal bruits
- Liver bruit (hepatoma; portal hypertension}

Extras, where appropriate
- PR, for unexplained weight loss, anaemia, altered bowel habit, bleeding
- PV, e.g. discharge, pelvic pain
- Genitalia, e.g. unexplained abdominal pain (testes), signs of immunocompromise (HIV)

5. Other systems
- Feet (peripheral oedema)
- Fundi (hyperlipidaemia)
- ABP, chest (renal failure)

Order:
1. Examine JVP at 45° recline
2. Sit patient forward to examine back and palpate cervical lymph nodes
3. Lie patient completely horizontal
4. Palpate, first light, then deep, in clockwise fashion

6. AND FINALLY...
Temperature chart
Weight chart, abdominal girth
Urine dipstick, β-HCG test

ABDOMINAL MASSES

Hepatomegaly

Hepatomegaly
Diffuse liver disease: **T.A.B.O.O^2.S^2.** – see p. 152
Nodular:
- Cirrhosis, esp. due to alcohol
- Neoplasia – 2°, 1°
- Cysts:
  - Benign, e.g. adult polycystic kidney disease
  - Abscess, incl. hydatid, gumma
  - Haemangioma (usually solid)
- Riedel lobe (apparent hepatomegaly)

Hepatomegaly and splenomegaly
As for causes of splenomegaly

Palpable gallbladder
Courvoisier's Law: Jaundice + palpable gallbladder = cancer of pancreas, common bile duct, or duodenum, but **not** chronic cholecystitis as gallbladder is fibrosed

Splenomegaly

Causes **B.I.G. S.P.A^2.N.**

Blood disorders: CML, CLL, myelofibrosis, myeloproliferative, haemolytic anaemia, ITP, sickle cell
Infection: Hepatitis, EBV, CMV, endocarditis, HIV, malaria, toxoplasmosis, leishmaniasis
Granulomatous: Sarcoid, primary biliary cirrhosis

Storage disease: Gaucher, Niemann–Pick disease
Portal hypertension, esp. 2° to cirrhosis
Autoimmune: Rheumatoid arthritis, SLE, Graves; **A**myloid
Neoplasia: Cysts, melanoma

Features:
Cannot get above
Superficial (dull on percussion)
Descends medially on inspiration
Medial notch

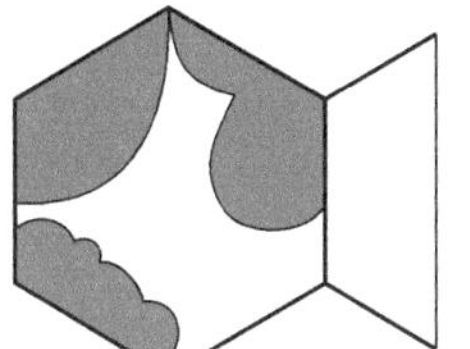

Other abdominal masses

I.N.V.I.S.i.**B.L.E.** *to the naked eye*

Infection: Abscess – appendicular, viral mesenteric adenitis, amoebic TB, *Actinomyces*, *Yersinia* (esp. RIF for all above)
Neoplasia: Gastric, pancreatic cancer or pseudocyst (epigastrium), colorectal, carcinoid (esp. right iliac fossa)
Vessel: Aortic or iliac aneurysm
Inflammatory: Crohn (esp. RIF), diverticular (esp. LIF)
Sex: Pregnancy, ovarian cyst or cancer
Bladder, pelvic kidney (e.g. transplant)
Lymphoma (esp. RIF, epigastrium)
Endocrine: Adrenal mass

Renal enlargement

P.H.O.N.E. – *shaped*

Polycystic kidneys
Hypertrophy 2° to contralateral renal agenesis
Obstruction/occlusion:
- Hydronephrosis
- Renal vein thrombosis

Neoplasia:
- Renal cell carcinoma
- Myeloma, lymphoma
- Amyloid

Endocrine: Diabetes mellitus

Features:
Can get above
Deep (tympanic on percussion)
Does not descend on inspiration
Bimanually ballotable, i.e. freely moving

OESOPHAGITIS

Causes

I.R.R.I.T.A.N.T.S.

Infection
Herpes (HSV, CMV, VZV), HIV, candida
Usually only occurs in immunocompromised, e.g. HIV, lymphoma

Reflux, gastro-oesophageal (GOR) – Structural
Lower oesophageal sphincter weakness may be 1° or due to:

- Hiatus hernia
  EPI: 10%, of which 10% are symptomatic – presents in infancy (congenitally short oesophagus), middle-age or elderly; female:male = 4:1
  Types:
  Sliding (95%) – along axis of oesophagus
  Rolling (5%) – greater curvature rolls over
- Pregnancy; multiparous women; obesity:
  - Pushes stomach up
  - Oestrogen relaxes oesophageal sphincter
  - Abdominal wall weakness
- Iatrogenic: cardia resection; nasogastric tube

Reflux, gastro-oesophageal (GOR) – Toxic
Smoking
Anti-cholinergics
Smooth-muscle relaxants: Calcium antagonists, aminophylline, sildenafil

Inflammatory bowel disease: Crohn

Toxins
Alcohol, hot tea, poisoning, e.g. caustic, corrosive
Drugs: Iron, aspirin, chemotherapy
Radiotherapy

Autoimmune
Vasculitis, incl. Behçet: Pemphigus, pemphigoid, epidermolysis bullosa

Neurological
All cause disordered motility, incl. food stasis and reflux:

- Achalasia causes food stasis
- Scleroderma
- Visceral myopathy

Trauma
Endoscopy/severe vomiting

Systemic
Uraemia
Hypothyroidism

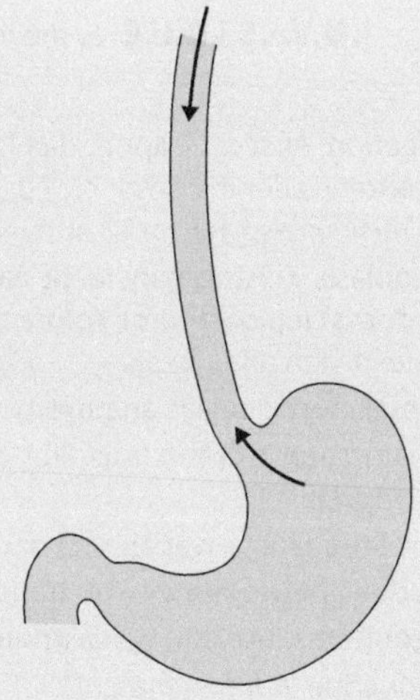

Lower oesophageal sphincter mechanisms
Oesophageal smooth muscle sphincter
Right crus diaphragm
Abdominal wall – increases intra-abdominal pressure
Acute angle of junction
Tall mucosal folds

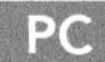

PC

B.U.R.N.S³.

Burning pain, heartburn
- Retrosternal or epigastric; radiates to arm + jaw
- Relieved by GTN (oesophageal spasm), sitting up, alkali (milk)

Ulceration
- Haematemesis, melaena, iron-deficiency anaemia

Reflux
- Acid regurgitation, water-brash (sour taste), halitosis, dental caries

Neoplasia
- Pre-malignant: Barrett oesophagus = columnar metaplasia within normal stratified, squamous epithelium of lower oesophagus (appear as red-brown, velvety islands among pink oesophageal mucosa); develops in 10% GOR
- Malignant: Adenocarcinoma; develops in 10% Barrett oesophagus

Stricture
- Dysphagia

Spasm
- Severe, acute, crushing (also caused by rolling hiatus hernia)

SOB, wheeze, palpitations, hiccoughs
- Due to reflex bronchospasm, hiatus hernia, aspiration pneumonitis

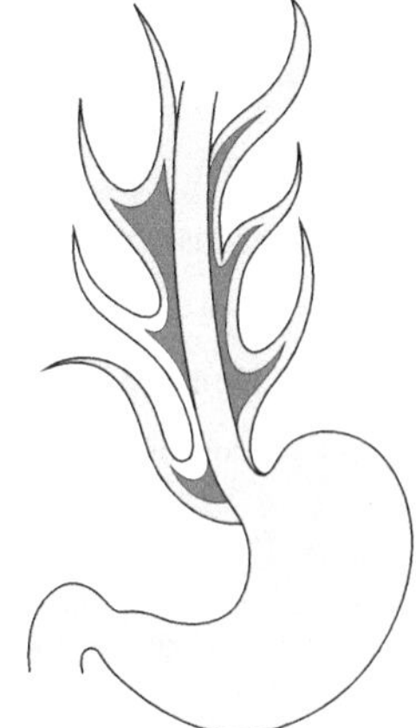

Ix

Bloods: FBC/ferritin: Iron-deficiency anaemia

Radiol: CXR:
- Hiatus hernia seen as gas bubble and fluid level in chest
- Aspiration pneumonitis, esp. right-middle lobe

Barium swallow: Reflux, spasm, mucosal irregularity

Special: OGD + biopsy
Oesophageal manometry: Propulsive motion, sphincter tone
Nasogastric tests: 24-hour ambulatory pH – 2× intraluminal electrodes records diurnal variation

Rx

Conservative S.O.S³.
- **S**moking
- **O**besity (+ loose clothing around waist)
- **S**mall **S**nacks and **S**leep upright

Medical:
- Mucosal protectants: Antacids ± alginates (Gaviscon) – forms viscous 'raft' on gastric contents
- Secretion suppression: Proton-pump inhibitor, e.g. omeprazole or H^2 receptor blocker, e.g. ranitidine
- Pro-kinetic: Domperidone or metoclopramide: ↑ LOS tone and gastric emptying:
  ☠ Extrapyramidal symptoms incl. acute dystonic reaction

Surgical:
- Hiatus hernia repair
- Nissen fundoplication: Gastric fundus mobilized and sutured around LOS, so that gastric contraction closes LOS

OESOPHAGEAL CARCINOMA

Epi

Inc: 1% of all cancers, but 5% of cancer deaths due to early spread to mediastinal structures
Age: Elderly (squamous cell carcinoma); middle-aged (adenocarcinoma)
Sex: men > women, esp. adenocarcinoma

Causes

Any cause of chronic oesophagitis or stricture

Upper oesophagus – Squamous cell carcinoma (10%)

Pharyngeal pouch
PC: Elderly person with dysphagia, regurgitation
Post-cricoid web (Plummer–Vinson syndrome)
PC: Middle-aged woman with chronic iron-deficiency anaemia, dysphagia

Middle oesophagus – Squamous cell carcinoma (40%)

Toxins
- Nitrites, nitrosamines – environment, food
- Alcohol, smoking, hot liquids, caustics
- Proton-pump inhibitor: i.e. *H. pylori* eradication

Nutrition
- Vitamin A, B, C, Zn deficiency; poor oral hygiene

Infection
- *Aspergillus flavus* contamination of grain
- Human papillomavirus

Inflammation
- Coeliac, achalasia (food stasis leads to chronic inflammation)
- Epidermolysis bullosa
- Tylosis (palmar keratosis) – autosomal dominant: 40% get cancer

Lower oesophagus – Adenocarcinoma (50%)

Gastro-oesophageal reflux (GOR)
- 'Barrett oesophagus' refers to columnar metaplasia at the lower oesophagus
- Metaplasia occurs in 10–15% of reflux patients
- Adenocarcinoma occurs in 10% of metaplasia

Predisposing: Obesity, hiatus hernia, cardiac surgery

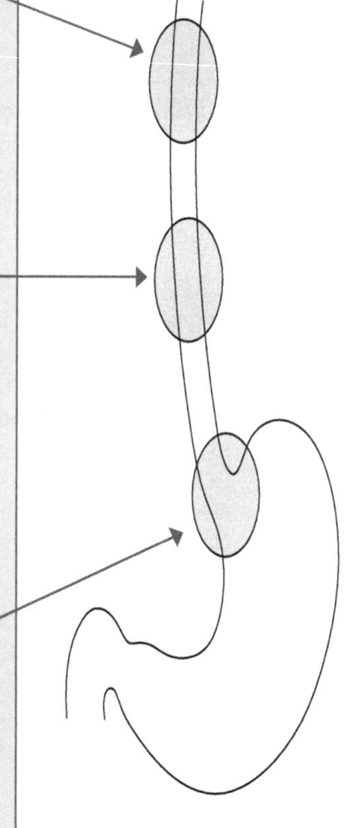

Rare oesophageal tumours

Benign: Mesenchymal leiomyoma, polyp, squamous papilloma

Malignant: Metastases or direct invasion (bronchial, gastric); Kaposi's sarcoma

PC

Polypoid or constrictive

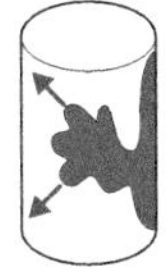

Pain: Retrosternal, due to direct pressure
Obstruction:

- Dysphagia (poorly localized), odynophagia
- Anorexia: LOW, malnutrition

Regurgitation: Heartburn, water-brash (sour taste), halitosis,dental caries, cough due to aspiration pneumonitis

Ulceration

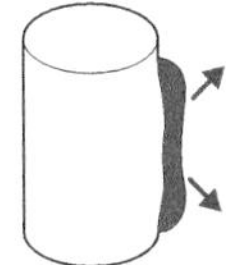

Pain: Mediastinitis; pleuritis
Haematemesis, melaena, iron-deficiency anaemia; catastrophic exsanguination (aorta-oesophageal fistula)
Perforation; infection: Mediastinitis, peritonitis

O/E

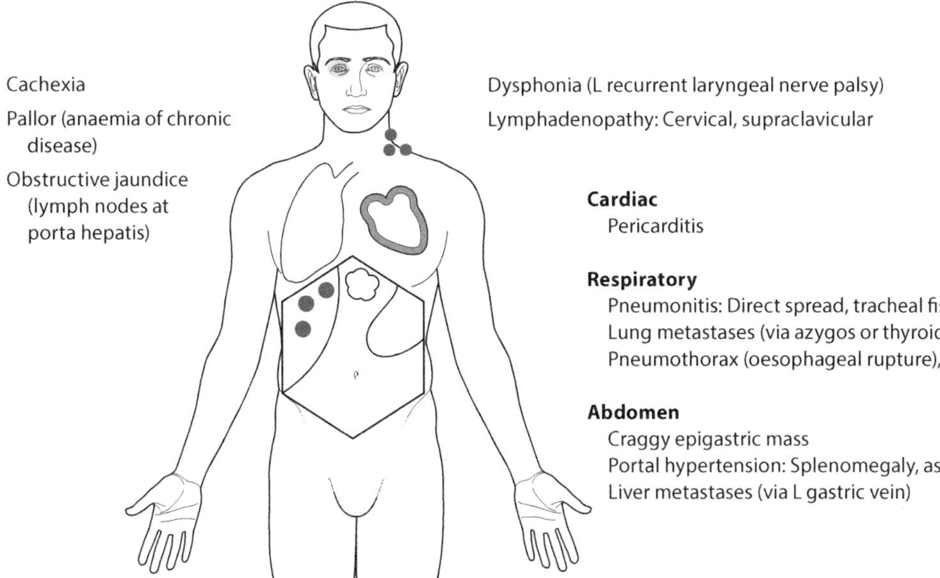

Ix

Bloods: FBC (iron-deficiency anaemia); ESR; U&E (vomiting); LFT (biliary obstruction, liver metastases)
Urine or faeces: Faecal occult blood
Radiol: CXR: Aspiration pneumonia, thoracic invasion, pulmonary metastases
Barium swallow: Irregular filling defect, stricture
CT, MRI
Special: OGD with biopsy – ulcerated mucosa, friable, oedematous, haemorrhagic

Rx

Curative: Total or subtotal oesophagectomy
Palliative if evidence of local or systemic spread:

- Endoscopic pulsion intubation
- Endoscopic laser photocoagulation or alcohol injection

Prog

5-year survival rate = 5% due to early spread (75% if resected before it spreads)

PEPTIC ULCERS

Locations

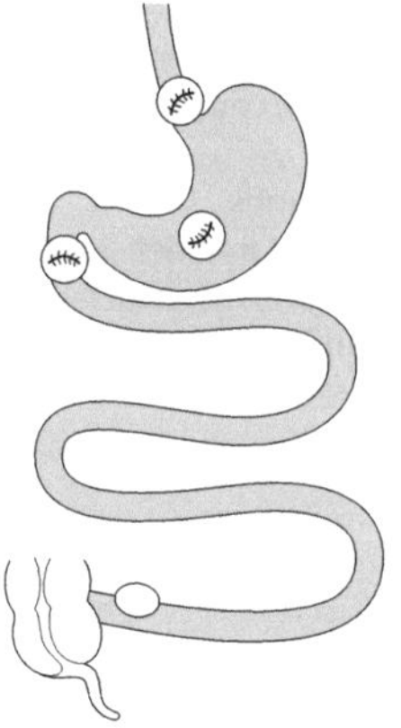

Locations listed in order of frequency

Causes

G.I.T. S.C³.A.R.S.

Genetic
- A family history often exists
- Blood group O (duodenal ulcers)

Infection – *Helicobacter pylori*

PATH:
- Antral infection: Inhibits somatostatin-secreting D-cells, which in turn disinhibits gastrin-secreting G-cells. Bacteria produce urease that ↑ local ammonia and ↑ mucosal IL-8 and TNF-α
- Duodenal infection: Causes gastric metaplasia, inflammation and HCO_3^- secretion ↓
- Corpus infection: Causes parietal cell atrophy, achlorhydria and resultant chronic gastritis

Toxins
- NSAIDs: 25% of all drug side-effects; 25% of all long-term NSAID users get PUs – inhibit COX-1 → prostaglandins E_2, I_2↓→ mucosal + HCO_3^- secretions ↓; HCl secretion ↓; mucosal blood flow ↓
- Steroids
- Chemotherapy, e.g. doxorubicin
- Smoking (duodenal ulcers); alcohol (acute gastritis and gastric erosions); salt

Surgery
- Antrectomy or gastro-enterostomy: Causes duodeno-gastric reflux of bile salts
- Extensive small-bowel resection: Disinhibition of gastrin secretion

Calcium ↑; **C**irrhosis; **C**RF

APUDoma – gastrinoma
- Zollinger–Ellison syndrome = non-islet cell pancreatic gastrinoma → gastrin ↑
- PC: Multiple, refractory peptic ulcers; diarrhoea; steatorrhoea; malabsorption, incl. vitamin B12 deficiency

Reflux, gastro-oesophageal

Stress
- Anxiety
- 'Stress ulcers': Ischaemia secondary to shock from sepsis, burns, ↑ICP

Epi

Inc: Life-time risk = 20% (males), 10% (females)
Age: 20–30s first presentation
Geo: Japan-China, South America more common and higher risk of carcinoma

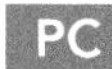

Pain

Epigastric-left upper quadrant, back, chest-shoulder
Recurrent (every 2 months; lasts 2 months), but when occurs is constant and burning
Relieved by milk or antacids
Assoc. bloating, abdominal distension, N+V

Duodenal ulcer
Dozy Fat Man

- Kept awake at night, as pain ↑ by lying flat and fasting ('hunger pains')
- Pain relieved by eating
- Men > women

Gastric ulcer
Anorexic **G**irls

- Thin as pain ↑ by eating
- Women > men

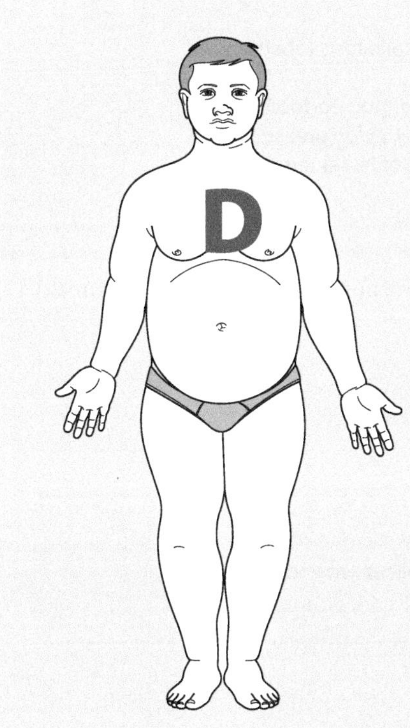

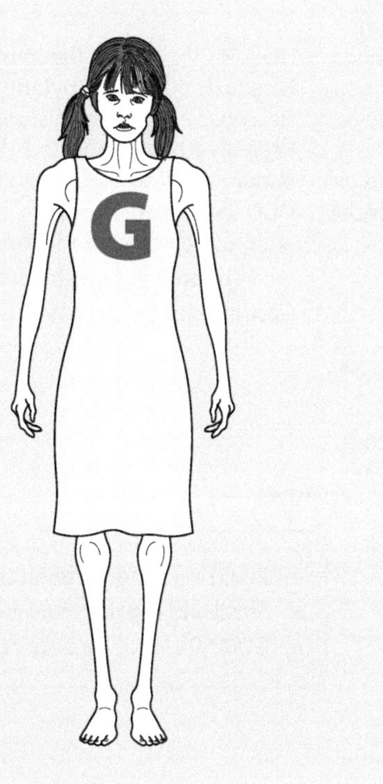

Comps

H.O.P.I.N.G. .... *I won't have!*

Haemorrhage
- Acute: Haematemesis, melaena
- Chronic: Iron-deficiency anaemia

Obstruction
- Vomiting, copious, projectile, stale-food (i.e. non-bilious), tetany due to alkalosis
- Constipation
- Colic, visible peristalsis
- Distension, succussion splash

Perforation
- Acute abdomen due to peritonitis, or back pain due to retroperitoneal perforation

Infection: Septic shock
Neoplasia: Gastric carcinoma, esp. if chronic, atrophic gastritis
Gas: Pneumatosis coli or pneumatosis cystoides intestinalis indicate necrotising fasciitis

Ix

Bloods: Hb ↓, MCV ↓; urea ↑ (haemorrhage); hypochloraemic alkalosis (obstruction)
Urine: Paradoxical aciduria (pyloric obstruction)
Micro: *Helicobacter pylori* from stool test or direct sampling during endoscopy
Urea-breath test: Ingested ^{13}C-urea is catabolised by *H. pylori* urease to CO_2
Radiol: Barium swallow: 'Hour glass' deformity due to fibrosis of lesser curvature
Special: OGD–endoscopy:
- Brush cytology and biopsy of rim + base
- *H. pylori* urease test: Gastric biopsy incubated with urea → NH_4^+ → pH ↑

Gastrin tests: Serum gastrin – fasting, post-prandial and post-secretin (gastrin ↓ in normals)

Rx

Conservative:

- Avoid smoking, alcohol, caffeine, NSAIDs, steroids
- Small and regular snacks; at night, take biscuits, milk or antacids to bed
- GORD Rx for oesophageal ulcers: Lose weight, Gaviscon, pro-motility drugs

Medical:

- *Helicobacter pylori* treatment

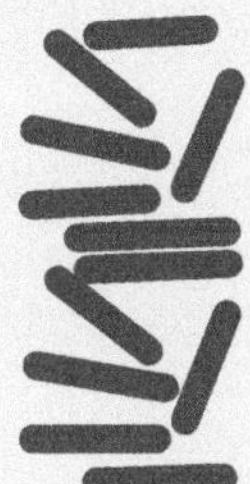

H. pylori eradication regime ('triple therapy') = 1 week course of:
Amoxicillin 1 g bd + clarithromycin 500 mg bd + lansoprazole 30 mg bd

or if penicillin allergic:
Metronidazole 400 mg bd + clarithromycin 250 mg bd + lansoprazole 30 mg bd

- Acid-suppression:
  - Proton-pump inhibitors – omeprazole, lansoprazole

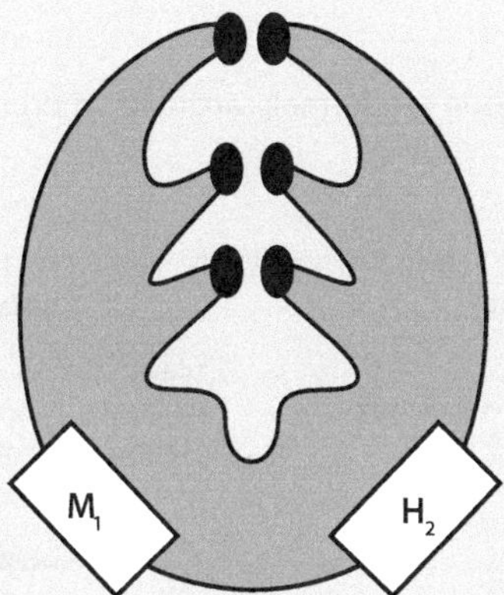

    - Irreversible inhibitors of H^+–K^+-ATPase pump in apical parietal cell membrane
    - Require acidification for activation (rabeprazole not as pH-dependent)
    - Decreases *H. pylori* infection of antrum, but increase corpus–fundus infection
    ☠ Diarrhoea, N+V, gastroenteritis by decreasing gastric protection; transaminitis (esp. lansoprazole); anaemia; headache; cytochrome p450 inhibitor (esp. omeprazole)
  - Histamine (H_2) receptor antagonists – ranitidine, cimetidine
    - Competitive inhibitors of parietal cell H_2 receptor: H^+ and pepsin secretion ↓
    ☠ Diarrhoea, bradycardia
    Cimetidine only: Gynaecomastia, decreased libido, cytochrome p450 inhibitor

GASTRIC NEOPLASIA

1% of all cancers, but 3% of cancer deaths due to gastric cancer presenting late

Risk factors **'7 As'**

Androgen (male)
Atrophic gastritis (due to *H. pylori* infection)
AIDS
Ash (smoking)
Adiposity (obesity)
Group **A** blood type
Anaemia (pernicious)

Types

Malignant
Adenocarcinoma
APUDoma: Gastrinoma (Zollinger–Ellison syndrome); carcinoid syndrome
Lymphoma
Secondaries: Carcinoma, melanoma

Microscopic	**Macroscopic**
Intestinal metaplasia Formation of intestinal glands	Excavated ulcer Irregular, heaped-up borders; shaggy, necrotic base
Diffuse infiltration Mucin stored intracellularly ('signet-ring cells') or secreted into extracellular stroma ('colloid carcinoma')	Flat or linitis plastica Broad infiltration of entire wall depth Rigid, thick + fibrotic walls

Pre-malignant
Adenomatous polyp: 30% have carcinoma within or in adjacent mucosa
Ménétrier disease: Rugal thickening due to glandular hyperplasia and mucin hypersecretion

Benign
Leiomyoma (mesenchymal)

PC

Anorexia, cachexia,
dyspepsia,
dysphagia (cardia cancer)

Projectile vomiting, stale-food (outlet obstruction – non-bilious), haematemesis

Pain – epigastric or back, early satiety

Obstruction – constipation, malnutrition
Haemorrhage – melaena, anaemia
Gastrocolic fistula – diarrhoea

O/E

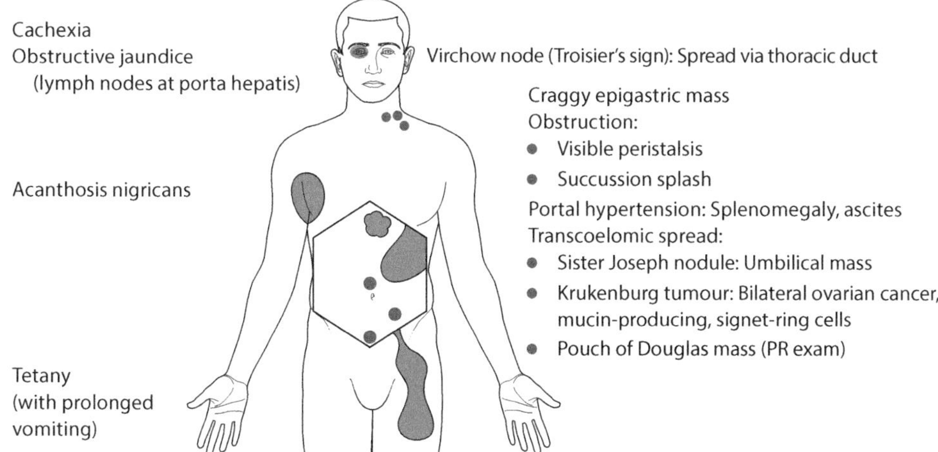

Metastases: Left hepatic lobe → bone, lung

Ix

Bloods: FBC, ferritin: Iron-deficiency anaemia, ESR↑
U&E: Pre-renal renal failure; hypochloraemic alkalosis (vomiting)
LFT: Biliary obstruction, liver metastases

Urine + faeces: Aciduria (with outlet obstruction); faecal occult blood

Radiol: CXR: Aspiration pneumonia, lung metastases
Barium meal + double contrast: Ulcers; polyp; generalized narrowing (linitis plastica)
CT/MRI: Staging

Special**:** OGD + brush cytology + biopsy: Lesser > greater curvature stomach
Endoscopic ultrasound: Allows staging (**T**umour, **N**odes, **M**etastases in liver)
Laparoscopy/laparotomy

Rx

Curative: Radical gastrectomy, node removal and adjuvant chemotherapy:

- Polya-type gastrectomy (distal 3/4) for antral cancer
- Total gastrectomy and distal oesophagectomy for gastric body cancer

Palliative: If evidence of local or systemic spread:

- Gastrectomy, gastroenterostomy (for pyloric obstruction), endoscopic laser photocoagulation, alcohol injection

Prog

5-year survival rate = 10% (95% if detected + resected early, e.g. by screening, as in Japan)

INFLAMMATORY BOWEL DISEASE

Epi

	Ulcerative colitis	Crohn disease
Inc	10/100,000 p.a.	5/100,00 p.a. (rising)
Age	Bimodal: 20s and 60s	Bimodal: 20s and 60s
Sex	Females predominantly	Males predominantly
Geo	Ashkenazi Jews↑; Africans↓, Asians 0	As for UC
Aet	Genetic: MZ concordance = 10%	Genetic: MZ concordance = 70%
Pre	Smoking *protects*	**C**igarettes and **C**ontraceptive pill **C**ause **C**rohn

PATH

	Ulcerative colitis	**C**rohn disease
Macro	Restricted; always in the following order: Rectum → colon → terminal ileum (proctitis) (colitis) ('backwash ileitis')	Global, but occurs as 'skip lesions' anywhere between mouth ↔ anus
Micro	Restricted: **U**lcers limited to m**U**cosa **U**ndermining ulcers	Transmural: **C**lefts + fissures **C**obblestone appearance non-**C**aseating granulomas→ lymphadenopathy
	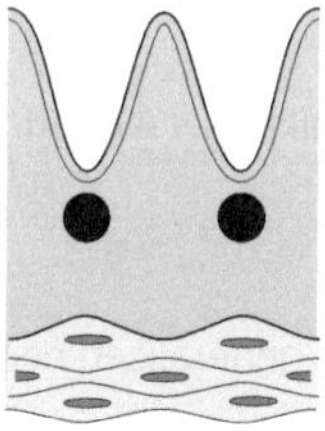 *Lumen* *Cryptitis and crypt abscesses* *Muscular wall*	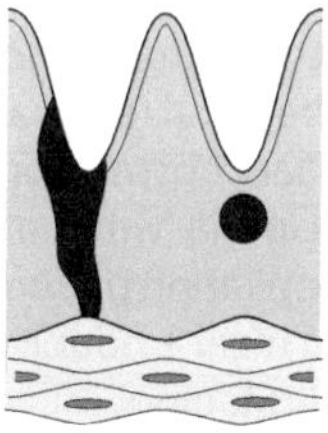
	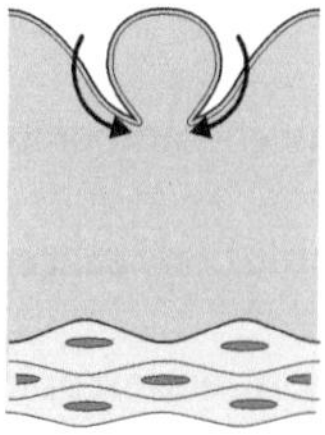 *Inflammatory pseudopolyp*	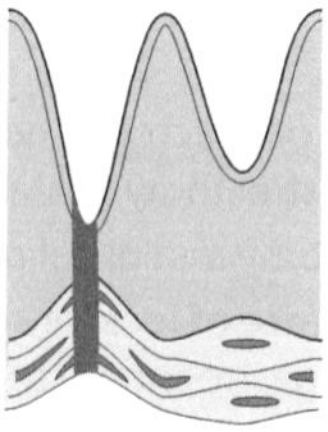 *Fibrosis, stricture, adhesions, fistula*

PC

	Ulcerative colitis	Crohn disease
Abdomen	**Colon–rectum** Diarrhoea, blood or mucus PR, tenesmus; faecal urgency *Less common*: Constipation, pain, abdominal distension (colon)	**Mouth** Aphthous ulcers, glossitis, cheilitis, granulomatous swollen lips **Ileum** Diarrhoea, colic, flatus **Terminal ileum** RIF pain, mass **Colon–rectum** As for UC **Anus** Piles, tags, fissure, fistula, dusky, blue colouration

Abdomen complications	**A.B.C.**
	Acute colitis
	PC: Toxic megacolon; mortality rate 10%, or 50% if bowel perforates
	Bleeding – massive
	Carcinoma:
	• Ascending colon commonest site
	• Risk = 10% every 10 years
	• Dep. on:
	  • Age at onset <25 y
	  • Unremitting Sx
	  • Pancolitis (40% risk)
	Less common:
	Obstruction: Benign strictures of sigmoid–rectum
	Protein-losing enteropathy
		F.O.A.M. B.C.
		Fistula
		Entero-enteric or colonic. PC: Diarrhoea
		Vesical: PC: Frequency, pneumaturia
		Vaginal, perianal, abdominal wall skin
		Obstruction: Benign strictures anywhere in GIT
		Abscess
		Bowel, psoas, subclinical perforation
		PC: Diarrhoea
		Malabsorption
		Fat: Steatorrhoea; gall, renal stones
		Protein: Oedema (also 2° protein loss)
		Vitamin B12: Megaloblastic anaemia
		Vitamin D: Osteomalacia
		Less common
		Acute colitis or ileitis: → toxic megacolon + perforation
		Bleeding – massive
		Carcinoma/lymphoma

Extra-abdominal	**H.A.S.S.L.E.S.** **H**aematology: Anaemia of chronic disease, DVT **A**rthritis: Enteropathic athropathy **S**ystemic: Fever, weight loss, anaemia of chronic disease, DVT, AA amyloid **S**pondylosis **L**iver: Sclerosing cholangitis, cholangiocarcinoma, chronic active hepatitis **E**yes: Iridocyclitis, phylectenular conjunctivitis, episcleritis **S**kin: Pyoderma gangrenosum, erythema nodosum or multiforme, vasculitis	

Ix

Bloods: Biochemistry:

- U&Es: Urea ↑, Na ↓, K ↓, Ca ↓, vitamin D ↓, Mg ↓ LFT: ALT ↑, ALP ↑, PT ↑, albumin ↓
- ABG: Metabolic acidosis, HCO_3 ↓

Haematology: Hb – microcytic anaemia; WCC – neutrophils ↑; ESR, CRP ↑

Urine: MSU: Faecal flora if entero-vesical fistula

Micro: Blood culture

Stool culture: Exclude *Campylobacter, Salmonella*, amoebiasis ('hot' specimen)

Crohn disease: Exclude infectious causes of right-iliac fossa mass – TB, *Yersinia*, actinomycosis (biopsy + stain)

Monitor: Tachycardia, temperature, tenderness (>5 days)

Stool count, daily (>6 BO at day 3)

Radiol: Erect CXR: Perforation

AXR:

- Transverse colon dilatation
- Sacro-iliitis
- Biliary or renal stones (Crohn disease)

Barium enema (Crohn: barium meal and follow-through) – see below

Special: Endoscopy + mucosal biopsies:

- UC: Granular mucosa; superficial ulcers; pseudopolyps; Crohn; granuloma
- UC: Perform annual check-up >10 years disease to detect dysplasia or neoplasia

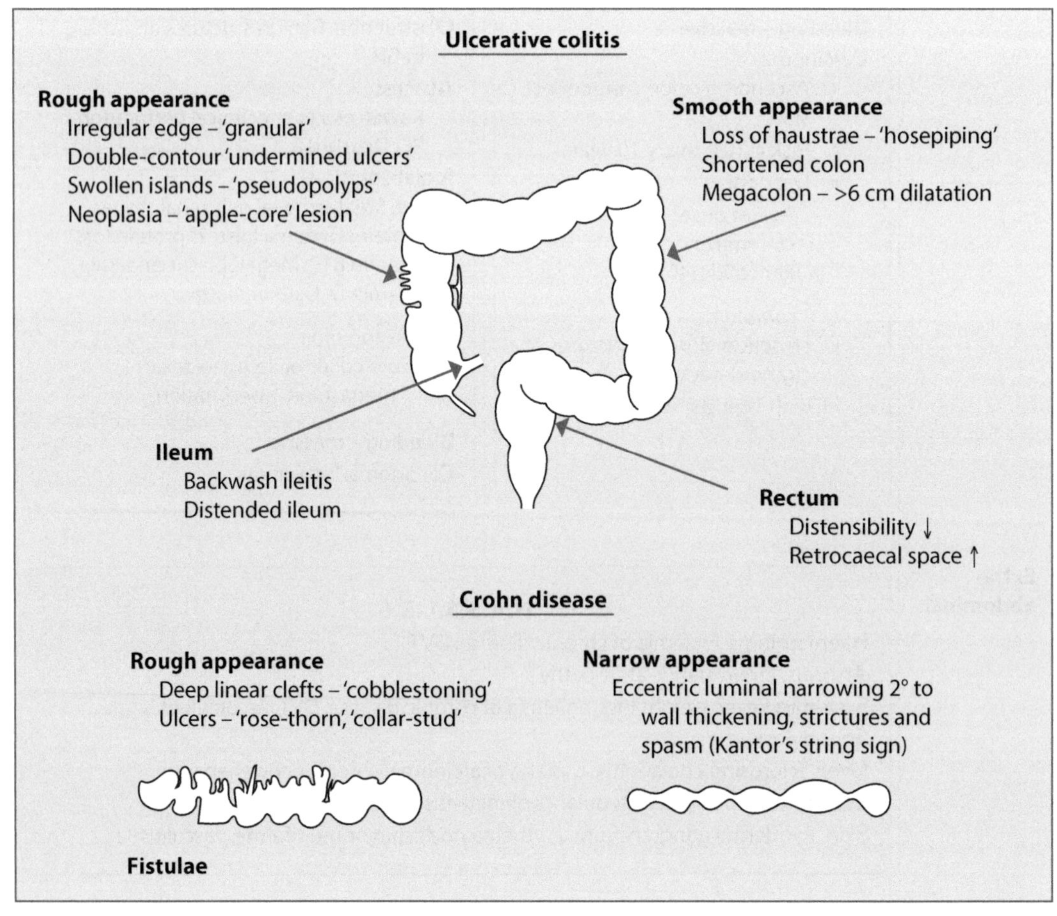

Rx

S.N.A.C.K.S.

Supportive:

Anti-diarrhoeal and anti-motility Rx:

- Mebeverine, buscopan, codeine
- Cholestyramine, hydrophilic colloid preparation (for bile-salt malabsorption in Crohn)

Smoking: Stopping causes 30% ↓ in risk of relapse over 5 years

Nutrition

Nutrient replacement: Protein; vitamins and haematinics (esp. Crohn); TPN if obstruction

Crohn:

- Acute relapse: Give liquid-formula diet to 'rest' bowel; elemental (amino acids); oligomeric (peptides); polymeric (protein) course = 4–6 weeks as sole nutrition (as effective as steroids)
  ☠: Unpalatable (can use NGT/PEG); high relapse rate afterwards
- High-carbohydrate refined sugars; avoid dairy products (lactose-intolerant)

Aminosalicylates:

Mesalazine, olsalazine, sulphasalazine (more side-effects):

- Activated by colonic bacteria: Use laxatives to ↓ faecal loading of colon
- Oral (ileum–colon); retention enema (desc. colon); suppository (proctitis)
- Indications: Acute disease if mild; chronic disease – maintains remission
  ☠: Headache, abdo pain, diarrhoea, rash, interstitial nephritis, megaloblastic anaemia

Corticosteroids/other imunosuppressants:

- Steroids:
  - Systemic: Prednisolone: 30–60 mg od, ↓ 5 mg/week; IV hydrocortisone
  - Topical: Hydrocortisone by retention or foam enemas
  - Budesonide PO: Minimal absorption; high 1st-pass metabolism; activated in ileum–colon
- Cyclosporin (IV or enema), tacrolimus, mycophenolate – acute relapses
- Methotrexate, azathioprine, thalidomide – chronic disease, esp. perianal Crohn
- Infliximab: Mouse–human chimeric anti-TNFα monoclonal antibody:
  - Used for refractory disease (65% improve) or fistulae; good in Crohn and maybe UC
    ☠: Headache, SLE-like syn.; lymphoma; obstruction due to rapid healing with fibrosis

Kill bacteria if signs of sepsis or infection (IV antibiotics)

Surgery

UC – *30% require at some time:*

- Types: Panproctocolectomy; permanent ileostomy and ileoanal anastomosis with ileal pouch
- Indications: Toxic megacolon; steroid-resistant disease; chronic (>10 y) or dysplasia

Crohn – *70% require at some time*:

- Types: Limited resection; endoscopic balloon dilatation; abscess drainage
- Indications: Resistant disease; stricture; fistula; tumour
  ☠: Recurrence occurs in 50% by 10 y

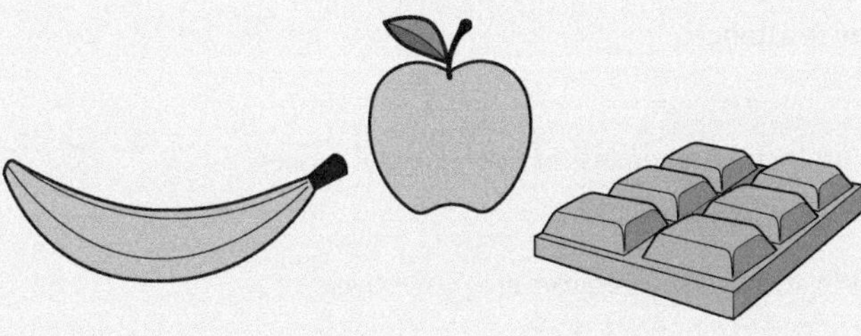

COLORECTAL CARCINOMA

Aet

Most colorectal cancers arise from adenomatous polyps, via a succession of mutations:

- K-ras proto-oncogene →
  APC (adenomatous polyposis coli) gene
  - *DCC* (deleted in colon cancer) gene
    → *p53* tumour-suppressor gene

Assoc

Colorectal cancer is often **H.I.D.D.E.N.**

Hereditary

The lifetime risk of developing colorectal cancer is 10% if one first-degree relative <50 y is affected, and 5% if one first-degree relative >50 y is affected. The background risk is 2%.

Familial syndromes (all autosomal dominant)

Hereditary polyposis coli:

- Adenomatous polyposis coli (APC, or familial adenomatous polyposis):
  - 100% patients get carcinoma by 40 years old
  - Due to tumour-suppressor gene (5q-), involved in sporadic cases of adenomatous polyp transformation
- Gardner syndrome
  PC: Colonic polyps + bone tumours (osteomas; sarcomas) + soft tissue tumours (lipomas, sebaceous cysts, dermoid cysts)
- Turcot syndrome:
  PC: Colonic polyps + brain tumours

Hereditary non-polyposis colon cancer (HNPCC)= Lynch syndrome

Def = 3 cases colorectal cancer over 2 generations with at least 1 case <50 years old; Type 1 = colorectal cancer only: <50 years old; usually R-sided; good prognosis; Type 2 = colorectal, gastric, ovarian, endometrial cancer

- 5% of all colorectal cancer; 1/200 population
- Due to mismatch repair gene mutation → microsatellite instability

Hamartomatous polyps syndromes: Polyps affect entire bowel + stomach

- Juvenile polyposis = assoc. various congenital abnormalities
- Peutz–Jeghers syndrome = mucocutaneous pigmentation
  Complications: Obstruction, intussusception → PR bleed, adenoma → carcinoma

Inflammation

Ulcerative colitis: 10% per 10 years; 30% lifetime risk (Crohn disease = less risk)

Coeliac

Infection: *Streptococcus bovis* endocarditis or septicaemia

Diet: Obesity is a risk factor, whereas high fibre diets protect

Diabetes and insulin resistance

Endocrine

Acromegaly

Oestrogen: HRT protects; women less at risk for rectal cancer

Nicotine and alcohol: Both increase risk

NB: NSAIDs, aspirin and COX-2 inhibitors are protective

PC

Approx. relative incidence in each site indicated:

Transverse + descending colon

(15%)

Abdominal pain, lower:

- Constant, gnawing: Invasion
- Colic: Obstruction

Obstruction

Perforation→ peritonitis

(stool solidifies + ∴ gets stuck)

Constitutional weight loss

Sigmoid

(30%)

Caecum + ascending colon

(15%)

Iron-deficiency anaemia:

- Fatigue, palpitations, angina (stool is liquid + ∴ slips past luminal narrowing)

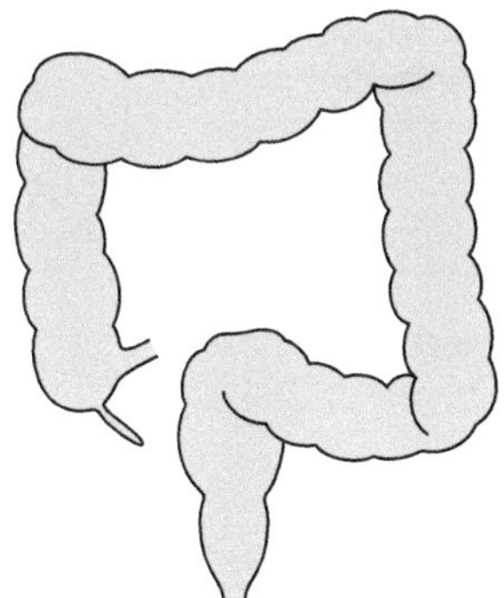

Rectum

(40%)

Bowel habit alteration and narrowing of stool caliber

Tenesmus (rectal discomfort, 'incomplete emptying')

Rectal bleeding:

Bright = distal colon–rectum

Dark = proximal colon

O/E: PR mass (rectal–anal cancer)

Anus

(2%)

Painful mass, pruritus, bleeding

Complications

Fistula, e.g. colonic–vesical, colonic–vaginal

Metastases: Liver, bone, lung

Ix

Bloods: FBC: Hb ↓, ferritin ↓, ESR ↑

Urine + faeces: Faecal occult blood – poor sensitivity (intermittent bleeding) + poor specificity (benign polyps)

Monitor: Plasma CEA (carcinoembryonic antigen) – increases on tumour recurrence

Radiol: Double-contrast barium enema: Annular, constricting 'apple-core' lesion
CT pneumocolon: Non-invasive alternative to colonoscopy
CT, liver USS: Staging

Special: Proctosigmoidoscopy (<60 cm) + biopsy
Colonoscopy + snare-biopsy: >95% sensitivity + specificity
Entire colon must be visualized due to risk of >1 polyp

Rx

Surgical:

- Anterior resection: Proximal tumours – colorectal anastomosis with staple gun
- Abdominoperineal (AP) resection : Distal tumours – end-sigmoid colostomy fashioned

Radiotherapy: Given pre-operatively in rectal cancer (recurrence ↓; survival rate ↑)

Chemotherapy: Adjuvant therapy with oxaliplatin or 5-fluorouracil

Palliative: Laser therapy, radiotherapy, chemotherapy

MALABSORPTION

Causes

Wall disease

C^2.R.A.G^2.G.Y^3.

Coeliac disease/**C**rohn disease; other autoimmune – collagenous sprue; scleroderma
Radiation enteritis
Arterial/venous
Arterial: Mesenteric ischaemia, e.g. AAA, vasculitis
Venous hypertension: CCF, constrictive pericarditis
Giardiasis/**G**astroenteritis, other infection
Salmonella, HIV, TB, protozoa
Whipple disease (lymphatic infection)
Genetic
Brush-border disaccharidase deficiency (lactase, maltase)
Agammaglobulinaemia
Y
Am**Y**loid
L**Y**mphoma (incl. coeliac disease); a-heavy-chain disease
L**Y**mphangectasia

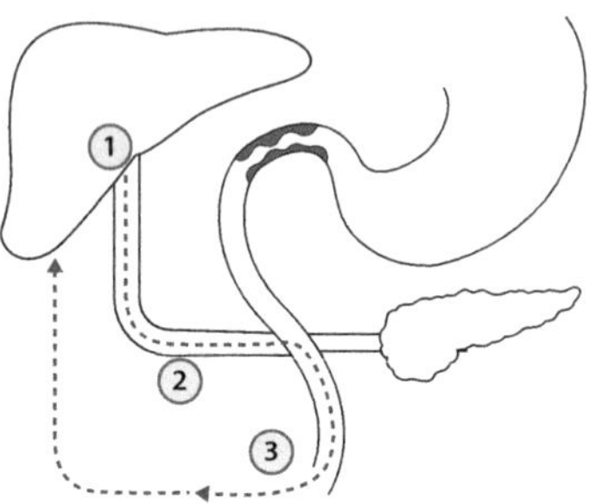

Bile salt circulation ↓

Bile salts combine with fatty acids to form micelles that are essential for fat absorption

1. Liver disease
Hepatocellular failure
Cholestasis

2. Bacterial overgrowth (bacteria deconjugate bile salts)
Structural:
- Strictures, adhesions, fistulae, e.g. Crohn, ischaemia
- Small bowel diverticulae
- Pneumatosis cystoides intestinales
- Blind loops, e.g. gastrojejunostomy

Motility ↓, e.g. scleroderma
Defence impairments:
- Achlorhydria (e.g. long-term PPI)
- Nodular lymphoid hypoplasia
- Agammaglobulinaemia

3. Terminal ileal disease
Crohn, TB, radiation

+ Drugs
Cholestyramine, neomycin, $CaCO_3$

Pancreatic disease

Chronic pancreatitis
Cystic fibrosis
Carcinoma of the pancreas, surgical resection

Other

Endocrine
Gastrinoma, or other APUDoma:
- H^+↑↑ inactivates pancreatic lipase
- Rapid intestinal transit

Systemic**:** Hyper- or hypo T4ism, Addison, DM

Diarrhoea
Any cause of rapid transit, e.g.
Gastroenteritis
Drugs: Laxatives
Surgery: Gastrectomy, duodenojejuno-ileal bypass

PC

Malabsorption symptoms: Carbohydrate, fat, protein, haematinics, vitamins (see p. 132)
Symptoms associated with cause, e.g. abdominal pain due to chronic pancreatitis or strictures

Ix

Bloods: U&Es: Ca, PO_4, Mg, vitamin D ↓
LFT: ALP ↑, albumin ↓, PT ↑
Glucose ↑: Pancreatic or coeliac disease (assoc. DM)
FBC: Micro- or macrocytic anaemia
Film: Megaloblastosis; hyposplenism (e.g. Howell–Jolly bodies) – coeliac disease
Haematinics: Ferritin ↓, Fe ↓, TIBC ↑
Folate ↓ (↑ in bacterial overgrowth due to bacterial synthesis)
Vitamin B12 ↓: Bacterial overgrowth; terminal ileal or pancreatic disease
Special: Amylase ↑ – pancreatic disease; anti-endomysium – coeliac; serum electrophoresis

Urine, faeces: Hyperoxaluria: Bile salt malabsorption
Faecal fat estimation: >6 g/day (pre-treat with 100 g fat/day for 2 days)

Micro: Exclude *Giardia*: Stool cysts, faecal antigen; duodenal aspirate – trophozoites

Monitor: Weights, vitamins

Radiol: Bone X-ray: Looser zones (OM); subperiosteal erosions (2° hyper-PTHism)
Small-bowel enema:

- Jejunal dilatation + flocculation ('snowflakes')
- Blind loops; strictures – bacterial overgrowth

AXR, CT, USS, ERCP – pancreatic disease

Special:

Wall disease

Biopsy, duodenal–jejunal, via OGD, or push enteroscopy:

- Sub-total villous atrophy present in most wall diseases, bacterial overgrowth, gastrinoma
- Other: Amyloid; Whipple (PAS +ve macrophages)

Absorption tests:

- Administer oral D-xylose, lactose or ^{14}C-labelled triolein (triglyceride)
- Measure urine xylose; exhaled H_2 (↑ in lactase deficiency) or CO_2 (↑ in lipase deficiency)

Bile salt circulation ↓

Breath tests

- ^{14}C-labelled-glycholate bile salt breath test:
  - Small-bowel bacteria deconjugate glycholate, with resultant CO_2 detectable in breath
  - Terminal ileal disease: Bile salt not absorbed; colonic bacteria deconjugate it to CO_2 in faeces
- H_2 breath test: Bacterial overgrowth: ↑ with fasting; oral glucose – early peak

Duodenal–jejunal aspirate: Shows $>10^5$ microorganisms/ml and polymicrobial flora
Empirical antibiotics: Coamoxiclav, metronidazole

Pancreatic disease

Faecal elastase – pancreatic exocrine insufficiency

COELIAC DISEASE

Epi

Inc: 1/2000, ↓ due to later introduction of cereals
Age: Any age, but esp. 1–5 y and 20–30 y
Sex: F>M
Geo: Common in West Ireland (1/300); rare in Afro-Caribbean and Japanese
Aet: Genetic: HLA-B8, DR3 in 80% (cf. 20% general population)
Enzyme deficiency: Pancreatic peptidase; brush border membrane disaccharidase
Mucosal absorption deficit

PC

*Anti-***G.L.I.A.D.I.N.S.**

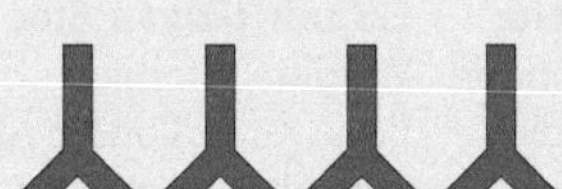

Gastrointestinal: malabsorption

Carbohydrates:

- N+V; watery diarrhoea
- Abdominal distension + colic
- Flatus, borborygmi (lactose intolerance)

Fat: Due to ↓ bile salt secretion (as cholecystokinin ↓) and bile salt malabsorption

- Steatorrhoea
- Renal stones (hyperoxaluria)

Protein: Due to peptidase deficiency, malabsorption, protein-losing enteropathy (ulcerative jejuno-ileitis)

- Oedema, ascites
- Weight loss, muscular atrophy
- Leuconychia

Haematinics:

- Folate, Fe: Dimorphic anaemia (vitamin B12 deficiency – only occurs late)
- Epithelial atrophy (cheilitis, glossitis, gastric atrophy, koilonychia, alopecia, pruritus)

Vitamins:

- D, Ca, Mg: Tetany, osteomalacia, osteoporosis
- A: Night blindness
- K: Petechiae
- B1 (thiamine): Wernicke encephalopathy; niacin: pellagra

Lymphoma and carcinoma
Lymphoma: Small bowel > other MALToma > extra-intestinal
Adenocarcinoma: Small or large bowel; breast
Squamous cell carcinoma: Oesophageal, oropharynx

Immune abnormalities
Type 1 DM, rheumatoid arthritis, thyroiditis
Infertility: Amenorrhoea, impotence
Inflammatory bowel disease (UC), PBC, PSC

Anaemia
Micro- or macrocytic anaemia + reticulocytosis
Splenic atrophy: Blood film shows Howell–Jolly bodies, acanthocytes, target cells, siderocytes

Dermatological
Dermatitis herpetiformis (IgA deposits in upper dermis and dermo-epidermal junction)
Follicular hyperkeratosis, pigmentation, aphthous ulcers, clubbing

Ig A mesangial nephropathy (and Ig**A** deficiency)

Neurological: Cerebral calcification (epilepsy), spinocerebellar degeneration, peripheral neuropathy

Systemic: Fatigue – 90%

Ix

Bloods: Biochemical: **R.E.A.L.M.S.**

Renal
Electrolytes: Ca, PO_4, Mg, vitamin D ↓
ABG
LFT: ALP ↑, albumin ↓, PT ↑
Metabolic: Glu (DM)
Special: Haematinics: Ferritin ↓, Fe ↓, TIBC ↑, folate ↓

Haematological:

- FBC: Micro- or macrocytic anaemia
- Film: Features of hyposplenism (e.g. Howell–Jolly bodies)
- ESR ↑ or normal

Immune:

- Tissue transaminase
- Anti-endomyseal abs: False –ve: IgA deficiency, adoption of gluten-free diet
- IgA: Majority ↑ (but may be ↓); IgM ↓

Urine: Haematuria: IgA mesangial glomerulonephritis
Hyperoxaluria: Bile salt malabsorption

Micro: Exclude *Giardia* with: Stool cysts, faecal antigen; duodenal aspirate

Monitor: Weight; new bowel symptoms (risk of neoplasia)

Radiol: Bone X-ray: Looser zones (osteomalacia); subperiosteal erosions (2° hyper-PTHism)
Small-bowel enema: Jejunal dilatation + flocculation ('snowflakes')

Special: OGD-endoscopy: 'scalloping' of duodenal valvulae conniventes; loss of Kerkring duodenal folds
Small-bowel biopsy (via OGD; push-enteroscopy or Crosby capsule) subtotal/total villous atrophy, reversible after 3–6 month gluten-free diet

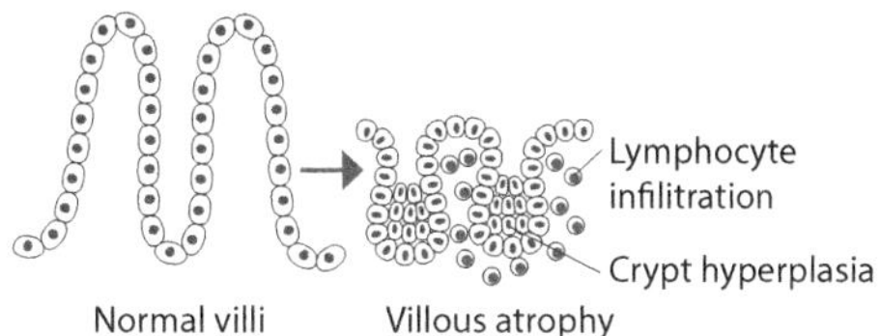

+ permeability test, tissue transglutaminase, disaccharidase activity

Pancreatic function tests deranged; bacterial overgrowth test normal

Rx

Diet: Gluten-free diet

AVOID flour from:

B.R.O.W.

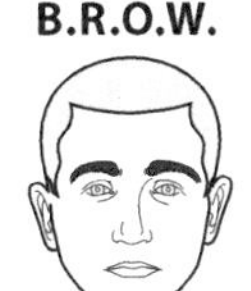

Barley (hordein)
Rye (secalin)
Oats (avenin)
Wheat (α-gliadin)

ACCEPTABLE

M.O.R.E.

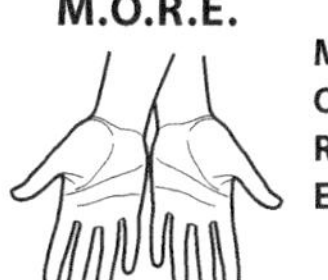

Maize
Oats (some tolerated)
Rice
Extra: Fibre
Vitamins, Ca, Fe, folate

Failure to respond (Ix: Repeat Bx after 3 months):

- Non-compliance (lesions return within 8–12 h of gluten-diet resumption)
- Resistant coeliac
- Complication: Lymphoma, ulcerative jejuno-ileitis, intestinal stricture
- Wrong diagnosis, e.g. hypolactasia

Medical:

- Corticosteroids, azathioprine – for those who have a poor response to gluten-free diet
- Dapsone – for dermatitis
  ☠ Herpetiformis; headache; haemolysis; methaemoglobinaemia

Surgical: For lymphoma or ulcerative jejuno-ileitis

ACUTE PANCREATITIS

PATH

Pancreatic duct blocks off, causing activation of proteases and lipases within pancreas
Histology shows oedema, fat necrosis and haemorrhage

Causes

A.G.I.T.A².T.E.S. M.E.

Alcohol
- Increases viscosity of pancreatic juice, thereby forming inspissated protein plugs in ducts
- Can occur with chronic consumption or one-off binge

Gallstones
- Large stones (wide cystic duct) block common biliary–pancreatic duct
- Stones may be recovered in faeces, several days after
- So-called 'idiopathic' pancreatitis may be caused by transient biliary sludge

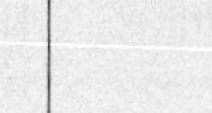

Iatrogenic or trauma
- ERCP
- Surgery: May occur after any operation, but especially Polya gastrectomy
- Trauma – blunt abdominal

Triglyceridaemia, hyper
- Triglycerides >10 mol/l, incl. DM

Autoimmune or **A**rterial
- Autoimmune: Vasculitis, Sjögren
- Arterial: Atherosclerosis, hypotension

Toxin
- Azathioprine, anti-HIV, tetracycline, valproate

Electrolytes
- Hypercalcaemia

Structural
- Pancreatic carcinoma, sphincter of Oddi dysfunction, pancreas divisum

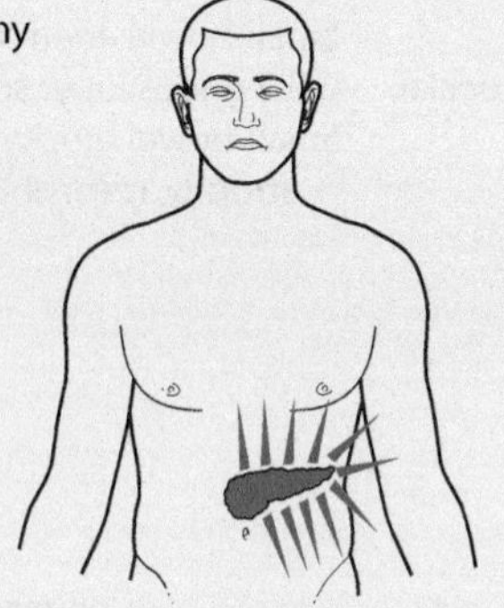

Mumps
- Or viral hepatitis, EBV, CMV, enteroviruses, mycoplasma

O**E**strogens – oral contraceptive pill

PC

P.A.N.C.R³.E.A.S.

Pain
Acute, severe, epigastric pain, radiates to back
Relieved by sitting up and flexing trunk
Assoc. N+V, abdominal distension, jaundice (pancreatic head compresses bile duct)
ABP ↓
Third-space sequestration: Blood and plasma protein accumulate retroperitoneally
Vasodilator release: Kinins, proteases, lipases
Septic shock: Coliforms, *Candida*
Haemorrhage: Gastritis, varices from portal vein thrombosis, DIC
Necrosis
Pancreatic necrosis:
- Cullen's sign = faint blue umbilicus (haemoperitoneum)
- Grey-Turner's sign = purple-brown flanks due to catabolism of tissue Hb

Panniculitis = subcutaneous nodules due to fat necrosis
Calcium and **C**ardiac arrhythmias, due to Ca↓, 2° to fat necrosis
Renal: Acidosis, AKI
Respiratory: Hypoxia, left-sided pleural effusion, ARDS
Retinopathy or encephalopathy
Endocrine: Hyperglycaemia
Abscess or pseudocyst
Occurs after 4 weeks
Pseudocyst = necrotic fluid in lesser sac (fistula with pancreas)
Complications: Rupture (MR = 15%) or haemorrhage (MR = 60%)
Stricture

Ix

Bloods: Amylase >1000 iU/l: Non-specific and may normalize after few days
Pancreas-type isoamylase, lipase, trypsin elevation: More specific and remain high for weeks
Radiol: Contrast-enhanced CT

Poor prognostic features

A.C.U.T.E.

ABGs: pO_2 <8 kPa	**A**lbumin <30 g/l
Ca^{2+} <2 mmol/l	**C**RP > 150 mg/l; WBC ↑↑
Urea >16 mmol/l	**U**rine output <50 ml/h
Transaminases (AST >200 U/l)	**T**rypsinogen activation pepetide (urine) ↑
Elderly, obese	**E**xtra: LDH, haematocrit ↑

Rx

Routine:
- NGT: 'Drip + Suck'
- IV cefuroxime + metronidazole
- Analgesics
- Bowel rest

Surgical: Debridement for necrosis

CHRONIC PANCREATITIS

PATH

Caused by recurrent clinical or subclinical episodes of acute pancreatitis

Similar causes to acute pancreatitis, **except that** gallstones do not cause it because cholecystectectomy is normally performed after 1st attack!

Causes

A.G.I.T.A.T.E.S.

Alcohol
Genetic
- Hereditary pancreatitis (autosomal dominant)
- Cystic fibrosis
- Haemochromatosis
- α_1-antitrypsin deficiency

Iatrogenic
- Gastrectomy

Triglyceridaemia
Autoimmune
Toxin
- Excess cassava (tropical)
- Protein–calorie malnutrition

Enzyme deficiency, isolated
- Trypsinogen, enterokinase, lipase, amylase
- Results in specific nutrient malabsorption

Strucural
- Stricture
- Pancreatic or duodenal cancer
- Congenital: Pancreas divisum, choledochal cyst

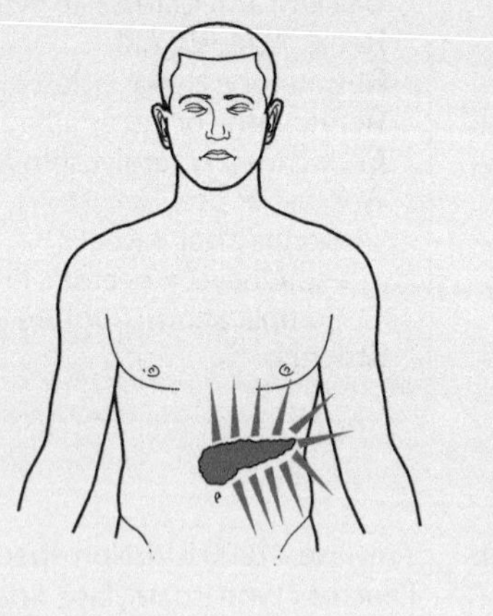

PC

Abdominal pain
Timing: Intermittent (due to duct obstruction) or constant (due to inflammation or duodenal ulcers secondary to ↓ HCO_3 secretion)
Location: Epigastric radiating to back; may present as chest or flank pain
Severity: May be severe enough to result in opiate abuse
Exacerbation: ↑by fatty food or alcohol (therefore encouraging anorexia)

Steatorrhoea
Stool pale, offensive, bulky, doesn't flush
Profuse: >35 g/day (cf. coeliac: 20–30 g/day; normal <6 g/day)
Malabsorption of fat-soluble vitamins + protein less problematic

O/E

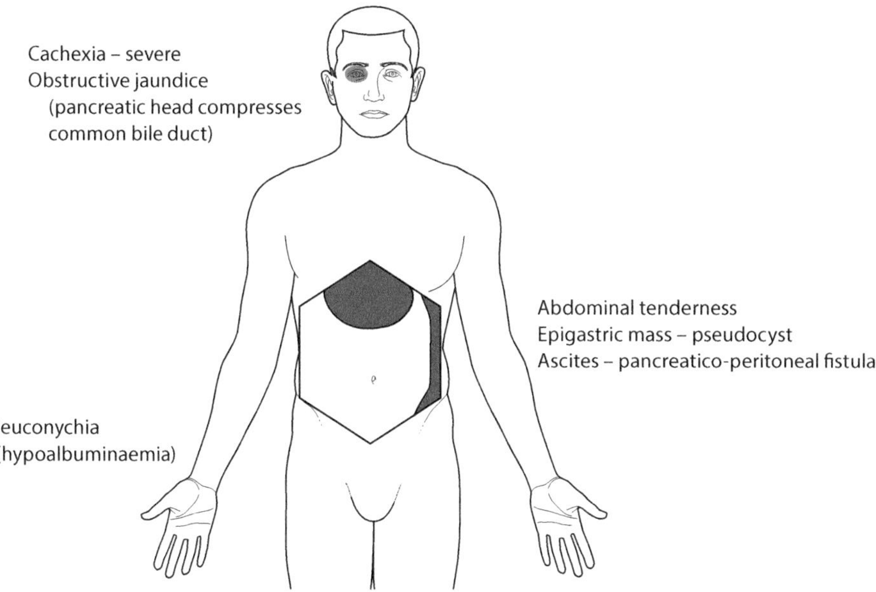

Ix

Bloods: CRP, WBC, ALT ↑↑
Urine or faeces: Faecal elastase <100 mm/mg stool; faecal fat collection >6 g/day
Radiol: PAXR, USS: Calcification
CT: Pseudocyst
ERCP: Differentiates pancreatitis from carcinoma but 3% risk of acute pancreatitis!
Special: Duodenal aspirate following 'Lundh meal' or secretin stimulation

Rx

Diet:

- Low-fat; high-carbohydrate; protein supplements; fat-soluble vitamins
- Alcohol abstinence

Medical:

- Pancreatic enzyme supplements
- Proton-pump inhibitor due to risk of duodenal ulcers
- Oral hypoglycaemics or insulin

Surgical:

- Sphincteroplasty
- Lateral pancreatico-jejunostomy
- Pancreatectomy – distal or Whipple, with coeliac ganglion block

JAUNDICE

Causes

Pre-hepatic	**Excess bilirubin production** Haemolytic anaemia Inefficient erythropoiesis, e.g. pernicious anaemia, thalassaemia Haematoma	

Hepatic	**Unconjugated hyperBRaemia**
	Bilirubin uptake
	Hereditary: Gilbert syn. (AD)
	• EPI: 5% pop., esp. young men
	• PC: Malaise on fasting or illness
	• Rx: Phenobarbitone (liver inducer)
	Fasting, acidosis
	Toxins: Rifampicin, aspirin
	↓Conjugation
	(BR-UDP-glucuronyl transferase ↓)
	Children:
	• Crigler- Najjar syndrome:
	  ◦ Type I severe (AR); II mild (AR)
	Neonates/breast milk
	Hypothyroidism
		Conjugated hyperBRaemia
		↓ Bilirubin excretion
		Hereditary
		• Dubin–Johnson syndrome (AR):
		  ◦ Canalicular membrane carrier defect
		  ◦ Black liver due to catecholamine metabolite accumulation
		  ◦ PC: Recurrent jaundice, asymptomatic
		• Rotor syndrome (AD):
		  ◦ Decreased uptake, storage, conjugation
		  ◦ Normal liver colour
		  ◦ Much rarer
		• Diffuse hepatocellular disease (can also cause unconjugated hyperBRaemia)

Post-hepatic	**Intrahepatic obstruction** **I.N.T.R.A.H.E.P.A.T.i.C.** **I**nfection: Systemic, HIV, abscess **N**eoplasia: 1° or metastases **T**oxins: Chlorpromazine (+ tricyclic antidepressants) Chlorpropamide, carbimazole, Ca-antagonists, carbamazepine Cloxacillin (+ erythromycin estolate, augmentin, rifampicin) Cyclosporin (+ azathioprine) **R**oids - steroids: Anabolic steroids, contraceptive pill **A**utoimmune: PBC, UC, coeliac **H**epatitis – icteric stage **E**ndocrine: Thyrotoxicosis/DM Obesity/malnutrition/TPN **P**regnancy **A**myloid **T**ransplant **C**holangitis, sclerosing	**Extrahepatic obstruction** **Biliary system** Stricture: Post-cholecystitis (Mirizzi's syn.) or ERCP Carcinoma: • Cholangiocarcinoma, incl. Klatskin ca. (bifurcation of common hepatic duct) • Gall bladder carcinoma Calculus Congenital: • Choledochal cyst • Caroli's disease **Stomach-duodenum** Gastric carcinoma porta hepatis lymphadenopathy Ampullary/duodenal carcinoma **Other** Retroperitoneal fibrosis **Pancreas** Carcinoma Pancreatitis or pseudocyst

Physiology

Normal bilirubin (BR) = 3–17 μmol/l. Jaundice occurs with levels >51 μmol/l (i.e. 3× ULN)

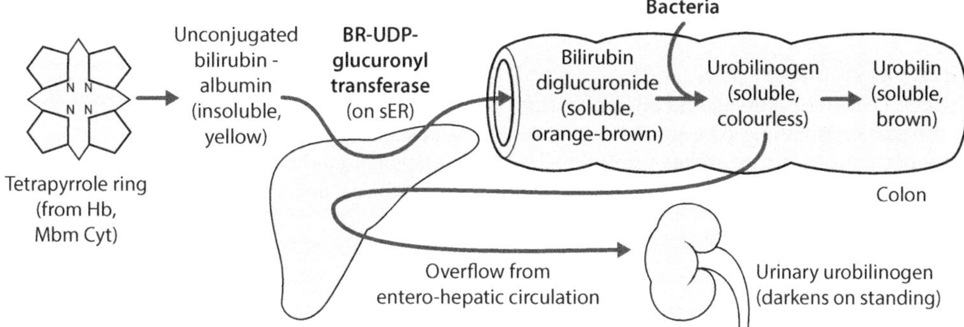

PC

	Urine	Stool	Other
Pre-hepatic	Dark: • Urobilinogen ↑ • Haemoglobinuria (if intravascular haemolysis)	Dark: Urobilin ↑	Pale conjunctivae; leg ulcers
Hepatic	Dark: Conjugated BR ↑ *(not Unconjugated hyperBRaemia)*	Pale: Urobilin ↓ due to partial cholestasis	Portal hypertension: Varices, ascites, encephalopathy
Post-hepatic	Dark: Conjugated BR↑	Pale: Urobilin ↓ fat malabsorption (steatorrhoea)	Pruritus; abdominal pain

Ix

	Urine	LFTs	Other
Pre-hepatic	BR nil ('acholuric') Urobilinogen ↑ Intravascular haemolysis: • Haemoglobinuria • Haemosiderinuria • Methaemalbuminuria	BR unconjugated↑ AST↑ LDH↑	FBC and film Reticulocytes: Normal – 1–2% a_2-haptoglobin (intravascular) Causes: • Hb electrophoresis • Direct Coombs' test
Hepatic	BR ↑ Urobilinogen ↓ Unconjugated hyperBRaemia: As for Pre-hepatic, except urobilinogen ↓	BR conjugated ↑ ALT ↑ ↑ ALP ↑ icteric stage GGT ↑ ↑ Function: Alb ↓, PT ↑ Unconjugated hyperBRaemia: BR unconjugated ↑	Anaemia: Normocytic, chromic Film: Target, spur, burr cells Causes: MCV↑; paracetamol levels; anti-LKM, ANA, ANCA; serology; liver USS + Doppler a_1,-AT, caeruloplasmin, ferritin
Post-hepatic	BR↑ Urobilinogen↓	As for Hepatic, except ALP ↑ ↑ greater than ALT ↑	Abdominal USS, ERCP, CT AMA, ANCA

LIVER FAILURE

PC

Jaundice + its associated features:

Hepatic: Dark urine (conjugated BR↑), pale stool (urobilin ↓ due to partial cholestasis)

Post-hepatic: Dark urine, pale stool-steatorrhea (fat malabsorption), pruritus

Portal hypertension: Varices, ascites – peripheral oedema, encephalopathy

Underlying cause features, e.g. nausea, fever (hepatitis); paraesthesia, delusions (alcoholism)

O/E

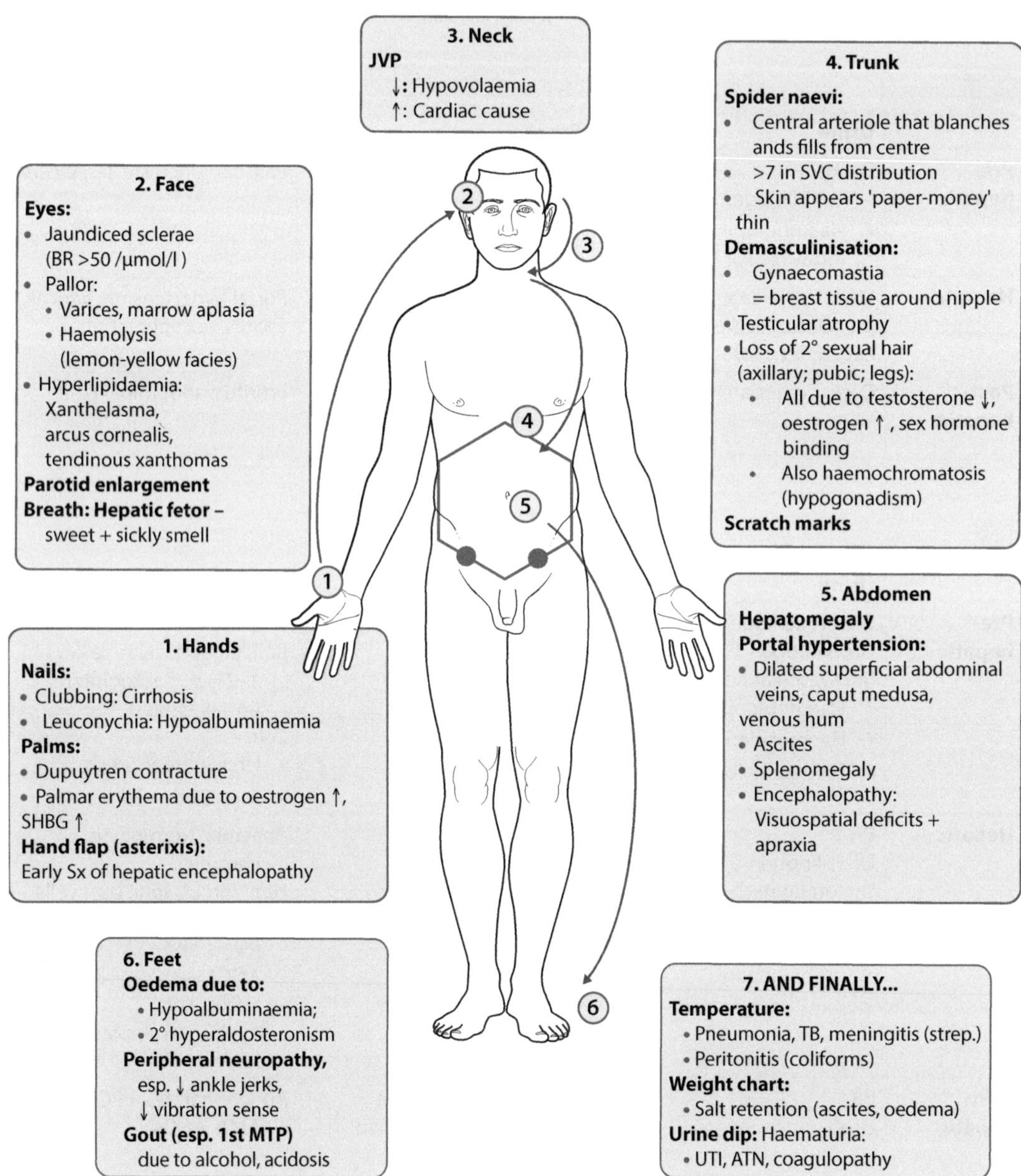

3. Neck
JVP
↓: Hypovolaemia
↑: Cardiac cause
4. Trunk
Spider naevi:
• Central arteriole that blanches ands fills from centre
• >7 in SVC distribution
• Skin appears 'paper-money' thin
Demasculinisation:
• Gynaecomastia = breast tissue around nipple
• Testicular atrophy
• Loss of 2° sexual hair (axillary; pubic; legs):
• All due to testosterone ↓, oestrogen ↑, sex hormone binding
• Also haemochromatosis (hypogonadism)
Scratch marks
2. Face
Eyes:
• Jaundiced sclerae (BR >50 /μmol/l)
• Pallor:
• Varices, marrow aplasia
• Haemolysis (lemon-yellow facies)
• Hyperlipidaemia: Xanthelasma, arcus cornealis, tendinous xanthomas
Parotid enlargement
Breath: Hepatic fetor – sweet + sickly smell
1
2
3
4
5
6
1. Hands
Nails:
• Clubbing: Cirrhosis
• Leuconychia: Hypoalbuminaemia
Palms:
• Dupuytren contracture
• Palmar erythema due to oestrogen ↑, SHBG ↑
Hand flap (asterixis):
Early Sx of hepatic encephalopathy
5. Abdomen
Hepatomegaly
Portal hypertension:
• Dilated superficial abdominal veins, caput medusa, venous hum
• Ascites
• Splenomegaly
• Encephalopathy: Visuospatial deficits + apraxia
6. Feet
Oedema due to:
• Hypoalbuminaemia;
• 2° hyperaldosteronism
Peripheral neuropathy, esp. ↓ ankle jerks, ↓ vibration sense
Gout (esp. 1st MTP) due to alcohol, acidosis
7. AND FINALLY...
Temperature:
• Pneumonia, TB, meningitis (strep.)
• Peritonitis (coliforms)
Weight chart:
• Salt retention (ascites, oedema)
Urine dip: Haematuria:
• UTI, ATN, coagulopathy

Ix

Bloods:

Biochemistry

R.E.A.L.M.S.

Renal: Urea ↓, creatinine ↑. Hepato-renal syndrome: due to impaired prostaglandin synthesis and over-activation of sympathetic system, RAAS and ADH → renal vasoconstriction and pre-renal renal failure

Electrolytes:

- Na^+, K^+ ↓: Secondary hyperaldosteronism due to hypovolaemia
- Ca^{2+} ↓, Mg^{2+} ↓, vitamin D ↓ due to vitamin D malabsorption; 0 25-*α*-hydroxylation of cholecalciferol
- Ammonium ↑: Hepatic encephalopathy
- Uric acid ↑ due to acidosis; purine metabolism ↑

ABGs: Metabolic acidosis, esp. with alcoholism, due to:

- NADH/NAD^+ ↑ → pyruvate converts to lactate
- Hypoglycaemia → lipolysis → ketoacidosis
- Hypoxia, due to pulmonary shunts → TLCO ↓

LFTs: BR ↑, ALT ↑, ALP ↑, GGT ↑, Alb ↓

Metabolic: Glucose ↓ due to:

- Glycogen storage ↓
- Gluconeogenesis ↓ (esp. alcoholism: NADH/NAD^+ ↑)
- Malnutrition:

Cholesterol ↑: Cholestasis; triglycerides ↑: alcoholism, hepatitis due to:

- Zone 3 necrosis;
- LCAT and TAG lipase ↓;
- Abnormal LDL (lipoprotein X) – cholestasis

Special: AFP ↑: Hepatoma

Causes of liver failure:

- Toxicology screen, esp. paracetamol; save serum; urine; gastric aspirate
- Transferrin saturation ↑ (haemochromatosis), caeruloplasmin ↓ (Wilson), α_1-AT ↓

Haematology Hb ↓ + macrocytosis + film: Target cells, acanthocytes, spur cells, ringed sideroblasts – anaemia due to:

- Marrow suppression + erythropoeitin insensitivity
- Haemolysis: Hypersplenism; alcohol ↑ cholesterol in RBC membrane
- Iron or folate deficiency, e.g. varices, malnutrition

WBC ↓, frequent infections – pneumonia, TB, spontaneous bacterial peritonitis

Plts ↓ due to hypersplenism, ITP (also, abnormal platelet function)

PT ↑ due to: vitamin K deficiency; synthesis ↓ + activation ↓; DIC

G&S; X-match if anaemic; varices; liver biopsy

Immunology: ANA, Rh factor, AMA, LKM – autoimmune hepatitis

Micro: Blood cultures:
MSU
Sputum
Ascitic tap
LP (stain for AA FB, for all)
Serology: HBV, HCV, HDV

Monitor: Glucose: 4 hourly if encephalopathic
Daily weights

ECG: Sx. of hypokalaemia
ECHO: Right-sided heart failure

Radiol: CXR: Pneumonia or TB; pulmonary oedema; cardiomegaly (RSH failure)
USS: Cirrhosis; hepatoma; ascites

Special Endoscopy: Varices
Liver biopsy

MANAGEMENT

Airway – Breathing

Airway:

- Clean vomit, loose teeth
- Cuffed endotracheal tube
- Nasogastric tube, if vomiting

Oxygen: 60%

Ventilation if comatose

Assessment

The three Gs

Glasgow coma scale
Glucose – BM stick
Group and save, X-match 4 units

C.O.A.T.

Cardiac monitor
O2 sats
ABP, CVP line
TPR

Investigations

Bloods, e.g. $K^+ \downarrow$, ABGs
Urine: Na, osmolality ↓
Micro: Blood cultures; serology
Monitor fluid balance: Daily weights, girth, urine catheter, NG-aspirate, ascitic taps
ECG
Radiology: CXR, Abdominal USS
Special: OGD, EEG, liver biopsy

1. Urgent endoscopy, if:
   - Varices suspected
2. ITU transfer, if:
   - Drowsy or comatose
   - Major haemorrhage
3. Liver transplant

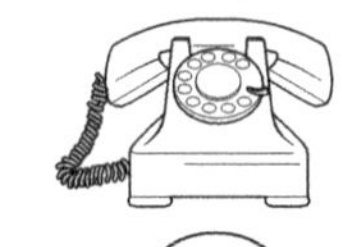
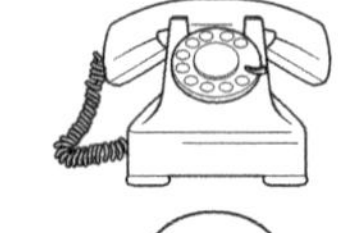
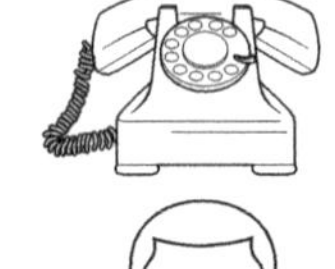
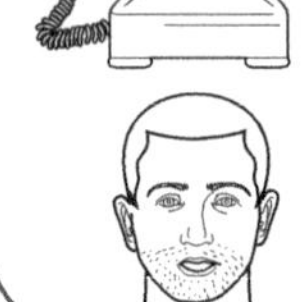
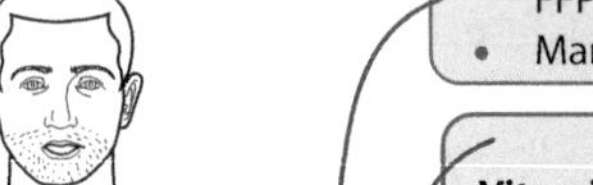

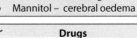

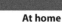

Hydration

Salt restriction and depletion:

- Fluid intake <1 l/day
- Spironolactone, furosemide
- Low-dose dopamine or haemodialysis if ARF

Fluids:

- Dextrose 5–50%, depending on BM, + KCl
- Salt-free albumin if ABP ↓
- Packed red cells, platelets, FFPs – if haemorrhage
- Mannitol – cerebral oedema

Drugs

Vitamins:

- Thiamine (B 1) – esp. alcoholics
- Vit B12, C – esp. alcoholics
- Vit K, FFP – for coagulopathy

Laxatives:

- Lactulose – lowers NH4
- MgS04 enemas – aim for 2 soft stools/day

Ulcer prophylaxis:

Omeprazole; sucralfate NGT

±

Broad-spectrum antibiotics,

e.g. ampicillin + gentamicin + metronidazole

Anti-convulsants:

Diazepam; phenytoin

Steroids based on Madri index,

i.e. give if bilirubin and PT ↑↑

Specific

Toxin overdose: Paracetamol – N-acetylcysteine
Autoimmune: Steroids, AZA
B: HBV, HCV – Interferon-α
Occlusive anti-coagulation
Syndromes:

- Haemochromatosis – venesection
- Wilson's – penicillamine

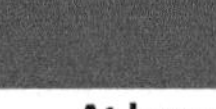

At home

Avoid alcohol;
refer for counselling
Avoid:
NSAIDs,
sedatives,
high-protein meals

LIVER TRANSPLANT

Indications

General

End-stage liver failure must be apparent, despite best medical therapy:

- Cholestasis: Pruritus, osteomalacia
- Portal hypertension: Varices, ascites
- LFTs: BR >150 µmol/l, albumin <30 g/l, PT >5 s

No other organ failure – i.e. patient survival is good if liver corrected. Hence, those with acute liver failure who are systemically unwell have a poorer 2-year survival rate (acute 70%, cf. chronic 90%)
Cause of liver failure does not predispose to recurrence in graft

Specific indications for liver transplant T.A.B.O^2.O^2.S.

Toxins
Drugs, e.g. paracetamol overdose, isoniazid or halothane idiosyncratic reactions
Chronic alcoholism, if:

- Child grade C cirrhosis
- Abstinent for >6 months

Autoimmune: Good survival rate due to disease not recurring (CAH) or uncommonly recurring (PBC)
B: Infections: Hep **B**, C, D:

- Hep B: Poor success rate (50%) due to extrahepatic replication and graft infection; must be e Ag –ve and HBV DNA –ve, and pre-treat with IFN + lamivudine
- Hep C: Good success rate due (90%) to recurrence of hepatitis being only mild
- Hep D: Intermediate success rate as Hep D prevents Hep B re-infection

Occlusive venous disease: Budd–Chiari syndrome
Obstetric: Fatty liver of pregnancy
Obstruction: PSC, biliary atresia; PSC has poor success rate due to infection and recurrent bile duct strictures
Oncology: Hepatoma – poor success rate due to tumour recurrence:
Indications:

- Fibrolamellar variant (metastasize late)
- Tumour size <5 cm
- AFP –ve

Syndromes **W.A.T.C.H.**
Wilson; α_1-**A**nti-trypsin deficiency; **T**yrosinaemia, galactosaemia, glycogen storage disease
Cystic fibrosis; **H**aemochromatosis (latter two are not cured by liver transplant)

Complications

Graft failure:

- Primary: Poor donor organ; hepatic vessel thrombosis <2 days: Rx = re-transplantation
- Acute: Immune 5–30 days: Rx = ↑immunosuppression
- Chronic: Shrinking bile ducts 1–3 months: Rx = re-transplantation

Infection:

- Opportunistic (from immunosuppression), e.g. PCP, *Candida*
- CMV or HSV reactivation from donor/host: Use prophylactic aciclovir

Recurrence of underlying condition, esp. infective hepatitis, hepatocellular carcinoma

PORTAL HYPERTENSION

Def

Resting portal venous pressure >12 mmHg (may be up to 50 mmHg)

Causes

Right-sided heart failure
Budd–Chiari syndrome (hepatic venous thrombosis)
Granulomas in hepatic veins:
- Schistosomiasis (Banti syndrome)
- TB
- Sarcoidosis

Cirrhosis or fatty infiltration (e.g. alcohol)
Acute liver failure
Hepatocellular carcinoma

Portal vein thrombosis due to:

P.I.N.C.H.E.S.

Pancreatic: Chronic pancreatitis, pseudocyst carcinoma
Inflammation: Diverticulitis, appendicitis, colitis, haemorrhoids
Neoplasia: GIT, pancreas, cholangiocarcinoma
Congenital: Atresia, AVM
Haematological: Prothrombotic state
Exogenous: Trauma, surgery
Splenomegaly, massive due to excess blood flow

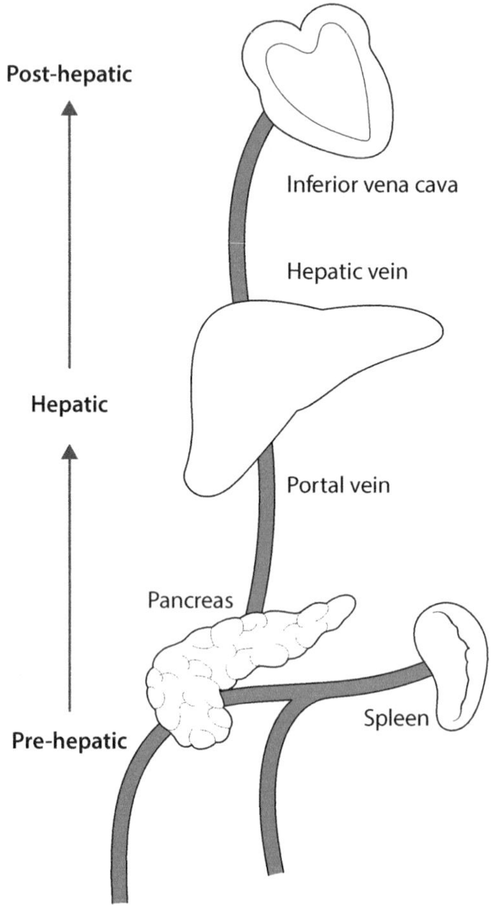

PC

Varices + other porto-systemic collaterals

Oesophageal varices
Occur in 2/3 of cirrhotics; 50% will die of them
Due to dilated venules between oesophageal (→ azygos vein) and left, and short gastric veins (→ portal vein)
Haemorrhoids
Worsens existing piles, but does not cause
Due to dilated venules between inferior, middle rectal (systemic) and superior rectal veins (portal)
Caput medusa
Dilated venules emerge radially from umbilicus, superficial abdominal veins enlarge, venous hum (Cruveilhier–Baumgarten syndrome)
Due to dilated venules between superficial epigastic, lateral thoracic (systemic) and umbilical (portal) veins
Surgical bleeding
Risk increased due to dilated venules between retroperitoneal, and diaphragmatic veins (systemic) and portal vein

Ascites + other oedema

Ascites, due to:
- Back-pressure → fluid exudation
- Hyperaldosteronism, due to hypoalbuminaemia and reduced aldosterone catabolism

Pleural effusion, esp. on R side
Ankle oedema

Splenomegaly

Due to back-pressure (congestive) or functional hypersplensim (i.e. cause of portal HT)

Hepatomegaly

If post-hepatic venous obstruction or hepatic inflammation or hepatic infiltration

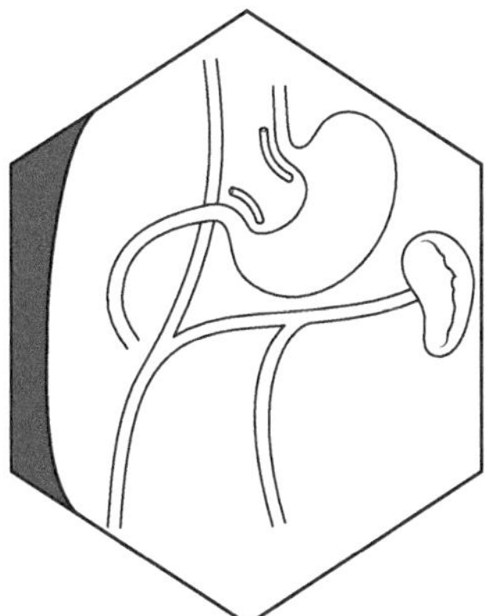

Cause

Encephalopathy

Diversion of GIT toxic metabolites, e.g. NH_4^+, cyclic amino acids, mercaptans, indoles away from liver into IVC directly

Precipitants:

H.E.I.G.h.T.e.N. *RISK*

Haemorrhage, e.g. varices
Electrolytes: Na^+↓, K^+↓
Infection: Spontaneous bacterial peritonitis, any other infection
Glucose↓, incl. low-calorie diet
Toxins: Diuretics, sedatives, anaesthetics, alcohol
Neoplasia: Hepatocellular carcinoma

PC

F.A.C².E².
Flap, dystonia
Ataxia, dysarthria, ophthalmoplegia
Confusion, **C**onstruction a praxia, inverted sleep pattern
Epilepsy; o**E**dema, cerebral

Ix

Bloods:	Elevated plasma ammonia Plasma bile acid ↑
EEG:	High-voltage, slow-wave form

Rx

- Remove cause, e.g. IV glucose if hypoglycaemic; IV colloid if hypovolaemic; IV antibiotics if sepsis
- Lactulose: Aim for bowel opening 2–3 times per day

OESOPHAGEAL VARICES

Def

Dilated venules between oesophageal (systemic) and gastic (portal) veins, due to portal hypertension (see p. 156 for causes)

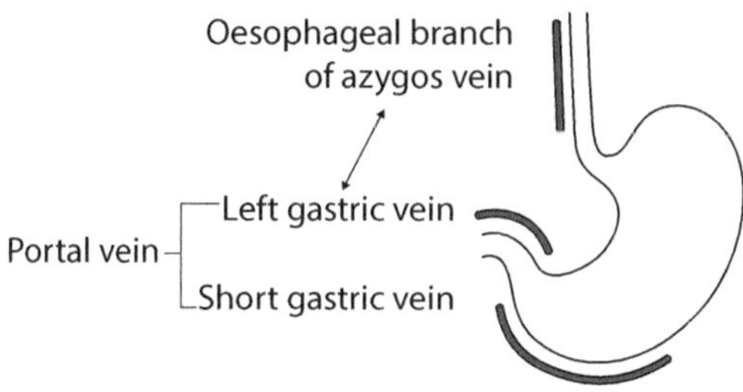

PC

Asymptomatic, e.g. identified on screening by endoscopy or barium meal
Massive haematemesis, hypovolaemic shock: Precipitated by erosion; food bolus; vomit; rise in portal venous pressure
Hepatic encephalopathy: Precipitated by GIT haemorrhage

Ix

Bloods: U&E: Urea↑ (blood digestion), creatinine↑ (AKI), Na↓ (RAAS activation)
LFT/clotting: Risk indicator (see below)
FBC: Hb↓ Plt↓
ABGs: Lactic acidosis
Glucose ↓

Urine: Na↓: Hepato-renal syndrome

Micro: Blood, urine and ascitic culture: Spontaneous bacterial peritonitis (Gram –ve)

ECG

Radiol: CXR: Aspiration pneumonitis
Abdominal USS: Ascites, hepatomegaly, hepatocellular carcinoma – hepatic or portal vein thrombosis (use duplex USS)
Tc-scintigram: In Budd–Chiari syndrome liver shows ↓ activity, except in the central caudate lobe due to different venous drainage

Special: OGD endoscopy

Severity markers (Child–Pugh Score)

I need **A.N. A.B.P.**:

Ascites
Neurological: Encephalopathy

Albumin ↓
Bilirubin ↑
Prothrombin time ↑

Used to assess operative risk

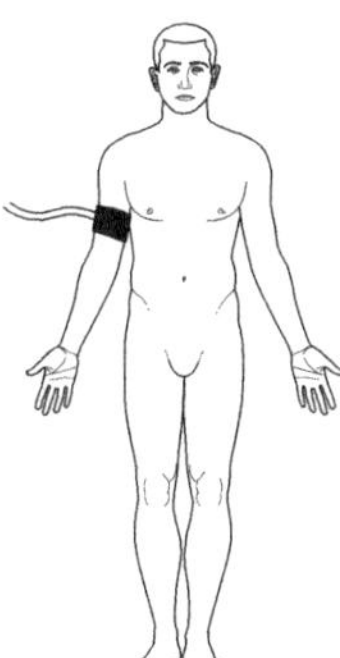

Rx

Airway – Breathing

Airway:
- Clean vomit, loose teeth
- Cuffed endotracheal tube,
- Nasogastric tube, if vomiting

Oxygen: 60%
Ventilation if comatose

1. Urgent endoscopy, if:
   - Varices suspected
2. ITU transfer, if:
   - Drowsy or comatose
   - Major haemorrhage
3. Liver transplant

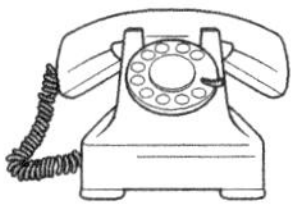

Hydration

- Dextrose 50%, 50 ml if 'hypo'
- Colloid, preferably salt-free
- Packed red cells:
  Initially: O Rhesus -ve or grouped blood
  Later: X-matched blood
  ☠: Ca ↓, K^+ ↑, pH ↑, temp. ↓
- Fresh frozen plasma (2 units), platelets (5 units), Vit K (10 mg IV)

Assessment

The three Gs
Glasgow coma scale
Glucose – BM stick
Group and save,
X-match 4 units

C.O.A.T.
Cardiac monitor
02 sats
ABP, CVP line
TPR

Investigations
Bloods: incl. FBC, clotting, urea ↑, K^+ ↓, ABGs
Urine: Na, osmolality
Micro: Cultures; serology
Monitor fluid balance:
CVP: Aim for 5-15 cm H_20
UO: Aim for >30 ml/h
ECG
Radiology: CXR, Abdominal USS
Special: OGO

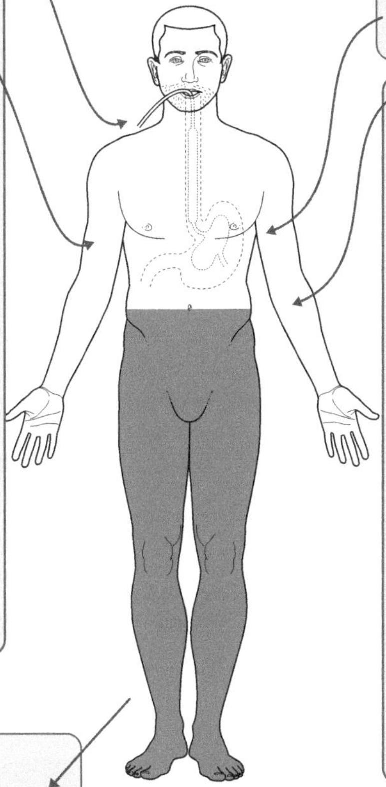

Drugs

Splanchnic vasoconstrictor
- Terlipressin (glypressin) IV or vasopressin IV: mortality rate ↓ by 1/3
  ☠: Coronary vasospasm, skin or gut necrosis, hypertension (for vasopressin: use GTN patch)
- Octreotide IV = (somatostatin analogue)

Laxatives
- Lactulose (laxative + probiotic) + $MgS0_4$ (oral + enemas) + neomycin (↓ NH_4^+ formation) ↓ 'blood meal' + encephalopathy

Metoclopramide 20 mg iv, ranitidine, PPI or sucralfate
Metoclopramide ↑ lower oesophageal pressure and ↓ azygos blood flow
Antibiotics: Ceftriaxone IV
Thiamine

Specific

Endoscopy: Injection sclerotherapy; ethanolamine or thrombin
Balloon tamponade: <12 h to avoid ischaemia
Radiological embolisation
T.I.P.S.S.:
Transjugular intrahepatic porto-systemic shunt
Surgical:
Transgastric oesophageal stapling; distal oesophagectomy

Prophylaxis

Propranolol or octreotide SC:
Reduce portal pressure by more than systemic
Endoscopy:
Rubber-band ligation
Surgery:
Gastric vein ligation; porto-caval shunt

ASCITES

Causes

P.A.T. P.I.N.T.S

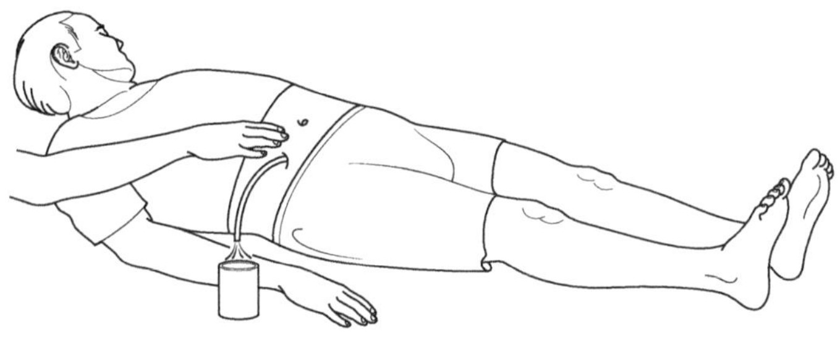

Transudate (protein <30 g/l):

Portal hypertension
- Pre-hepatic: Right-sided heart failure, schistosomiasis (NB: Budd–Chiari syndrome: exudate!)
- Hepatic: Cirrhosis, acute liver failure
- Pre-hepatic: Pancreatic disease, inflammation, neoplasia, congenital

Albumin ↓
- Malnutrition, malabsorption, protein-losing enteropathy
- Cirrhosis
- Nephrosis

Thyroxine ↓

Exudate (protein >40 g/l, plus WBCs, RBCs):

Pancreatitis
- Acute pancreatitis: Bloody and yellow-white flecks of fat necrosis
- Chronic pancreatitis: Purulent
- Ix: Amylase ↑

Infection
- TB (high protein content)
- Peritonitis (purulent)

Neoplasia
- 1° peritoneal: Mesothelioma, pseudomyxoma peritonei
- 1° visceral:
  - Colonic or ovarian cancer, ovarian fibroma (Meig syndrome)
  - Hepatoma
- 2°, e.g. breast. Ix: Cytology +ve

Thrombosis, hepatic vein: Budd–Chiari syndrome. Ix: Venography or Tc-scintigraphy showing caudate lobe sparing

Severe pain: Ectopic pregnancy, abdominal aortic aneurysm, trauma. Ix: Bloody tap on all of 3 attempts

PC

Weight + girth $\uparrow$
Peritonitis: Gram –ve, esp. if protein <10 g/l

O/E

Abdominal circumference
Shifting dullness
Fluid thrill

Bloods: Na, albumin $\downarrow$ (may precede oedema)
Urine: Na $\downarrow$
Monitor: Daily weights
Micro: Ascitic tap culture; also send for:
- Chemistry: Protein, glucose, lactate, amylase
- Cytology

Blood cultures
Radiol: USS – confirms diagnosis and allows drain site to be marked
CXR
MRI, MRV, hepatic and portal venography

Rx

General
Conservative:
- Salt (fluid) restrict
- Bed rest

Diuretic: Spironolactone ± loop
Drain (paracentesis) + IV albumin replacement

Specific
Portal hypertension: TIPSS
Malignant ascites:
- Intraperitoneal bleomycin
- Le-Veen shunt: Subcutaneous catheter connects to internal jugular vein, via 1-way valve

ACUTE LIVER FAILURE – CAUSES

T.A.B.O^2.O^2.S^2.!

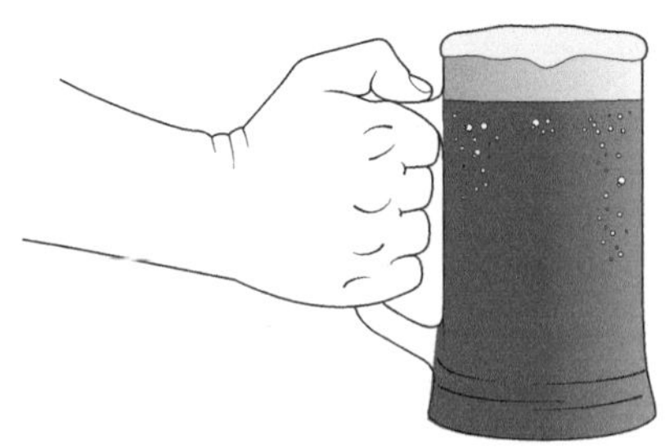

Toxins
- Alcohol, and other poisons
- Drug overdose
- Idiosyncratic

Autoimmune hepatitis
- Classical lupoid
- LKM +ve
- SLA +ve

B: hepatitis virus + other infections
- Viral: Hepatitis A–G, herpes group (esp. EBV, CMV), measles, yellow fever
- Bacterial: Leptospirosis
- Protozoal: Malaria, toxoplasmosis

Occlusion/**O**bstruction
- Hepatic vein thrombosis: Budd–Chiari syndrome
- Ischaemic hepatitis: Hepatic artery thromboembolism, or profound hypotension
- Obstructive jaundice

Obstetric
- Acute fatty liver of pregnancy
- Cholestasis of pregnancy
- HELLP syndrome (haemolytic anaemia + elevated liver enzymes + low platelets)

Oncology
- Massive malignant infiltration
- Lymphoma

Syndrome/**S**torage disease
- Reye syndrome
- Wilson disease

Toxins

Alcohol, and other poisons:

- Herbal tea
- CCl_4, trichloroethylene, yellow phosphorus (zone 1 necrosis)
- *Amanita phalloides* (Death cap mushrooms)

Drug overdose:

- Paracetamol: Saturation of conjugation reactions → P450 oxidation to NABQI → glutathione consumption
- Aspirin
- Iron sulphate (zone 1 necrosis)

Idiosyncratic – **M.A.I.N.**

Methotrexate + NSAIDs, esp. indomethacin, ibuprofen
Amiodarone + other cardiac: Methyl-dopa, Ca antagonists, enalapril
Isoniazid, esp. in fast acetylators, e.g. Inuits, other inducer, women >50 + other antibiotics, e.g. nitrofurantoin, flucloxacillin, AZT, fansidar, keto-/fluconazole
Neuro/psychiatric/anaesthetic:

- Anticonvulsants (phenytoin, CMZ, valproate)
- Antidepressants (TCA/MAOI/chlorpromazine – cholestasis)
- Psychostimulants: Ecstasy, cocaine, glue-sniffing (trichloroethylene, toluene)
- Halothane

Budd–Chiari syndrome

Causes

Thrombophilic state, esp. myeloproliferative disorders (60%), paroxysmal nocturnal haemoglobinuria, antiphospholipid syndrome, ulcerative colitis, oral contraceptive pill
Local tumour: Hepatocellular carcinoma, renal cell carcinoma, adrenal carcinoma
Congenital: Membranous obstruction of inferior vena cava (commonest cause in Japan)
Exogenous: Azathioprine, radiation, bone-marrow transplant, herbal bush teas (pyrrolidizine alkaloids = bush tea disease), trauma, hydatid cyst

PC

Abdominal pain – right upper quadrant (stretching of Glisson capsule)
Jaundice, liver failure
Ascites (exudate!)

Ix

Duplex scan: Cavernous transformation
Colloid scan: ↑ uptake caudate lobe
Venography with retrograde CO_2 portography
Liver Bx: Centrilobular congestion/sinusoidal dilatation/haemorrhagic necrosis/fibrosis

Rx

Medical: Anticoagulation, providing clotting initially normal

CHRONIC LIVER DISEASE – CAUSES

E.M.O².T.I.O.N².

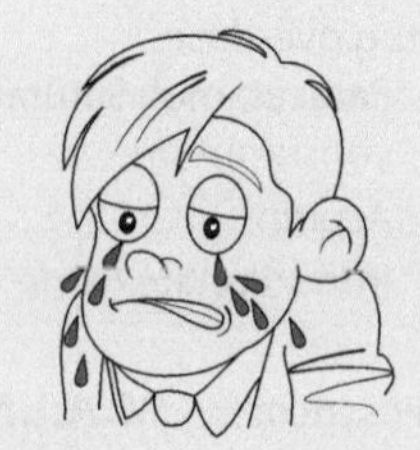

Errors of immunity
- Autoimmune hepatitis
- Primary biliary cholangitis
- Primary sclerosing cholangitis
- Lupus

Metabolic/inherited disorders: **W.A.T.C.H.**
- **W**ilson disease
- α_1-**A**ntitrypsin deficiency
- **T**yrosinaemia, galactosaemia, glycogen storage disease, fructose intolerance
- **C**ystic fibrosis
- **H**aemochromatosis

Occlusion/**O**bstruction
- Hepatic vein disease:
  - Hepatic vein thrombosis: Budd–Chiari syndrome or IVC web
  - Hepatic vein congestion: Right-sided heart failure, constrictive pericarditis
- Hepatic ischaemia: Sickle cell anaemia
- Obstructive jaundice: primary biliary cirrhosis, sclerosing cholangitis, biliary atresia

Toxins
- Alcohol, and other poisons
- Idiosyncratic

Infection: Hepatitis B and C
- Viral: Hepatitis B, C, D, G, herpes group (esp. EBV, CMV), measles, yellow fever
- Bacterial: Brucella, syphilis
- Nematode: Hydatid disease, schistosomiasis (pipe-stem fibrosis, pre-sinusoid portal hypertension)

Oncology
- Hepatocellular carcinoma
- Graft-versus-host-disease (GVHD)

NASH and **N**AFLD: Usually with concomitant diabetes and/or dyslipidaemia

Histology

Chronic persistent hepatitis (CPH): Lymphocytic infiltrate + fibrosis of portal tracts >6 months
Chronic active hepatitis (CAH): Piecemeal, bridging necrosis centred on portal tracts
Cirrhosis: Fibrosis + nodular regeneration + distorted lobular architecture

Toxins

Drugs may induce a wide range of liver diseases:

Hepatitis – cirrhosis
Alcohol, and other poisons:

- Alcohol: fatty change → hepatitis → cirrhosis
- Vinyl chloride

Idiosyncratic: **M.A.I.N.**

Methotrexate + other NSAIDs, e.g. diclofenac
Amiodarone + other cardiac: Methyl-dopa
Isoniazid (esp. fast acetylators) + nitrofurantoin, minocycline (+ isotretinoin)
Neuro/psychiatric/anaesthetic:

- Anticonvulsants: Valproate, phenytoin, carbamazepine
- Dantrolene

Fatty change
Valproate
Amiodarone
Asparaginase
Tetracycline

Hypersensitivity and granulomas
Carbamazepine
Allopurinol
Phenylbutazone
Sulphonamide

Veno-occlusion: Azathioprine, radiation

Tumour : Androgens, oral contraceptive pill

Biliary cholestasis: Androgens, oral contraceptive pill, rifampicin, gold
Calculi: Ceftriaxone
Sclerosing cholangitis: Fluorodeoxyuridine

INFECTIVE HEPATITIS

Types

	Spread	Virus type	Associated cause	Incubation (months)
A	FO	RNA ss+ve	**A**broad (esp. seafood); **A**utumnal peaks	1 (<2)
B	IV	DNA ds	**B**lood; **B**ody fluids; **B**abies (vertical transmission)	3 (<6)
C	IV	RNA ss+ve	As for Hep B, but ↑ blood and ↓ vertical risk	2 (<6)
D	IV	RNA ss+ve	**D**ependent on prior Hep B as envelope-**D**eficient	3 (<6)
E	FO	RNA ss+ve	**E**conomically-poor countries, e.g. post-flood	1 (<2)

FO: faeco-oral; IV: parenteral

Epi

Hep B Mediterranean, Far East – 30% carriers; Hep C: Middle East – 15% carriers

PC

Prodrome

Hep **A** associated with small-joint **A**rthritis
Hep **B** has a particularly **B**ad prodrome – high fever, flu-like, angioedema, arthritis

General PC
Fever, flu-like symptoms, headache, arthralgia
Lymphadenopathy, hepatosplenomegaly

Acute hepatitis

Hep A > B > C; in order of frequency of jaundice: 99%, 75%, 25%

PC

Hepatitis

Cholestasis (dark urine, pale stool) may precede jaundice by 5 days
Fulminant hepatic failure occurs in <1%; more in Hep D and E

Immune-complex reactions S.N.A.G.S.

Skin: Hep A = pruritus, urticaria, papular rash
Hep B, C = vasculitis (PAN, cryoglobulinaemia), lichen planus, porphyria cutanea tarda
Neurological: Peripheral neuropathy, transverse myelitis
Aplastic anaemia
Glomerulonephritis, membranous or membranoproliferative
Systemic: Pancreatitis, myocarditis, pneumonitis, thyroiditis

NB: Infectivity begins from 3 days pre-jaundice and lasts until 2 weeks post-jaundice

Chronic hepatitis

*Hep **C** and **C**hildhood Hep B are most **C**hronic, but Hep A may cause symptoms for <1 year*
Carrier is defined for Hep B as sAg +ve >6 months, or eAg +ve >2 months
Hep C as HCV RNA or ALT↑ >6 months

Risks

Carrier	Hep B: 10% (↑ if eAg +ve)	Hep C: 80%
Chronic active hepatitis:	Hep B: 10%	Hep C: 60%
Cirrhosis	Hep B: 5% (↑ by Hep D)	Hep C: 20%

Serology

Hep A

Anti-HAV: IgM occurs from 1–3 months post-infection; IgG predominates >3 months

Hep B

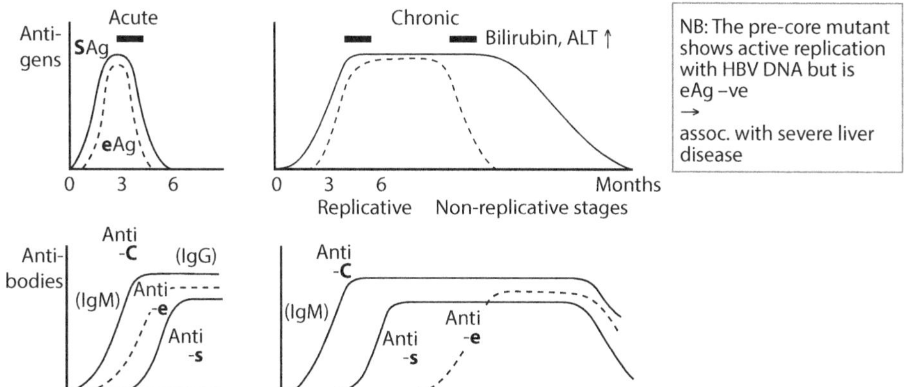

NB: In acute infection, order of antibody appearance is alphabetic; in chronic infection, anti-e appears late.

s**A**g = acute infection; reactivation; chronic carrier
Anti-c: **IgM** acute infection
IgG reactivation or past infection

NB: May be +ve even when HBsAg –ve and so more sensitive!

e**A**g = high level of virus replication (also indicated by HBV DNA and pre-S1, S2 proteins)
Anti-e –ve = high infectivity; **+ve** = low infectivity
Anti-s = past infection or immunized

Hep C

Anti-HCV: Pre-clinical (anti-C22 or C33); clinical (anti-C100-3)
HCV RNA PCR: Infectivity index

L.A.S.T.

Liver support: No aspirin or alcohol; manage liver failure (lactulose, low-protein diet)
Anti-viral

- PEGylated IFN. Indications: Recently acquired chronic infection (6 months–2 years); low HBV DNA or HCV RNA, mild hepatitis on biopsy.
  Response: Hep B = 40% seroconvert; Hep C =10% seroconvert
- Nucleotide analogues: Hep B, lamivudine; Hep C, ribavirin

Steroids. Indications: Prolonged cholestasis (esp. Hep A); prior to anti-viral (Hep B, C)
Transplant liver

Prophylaxis

Safe sex, needle exchange (Hep B, C); hygiene precautions (Hep A, E)
Vaccine: HAV; HBV sAg; human immunoglobulin

PRIMARY BILIARY CHOLANGITIS

Epi

Middle-aged Caucasian women
Predisposing:

- HLA-B8, -DR8
- Autoimmunity
  - Scleroderma, dermatomyositis, rheumatoid arthritis, Sjögren (in 80%)
  - Addison, coeliac, vitiligo, Hashimoto, pulmonary fibrosis

PATH

Non-suppurative destructive cholangitis

G*ot* P.B.C.?

Stages 1 **G**ranulomas (may also occur in other tissues)
2 **P**roliferation or disappearing bile ducts
3 **B**ridging septa + fibrosis
4 **C**irrhosis

$P^2.B^2.C^2.$

Pruritus: Excoriations, due to cholestasis. Also pale stool, dark urine, steatorrhoea, but jaundice occurs late. Can become unbearable
Pigmentation: Melanosis of face; Kayser–Fleischer rings may also occur in cornea
Bones: Osteomalacia, osteoporosis – due to poor vitamin D absorption; also arthralgia
Big organs: Hepatosplenomegaly; lymphadenopathy, incl. at porta hepatis
Cirrhosis: Clubbing ,varices, ascites
Cholesterol↑: Xanthomata

50% are asymptomatic at presentation (abnomal LFTs); but 50% of these have cirrhosis!

Ix

Anti-mitochondrial Abs, esp. PDH, E2 and E3 binding protein on inner mitochondrial membrane (95%)
Other autoantibodies: Anti-smooth muscle, ANA, ANCA; IgM ↑↑
Liver biopsy

Supportive
Pruritus: Cholestyramine, naltrexone, rifampicin
Nutritional: Vitamin A, D, E, K, Ca, medium-chain triglycerides
Disease-modifiying: Ursodeoxycholic acid slows disease progression, reduces cholestasis but has no effect on symptoms
Liver transplant: Disease may recur

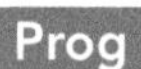

Normal LFTs 12 y   Abnormal LFTs 10 y   Symptomatic 8 y   Cirrhosis 4 y

Bilirubin >150 μmol/l predicts 18 months median survival

AUTOIMMUNE HEPATITIS

Epi

Middle-aged Caucasian women (ANA +ve)
Equal sex ratio and occurs more commonly in children (LKM +ve)
Predisposing:

- HLA-A1, B8, DR3 occurs in 40%, and is associated with more severe disease (ANA +ve)
- Autoimmunity common in patient and family (any form)
- Hepatitis C (LKM +ve)

PATH

Piecemeal bridging necrosis, and lymphocytic infiltrate, centred on portal tracts
Present for >6 months
LE cells in 10%

PC

Chronic **A**utoimmune **H**epatitis

Early:
- **C**onstitutional: Fatigue, nausea, pruritus
- **C**ushingoid: Striae, hirsute, acne
- **A**menorrhoea
- **A**rthralgia: May also develop rheumatoid or migratory arthritis
- **H**epatitis: Recurrent jaundice
- **H**epatosplenomegaly: Tender, lymphadenopathy

Complications:
- **C**irrhosis
  - Present in 70% at presentation; esp. LKM +ve
  - Spider naevi, palmar erythema, purpura (PT↑)
- **A**utoimmune
  - **C**olitis, ulcerative; **C**holangitis, sclerosing; **C**onjunctivitis or uveitis
  - **A**cidosis, renal tubular
  - **H**yperthyroidism (thyroiditis); **H**yperglycaemia – type 1 DM (LKM +ve)
- **H**aematological
  - Normocytic anaemia, Coomb +ve haemolysis
  - Pancytopenia due to hypersplenism

Ix

Auto-antibody patterns

ANA +ve (homogeneous immunofluorescent staining pattern): May occur with anti-dsDNA, anti-mitochondrial, anti-smooth muscle, p-ANCA
LKM Ab +ve (liver and kidney microsomal antigen = cytochrome P450)
SLA Ab +ve (soluble liver antigen = glutathione-S-transferase)

Rx

Immunosuppression: Prednisolone 60 mg od titrated according to ALT; can also use azathioprine. Response better for no autoAbs > ANA +ve >L KM +ve
Liver transplant: Disease does not recur in graft

HAEMOCHROMATOSIS

Epi

Inc: Prevalence: 1/3000, although 10% of population are gene-carriers
Age: Onset 40–60 years
Sex: Women present 10 years later due to menses
Geo: Celtic origin
Aet: 1°: ***HFE*** gene (esp. C282Y mutation), results in:

- Increased divalent-metal transporter (DMT-1) expression on brush border of enterocytes
- Reduced hepcidin expression in liver (hepcidin inhibits iron absorption from gut)

2°: Haemolytic anaemia, aplastic anaemia, sideroblastic anaemia, due to ineffective erythropoiesis and iron release, increased iron absorption, repeated blood transfusions

PC

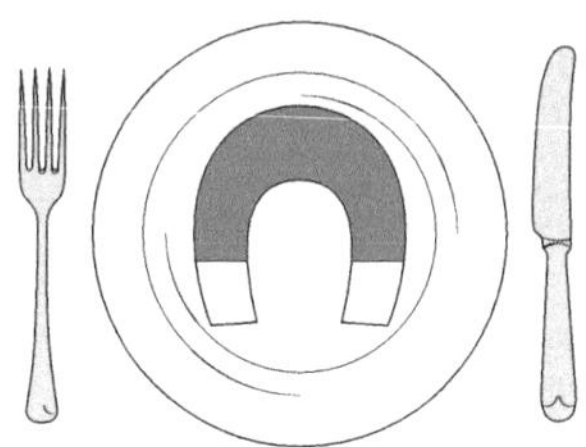

Iron **M.E.A.L.S^2.**

Myocardial: Arrhythmias, heart block, dilated or restrictive cardiomyopathy
Endocrine: **P**ancreas – diabetes (in 2/3)
Pituitary – amenorrhoea, infertility (hypogonadotrophic hypogonadism)
Parathyroid – hypocalcaemia; hypothyroidism
Arthritis: Calcium pyrophosphate deposition in joints
Liver: Chronic active hepatitis, cirrhosis, hepatocellular carcinoma (in 1/3 if untreated), abdominal pain, hepatomegaly
Skin: Bronzed appearance (due to melanosis and iron), porpyria cutanea tarda
Systemic: Fatigue

Ix

Bloods: Transferrin sat. ↑ (>60%); TIBC ↓; plasma Fe ↑; ferritin ↑
HFE genotype
Urine: 24-h urinary Fe ↑ (post-desferrioxamine injection)
ECG, **E**CHO
Radiol: Liver CT or MRI – detects increased Fe stores
Special: Liver biopsy; dry weight >2%: iron in hepatocytes

Rx

Iron removal
Venesection: initially, 1–2× per week for 1–2 years; then once every 3 months
Desferrioxamine
Liver transplant
Family screening and treatment

WILSON DISEASE

Epi

Inc: Prevalence: 1/50,000
Age: Presents between childhood and 30; never after mid-50s
Aet: Reduced copper excretion from hepatic lysosome into bile, due to mutant copper transporter ATPase 7B (chromosome 13; autosomal recessive)

PC

C^2.L.A.N.K.i.N.G^2.

Corneal/**C**ataracts
- Kayser–Fleischer rings: Grey-green copper deposits around rim of cornea
- Sunflower cataracts

Liver
- Acute: Hepatitis, fulminant hepatic necrosis
- Chronic: Fatty liver, chronic active hepatitis, cirrhosis

Arthritis
- Chondrocalcinosis
- Osteoporosis

Neurology
- Parkinsonism; tremor (intention, postural)/chorea/tics
- Spasticity, pseudobulbar dysarthria and dysphagia
- Dementia, psychosis – mania, headache

Kidney: Renal tubular acidosis/Fanconi syndrome, resulting in osteomalacia
Negative, Coombs' – haemolytic anaemia
Growth failure (puberty)
Gynaecological – amenorrhoea

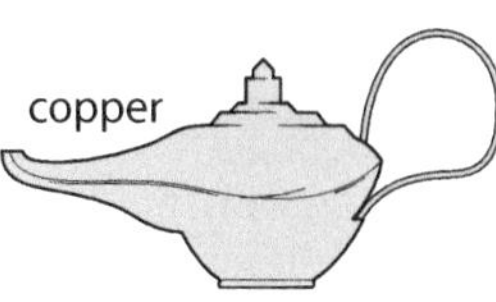

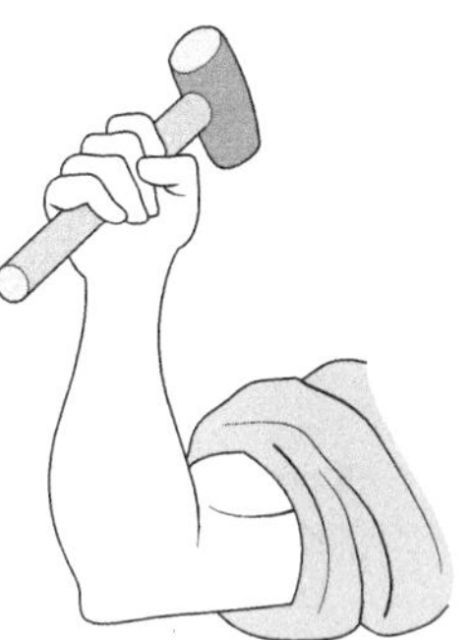

Ix

Bloods: Serum caeruloplasmin↓ (<20 mg/dl); serum Cu-free↑ (but total↓)
Urine: 24-h urinary Cu ↑ (esp. post-penicillamine)
Special: Slit-lamp exam for Kayser–Fleischer rings; sensitivity = 70%; false +ve in primary biliary cholangitis
Liver biopsy: Dry Cu weight increased; false +ve in primary biliary cholangitis

Rx

Copper-chelators
Penicillamine:
- Take for 2 years
- Adjuvant vitamin B6 and zinc ± steroids, e.g. for ITP, arthralgia

Trientine: If penicillamine worsens neuro Sx or intolerance
Dimercaprol
Plasmapharesis
Liver transplant: Curative

LIVER TUMOURS

Primary hepatocellular carcinoma

Causes

Cirrhosis, therefore **E.M.O^2.T.I.O.N^2.S.**

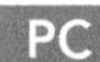

PC

Abdominal pain; **A**scites, blood-tinged; **A**cute decompensated liver failure (encephalopathy)

O/E

Abdominal mass
Liver bruit, friction rub

Complications

Paraneoplastic: Glucose ↓, cholesterol ↑, PTH-rp: Calcium ↑, polycythaemia, DIC
Metastases: Bone, lung

Ix

AFP ↑↑ (>500 μg/l); ALP ↑↑
USS or CT: Satellite lesions may be present
Angiogram + ^{131}I-lipiodol pre-injection – selectively retained within tumour (avoid biopsy due to vascularity, coagulopathy + risk of spread along needle tract!)

Rx

<5 cm
- Hepatic artery embolisation: Gel foam; alcohol; doxorubicin
- Liver transplant: Risk of recurrence if metastasized

>5 cm: Resection

Prog

Median survival: 4 months; prognosis better in fibrolamellar variant (no underlying cirrhosis)

Secondary – metastases

Breast; Bronchus
Intestinal: Colorectal, carcinoid, pancreas
Gastro-oesophageal

Melanoma
Endometrial
Testis
Special: Lymphoma

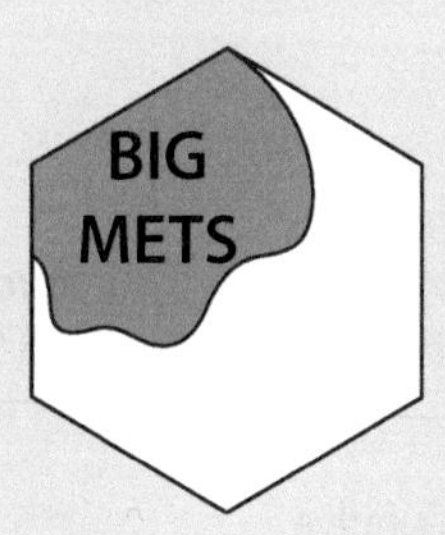

PANCREATIC TUMOURS

Exocrine – Ductal Adenocarcinoma (90%)

Causes

S.I.N.S.

Smoking: Risk increases three-fold
Inflammation: Chronic pancreatitis, esp. hereditary pancreatitis
Nutrition: High calorie intake, obesity, diabetes mellitus
Surgery: Partial gastrectomy leads to biliary reflux into stomach, and secondary cholecystokinin release

Abdominal – back pain
Anorexia – weight loss
Altered stool colour – pale (obstructive jaundice); silver (ampullary carcinoma)

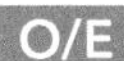

Abdominal mass
- Umbilical mass due to tumour
- Gallbladder due to bile duct compression (also causes jaundice)
- Splenomegaly, and umbilical mass due to portal vein compression

Lymphadenopathy: Troisier's sign (supraclavicular)

Complications

Local compression: Obstructive jaundice, portal hypertension, IVC obstruction
Pancreas failure: Diabetes mellitus
Paraneoplastic:
- Thrombophilia causes migratory thrombophlebitis (Trousseau's sign)
- Panniculitis: Fat necrosis

Metastases: Liver

Ix

Bloods: Amylase ↑
CEA, CA 19-9
FBC (anaemia), ESR↑, LFT changes
Radiol: CT
Angiography
Special: ERCP or endoscopic USS
Biopsy, via USS or CT guidance

Rx

Surgery (in only 10%): Whipple procedure – pancreatico-duodenectomy
Radiotherapy + 5-fluorouracil 'sensitizer': ↑ survival pre-operatively
Chemotherapy: Gemcitabine – for palliative use only

Prog

Median survival = 6 months if inoperable

Endocrine – Islet cell APUDomas (10%)

α: Glucagonoma; *β:* Insulinoma; δ: Somatostatinoma, **G**astrinoma, VIPoma; PPoma

GALLSTONES

Physiology

Normal bile content =

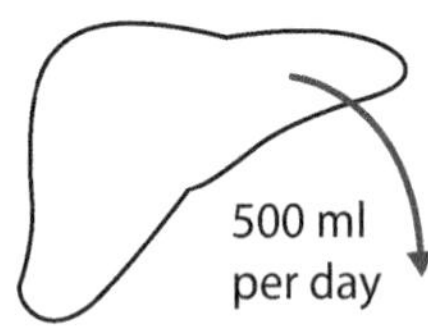

10%: Bile salts (cholic and chenodeoxycholic acid) = *stone-preventing*
conjugate with glycine or taurine
5%: Phospholipid
1%: **Cholesterol**
1%: **Conjugated bilirubin**
also protein, drugs

(Cholesterol and conjugated bilirubin: **Stone-forming**)

Types

Mixed cholesterol (75%)

Composition: Monohydrate cholesterol (70%) + variable calcium salts (only 10% show on X-ray) + bile acids

Cause: Bile becomes supersaturated with cholesterol, relative to bile salt, due to:

- Excess hepatic secretion, e.g. HMG CoA reductase activity ↑
- Gallbladder concentration

Predisposing:

A².F³.F².L.I.C.T.S².

Age (20% of females over 40) + **A**mericans (native USA, Chile)
Females (3:1 ratio), **F**ertile (multiparous), **F**emodene (i.e. oral contraceptive pill), HRT
Fatty foods
Family history
Liver disease, chronic**:** Bile salt production ↓
Ileum, terminal disease: Crohn, lymphoma – bile salt recycling ↓
Congenital: Choledochal cyst, cystic fibrosis
Toxins: Clofibrate, ceftriaxone, cholestyramine + octreotide
Surgery: Vagotomy – gallbladder contraction ↓
Somatostatinoma: Gallbladder contraction ↓

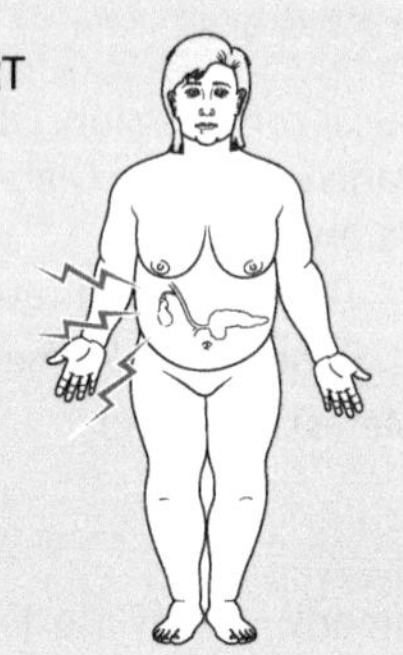

Pigment (25%)

Composition: Calcium bilirubinate + PO_4, CO_3 salts

Cause:

- Haemolytic anaemia: Sickle cell, hereditary spherocytosis, malaria. Path: Excess RBC turnover → black stones
- Helminths:
  - Nematodes – *Ascaris lumbricoides* (human roundworm)
  - Trematodes – *Cionorchis sinensis* (liver fluke; esp. Japan)

  Path: Supervening *E. coli* infection produces β-glucuronidase, which deconjugates bilirubin diglucuronide (soluble) to bilirubin (insoluble) → brown stones

PC

Gallstones solely within the gallbladder fundus are asymptomatic – problems arise when they move out! Presentation subsequently depends on site of gallstone occurrence:

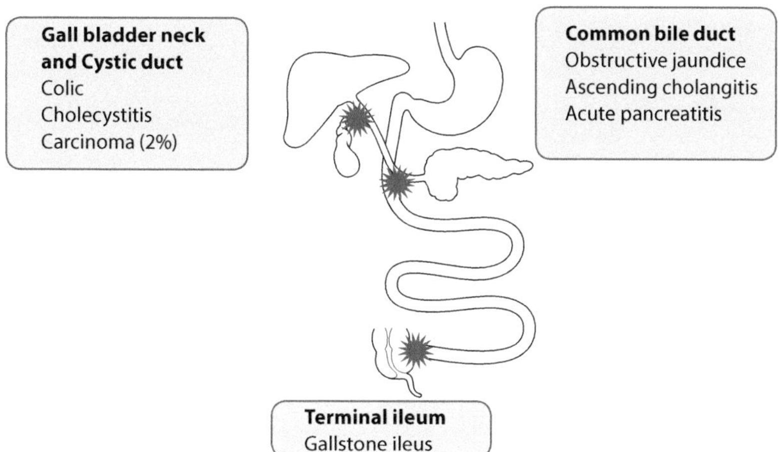

Cholecystitis

Acute

Path: Sustained blockage of gall-bladder neck or cystic duct + secondary bacterial infection of stagnant gallbladder fluid (enterococci, coliforms)

PC: Acute abdomen or chest pain, N+V, septic shock

O/E: Right-upper quadrant tenderness + guarding, mass; Murphy Sx (tender on inspiration); Boas Sx (R loin hyperaesthesia)

Ix: USS, ERCP – cholangiography

Rx: NBM + IV hydration; IV cefuroxime + metronidazole; early or late cholecystectomy

Chronic

Path: Fibrous contraction of gallbladder following repeated bouts of gallbladder neck blockage and failure of gallbladder to concentrate fluid and contract

PC: Episodic biliary colic; flatulent dyspepsia; fat intolerance

Rx: High-dose bile salts; cholecystectomy

Complications:

- Empyema (pus collection)
- Mucocoele (mucus collection)
- Gangrene → perforation

Obstructive jaundice

Usually painless, unless stone is at sphincter of Oddi

Ascending cholangitis

PC: Charcot triad = fever + colic + jaundice

Complications: Liver abscesses, septicaemia, ARF

Gallstone ileus

Stone erodes through gallbladder wall → penetrates duodenum → travels via small bowel to terminal ileum, i.e. narrowest point

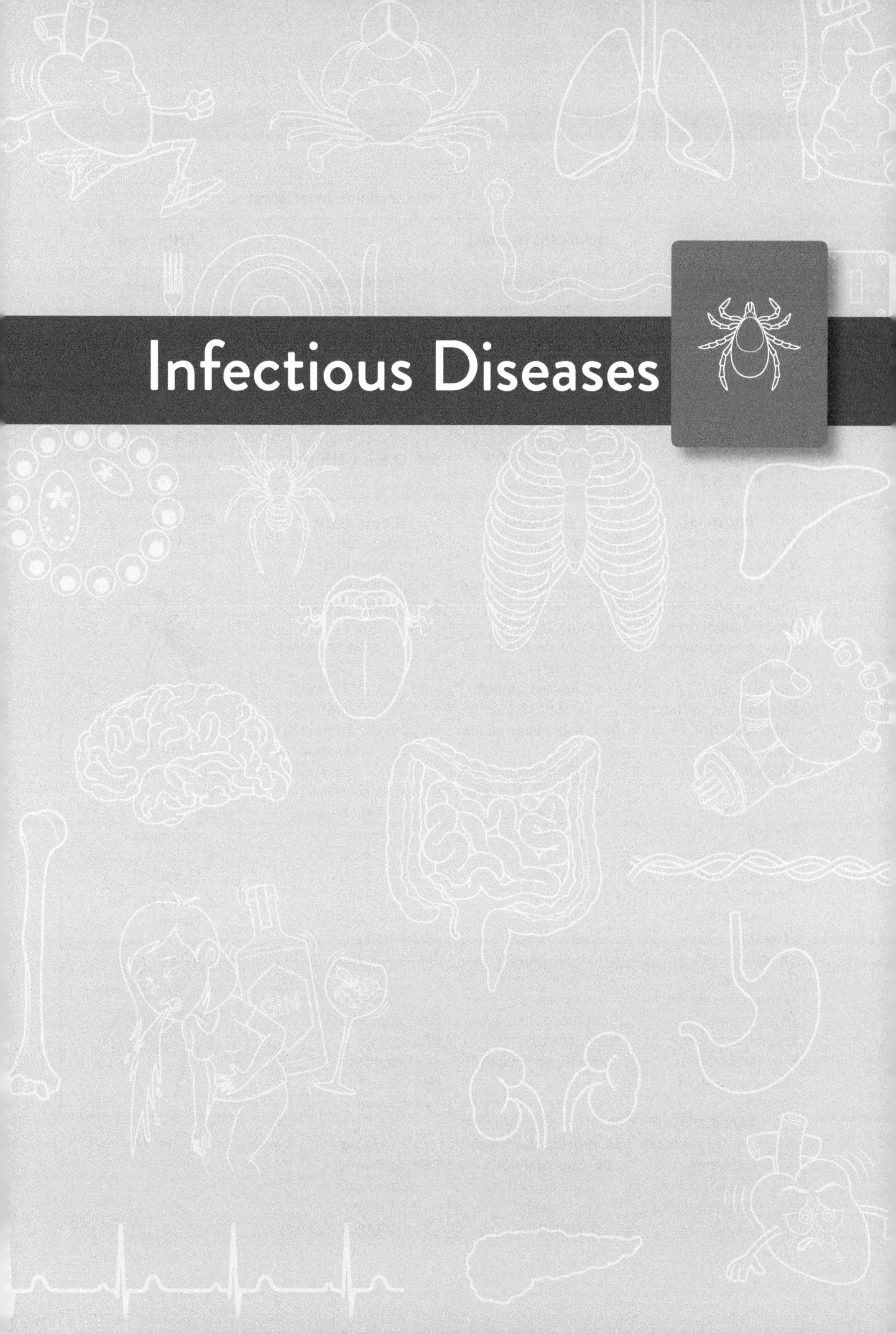

Infectious Diseases

INFECTIOUS ORGANISMS – 1

Multicellular: Invertebrates

Helminths (worms)

Nematodes

= roundworms

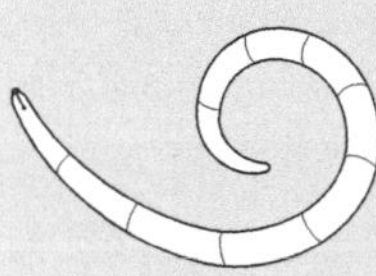

S.N.A^2.K.E^2. FI.G.h.T^2.S

Intestinal

***S**trongyloides stercoralis*
***N**ecator americanus/ **A**ncylostoma duodenale* (human hookworm)
***A**scaris lumbricoides* (human roundworm)
K: Anisa**K**iasis, capillarious
***E**nterobius vermicularis* (threadworm)
Extra: Whipworm – *Trichuris trichuria*

Tissue

FIlariasis
- *Onchocerca volvulus:* River blindness
- *Wuchereria bancrofti:* Elephantiasis
- *Loa loa*
- *Brugia malayi*

Guinea worm: *Dracunculus medinensis*
***T**oxocara canis*
***T**richinella spiralis*
Skin: Hookworm: Cutaneous larva migrans:
- Animal hookworm, e.g. *Ancylostoma brasiliense*
- Human hookworm

PC: Serpiginous rash

Cestodes

= tapeworms

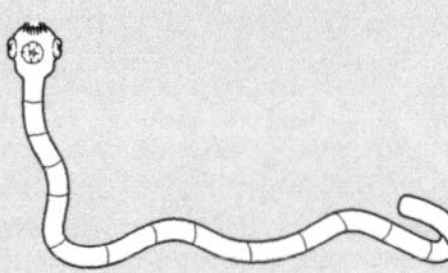

P.H.D. P.E.T.S.

Intestinal

Pork and beef tapeworms = *Taenia solium* and *T. saginata*
***H**ymenolepis:*
- *H. nana* (dwarf): Human-limited
- *H. diminuata:*
  - *Rodent-spread*
  - *Young children*

***D**iphyllobothrium latum:*
PC:
- Diarrhoea, wt. loss
- Vit B12 deficiency
- Cholangitis/cholecystitis

Tissue

Pork tapeworm:
T. solium = 'cysticercosis'
PC: Brain and cord inflammation → epilepsy, hydrocephalus
***E**chinococcus granulosus:* 'Hydatid disease'
PC: Lung + liver cysts
***T**. solium* (cysticercosis)
***S**pirometra:* 'Sparganosis'
PC: Subcutaneous tissue and orbital swelling and destruction

Trematodes

= flatworms

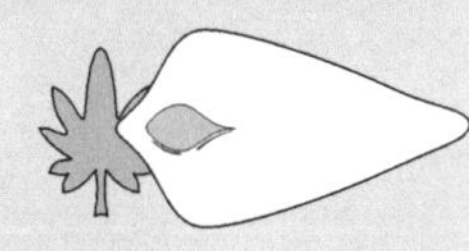

S.C.O.F.F.s HE.M.P.

Blood, veins

Schistosomiasis: Ova have characteristic shapes and organ sites
***S**chistosoma mansoni*: Colon, brain

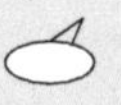

Dorsal spine: Charles Manson's knife

***S**. japonicum*: Ileum, cord
Japanese small willy!
***S**. haematobium*: Bladder

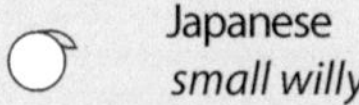

Terminal spine – terminal like the bladder

Liver

***C**lonorchis sinensis*
***O**pisthorchis*
***F**asciola hepatica*

Intestine

***F**asciolopsis buski*
***HE**terophyes heterophyes*
***M**etagoniums yokogawai*

Lung

***P**aragonimus westermani*
PC: Cutaneous nodules, epilepsy

Arthropods

Insect

Fleas
- Siphonaptera

Flies (Diptera):
- Anopheles
- Tsetse
- Midges
- Gnats

Lice, bugs
- *Pediculus* (hair + body)
- *Phthirus pubis* (pubic: 'crabs)

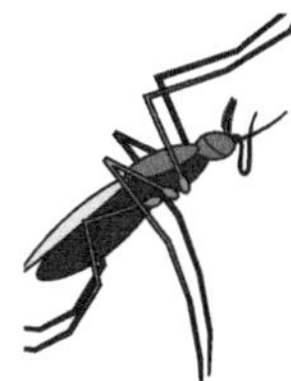

Arachnida

Spiders, scorpions
Ticks
Mites = microscopic:
- *Sarcoptes scabiei* (scabies)
- Chigger: red larvae

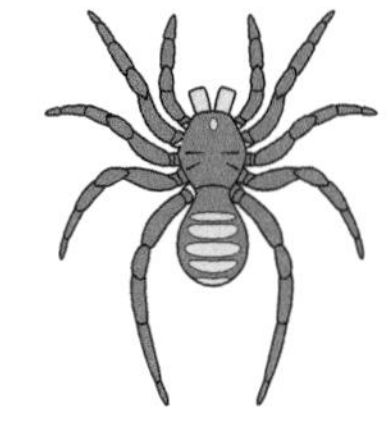

Unicellular: Eukaryotes (organelles, nucleus)

Fungi/yeasts (rigid cell wall)

Superficial

Dermatophytes:
Ringworm = tinea:
Trichophyton, Microsporum
PC:
- Tinea capitis, corporis, cruris or pedis – athlete's foot
- Onychomycosis

Malassezia furfur
= *Pityrosporum orbiculare*
PC: 'Pityriasis versicolor'; seborrhoeic dermatitis; dandruff

Subcutaneous:
Madura foot (mycetoma), sporotrichosis, chromoblastomycosis

Superficial + Deep

***Candida albicans*:**
Thrush: Oral, genital
Systemic (in immunocompromised)
PC:
- Meningitis
- Endophthalmitis
- Osteomyelitis
- Liver, spleen, kidney
- Endocarditis

Deep

Pneumonia:
Pneumocystis jirovecii
Aspergillus (neutropenics)
Pneumonia and/or meningitis:
Cryptococcus (AIDS)
Histoplasma capsulatum (endemic S. USA)
Coccidioides immitis
Blastomyces
Retro-orbital:
Mucormycosis (DM)

Protozoa

Sporozoa

= intracellular

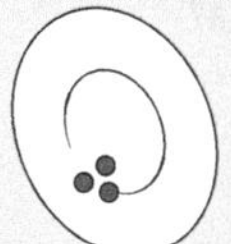

Prisoners of **T**he **B**lood **C**ell

Plasmodium – malaria:
Spread by Anopheles mosquito
Types:
- *P. falciparum*: Severe
- *P. vivax/ovale*: Benign, tertian
- *P. malariae*: Benign, quartan

Toxoplasma gondii:
Spread from cat and animal faeces
PC:
- Acute: lymphadenopathy
- Chorioretinitis
- Cerebral mass lesion
- Fetal malformation

Babesia – babesiosis:
Spread by ixodid tick similar to malaria
Types:
- *B. divergens*: cattle
- *B. microti:* rodents

Cryptosporidium + Microsporum
Isospora belli
PC: Chronic gastroenteritis in AIDS

Amoeboid

= simple

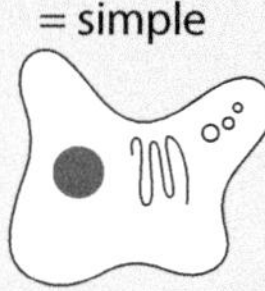

Entamoeba histolytica
PC:
- 'Amoebic dysentry', i.e. colitis
- Amoebic cyst

Acanthamoeba
PC:
- Contact-lens keratitis
- Cerebral abscess

Naegleria fowleri:
Found in swimming pools contaminated with soil, e.g. Roman baths
PC: Meningoencephalitis

Flagellate

= has flagellum

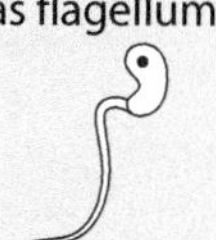

Looks like **T.**a.**G.L.**ia.**T.**elle

***T**rypanosoma brucei*
gambiense (W. Africa)
rhodesiense (E. Africa)
spread by *Glossina*, the 'tsetse fly'
PC: 'Sleeping sickness':
- Fever+ lymphadenopathy
- Encephalopathy

E**AS**t form: **A**cute, **S**evere
West form: Chronic, mild

***T**rypanosoma cruzi* – autonomic neuropathy:
Spread by reduviid bug in South America
PC: 'Chagas' disease':
- Myocarditis
- Achalasia
- Megacolon, constipation

***G**iardia lamblia*
PC: Duodena-jejunitis

***L**eishmania*: Spread by sandfly
Types:
- Cutaneous – oriental sore: *L. mexicania or L. tropica*
- Nasal mucosa – 'espundia': *L. brasiliensis*
- Visceral – 'kala-azar': L. donovani

***T**richomonas vaginalis*
PC: Vulvo-vaginitis

Ciliate

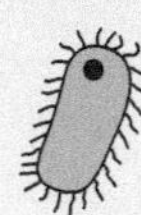

The only pathogenic ciliate is *Balantidium coli*, which causes an amoebic dysentry-like picture

INFECTIOUS ORGANISMS – 2

Unicellular: Prokaryotes (1 circular chromosome; no organelles)

Bacteria
(cell wall)

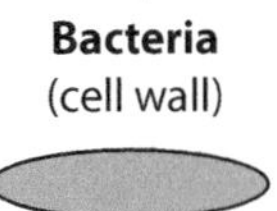

Mycoplasma/
Unreaplasma
(no cell wall)

Obligate intracellular parasites

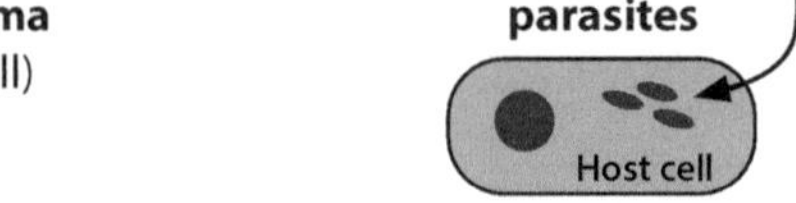

Typical bacteria (p. 172)

	Gram +ve	Gram –ve
Cocci	●	○
Rods (bacilli)	▬	▭
	Anaerobes	

Mycobacteria (pp. 202–4)

Weakly-staining Gram +ve rods
Facultative intracellular parasites

T.A.X. S.L.U.M

***T**uberculosis*
***A**vium intracellulare* (MAI); *cheloni*
***X**enopi; kansasii*
***S**crofulaceum*
***L**eprae:* Leprosy
***U**lcerans*: Buruli ulcer
***M**arinum*: Fish-tank granuloma

Spirochaetes (pp. 206–8)

Helical-shaped

BO.L.T.

***BO**rrelia:*
Lyme disease: *B. burgdorferi*
Relapsing fever:
- *B. recurrentis:* louse-borne (epidemic)
- *B. du**TT**oni:* **T**ick-borne (endemic)

Vincent's angina: *B. vincentii* – necrotising gingivitis

***L**eptospira interrogans:* Weil disease

***T**reponema:*
Syphilis: *T. pallidum*
Yaws: *T. pertenue*

Mycoplasma

M. pneumoniae:
Atypical pneumonia
M. hominis: UTI

Ureaplasma

U. urealyticum: UTI

NB:
Smallest free-living organism

Small genome – limits biosynthesis and *in vitro* culture

No cell wall – so penicillins and cephalosporins are ineffective!

Rickettsiae (p. 210)

- Characterized by mammalian reservoirs and arthropod vectors
- All are small Gram –ve bacilli

Q.ua.R.T.i.L.E.S.

Q-fever (*Coxiella burnettii*):
Epi: No vector required: spread by aerosol from uterus or mammary glands of peripartum farm animals, pets
PC: Atypical pneumonia

Rocky-mountain spotted fever:
Caused by *Rickettsia rickettsii* (tick-borne)

Tick-borne typhus – other:
- *Ehrlichia chaffeensis:* monocytes
- *E. phagocytophilia:* granulocytes
- 'Mediterranean spotted fever' – *Rickettsia conorii*

Louse-borne:
Epidemic and endemic typhus:
- 'Epidemic typhus' caused by *Rickettsia prowazekii,* humans are only host
- 'Endemic murine typhus' caused by – *Rickettsia typhi*

Scrub typhus: *Orientia tsutsugamushi* (chigger-borne)

Chlamydia

C. pneumoniae/C. psittaci:
Atypical pneumonia
C. trachomatis:
- PID/urethritis
- Lymphogranuloma venereum
- 'Trachoma': keratitis

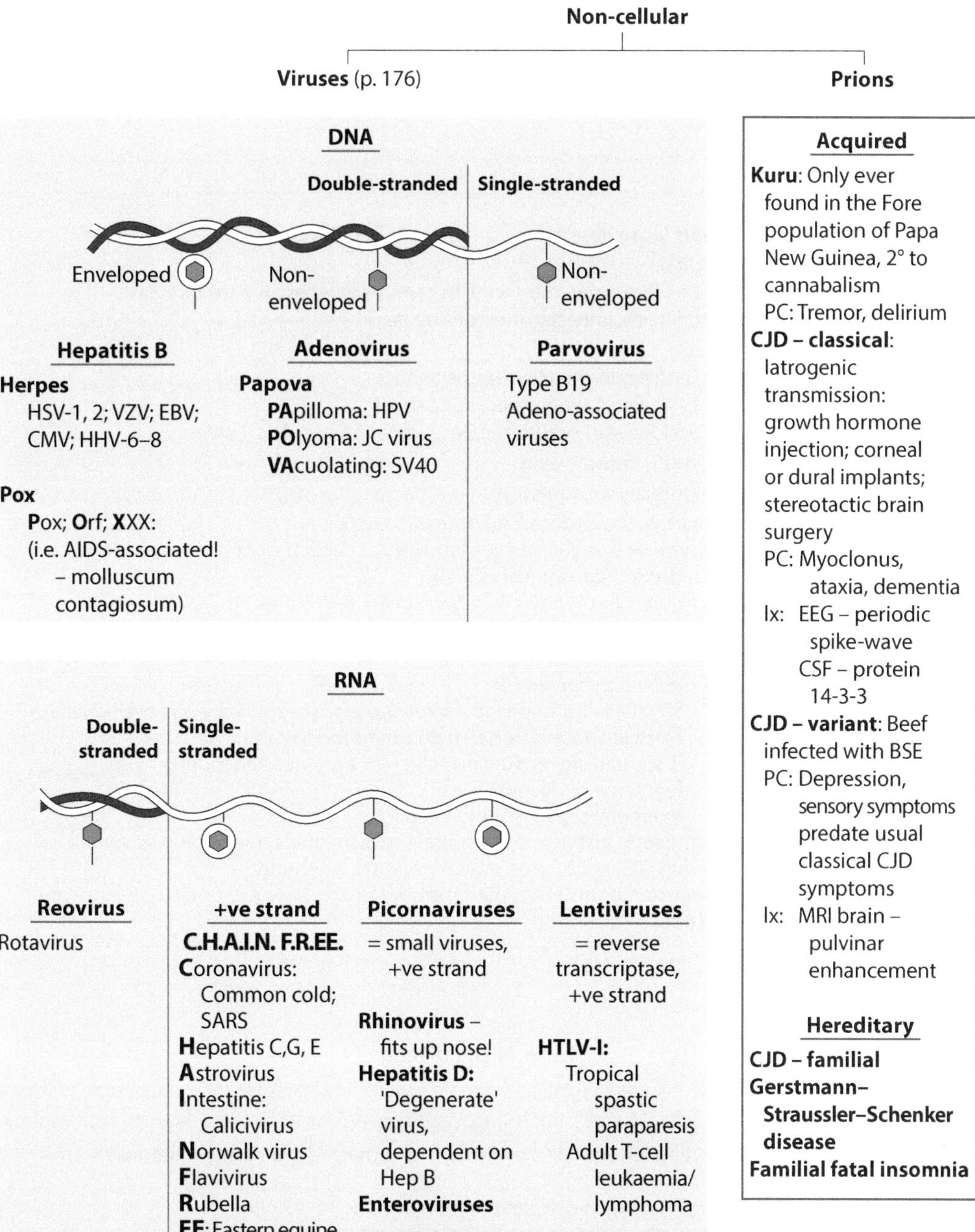
Non-cellular
Viruses (p. 176)
Prions
DNA
Double-stranded
Single-stranded
Enveloped
Non-enveloped
Non-enveloped
Hepatitis B
Herpes
HSV-1, 2; VZV; EBV; CMV; HHV-6–8
Pox
Pox; Orf; XXX: (i.e. AIDS-associated! – molluscum contagiosum)
Adenovirus
Papova
PApilloma: HPV
POlyoma: JC virus
VAcuolating: SV40
Parvovirus
Type B19
Adeno-associated viruses
RNA
Double-stranded
Single-stranded
Reovirus
Rotavirus
+ve strand
C.H.A.I.N. F.R.EE.
Coronavirus: Common cold; SARS
Hepatitis C,G, E
Astrovirus
Intestine: Calicivirus
Norwalk virus
Flavivirus
Rubella
EE: Eastern equine (alphavirus)
–ve strand
O.P.E.R.A. is –ve!
Orthomyxovirus
Paramyxoviruses
Ebola (arenaviruses)
Rabies
Arbovirus group C: Hantavirus
Picornaviruses
= small viruses, +ve strand
Rhinovirus – fits up nose!
Hepatitis D: 'Degenerate' virus, dependent on Hep B
Enteroviruses
ECHO, E.C.H.O, ...
ECHO: Meningitis
Enterovirus spp.
Coxsackie
Hepatitis A
O: pOliO
Lentiviruses
= reverse transcriptase, +ve strand
HTLV-I: Tropical spastic paraparesis
Adult T-cell leukaemia/ lymphoma
HTLV-II
HIV-1/2: AIDS
Acquired
Kuru: Only ever found in the Fore population of Papa New Guinea, 2° to cannabalism
PC: Tremor, delirium
CJD – classical: Iatrogenic transmission: growth hormone injection; corneal or dural implants; stereotactic brain surgery
PC: Myoclonus, ataxia, dementia
Ix: EEG – periodic spike-wave
CSF – protein 14-3-3
CJD – variant: Beef infected with BSE
PC: Depression, sensory symptoms predate usual classical CJD symptoms
Ix: MRI brain – pulvinar enhancement
Hereditary
CJD – familial
Gerstmann–Straussler–Schenker disease
Familial fatal insomnia

BACTERIA

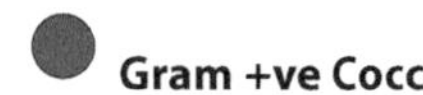

Gram +ve Cocci

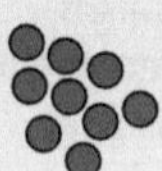

Staphylococcus – ***aureus*** (coagulase +ve): **S.T.A.P.H.**

Skin
- Boil (furuncle/carbuncle): Becomes walled off due to coagulase
- Cellulitis, impetigo, necrotising fasciitis

Toxin
- Gastroenteritis: Heat-stable toxin
- Toxic shock syndrome: Septic shock
- Scalded skin syndrome: Desquamation of palms + soles

Arthritis/osteomyelitis

Pulmonary: Lung abscess

Heart: Acute endocarditis/**H**epatic: Abscess

– ***epidermidis*** (coagulase –ve): Iatrogenic infection – line-associated sepsis

Streptococcus **α-haemolytic**: Plate appears green
- *S. viridans*, e.g. *S. bovis*, *S. mitior*: Subacute endocarditis
- *S. pneumoniae* (diplococci): Pneumonia, endocarditis, meningitis, otitis media

ß-haemolytic: Cause complete haemolysis – plate has 'punched-out holes'
- Group A: *S. pyogenes* **S.T.R².E.P.**
  - **S**kin: Cellulitis, impetigo – spreads due to streptokinase and hyaluronidase
  - **T**onsillitis: Quinsy, pharyngitis, otitis media, sinusitis (immune phenomena)
  - **R**heumatic fever; **R**enal: Proliferative glomerulonephritis (immune phenomena)
  - **E**rythema nodosum (immune phenomena)
  - **P**uerperal sepsis; wound infections
- Group B: *S. agalactiae*: Puerperal sepsis, neonatal meningitis
- Group G: *S. milleri*: Abscesses – cerebral, liver, lung

Enterococci: Endocarditis, peritonitis, UTI – non-haemolytic, lactose-fermenting

Anaerobic: Endocarditis

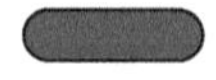

Gram +ve Rods

B.L.A.N.D. *bacteria*

***B**acillus cereus*: Food poisoning from reheated Chinese food

***L**isteria monocytogenes*: Meningoencephalitis in elderly, miscarriage, septic shock in immunocompromised

Anthrax (*Bacillus anthracis*): Cutaneous – eschar; pneumonia

***N**ocardia*: 'No heart' – occurs with heart transplant/immunosuppressed

Diphtheria (*Corynebacterium diphtheriae*): Pharyngitis ('bull neck'), myocarditis, bulbar palsy

Gram +ve Rods – Anaerobic

Clostridium:
- *C. perfringens*: Food poisoning, gas gangrene, puerperal sepsis
- *C. botulinum*: Botulism
- *C. difficile*: Pseudomembranous colitis
- *C. tetani*: Tetanus

Actinomycosis: Dental-cervical; ileocaecal abscess
PATH: Form yellow sulphur granules, granulomas

Gram –ve Cocci

***N**eisseria – meningitides*: Bacterial meningitis (types A, B, C)
– *gonorrhoeae*: Urethritis, arthritis, pharyngitis
***M**oraxella catarrhalis*: Community-acquired pneumonia

Gram –ve Rods

S^2.P.Y. S.E.E.K.S. G.B.H., P.V^2.C. + LEATHER!

Enterobacteria: All cause gastroenteritis (except where indicated)

Non-lactose fermenting (plates contain lactose + pH indicator that turns pink):
S**almonella*/S**higella*: Bacillary dysentery
***P**roteus mirabilis*: UTI
***Y**ersinia enterocolitica* or pseudotuberculosis: Ilieocaecal mass/*Y. pestis*: Plague

Lactose-fermenting ('coliforms'):
***S**erratia*
***E**scherichia coli*
***E**nterobacteria* spp.
***K**lebsiella*: UTI; neonatal meningitis, severe, nosocomial pneumonia
***S**higella sonnei*: Only *Shigella* sp. that ferments lactose

Parvobacteria (small size – **all end in 'ella', except *Haemophilus***):
***G**ardner**ella** vaginalis*: Vaginitis
*Francis**ella** tularensis*: Tularaemia: ulcers, lymphadenopathy, pneumonia – from rabbits, deer
*Pasteur**ella***: Localized or systemic infection from animal-bite
***B**ruc**ella** melitensis/B. abortus*: Pneumonia, meningitis, endocarditis – contracted from farm animals
*Bordet**ella** pertussis*: Whooping cough
*Barton**ella***: Cat-scratch disease (*B. henselae*), Oroya fever, bacillary angiomatosis
***H**aemophilus holeraa*: Pneumonia, epiglottitis, meningitis
H. ducreyi: Chancroid

Other
***P**seudomonas aeruginosa*: **P^2.S.E.U.D.O.**
Pneumonia in cystic fibrosis or ITU
Septicaemia
Ecthyma gangrenosum in immunocompromised
UTI
Dermatological: Wound infection
Ophthalmology: Endophthalmitis 2° to trauma

*Burkholderia **p**seudomallei* (related bacteria): Melioidosis; glanders – pneumonia
***V**ibrio cholerae*: Cholera
***V**. parahaemolyticus*: Food-poisoning
C*ampylobacteria jejuni*: Bloody diarrhoea
L*egion**ella** pneumophila*: Atypical, severe pneumonia

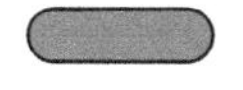

Gram –ve Rods – Anaerobic

Bacteroides: *B. fragilis*: Peritonitis 2° to bowel/gynaecological disease
B. oralis/Fusobacteria: Dental abscess-gingivitis/Lemierre disease
Helicobacter pylori: Peptic ulcer, gastric carcinoma, gastic MALToma

ANTIBIOTICS

Choice

Gram +ve Cocci

Staphylococci
Beta-lactams: Flucloxacillin, co-amoxiclav
Glycopeptides: Vancomycin, teicoplanin
Oxazolinedione: Linezolid
Special circumstances:

- Osteomyelitis: Clindamycin, fusidic acid
- Endocarditis: Gentamicin
- Penicillin-allergic: Macrolide – clarithromycin

Streptococci
Beta-lactams:
Penicillins:

- Benzylpenicillin (IV)
- Phenoxymethylpenicillin, 'Pen V' (PO)
- Amoxicillin, ampicillin

Cephalosporins:

- 1°: Cefalexin (PO)
- 2°: Cefuroxime (IV)

Carbapenems: Meropenem
Penicillin-allergic: Macrolide – clarithromycin

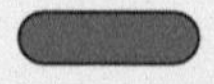

Gram +ve Rods

L.A.N.D.

***L**isteria*: Amoxicillin + gentamicin
***A**nthrax*: Penicillin/ciprofloxacin
***N**ocardia*: Cotrimoxazole
Diphtheria: Anti-toxin

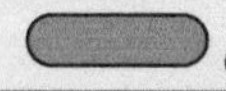

Gram +ve Anaerobes

Clostridia botulinum/C. perfringens: Benzylpenicillin, clindamycin, metronidazole
Clostridium difficile: Metronidazole, vancomycin
Actinomycoses: Co-amoxiclav

Gram –ve Cocci

Meningococci
Penicillins: Benzylpenicillin
Cephalosporin, 3°: Ceftriaxone, cefotaxime
Penicillin-allergic: Macrolide – erythromycin

Gonococci
Amoxicillin, ampicillin
Cephalosporins: 2°, 3°
Quinolone: Ciprofloxacin
Penicillin-allergic: Macrolide – erythromycin

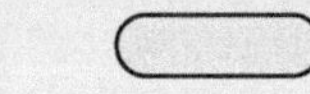

Gram –ve Rods

Enterobacteria, e.g. *Salmonella, E. coli*
Trimethoprim
Aminoglycosides: Gentamicin, amikacin
Quinolone: Ciprofloxacin

Parvobacteria, e.g. *Haemophilus, Bordatella pertussis*
Amoxicillin, ampicillin
Cephalosporins: 2°, 3°

Pseudomonas aeruginosa
Beta-lactams:

- Temocillin, piperacillin
- Ceftazidime
- Aztreonam (monobactam)

Aminoglycosides: Gentamicin, amikacin
Quinolone: Ciprofloxacin
Brucella: Doxycycline + gentamicin/rifampicin
Legionella: Clarithromycin, ciprofloxacin

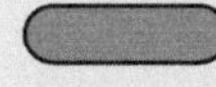

Gram –ve Anaerobes

Bacteroides: Metronidazole
Helicobacter: Metronidazole or clarithromycin, plus amoxicillin

Atypical bacteria

Mycoplasma, spirochaetes, Rickettsiae, Chlamydiae
Macrolides: Erythromycin, azithromycin, clarithromycin
Tetracyclines: Tetracycline, oxytetracycline

Mycobacteria
TB: **R.I.P.P.E.R.S^3.** (p. 203)
Leprosy: Rifampicin, clofazimine, dapsone
Atypical: Rifampicin, clofazimine, macrolide

Sites of action

Peptidoglycan cell-wall

Beta-lactams:
Binds to penicillin-binding protein
Inhibit transpeptidation cross-link between peptide backbones
Inhibit autolysis inhibitor: Osmotic pressure ruptures plasma membrane
Cycloserine: Inhibits addition of final 2 alanine amino acids
Glycopeptides, bacitracin: Inhibits release of peptidoglycan building block from lipid carrier
Polymixin: Cationic detergents disrupt lipid bilayer

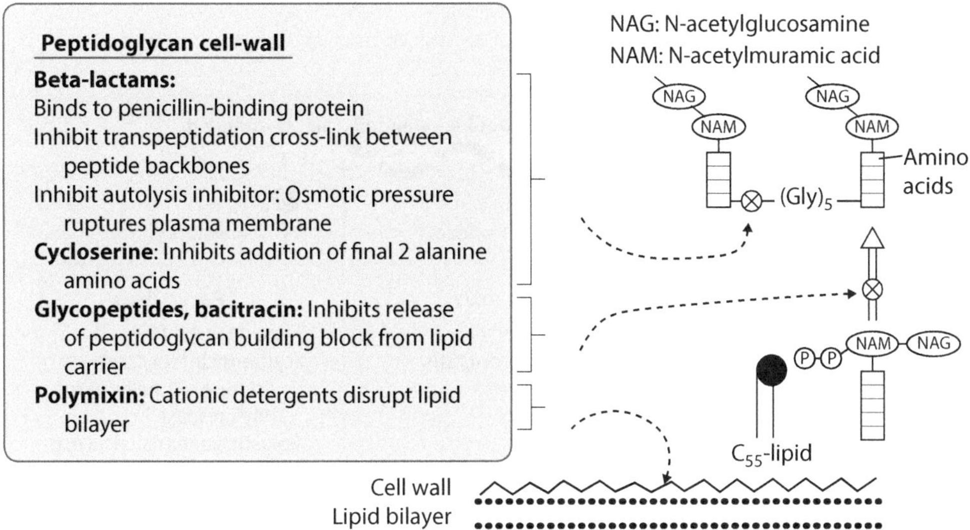

DNA/RNA synthesis

Quinolones (ciprofloxacin):
Inhibit DNA relaxation prior to transcription or replication
Inhibit DNA coiling prior to cell division
Metronidazole:
Fragments DNA via free-radicals
Inhibits nucleic acid synthesis
Inhibits reductase enzyme in anaerobic respiratn pathway
Rifampicin: Inhibits prokaryote RNA polymerase

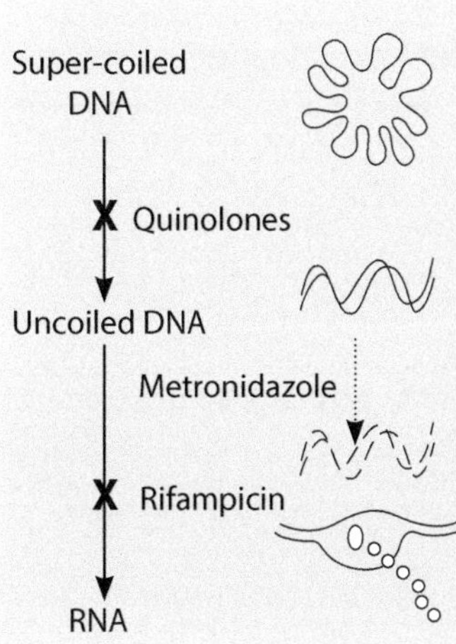

Protein synthesis

Tetracyclines:
Selective uptake into bacteria
Competitive inhibitors with incoming tRNA for amino site
Aminoglycosides:
Selective uptake
Causes misreading of codon (mRNA) anticodon

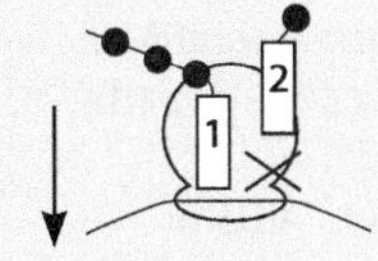

Chloramphenicol, clindamycin:
Inhibit transpeptidation

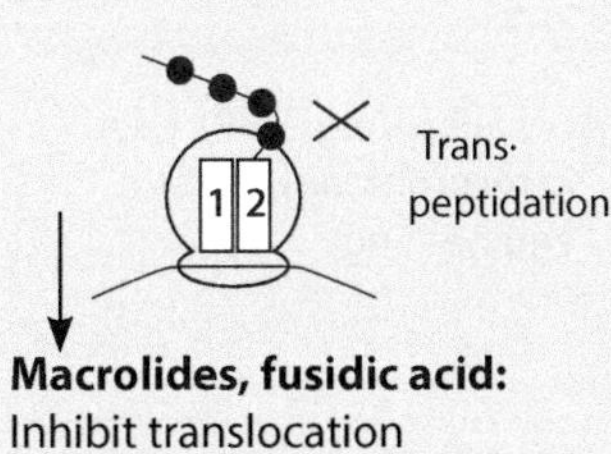

Macrolides, fusidic acid:
Inhibit translocation

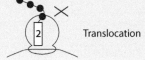

Folate synthesis

Sulphonamides:
Competitive inhibitors of dihydropteroate synthetase
Trimethoprim:
Competitive inhibitor of bacterial DHFR (dihydrofolate reductase)

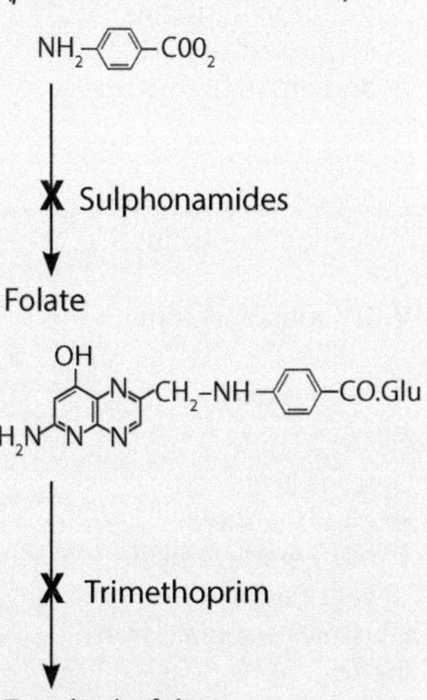

VIRUSES

DNA

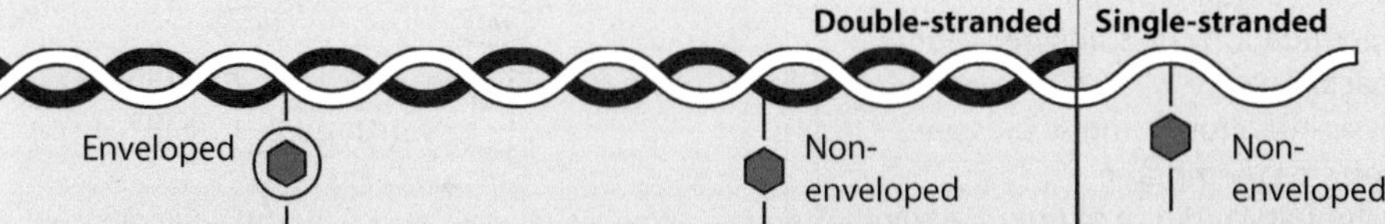

Hepatitis B (p. 152)

Herpes (pp. 193–5)

HSV-1:
- Labial herpes
- Encephalitis

HSV-2:
- Genital herpes
- Meningitis, recurrent

VZV:
- Chicken pox (varicella)
- Zoster
- Brainstem encephalitis, myelitis

EBV:
- Glandular fever
- Lymphoma (esp. Non-Hodgkin)
- Nasopharynx carcinoma

CMV:
- Retinitis
- Colitis/hepatitis
- Pneumonitis (disease only occurs in immuno-supressed, esp. AIDS and organ transplant)

HHV-6:
- Roseola infantum (exanthema subitum)
- Meningoencephalitis

HHV-7

HHV-8: Kaposi's sarcoma

Pox

Pox:
- Cowpox (vaccinia)
- Smallpox (variola) both eradicated by vaccination

Orf: Pustules, acquired from sheep

XXX (assoc. with HIV) molluscum contagiosum: Pearly, umbilicated pustules

Adenovirus

Types 1-30:
- Pharyngitis – bronchitis
- Conjunctivitis
- Meningitis

Types 40, 41: Diarrhoea

Papova

PApilloma:

Human papillomavirus (HPV)

Types 6, 11:
- Warts, condylomata acuminata

Types 16, 18:
- Carcinoma of cervix, vulva, penis, rectum

POlyoma

JC virus:
- Progressive multifocal leucoencephalopathy (PML)
- Occurs in AIDS or pts. given integrin inhibitors. e.g. as Rx for multiple sclerosis

BK virus

VAculating, e.g. SV40: Used in recombinant genetic engineering

Parvovirus

Type 819: (p. 193)
- Erythema infectiosum ('slapped cheek syn.' or 'fifth disease')
- Aplastic anaemia crisis esp. in hereditary haemolytic anaemias, e.g. sickle cell disease

Adeno-associated viruses

RNA

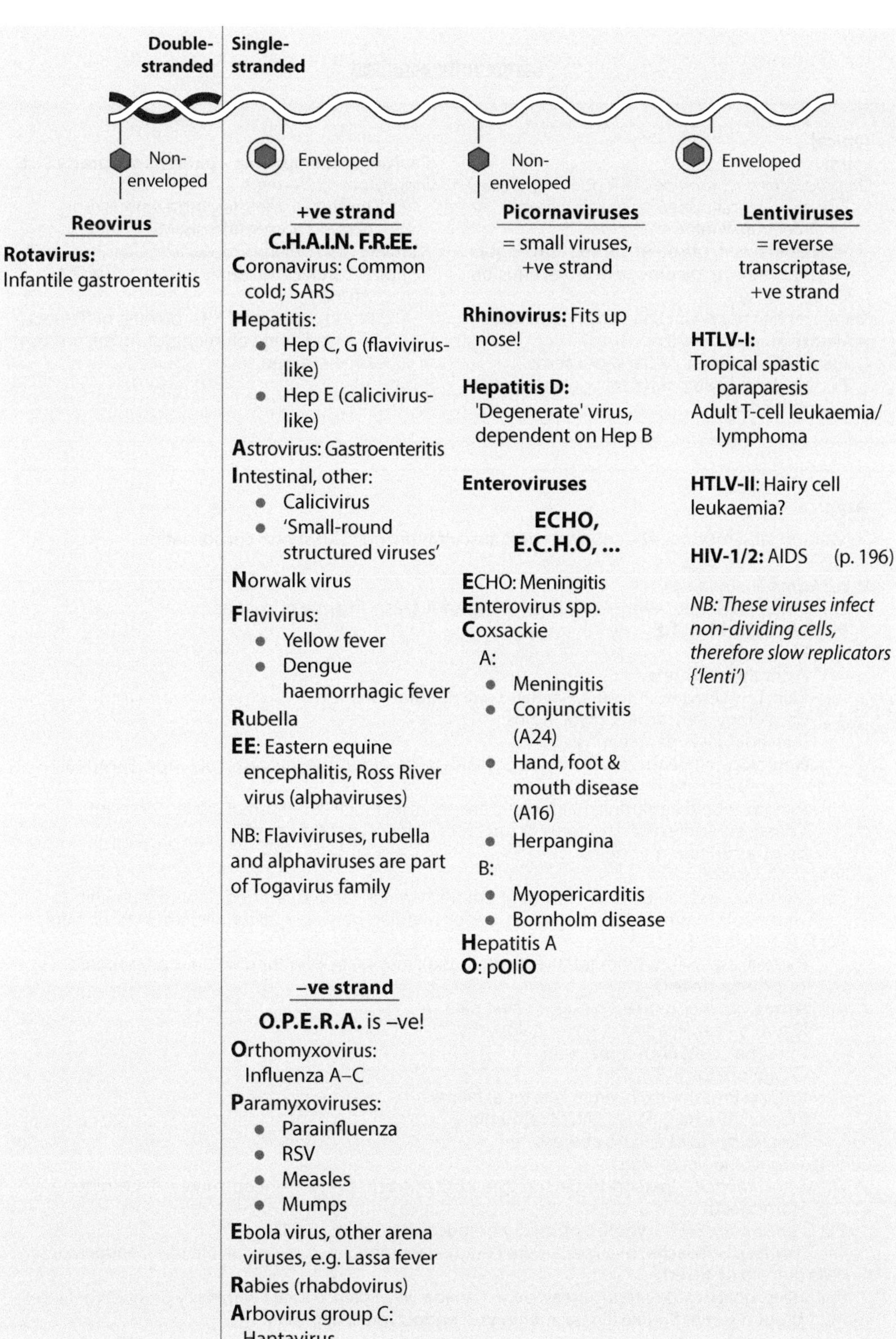

Reovirus

Rotavirus:
Infantile gastroenteritis

+ve strand

C.H.A.I.N. F.R.EE.

Coronavirus: Common cold; SARS

Hepatitis:
- Hep C, G (flavivirus-like)
- Hep E (calicivirus-like)

Astrovirus: Gastroenteritis

Intestinal, other:
- Calicivirus
- 'Small-round structured viruses'

Norwalk virus

Flavivirus:
- Yellow fever
- Dengue haemorrhagic fever

Rubella

EE: Eastern equine encephalitis, Ross River virus (alphaviruses)

NB: Flaviviruses, rubella and alphaviruses are part of Togavirus family

–ve strand

O.P.E.R.A. is –ve!

Orthomyxovirus: Influenza A–C

Paramyxoviruses:
- Parainfluenza
- RSV
- Measles
- Mumps

Ebola virus, other arena viruses, e.g. Lassa fever

Rabies (rhabdovirus)

Arbovirus group C: Hantavirus

Picornaviruses

= small viruses, +ve strand

Rhinovirus: Fits up nose!

Hepatitis D: 'Degenerate' virus, dependent on Hep B

Enteroviruses

ECHO, E.C.H.O, ...

ECHO: Meningitis
Enterovirus spp.
Coxsackie

A:
- Meningitis
- Conjunctivitis (A24)
- Hand, foot & mouth disease (A16)
- Herpangina

B:
- Myopericarditis
- Bornholm disease

Hepatitis A
O: pOliO

Lentiviruses

= reverse transcriptase, +ve strand

HTLV-I:
Tropical spastic paraparesis
Adult T-cell leukaemia/lymphoma

HTLV-II: Hairy cell leukaemia?

HIV-1/2: AIDS (p. 196)

NB: These viruses infect non-dividing cells, therefore slow replicators ('lenti')

PNEUMONIA – PATHOGENS

Community-acquired

Typical

Lobar

Streptococcus pneumoniae (AKA pneumococcus)
Epi: Recent viral upper-respiratory tract infection, winter
PC: **R**apid onset, offset; **R**usty sputum; **R**igors (septicaemia); pleural, pericardial effusion; MR = 20%

Gram –ve: *Haemophilus influenzae* type b (rods) or *Moraxella catarrhalis* (cocci)
Epi: COPD, elderly, infants, septicaemic
PC: Insidious onset; purulent sputum; cor pulmonale

Cavities and empyema – patients are pretty SicK

***S**taphylococcus aureus*
Epi: Influenza; measles; intravenous drug abusers; cystic fibrosis; MR = 30%

***K**lebsiella* (short, plump, capsulated, Gram –ve bacilli)
Epi: Alcoholics, diabetes mellitus, COPD; S. Africa
PC: Bloody sputum; CXR – bowing of fissures; reduced lung volume; sputum microscopy +ve for organism

Atypical – 1

Constitutional symptoms with normal chest auscultation, but CXR shows consolidation

Mycoplasma pneumoniae
Epi: Winter epidemics every few years; young adults, esp. in army or college
PC: **F.A.S.C.I.N.A.T.E.**
- **F**lu-like: Fever
- **A**rthralgia, arthritis
- **S**kin: Erythema multiforme, Raynaud (cold agglutinins)
- **C**ardiology: Pericarditis, myocarditis;
- **I**ntestinal: D+V, pancreatitis
- **N**eurological: Headache common; Guillain–Barré syndrome, myelitis, meningo-encephalitis, cerebellar ataxia
- **A**naemia: Cold agglutinin haemolytic anaemia; jaundice (NB: Normal white cell count)
- **T**hroat, sore, injected; laryngitis or tracheitis – dry or mucoid cough
- **E**arache: Bullous myringitis

Legionella pneumophila
Epi: Outbreaks, esp. on contact with stagnant fresh-water supply, air-conditioning, humidifiers, whirl-pools; summer; Mediterranean travel; middle-age, obese, alcoholic, smokers, diabetes
PC: **P.A.N.I.C.K.E.R.**
- **P**yrexia, esp. >40°C (with relative bradycardia); may be self-limiting without pneumonia ('Pontiac fever')
- **A**rthralgia, incl. marked pleuritic chest pain
- **N**eurological: Headache, encephalopathy
- **I**ntestinal: D+V, abdominal pain
- **C**oagulopathy (DIC), CK ↑
- **K**idney: Proteinuria, haematuria, renal failure
- **E**lectrolytes: Na ↓, PO_4 ↓, ALT ↑, albumin ↓
- **R**espiratory failure, lung abscess

Chlamydia pneumoniae/psittaci
Epi: *C. pneumoniae* – person-to-person spread; *C. psittaci* – parrots; sheep, turkey, duck, pigeon (ornithosis)
PC: *C. pneumoniae*: Pharyngitis, otitis; dry or mucoid cough occurs late
C. psittaci: Headache, myalgia; severe cough, haemoptysis, 2° bacterial infection; endocarditis

Coxiella burnetti (Q-fever)
Epi: Sheep, goats, cattle-rearing areas, e.g. E. Canada, NW. Spain; contact with dairy products or faeces
PC: Abrupt onset of flu-like illness; meningitis; endocarditis; hepatitis

Atypical – 2

Bacteria
- TB
  - Epi: Alcoholics, debilitated, Indian
  - PC: Insidious symptoms – chronic cough, haemoptysis, weight loss
- Meliodiosis; *Actinomyces israelii*; Tularaemia; plague; anthrax

Viruses:
- Adenovirus, influenza, parainfluenza, RSV, measles – mainly children; causes interstitial pneumonitis
- Hantavirus: rodents, deer in USA

Fungi
- Histoplasmosis – Mid-west or SE. USA: bats, soil; coccidioidomycosis – SW. USA deserts; blastomycosis
- Cryptococcosis – pigeon droppings

Nosocomial

Def

Pneumonia acquired in hospital ≥2 days after admission

Causes

C.I.R.C.U.L.AR. … *like the treatment of them*
- **C**ontact with other patients
- **I**mmunocompromise
- **R**ecumbency (basal atelectasis)
- **C**atheters, incl.:
  - **U**rinary
  - **L**ines and ET tubes
- **A**ntibiotic **R**esistance

Organisms:

Gram +ve (30%)

Staphylococcus aureus, esp. MRSA

Streptococcus faecalis incl. vancomycin-resistant enterococci (VRE)

Streptococcus pneumoniae

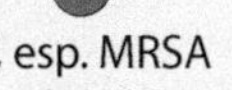

Gram –ve (50%)

Pseudomonas aeruginosa – tubes

Acinetobacter

Legionella – nebulizer, ventilators

Enterobacteria: *Proteus, Serratia, Enterobacter*

Anaerobes: *Bacteroides, Fusobacterium*

Fungi

Immunocompromised

Innate

Aspiration, e.g. alcoholics, drug overdose, bulbar weakness incl. stroke, seizure: Anaerobes, e.g. *Bacteroides, Streptococcus milleri*

Cystic fibrosis: *Haemophilus, Staphylococcus, Pseudomonas aeruginosa/P. cepacia*

Bronchial obstruction, e.g. foreign body; carcinoma; lymph node, bronchopulmonary sequestration: Anaerobes, e.g. *Bacteroides, S. milleri*

Neutropenia: Coliforms, *S. aureus, Aspergillus*

B cell, e.g. splenectomy, hypogammaglobulinaemia: *S. pneumoniae, Haemophilus* (both encapsulated bacteria), *Mycoplasma*

T cell, e.g. AIDS:

Aspiration, e.g. alcoholics, drug overdose, bulbar weakness incl. stroke, seizure:
- Bacterial:
  - Community-acquired pneumonia – occurs early in AIDS; more severe
  - TB, MAI
- Fungi: PCP – 80% develop without prophylaxis; *Cryptococcus* – mild pneumonia
- Viruses: Herpes viruses: CMV, EBV, HSV, VZV, HHV-8 (Kaposi's sarcoma)
- Toxoplasmosis

B + T cell, e.g. post-transplant immunosuppression:

Nosocomial, e.g. *Legionella*

Nocardia (esp. heart transplant)
- PC: Pleurisy, cavitates, metastases
- Ix: Acid-fast hyphae

Candida; *Aspergillus*

CMV: Systemic disease

FOOD POISONING

Def

Caused by bacteria or toxin residing in food source
Derives from infection within animal, or contamination during food storage or preparation

Causes

Classified by:
Cause: Pre-formed toxin vs. bacterial multiplication (often with toxin secretion)
Incubation time: Hours (pre-formed toxin)–days (bacterial multiplication within gut)

Pre-formed toxin: 1–6 hours **S.i.C.k.**

S*taphylococcus aureus*: Heat-stable enterotoxins A–E
Food: Contaminated dairy or meat; septic lesion on hand of food-handler
PC: Vomiting (± diarrhoea)
Rx: Flucloxacillin if bacteria isolated
C*lostridium botulinum*: Heat-labile toxin (blocks pre-synaptic release of Ach)
Food: Tinned foods kept in anaerobic conditions, esp. home-canners, canned fruit
PC: Vomiting (± constipation); descending paralysis (ophthalmoplegia, ptosis, bulbar weakness)
Rx: Anti-toxin; nerves resprout in 2–3 months

Toxin/cell multiplication: 8–24 hours **S.i.C.k.**

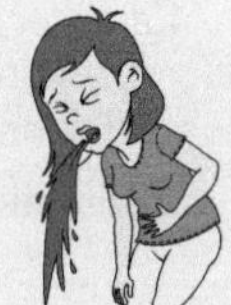

Special foods:
Seafood, raw – *Vibrio parahaemolyticus*
Micro: Forms blue-green colonies on thiosulphate agar
PC: Vomiting; diarrhoea; abdominal pain
Rx: Tetracycline
Soups, sauces; or reheated, fried rice – *Bacillus cereus*
Micro: Forms 'curled hair' colonies on agar
PC: Early vomiting (rice); diarrhoea, abdominal pain (soup, sauce)
C*lostridium perfringens* (heat-labile toxin + bacterial multiplication)
Food: Reheated meat, e.g. meat pies, mincemeat, stew
Micro: Nagler reaction detects toxin (half the plate has anti-toxin, which inhibits growth)
PC: Colic (gas-producing –same organism as in gas gangrene!)

Cell multiplication: 1–10 days **S.i.C.k.**

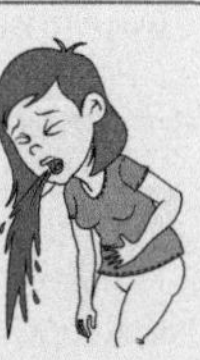

S*almonella* spp. (2000 serotypes, incl. S. *enteritidis* phage type 4)
Food: Eggs, chicken, milk stored at room temp./nursing home outbreaks
Micro:
- Non-lactose fermenting on MacConkey medium
- Serotyped by antigens O (lipopolysaccharide) and H (flagella)

PC:
- Vomiting; diarrhoea (profuse, watery ± blood in 25%); abdominal pain
- Fever; septicaemia, due to invasion of wall; esp. immunocompromised, *S. virchow*
- Asymptomatic carriage

Rx: Ciprofloxacin or amoxicillin – only if septicaemia due to risk of prolonged carriage
C*ampylobacter jejuni* (cholera-like heat-stable toxin)
Food: Cooked meat, heated milk
Micro: Motile, curved spiral-shaped rods – like seagulls
PC:
- Prodrome: Fever, vomiting, headache, generalized aches
- Profuse watery, bloody diarrhoea (± mucus, pus); abdominal pain

Rx: Erythromycin (decreases excretion rate), ciprofloxacin

GASTROENTERITIS

Def

Bacteria spread between people, via faecal–oral route, e.g. food handling by case; in water supply
Bacteria cause colitis – except for *Vibrio cholerae* and *Salmonella typhi*, which cause ileitis

Causes

V.E.R.Y. S^2.i.C^2.k.

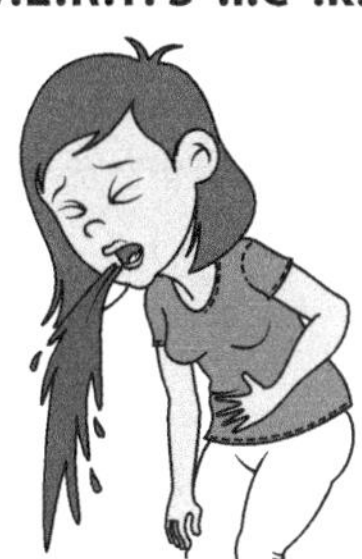

V*ibrio cholera*
E*scherichia coli*: **P.I.T.H.y.:**
- **P**athogenetic – paediatric (neonatal and infantile gastroenteritis)
- **I**nvasive (*Shigella*-like dysentery)
- **T**oxicogenetic – traveller's diarrhoea (cholera-like)
- **H**aemorrhagic – haemorrhagic colitis/haemolytic–uraemic syndrome

Rotavirus, and other viruses:
- Rotavirus (esp. group A) – double-stranded RNA
  - Epi:
    - Occurs in infants or elderly in institutions (outbreaks), esp. in winter
    - Spread via respiratory secretions, as well as faecal–oral route
  - PC: May cause respiratory symptoms, as well as D+V + abdominal cramps + fever
  - Electron microscopy: Spherical particles with spoke-like surface
- Astrovirus, calicivirus, Norwalk-like viruses – single-stranded +ve RNA
  - Epi: Outbreaks among children (esp. caliciviruses) or families
  - Electron microscopy: 6-pointed star, small-round structured viruses (SRSVs)
- Adenovirus (esp. serotypes 40, 41) – DNA virus
  - Epi: Endemic, due to prolonged faecal excretion by cases
  - Electron microscopy: Icosahedral symmetry with round capsomeres
- CMV – DNA virus
  - Epi: Immunocompromised, e.g. HIV

Y*ersinia enterocolitica/pseudotuberculosis*
S*almonella typhi* – 'typhoid fever'
S*higella dysenteriae* – 'bacillary dysentry'
C*lostridium difficile* – 'pseudomembranous colitis'
- Also *Clostridium septicum*: Neutropenic enterocolitis

C*ryptosporidium*, and other protozoa:
- Sporozoa: *Cryptosporidium*, *Microsporidium*, *Isospora belli* – HIV-related
  Plasmodium – malaria
- Amoeba: *Entamoeba histolytica* – 'amoebic dysentry'
- Flagellate: *Giardia lamblia*
- Ciliate: *Balantidium coli*

GASTROENTERITIS – ILEAL-BASED

Salmonella – 'Typhoid' or 'Enteric fever'

Salmonella typhi – severe; *S. paratyphi* – asymptomatic or mild, and less carriership

Epi

- Spread by cases <2 months post-infection, OR chronic carriers (2%), who excrete bacteria indefinitely
- Carriage assoc. with elderly women, gallstones, *Salmonella* Vi antigen +ve (capsule)
- Medium of spread: Water supply (excreted by faeces, urine), or carriers' hands on meat, eggs, milk
- Sporadic: 3/4 in UK acquired abroad; OR outbreaks, e.g. Croydon 1937; food-borne, e.g. Typhoid Mary
- Risk factors: Achlorhydria ↑ risk; sickle cell ↑ septicaemia

PATH

Bacteria cross ileal epithelium (cf. *Shigella* – remains within colonic epithelium)

Weeks 1–2

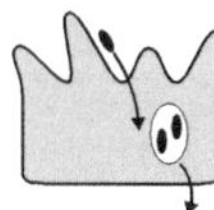

- Binds to mannose
- Distorts microvilli – 'actin splash'
- Transcytosis via endosome
- Transient bacteraemia

Weeks 2–3+

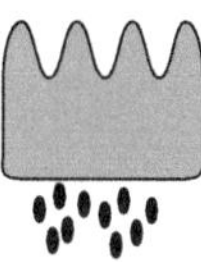

- Proliferates in lamina propria
- Spreads to lymph nodes

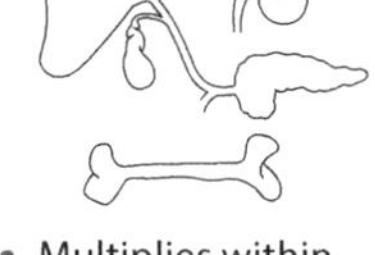

- Multiplies within macrophages of reticuloendothelial systems

Chronic cholecystitis reinfects bowel in Peyer patch

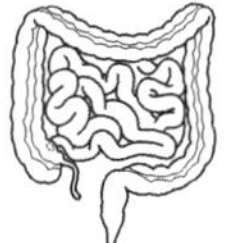

Bacteraemia

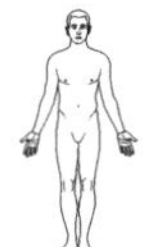

PC

G.O. S.A.L.M.O.N^2.E.L.LA.

GIT: 1st week – constipation; abdominal pain, distension, 3+ week – infectious diarrhoea
Complications: GIT haemorrhage; ileal ulceration, perforation
Organomegaly: Hepatosplenomegaly
Systemic: Fever (transient bacteraemia)/**S**kin: Rose spots
Arthralgia, arthritis; myalgia, myositis, necrosis
Lungs: Pneumonitis/URTI symptoms common, e.g. sore throat, epistaxis
Myocarditis: Bradycardia common
Osteomyelitis
Neurological: Headache common, meningo-encephalitis
Nephritis: Glomerulonephritis, pyelonephritis
Extra: DVT
Lymphocytes ↑; WBC ↓
LAte: Mortality 10% without Rx; 0.1% if treated

Ix

Culture
1st 10 days: Blood or bone marrow culture
2nd 10 days: Stool or urine culture
Non-lactose fermenting on MacConkey medium

Serology Widal test: Diluted patient's serum (Ig) + killed test bacteria in visible clumps

Rx

Amoxicillin, trimethoprim, ciprofloxacin, ceftriaxone (IV) – resistance common
Cholecystectomy: Cures carriage in 75%, but small risk of death
Vaccine: Killed monovalent IM or Vi-capsular polysaccharide Ag, live oral – 3 years' protection

Cholera

Vibro cholerae

Type 01; biotype classical (severe); serotype Ogawa, Inaba, Hikojima
Type 01; biotype El-Tor (mild)

Epi

Spread by cases, and asymptomatic carriers that occur commonly in outbreaks
Medium of spread: Water supply, seafood, flies – but cooking destroys bacteria
Risk factor: Achlorhydria; epidemics and pandemics

PATH

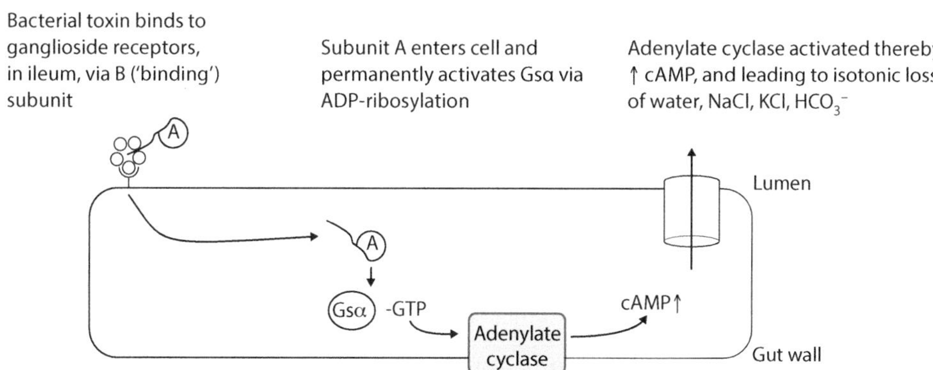

Bacterial toxin binds to ganglioside receptors, in ileum, via B ('binding') subunit
Subunit A enters cell and permanently activates Gsα via ADP-ribosylation
Adenylate cyclase activated thereby ↑ cAMP, and leading to isotonic loss of water, NaCl, KCl, HCO_3^-
A
A
Gsα
-GTP
Adenylate cyclase
cAMP↑
Lumen
Gut wall

PC

Incubation period 5 hours – 5 days
D+V:

- Profuse, 'rice-water' stool (turbid, due to flecks of mucus and shed epithelium)
- Severe dehydration: 'Choleraic facies' = sunken eyes and cheeks; hypovolaemic shock, acute tubular necrosis

Ix

Bloods: Na^+ normal; K^+ ↓ (muscle cramps)
Metabolic acidosis

Stool microscopy/cultures:
No WBCs or RBCs seen
Culture: Sucrose-fermenting
Bacteria appear as small curved, comma-shaped , motile Gram –ve rods

Type, e.g. 01; biotype: Classical or El-Tor; serotype: slide agglutination; phage type

Rx

Tetracycline (PO/IV): ↓ fluid loss and ↓ infectivity
Killed vaccine: Only protects 50% (not 0139)

BACTERIAL GASTROENTERITIS – OTHER

Escherichia coli

Types

P².I.T².H.Y.

Paediatric

Entero**P**athogenetic: Infantile gastroenteritis (0–2 years)

Epi:

- Sporadic, or outbreaks in nurseries and resource-poor countries
- Breast-feeding protects

PATH: Acts by combination of invasion and toxins

PC:

- Profuse watery diarrhoea, dehydration, metabolic acidosis
- High mortality rate

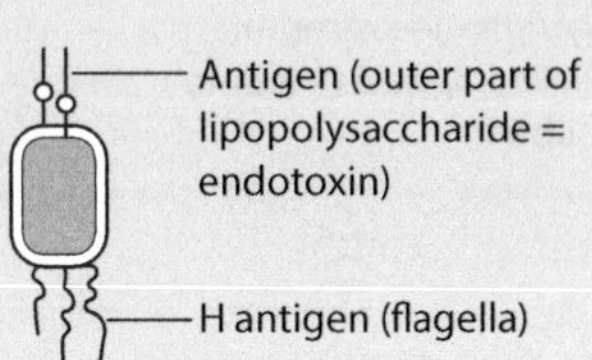

Entero-aggregative: Neonatal gastroenteritis (0–6 months)

Invasive

Entero**I**nvasive

Epi: All ages

PATH: Shiga-like toxin causes *Shigella*-like dysentry in colon

Ix: Stool microscopy – RBCs and WBCs

Traveller's diarrhoea

Entero**T**oxicogenic: Travellers' diarrhoea, e.g. O6 type (local *E. coli* possess different antigen types to commensal bacteria)

Epi:

- Adults recently arrived in foreign country ingesting contaminated water/food
- Infants in resource-poor countries

PATH:

- Colonisation factor antigen = special fimbriae or pili that allow ileal adherence
- Heat-labile toxin or heat-stable toxin (activates guanylate cyclase)

PC:

- Cholera-like: profuse watery diarrhoea, vomiting, abdominal pain, mild fever
- Lasts for a few days, or rarely weeks

Rx: Doxycycline or ciprofloxacin in severe cases

Haemorrhagic

Entero**H**aemorrhagic (Veroc**Y**totoxicogenic):

- Haemorrhagic colitis
- Haemolytic–uraemic syndrome

e.g. 0157 antigen type, H7 serotype (as in the USA hamburger outbreak)

Epi:

- All ages susceptible, but children and elderly most at risk
- Sporadic (through contact with cattle that act as carriers)
- Outbreaks, e.g. undercooked hamburgers, unpasteurized milk, nursing homes

PATH:

- Attachment–effacement (eae)' gene = pilus that allows colonic binding via mannitol
- Verocytotoxins' (VT1,2) = Shiga-like toxins

PC: Haemorrhagic colitis:

- Profuse bloody diarrhoea with red and white blood cells in stool
- Thrombotic thrombocytopenic purpura
- Usually apyrexial

Haemolytic–uraemic syndrome (in 10%):

- Haemolytic anaemia or thrombocytopenia
- Uraemia (red blood cells crenate and block glomeruli)
- 5% die!

Rx: Fosfomycin?

Shigella – 'Bacillary dysentery'

(in order of decreasing severity):
S. dysenteriae (epidemics) → *S. flexneri/S. boydi* (endemic in resource-poor countries) → *S. sonnei* (UK nursing home outbreaks)

Epi

Faecal–oral route. NB: Only a small infective dose is required, and cases continue to excrete for several months after infection

PATH

Infection confined to epithelium of terminal ileum and colon (as opposed to *Salmonella*)

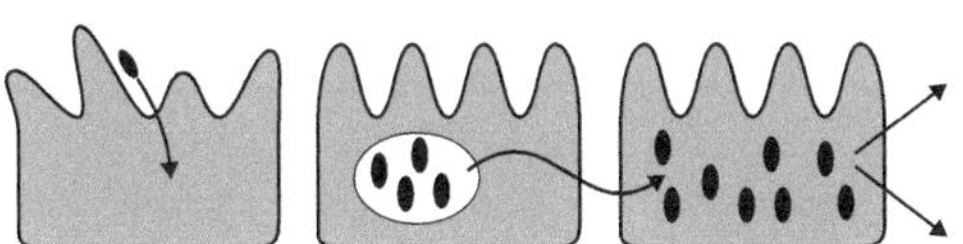
Shiga toxin: Inhibits ribosomal function and protein synthesis
Apoptosis: Epithelial sloughing, ulceration and haemorrhage (sigmoidoscopy: denuded mucosa)
Adhesion + formation of 'actin splashes'
Intracellular replication
Neighbouring cell invasion

PC

Incubation period 1–7 days

S.H.I.G.A.

Systemic:
- Abrupt fever
- Septicaemia in 10%, esp. with *S. dysenteriae* in immunocompromised

Headaches: Meningism (but sterile CSF)

Intestinal:
- Diarrhoea – frequent, but scanty volume, with multiple white and red cells and mucus
- GI haemorrhage
- Abdominal pain and cramps

Glomerulonephritis: Haemolytic–uraemic syndrome

Arthralgia incl. reactive arthritis

Ix

Bloods: Haemolytic–uraemic syndrome; Na ↓, glucose ↓

Stool: Microscopy: ↑ ↑ WBC (cf. amoebic dysentry), ↑ RBC, ↑ mucus
Culture: Non-lactose fermenting (except *S. sonnei*)

Rx

Amoxicillin, trimethoprim, ciprofloxacin; avoid anti-diarrhoeals

Yersinia enterocolitica/pseudotuberculosis

Epi: Milk, unpasteurized cheese, tofu; Fe-overload, e.g. thalassaemia, haemochromatosis; pets act as reservoirs

PATH: Terminal ileitis with local mesenteric adenitis (right iliac fossa mass)

PC:
- Early diarrhoea (incubation period 1–7 days)
- Immune reactions (erythema nodosum, reactive arthritis)
- **S.A.L.M.O.N.**ella-like systemic symptoms (**S**kin – cellulitis, **A**rthralgia, **L**ung, **M**yoendocarditis, **O**steomyelitis, **N**eurological)

Rx: Tetracycline, ciproflocxacin (PO); ceftriaxone or gentamicin (IV)

Clostridium difficile – 'pseudomembranous colitis'

Epi: Antibiotic therapy within 24 hours starting to 6 weeks after stopping; elderly, debilitated

PATH: Proctitis, later colitis; may progress to toxic megacolon with perforation; toxin-mediated

PC: Abdominal pain, tenderness; profuse diarrhoea; fever; neutrophilia

Rx: Vancomycin or metronidazole (PO)

PROTOZOAL GASTROENTERITIS

Sporozoa – intracellular organisms

Plasmodium falciparum – acute malaria
Cryptosporidia; Microsporidia; *Isospora belli*

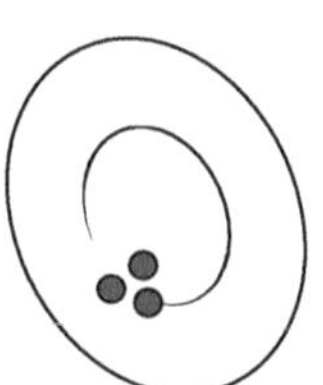

Round, circular, organisms

PC

Immunocompetent: Self-limiting diarrhoea
Immunocompromised, incl. AIDS:

- Chronic diarrhoea
- Wasting

Ziehl–Nielsen staining (Cryptosporidia)
Electron (Microsporidia)
Bowel biopsy:

- Ileal (Cryptosporidia)
- Jejunal (Microsporidia)

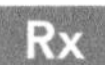

Chemotherapy: Nitazoxanide (Cryptosporidium), albendazole (Microsporidium)
Supportive: Rehydration, electrolyte correction

Amoebae – simple unicellular organisms

Entamoeba histolytica – 'amoebic dysentery"

PATH

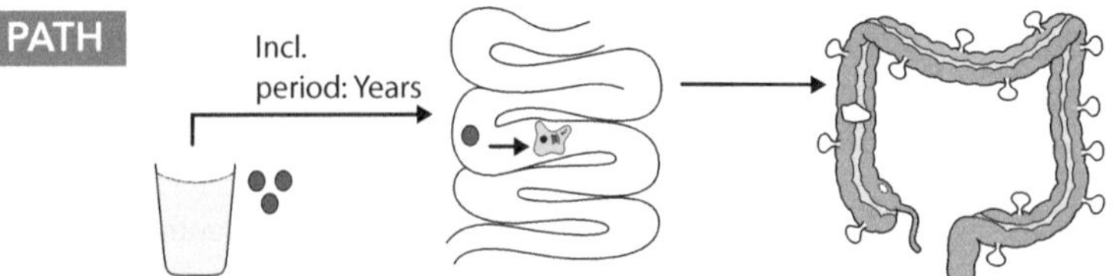

Cysts in uncooked food or water (survive for weeks)

Trophozoites emerge in duodenum-ileum ("excystation')

Trophozoites invade colon via flask-shaped ulcers ('encystment')

Feet-like 'pseudopodia'

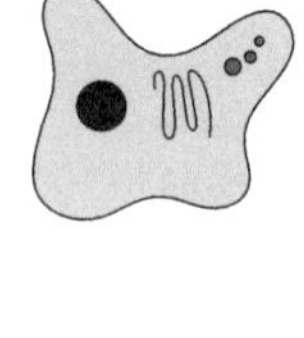

PC

Amoebic colitis (variable):

- Asymptomatic carriage
- Mild, relapsing-remitting diarrhoea, rectal bleeding, colic, fever
- Acute, fulminant → toxic megacolon, perforation

Amoebic liver abscess (esp. men)

- Acute RUQ/R shoulder pain
- ↑ with inspiration, alcohol
- Perforation into cavities – peritoneal, pleural, pericardial, with high mortality
- Diarrhoea in only 10%

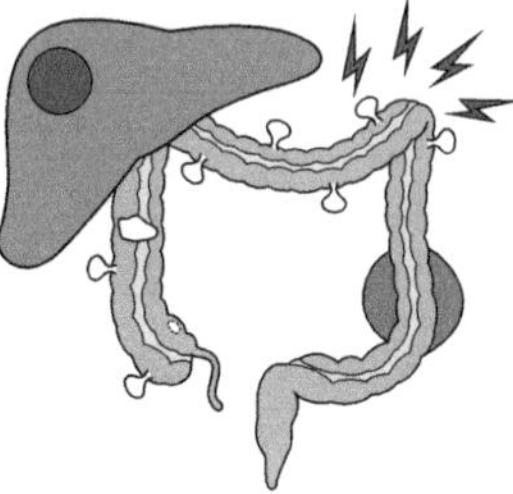

Amoeboma
Colonic or caecal inflammatory mass

Ix

Bloods: Serology: Immunofluorescence or ELISA +ve in 90%, WBC ↑ (not eosinophilia), LFT normal unless abscess causes cholestasis

Micro: Fresh stool micro – cysts, trophozoites found in <40%; WBCs less than in bacillary dysentery

Radiol: USS or CT abdomen – liver abscess esp. right lobe

Special: Colonoscopy: Ulcer biopsy

Rx

Metronidazole (tissue amoebicide) – first 10 days; diloxanide (luminal amoebicide) – second 10 days

Abscess: Aspiration, fluid appears like fish sauce!

Flagellata – motile unicellular organisms

Giardia lamblia (also called *G. intestinalis*) – giardiasis

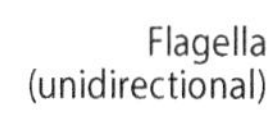

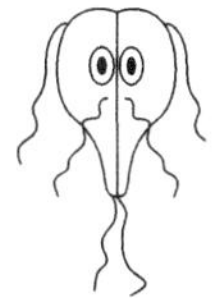

PATH

Cysts in unboiled water (tropical or temperate zones); survive for 2 months

Faecal-oral contact:
- Men who have sex with men
- Nurseries

Immunodeficiency:
- Achlorhydria
- Hypogammaglobulinaemia

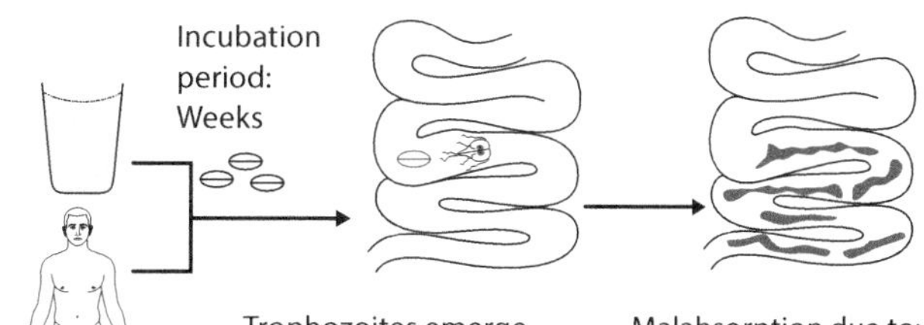

Trophozoites emerge in duodenum-jejunum ('excystation')

Malabsorption due to:
- Functional disaccharidase and bile salt deficiency
- Sub-total villous atrophy and mucosal inflammation

PC

Patient may carry asymptomatically or present with malabsorption:
- Anorexia, weight loss
- Epigastric cramps, flatulence
- Chronic diarrhoea – pale stool, steatorrhoea

Ix

Stool – fresh microscopy: Cysts or trophozoites; 75% sensitivity if sample repeated; no WBCs or RBCs
– stool antigen test (ELISA): Sensitivity 90%, specificity 99%

Duodenal aspirate and/or biopsy: Demonstrates trophozoites with 90% sensitivity

NB: Treatment is often given empirically without need for +ve microscopy, on basis of travel history

Rx

Avoid milk; metronidazole

Ciliate – motile unicellular organisms

Balantidium coli – balantidiasis

Cilia (multidirectional)
Largest protozoan pathogen (100–200 μm)

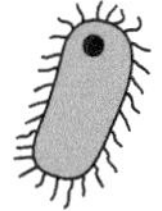

Epi

Transmitted from pigs

PC

Resembles amoebic colitis

Ix

Fresh stool microscopy

Rx

Tetracycline

GENITAL DISCHARGE

Genital discharge

Causes

The following cause urethral or vaginal discharge:

G.U.C.C.I.'S. V.A.G.I.N.A.

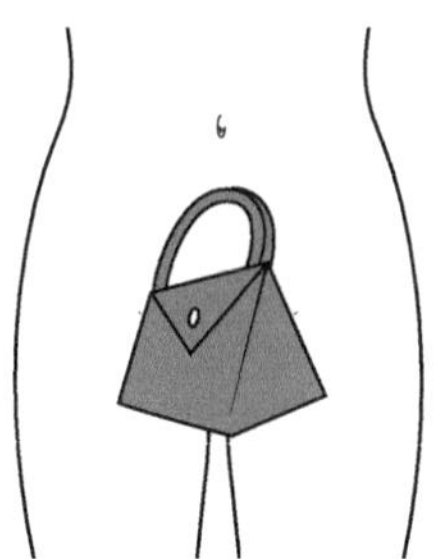

Gonorrhoea
Ulcers, e.g. HSV, syphilis chancre
Chlamydia
Candida
Infections – other:
UTI – Mycoplasma, Ureaplasma, enterobacteria, incl. 2° to pyelonephritis
***S**taphylococcus aureus* ('toxic shock syndrome')
Streptococcus pyogenes (scarletina vulvovaginitis)

***V**aginalis, Trichomonas* = flagellate protozoa:
O/E: Frothy green discharge, strawberry spots in vagina, vulval excoriation
Allergy, foreign body
***G**ardnerella vaginalis* = Gram –ve bacillus
O/E: Thin grey discharge, with fish-like odour after sex
Inflammatory: Crohn fistula
Neoplasia:

- Carcinoma of vulva, vagina, cervix/penile
- Wart (HPV)

Age (physiological): Post-menopausal – atrophic vaginitis

Gonorrhoea *(Neisseria gonorrhoeae)*

Epi Women > men (5:1)

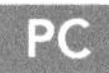

PC

C.R.A.P^2.P^2.E.R.S.!

Conjunctivitis
Rash:

- Maculopapular; vesicular; haemorrhagic; vasculitic-necrotic
- Limbs, esp. on same limb as arthritis

Arthritis (septic or reactive): Migratory polyarthritis or monoarthritis, tenosynovitis, e.g. wrist extensors
Pharyngitis
Penis – **P**rostatitis: Urethral gland and vesiculitis infection → discharge or stricture
Pelvic inflammatory disease – bartholinitis: Often asymptomatic, and so in women, initial infection goes untreated and so septicaemia is more likely
Epididymo-orchitis
Rectum: Asymptomatic; painful defaecation; bloody–purulent discharge
Septicaemia: Meningitis; perihepatitis with adhesions; carditis

Chlamydia *(Chlamydia trachomatis)*

Epi Men > women

PC

a real G.O.A.

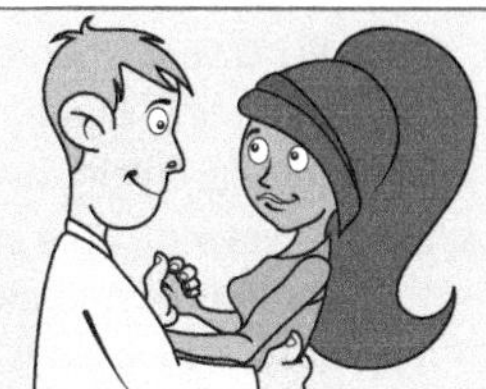

Genital:

- Urethritis (discharge); prostatitis
- Pelvic inflammatory disease; cervicitis

Ophthalmic: Conjunctivitis; anterior uveitis
Arthritis: Lower limb; mono- or oligoarthritis

+ S.C.A.R.E.D. S.L.O.U.C.H.E.R.S.

Spondylosis
Chest: Thoracic spondylosis
Arthritis
Respiratory: Pulmonary infiltrates
Enthesopathy
Dactylitis

Systemic: Fatigue, low-grade fever, anorexia – weight loss
Liver: Fitz–Hugh–Curtis syndrome (perihepatitis + pleural effusion)
Ophthalmic: Conjunctivitis, iridocyclitis, episcleritis
Ulcers: Orogenital, incl. circinate balanitis
Cardiac: Aortic root fibrosis and regurgitation; pericarditis
Haematological: Anaemia of chronic disease
Extra: Meningo-encephalitis, peripheral neuropathy, lymphogranuloma venereum
Respiratory: Chest wall ankylosis, apical fibrosis
Skin: Keratoderma blenorrhagicum; nail ridging, onycholysis

GENITAL ULCERATION

Genital ulceration

Causes

S.H.A.G.G.I.N.' S.C.A.R.S.!!

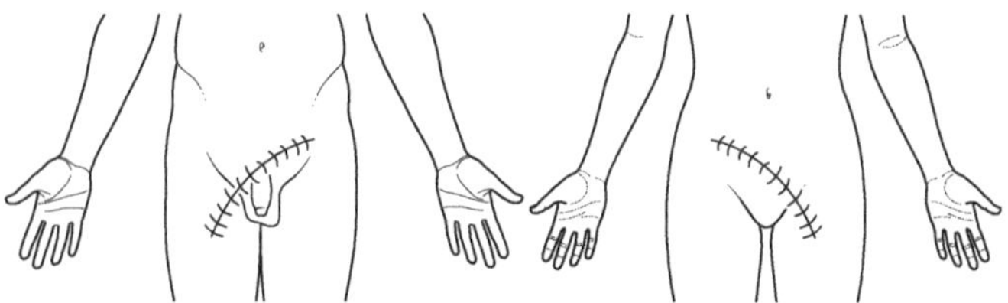

Syphilis (p. 206)
  Primary chancre – single, painless ulcer
  Secondary – multiple, painful ulcers
  Gumma (latency stage between 2° and 3°) – single, painless ulcer
Herpes simplex virus-2/(rarely VZV)
Autoimmune:
  Behçet syndrome
    PC: Orogenital ulcers, uveitis, CNS disease
  Reactive arthritis
    PC: **G.O.A.** – genital (circinate balanitis – single, painless ulcer), ophthalmic, arthritis
  Crohn – single, painless ulcer
Gonorrhoea, chlamydia, candida, trichomonas – causes of urethritis
Granuloma inguinale and other granulomatous:
  Granuloma inguinale (Donovanosis) – *Klebsiella granulomatis*; tropical infection (esp. Papua New Guinea, Durban) – solitary or multiple painless ulcers
  Lymphogranuloma venereum – *Chlamydia trachomatis*; tropical infection (esp. Africa, Caribbean) – painless anal ulcer with inguinal lymphadenopathy
  Tuberculosis – single, painful ulcer
Injury: Trauma
Neoplasia: Squamous carcinoma; associated HPV; single, painless

Scabies, pubic lice; pediculosis; tinea cruris
Chancroid: *Haemophilus ducreyi* ; tropical infection, causing multiple, painful ulcers and inguinal lymphadenopathy ('buboes')
Allergy, e.g. drug reaction, erythema multiforme, Stevens–Johnson syndrome, contact dermatitis – history of particular soap or underwear
Rash – dermatological:
- Lichen sclerosus et atrophicus/leukoplakia – painless
- Lichen planus – itchy mauve papules or annular lesions
- Psoriasis – red + shiny patches, or scaly
- Seborrhoeic dermatitis – scalp, nose, chest also involved

Staphylococcus: Folliculitis, impetigo, *Borrelia vincentii*

Herpes simplex virus-2

Types:
- 1° infection: Extensive lesions, fever, malaise, meningism
- Recurrence: Milder and shorter course; no systemic symptoms; due to stress, illness, menses

PC:
- 1° infection: Extensive lesions, fever, malaise, meningism
- Prodromal symptoms: Tingling 1–2 days before painful ulcers appear
- Superficial dyspareunia: Cervical and vulval lesions
- Dysuria → urinary retention: Urethral; sacral autonomic plexus lesions
- Painful defaecation → constipation: Ano-rectal lesions

O/E:
- Erythema → pustular vesicle in centre → wet ulcer → dry crust
- Inguinal lymphadenopathy

Rx:
- Warm saline baths
- Antibiotics for 2° bacterial infection
- Aciclovir – effective only in 1st week

Granuloma inguinale and other tropical genital ulcers

Granuloma inguinale (Donovanosis) – *Klebsiella granulomatis* = intracellular Gram –ve rod
PC: Genital, anal, inguinal ulceration – deep red ' beefy', contact bleeding, well-circumscribed, painless

Lymphogranuloma venereum – *Chlamydia trachomatis* = obligate intracellular bacteria
PC:
- Commonly presents as painful inguinal lymphadenopathy (buboes), with 'groove sign' due to inelastic inguinal ligament
- Haemorrhagic proctitis, stricture or fistula
- Conjunctivitis, meningoencephalitis

Chancroid: *Haemophilus ducreyi*
PC: Tender, sharply demarcated ulcer, usually on prepuce or coronal sulcus in men, or fourchette or labia majora in women

Scabies and other infestations

Scabies: *Sarcoptes scabiei*
PC: Intense itching, worse at night
O/E: Red papules, scaling, ulceration, bleeding
Ix: Scrape a burrow with a scalpel blade → 10% KOH → microscopy to look for mite
Rx: BHC (benzene hexachloride); malathion; permethrin

Pubic lice/pediculosis (*Phthirus pubis*)
PC: Itch, but no direct rash
Ix: Microscopy
Rx: BHC, carbaryl shampoo

Tinea cruris (fungus: *Trichophyton/Epidermophyton*)
PC: Erythematous, scaly rash with distinct margin, in groin of men
Ix: Scrapings under microscope reveal mycelium
Rx: Benzoic acid ointment, clotrimazole cream

Lichen sclerosus et atrophicus/Leukoplakia

PC:
- White-purple plaques on thin, shiny, atrophic skin, with skin contraction
- Men: BXO (balanitis xerotica obliterans) – urethral pain; phimosis; urinary obstruction
- Women: Pruritus vulvae; superficial dyspareunia
- Complication: squamous cell carcinoma

Ix: Skin biopsy

Rx
Medical: Potent corticosteroid cream
Surgical: Meatal dilation, circumcision

VIRAL EXANTHEMA AND RELATED

Measles

PC Incubation period 2 weeks

M.E.A.S.L.E.S.

Mouth:
- Koplik spots – day 2: Salt-grain spots on buccal mucosa opposite molars
- Stomatitis (primary or secondary to herpes), gingivitis, cancrum oris

Eye:
- Keratoconjunctivitis – glassy red eye, swollen semilunar folds (Meyer's sign)
- Corneal scarring, xerophthalmia, vitamin A deficiency

Abdomen:
- Gastroenteritis: D+V
- Malabsorption from villous atrophy, esp. protein and energy

Skin (day 4):
- Maculopapular rash: post-auricular → face → descent over trunk until 7th day
- Confluent, blotchy; stains, doesn't blanch; peels with healing
- DIC: Purpura – rare complication
- Coincides with peak fever (40°C)

Lung:
- Bacterial pneumonia, esp. staphylococcal, pneumococcal, due to lymphopenia
- Giant-cell pneumonitis: High mortality

Ears: Sinusitis, otitis media

SSPE etc.:

Acute meningo-encephalitis: Autoimmune demyelination post-infection (0.1%)
PC: Deafness; cognitive impairment in 25%; death in 10%
SSPE (subacute sclerosing panencephalitis): Due to persistent viral replication (rare)
PC: 3–12 years post-infection – cognitive impairment, ataxia, myoclonus, seizures

Mumps

PC Incubation period 2–3 weeks

M.U.M.P.S.

Mouth: Bilateral parotitis
Uro-genital: Orchitis, oophoritis (both associated with infertility), mastalgia
Meningo-encephalitis (lymphocytic CSF), deafness, otalgia
Pancreatitis, or just elevated serum amylase
Severe: Myocarditis

Rubella

PC Incubation period 2–3 weeks

R.U.B.E.L.I.A.

Rash:
- Discrete, pink, punctate macules that become confluent; spread from face to trunk
- Purpura: Due to thrombocytopenia

Unnoticed: Often asymptomatic, or only mild 'cold'-like symptoms in children
Babies – congenital infection: Cataracts, cardiac, deafness, microcephaly
Eyes: Conjunctivitis; pharyngitis – usual first symptoms
Lymphadenopathy: Suboccipital
Arthralgia: Rheumatoid pattern

Varicella (chicken pox)

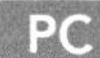

Incubation period 2 weeks

S.O.R.E.

Skin – vesicular rash:

- Day 0: Sparse, erythematous, maculopapular rash; coincides with low-grade pyrexia
- Day 2: Central distribution of itchy, elliptical vesicles and pustules, in 'crops', i.e. different areas at different stages of development
- Day 5: Crusts – separates from lesion without scarring, by 10th day temperature recedes
- Complications: Haemorrhagic rash scarring due to scratching or secondary staphylococcal infection

Oral ulcers: Pharynx and oesophagus – dysphagia

Respiratory: Pneumonitis due to ulcers spreading to upper respiratory tract

PC: Acute: Severe pulmonary oedema, chest pain, haemoptysis

Chronic: Lung fibrosis (CXR – diffuse nodular opacification)

Encephalitis, meningo:

- May just present as headache (common)
- Associated with cerebellar ataxia that recovers

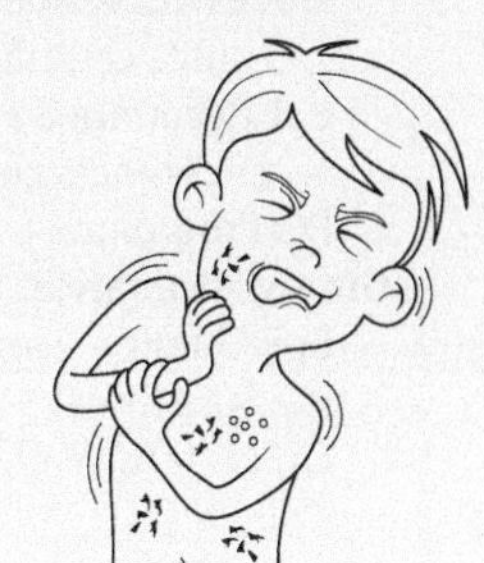

NB: More severe in adults, neonates and immunocompromised

Rx

Supportive: Avoid scratching; daily chlorhexidine washes; flucloxacillin if spots are infected
Aciclovir or famciclovir: For adults or infants, within 24 hours of rash
VZV Ig: For exposed non-immune pregnancies and to subsequent newborns; immunocompromised

Parvovirus B19 (erythema infectiosum)

Epi

Occurs in 2-yearly epidemics, every 4 years, during winter–spring
Immunity occurs in 70% of population (one attack confers lifelong immunity)

Incubation period 2 weeks

F.A.C.E. *(cheeks)*

Fever, mild and 'cold'-like symptoms during 1st week of infection

Arthralgia: Commonest symptom in adults, esp. women; lasts weeks

Cheeks: 'Slapped-cheek' syndrome – lacy, reticular erythema over face

Extreme:

Aplastic crisis or chronic anaemia:

- Esp. in sickle cell disease, thalassaemics, immunocompromised
- Due to viral replication in erythroid progenitor cells
- Rx: IVIg

Miscarriage or hydrops fetalis if acquired *in utero*: Rx: Intrauterine blood transfusion

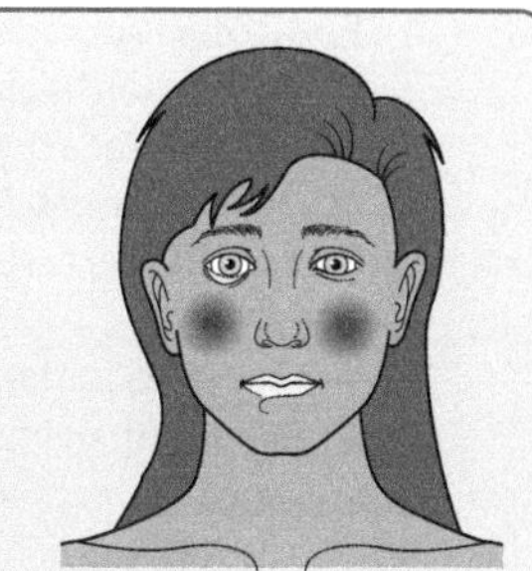

HERPES SIMPLEX VIRUS

PC

G.O. S.O.O.N.

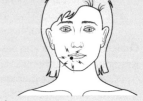

Genital/anal, cervical ulcers usually HSV-2 (unless oral sex with HSV-1 carrier) – see p. 191

Oral: Usually HSV-1

Herpes labialis ('cold sore'):
- PATH: Virus resides in trigeminal dorsal root ganglion; reactivation causes centrifugal migration to skin
- Epi: Recurrence assoc. with stress, menses, infections (e.g. pneumococcus, malaria), UV-light
- PC: Prodrome of skin tingling 1–2 days pre-eruption

Gingivostomatitis:
- Epi: Children – severe disease; adults – mild
- PC: Sore throat → drooling; perioral vesicles; fever, lymphadenopathy
- O/E: Extensive ulcers with yellow slough over entire oral cavity

Skin

Herpetic whitlow:
- Epi: Children, medical personnel (due to excretion from ill patients)
- PC: Minor trauma to hand results in painful, red finger; vesicles; fever, lymphadenopathy; may recur with pain and oedema

Herpes gladiatorum:
- Epi: Contact sports players
- PC: Virus pressed into skin by force, similar to whitlow

Eczema herpeticum, or superinfection of other skin disease (e.g. burns):
- Epi: Children or immunosuppresssed (incl. steroid Rx)
- PC: Extensive, painful vesicles occur on eczema

Erythema multiforme

Ophthalmic

Keratoconjunctivitis:

PC:
- Acute: Painful, red eye; lacrimation, photophobia; chemosis (subconjunctival oedema)
- Chronic: Corneal 'dendritic' ulcers (appear as many branches under fluorescein staining)

Organs: Pneumonitis, hepatitis, oesophagitis, DIC – in immunocompromised

Neurological:

Encephalitis:
- Epi: Occurs sporadically without apparent risk factors
- PATH: Haemorrhagic necrosis of temporal lobes, orbitofrontal cortex, due to HSV-1
- PC: Fever, headache, N+V; complex partial seizures; confusion; coma
- Ix: MRI – temporal lobe oedema; CSF – lymphocytes, PCR; EEG – periodic lateralized discharges
- Rx: IV aciclovir; carbamazepine or other AEDs

Meningitis:
- Occurs as part of 1° HSV-2 infection with genital ulcers
- Recurrent, mild, self-limiting, Mollaret's meningitis (probably HSV-2-mediated)

Bell's palsy

EPSTEIN–BARR VIRUS

PC

G.O.E.S. S.L.O.W.L.Y[5].

Glandular fever
Oral: Pharyngo-tonsillitis – pearly, white **E**xudate, with petechiae at junction of hard and soft palate (oral hairy leukoplakia – white plaques that form on side of tongue in AIDS)
Systemic: Fever

Skin:

- Maculopapular rash esp. if patient inadvertently given amoxicillin (90% pts. get in this case)
- Periorbital oedema

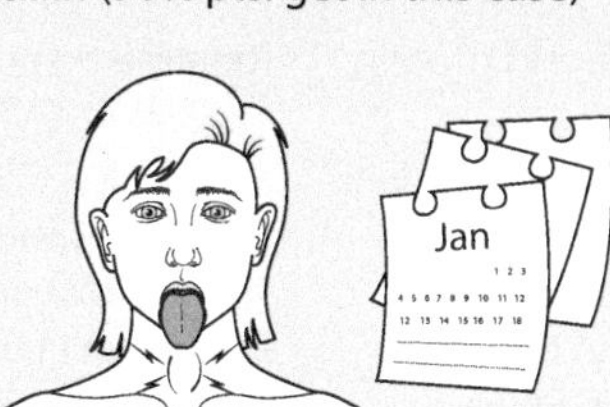

Lymphadenopathy: Generalized
Organomegaly: Hepatosplenomegaly (± splenic rupture)
White blood cell count:

- Lymphocyotsis: WCC = 10–50 × 10^9/l
- 'Atypical lymphocytes' on blood film – also seen in:
    - Other infections: CMV, hepatitis A, HIV, rubella, brucella, toxoplasmosis
    - Non-infective: CLL, mycosis fungoides; drug reaction

Liver: Hepatitis (jaundice may occur due to both hepatitis and haemolytic anaemia)
Y: c**Y**topenias:

- Thrombocytopenia – due to splenomegaly
- Autoimmune haemolytic anaemia (IgM cold agglutinins)

m**Y**elitis, transverse + other neurological: Menigoencephalitis; peripheral neuropathy; Guillain–Barré syndrome
ps**Y**chiatric: Prolonged malaise for several months post-infection, or rarely, 'chronic fatigue syndrome'
m**Y**ocarditis, pericarditis, pneumonitis
l**Y**mphoma: Associated with EBV esp. Burkitt lymphoma (occurs in African children immunosuppressed with malaria. PC: jaw mass)
EBV is also associated with nasopharyngeal carcinoma

Ix

Heterophile antibodies, e.g. Monospot – relies on differential absorption of antibodies by different test cells:

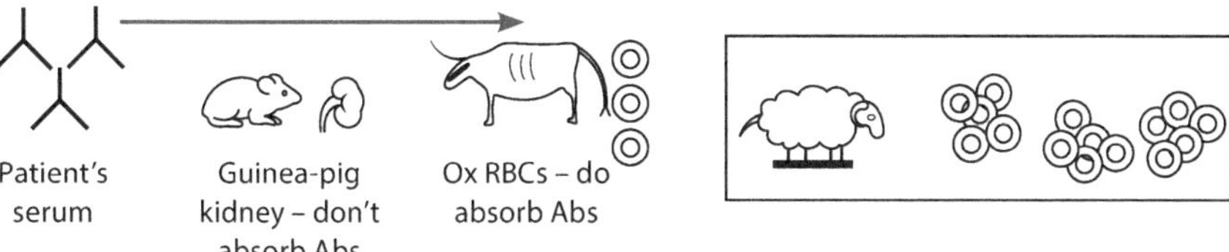

(also seen in: rubella, malaria; hepatitis; SLE; lymphoma, adenocarcinoma)

HIV – PATHOGENESIS

PATH

The RNA genome of HIV is converted to dsDNA within the host cell, and is there integrated within the host genome to form a DNA 'provirus'

This may later be transcribed and translated back to form numerous virions

The genome codes for 3 structural/enzyme proteins and 3 regulatory proteins:

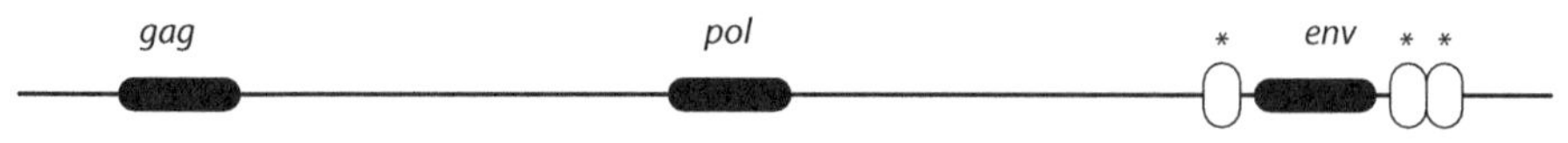

Nucleocapsid	Polymerase enzymes etc.	Envelope	Regulatory proteins*
p24 capsid protein + p17 matrix protein + nucleocapsid protein that coats diploid RNA	**Reverse transcriptase:** Converts viral RNA into dsDNA **Integrase:** Integrates dsDNA into host genome **Protease:** Enables budding of new virion from host cell	Gp120 = surface glycoprotein gp41 = transmembrane glycoprotein	Tat: ↑ transcription Rev: ↑ transfer to cytoplasm Nef (negative factor): ↓ CD4, MHC-I

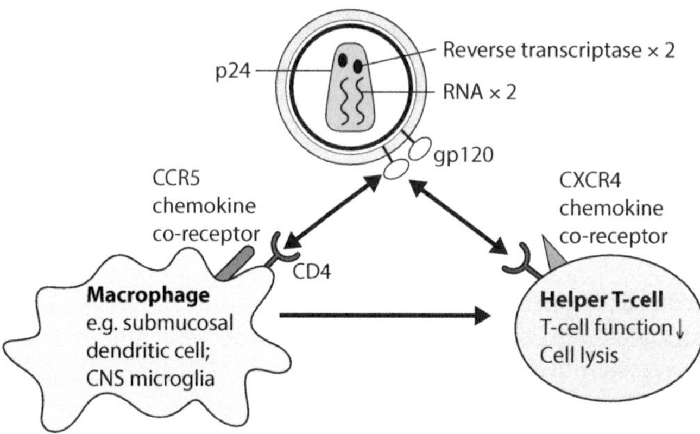

Entry

- Virus enters macrophages or helper T cells via gp120–CD4 interaction, facilitated by co-receptor
- HIV genome evolves to use CXCR4 co-receptor more efficiently, during course of infection

Integration

- RNA homes in on nucleus via nuclear transport signals, e.g. p. 177
- Integration of viral RNA into host genome enabled via viral 'integrase', even in cells not actively dividing

  Latency: Viral DNA remains inactive for a variable period, depending on immune surveillance

Transcription–translation

- Cellular DNA polymerase begins transcription of 'instability' sequences that code for Tat regulatory protein
- Tat re-enters nucleus and binds to specific Tat-responsive elements, which amplifies transcription

Capsid assembly – budding

- Proteins assembled on rough ER and free ribosomes before being packaged
- Incorporates host protein called 'cyclophilin' (essential for replication); protease required for budding

HIV – NATURAL HISTORY

1. Inoculation: 3 weeks – 3 months

2. Seroconversion (70% are symptomatic): **G.A.I.N.**

Glandular-fever-like: Maculopapular rash, sore throat, aphthous ulcers, fever, lymphadenopathy
Arthralgia, myalgia
Intestinal: Diarrhoea, weight loss
Neurological: Meningo-encephalitis, retro-orbital pain, peripheral neuropathy, myelopathy

Ix: p24 antigenaemia, lymphopenia (initially all lymphocyte types; later CD4 ↓, CD8 ↑)

90% enter asymptomatic stage; 10% progress immediately and rapidly

3. Latency stage: 1–5% patients are long-term non-progressors = up to 8 years without symptoms or drop on CD4 count

4. Persistent generalized lymphadenopathy (PGL): Enlarged lymph node (>1 cm), in 2 or more extra-inguinal sites for >3 months, without obvious cause

AIDS-related complex (ARC) – early symptomatic disease: **G.O.S.H.**

General: Wasting, fever, diarrhoea
Oral: Candida, oral hairy leukoplakia (EBV), aphthous ulcers
Skin: Molluscum contagiosum, shingles, HSV, seborrhoeic dermatitis, psoriasis, condylomata accuminatum
Haematology: ITP (assoc. anti-gpl20), anaemia

5. AIDS

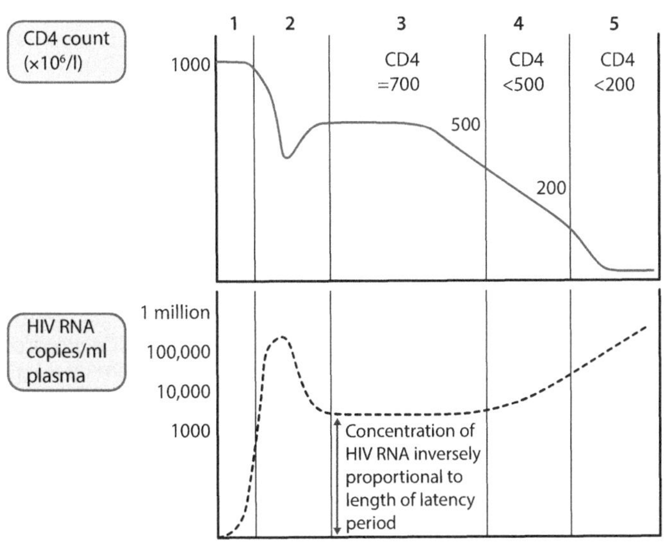

HIV – CLINICAL

PC

Neurological – ophthalmological

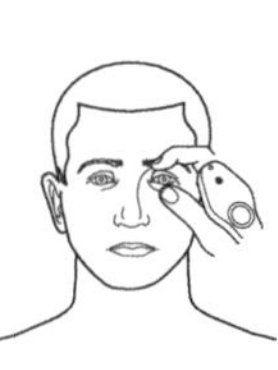

CNS:
- Meningitis: HIV ('aseptic') – at seroconversion or during early AIDS
- Cryptococcus, TB, histoplasmosis, coccidioidomycosis, syphilis
- Mass lesion: Toxoplasmosis, lymphoma, Kaposi's sarcoma, tuberculoma, cryptococcoma
- Cerebral atrophy: HIV-dementia complex in 25% AIDS
- White-matter: Progressive multifocal leucoencephalopathy (PML) – polyoma JC virus
- Cord: HIV vacuolar myelopathy (dorsal columns), HtLV-I, HSV, VzV, CMV, syphilis, TB

PNS:
- Roots: CMV polyradiculopathy, esp. lumbosacral – sacral pain, incontinence, paraparesis
- Peripheral nerves: Guillain–Barré syn.; glove and stocking or mononeuritis multiplex due to HIV, e.g. facial nerve palsy
- Myopathy

Retinitis:
- HIV 'cotton wool spots'; CMV retinitis – 'cheese + tomato pizza'; HSV, VZV – necrosis
- Toxoplasmosis, *Pneumocystis carinii*, candida, syphilitic papillitis

Respiratory

Bacterial:
- Community-acquired pneumonia, sinusitis
- TB, multidrug-resistant TB, MAI

Fungal:
- *Pneumocystis jirovecii* pneumonia – 80% develop without prophylaxis
- *Cryptococcus, Candida, Histoplasma, Aspergillus*

Viral: CMV; HSV, VZV, EBV – lymphocytic pneumonitis
Neoplasm: Kaposi's sarcoma (HHV-8), lymphoma
Pulmonary hypertension

Cardiac

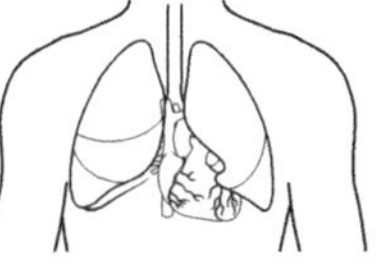

Pericardial effusion
Myocarditis:
- Due to HIV or *Cryptococcus*
- Results in arrhythmias, dilated cardiomyopathy

Marantic endocarditis

GIT

Mouth: Aphthous ulcers, HSV, VZV
Oesophagitis: *Candida,* CMV, HSV, VZV
Gastroenteritis:
- HIV enteropathy = diarrhoea >1 month, no other cause
- *Cryptosporidium/Microsporidium/Isospora belli*
- *Entamoeba histolytica*/giardiasis
- *Shigella, Salmonella, Campylobacter,* atypical TB (MAI)
- CMV colitis

Neoplasia: Kaposi's sarcoma (HHV-8), lymphoma

Abdominal – other

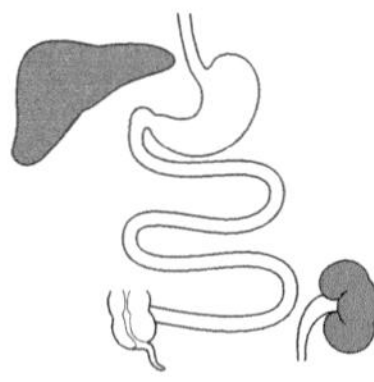

Liver – MAI: Hepatitis; ALP ↑
Pancreas: Acute pancreatitis (often 2° to Rx)
Renal: Focal segmental glomerulosclerosis – nephrotic syndrome

Skin/Genito-urinary

Skin:
- Viral:
  - VZV: severe chickenpox, multifocal zoster
  - HHV-8: Kaposi's sarcoma
- Bacteria: *Bartonella henselae* – bacillary angiomatosis
- Fungi: Umbilicated rash (cryptococcosis), tinea

Mucosa (penis, vagina, cervix, anus):
- HSV, HPV: Cervical or anal carcinoma, esp. invasive
- Other STDs: *Candida, Chlamydia, Trichomonas*

Other

Arthritis: HIV, *Cryptococccus*, reactive, Sjögren
Endocrine: Primary weight loss, hypogonadism
Cytopenias due to:
- Bone marow suppression due to HIV, TB, MAI
- Autoimmune: ITP, haemolysis
- Lymphoma, drug-related

Rx

Highly-active anti-retroviral therapy (HAART)

NARTIs (nucleoside analogue reverse transcriptase inhibitors):
- Drugs: Zidovudine (AZT), didanosine (ddI), zalcitabine (ddC), lamivudine (3TC), stavudine
- Mechanism: Phosphorylated to triphosphate, and are then incorporated into growing DNA chain, thereby blocking further chain extension

NNARTIs (non-nucleoside analogue reverse transcriptase inhibitors):
- Drugs: Nevirapine, efavirenz
- Mechanism: Do not require phosphorylation

PIs (protease inhibitors):
- Drugs: Indinavir, ritonavir, saquinavir
- Mechanism: Prevent viral budding

Combination: (2 NARTIs and 1 NNARTI) or (2 NARTIs and 1 or 2 PIs)

Indications:
Primary infection (i.e. within 6 months of contracting)
CD4 count <500/µl, or viral load >30,000 copies/ml
Symptoms, esp. dementia
Pregnancy: ↓ risk of transmission (also use caesarean, formula-feed)

Side-effects:

A.N.G.R^2.Y.

Anaemia macrocytic (+ other cytopenias); Acidosis, lactic
Neurological: Peripheral neuropathy, myopathy (lamivudine), cognitive (efavirenz)
GIT: Anorexia, N+V, diarrhoea (ritonavir); renal stones (indinavir); pancreatitis (ddI)
Resistance: With NNARTI, cross-resistance occurs between drugs
Reconstitution: Immune syndrome – flare-up of subclinical infection on starting or on withdrawal, e.g. hep B with lamivudine
Y: lipod**Y**strophy syndrome: Fat redistribution

Opportunistic infection – Treatment

Neurology:
- TB meningitis: As for pulmonary TB, but for 1-year duration
- *Cryptococcus*: Amphotericin + 5-flucytosine IV, fluconazole
- *Toxoplasma*: Pyrimethamine + sulphadiazine, or clindamycin
- Lymphoma: Dexamethasone and radiotherapy
- CMV retinitis: Ganciclovir IV (Ix: FBC, LFT), foscarnet IV (Ix: U&E)

Pneumonia:
- TB: **R.I.P.E.** (p. 203) – NB: Interaction with HAART; multi-drug resistance common
- *Pneumocystis*: Co-trimoxazole (trimethoprim + sulphamethoxazole)/dapsone + pentamidine

GIT:
- Oesophagitis: *Candida* – fluconazole; CMV – ganciclovir; HSV – acyclovir
- *Cryptosporidium*: Paromomycin – decreases stool volume, but doesn't eradicate
- *Salmonella* or *Campylobacter*: Ciprofloxacin
- MAI: Azithromycin or clarithromycin

Opportunistic infection – Prophylactic

Pneumocystis: Cotrimoxazole or dapsone
Candida: Amphotericin lozenges or oral fluconazole
TB/MAI: Rifabutin

Other

Aphthous ulcers of mouth and oesophagus: Corticosteroids, thalidomide
Weight loss: Testosterone or anabolic steroids, growth hormone

TUBERCULOSIS – CLINICAL

Epi

Inc: Resource-rich countries: 5/100,000 p.a.; resource-poor: 500/100,000 p.a.
Most important disease in world: Prevalence: 1/3 world population; 3 million die of TB p.a.
Increasing incidence, due to AIDS; drug resistance ↑ ; vaccination ↓
Age: Children and elderly most at risk, as cell-mediated immunity impaired
Geo: Asian immigrants: Come from endemic areas
Inner city homeless: Due to malnutrition, alcohol; overcrowding; BCG uptake ↓
Black ethnicity: Genetic predisposition?
Aet: *Mycobacterium tuberculosis:* Spread by aerosol or dust
M. bovis: Spread by unpasteurized milk (mainly children) – GIT, bone, renal disease
Pre: Any impairment of cell-mediated immunity – **5 Ds**:
Drugs: Steroids, chemotherapy/BCG not given
Drug addicts, intravenous, esp. because of AIDS; alcoholics
Debility: Dementia, diabetes, renal failure
Deficiency: Malnutrition, esp. vitamin D deficiency; malabsorption, e.g. post-gastrectomy
Dust: Silicosis (metal or quarry workers); medical personnel

PATH

1° infection

Ghon focus = midzone, subpleural, acute inflammatory lesion
Regional hilar lymph nodes → may cause obstruction and lobar collapse

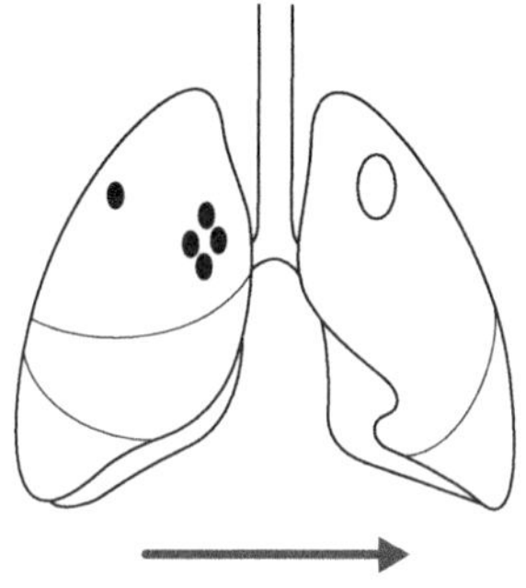

Post-1° infection

Assmann focus = caseating granuloma
Granuloma may:

- Fibrose and simply calcify, or
- Cavitate (coalesces with others)
- Invade lung

PC

Asymptomatic or self-limiting, e.g. slight cough, fever, fatigue
Delayed type hypersensitivity (2–3 weeks post-infection):

- Phylectenular conjunctivitis
- Erythema nodosum
- Lymphadenopathy

Lung invasion or miliary spread occurs in only 5% at this stage

Reinfection or reactivation due to:

- Genetic predisposition
- Virulent strain
- Cell-mediated immunity ↓, e.g. steroid therapy

Epithelioid cells (plump macrophages) or Langhan's giant cells in centre of granuloma)

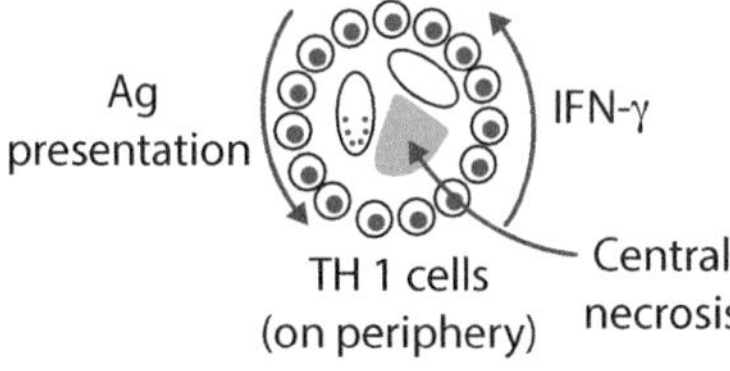

PC

Constitutional: Due to cytokines:

- Fatigue, malaise (IFN-γ)
- Anorexia, weight loss (TNF-α)
- Fever, night sweats (IL-1)

Lung invasion:

- Due to granuloma invasion of bronchus or pulmonary artery, or lymphatics (→ SVC)
- Presents as cough, esp. with green sputum or haemoptysis; chest pain

Miliary spread due to granuloma invasion of pulmonary vein

PC

R.A^7.N.S.A.C.K.S. *the whole body!*

Respiratory **P.O.P^2.U.L.A.r. presentations!**

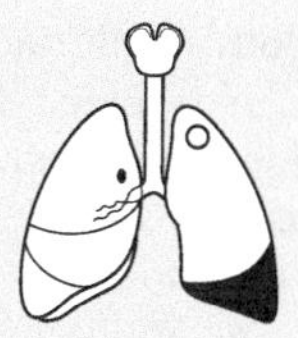

Pneumonia: Lobar or bronchial

Obstruction, bronchial:

- Lobar collapse (1° infection)
- Bronchiectasis (post 1°)

Pleurisy/**P**leural effusion/empyema; if left for long, forms chest wall sinus ('empyema necessitans')

Upper respiratory tract: Laryngitis, tonsillitis, otitis media

Lymphadenopathy, cervical

Abscess, upper zone:

- Cavitation → massive haemoptysis/mycetoma
- Fibrocalcification: tracheal deviation

Abdominal

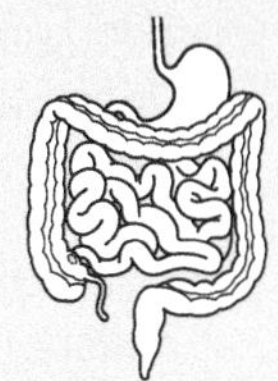

Acute peritonitis: Diffuse, abdominal pain, due to disseminated miliary tubercules

Adenitis, mesenteric: Right iliac fossa pain and mass (ileo-caecal lymph nodes)

Abscess, psoas: Painful or painless groin swelling; femoral neuropathy

Ascites: High protein content

Adhesions: Bowel obstruction

Addison crisis: Due to adrenal granulomas

PATH: Colonisation occurs via:

- Swallowing sputum or milk *(M. bovis)*
- Blood or transcoelomic spread (i.e. from ovaries)

Neurological

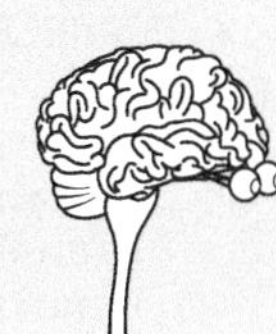

Basal meningitis-encephalitis:

- Headaches, confusion, hydrocephalus, SIADH
- Focal neurology (cranial neuropathy), tuberculoma, infarct

Fundus: Choroiditis (miliary tubercles), papilloedema

Cord: Spinal meningitis, block

Skin

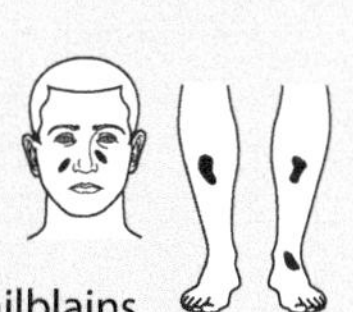

Lupus vulgaris: Red-brown scaly plaques, scars

Erythema nodosum: Tender

Erythema induratum (Bazin disease): Deep purple, ulcerating nodules; assoc. chilblains

Papulo-necrotic tuberculides: Firm, dusky, ulcerating papules on elbows, knees

Arthritis-osteomyelitis

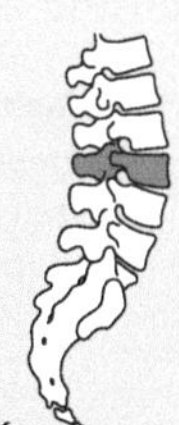

PATH: Subchondral osteomyelitis → cartilage invasion: synovitis → may form sinus

Types:

- Spine: Discitis, vertebral collapse (kyphosis or 'gibbus') – esp. children
- Knee, hip, ankle, esp. adults

Cardiac

Pericardial effusion, constrictive pericarditis; O/E: Pulsus paradoxus; Kussmaul's sign; knock

Kidney

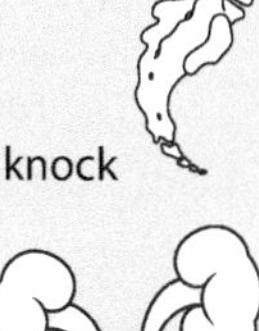

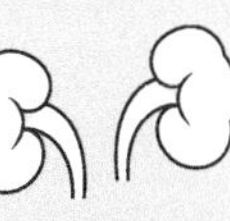

Nephritis – cortex granulomas: PC: Painless haematuria, loin pain

Ureter blockage → hydro- or pyonephrosis; chronic renal failure

Cystitis

Sexual organs

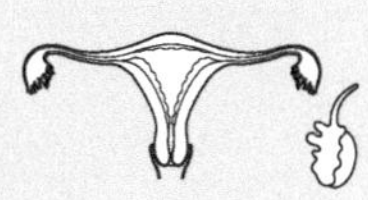

Salpingitis: PC: Fever, peritonitis, cervical excitation, amenorrhoea, infertility

Complications: Endometriosis, oophoritis, vulvitis

Epididymo-orchitis: Unilateral, hard painless testis swelling; 'string of beads' vas

TUBERCULOSIS – IX AND RX

Ix

Bloods: FBC: Monocytosis
ESR: ↑↑
Urine: 3× early-morning urines (EMUs) – see Micro
Micro:
Pulmonary:
- Sputum, early morning: Induce with hypertonic saline or gastric lavage, ×3
- Bronchoscopy: Bronchoalveolar lavage (BAL), transbronchial biopsy (TBB)
- Pleural: Aspirate, biopsy
- Mediastinal lymph node biopsy, via mediastinoscopy or thoracotomy

Extrapulmonary:
- Skin: Lymph node, rash, sinus
- Urine: Early morning ×3
- Blood (special culture bottles); bone marrow biopsy

Laboratory:
- Staining: Alcohol + acid fast bacilli – Ziehl-Nielsen/auramine stain
- Culture: Lowenstein–Jensen medium:
  - Slow growth: 1–8 weeks (each round of replication takes 24 h)
  - Cultures appear 'rough, tough + buff': Dry, crumbly, not easily smeared
- Serology (ELISA/haemagglutination): Protein Ags 5, 6; plasma membrane Ag
- PCR/RFLP: Tracks different strains, e.g. outbreaks, multi-drug resistance

Radiol: CXR

1° infection:
Mediastinal lymphadenopathy
Bronchial obstruction:
- Lobar collapse
- Bronchiectasis (long-standing)

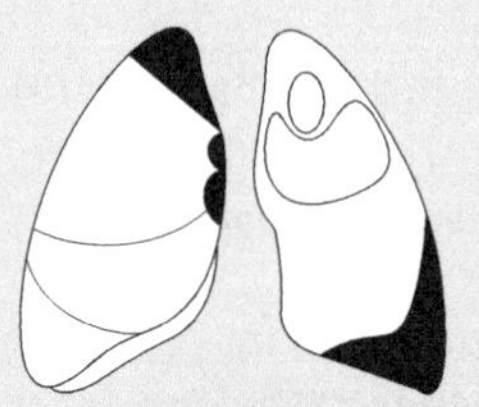

Pleural effusion

Post-1° infection:
Fibrocalcification
Cavitate
Invasion: Pneumonia

Skin test – Tuberculin:

Mantoux: Needle injection
Heaf: Circle of needles
Ingredient: Intradermal injection of PPD (purified protein derivative)
Dose: 1 unit if TB expected, or 10 units if high sensitivity required

Mantoux: Disc diameter >10 mm = +ve or >15 mm if previous BCG)
measure induration, not erythema
Heaf: Ring of induration = +ve (or confluent disc if previous BCG)

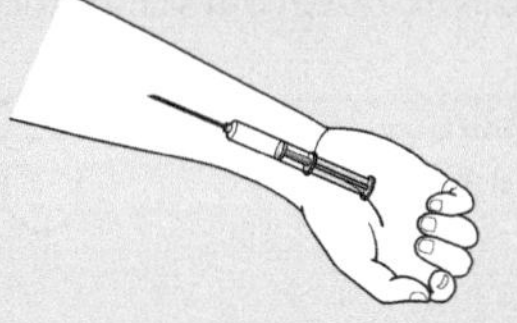

48–72 hours
i.e. time for
delayed-type
hypersensitivity

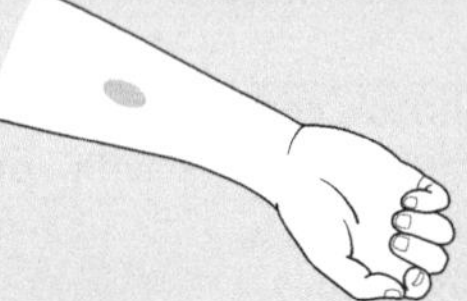

False –ve ('anergy'): Miliary TB; co-existent HIV, measles, EBV
False +ve: Previous BCG/infection; atypical mycobacteria
Side-effect: Ulceration, abscess, lymphadenopathy

Rx

R.I.P.P.E.R.S^3.!!

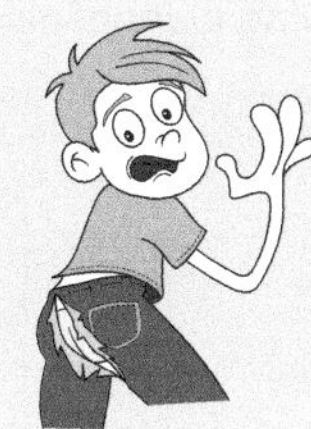

Rifampicin: RNA polymerase inhibitor
Isoniazid: Mycolic acid + metabolism inhibitor
+ **P**yridoxine (vitamin B6): Protects against isoniazid-induced, neuropathy esp. in alcoholics, diabetics
Pyrazinamide
Ethambutol

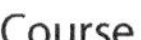

Course

6 months: **R.I.P.E.** for 2 months → **R.I.** for further 4 months (as these 2 drugs are bacterio**cidal**)
9 months: Immunocompromised or multi-drug-resistant TB
12 months: Extrapulmonary or miliary TB
Compliance must be ensured: Check urine is orange; use 'directly-observed therapy' (DOTS)
☠ TB drugs can cause rash, N+V and hepatitis, but the following side-effects are drug-specific:

Rifampicin:	Diarrhoea, stains bodily fluids orange, incl. contact lenses, liver inducer (e.g. reduces effectiveness of some medications)
Isoniazid:	Fulminant liver failure, peripheral neuropathy, optic neuritis, SLE, ITP (NB: If patient has slow-acetylator status then ↑ efficacy, but ↑ side-effects)
Pyrazinamide:	Vomiting prominent, gout (↓ urate excretion), sideroblastic anaemia
Ethambutol:	Optic neuritis (colour vision must be checked at start and during follow-up), gout

Resistant TB (multi-drug resistant TB [MDR-TB]):

High-risk groups:

- AIDS or IVDU; alcoholics; children
- Travel from MDR-endemic area, e.g. Africa, Korea; or nosocomially acquired
- Inadequate previous anti-TB Rx , esp. if prolonged

Rx: **R.I.P.E.** + **M**acrolide: Azithromycin, clarithromycin
Aminoglycoside: Capreomycin ☠ Vertigo, deafness, renal toxicity
Cycloserine (+ pyridoxine) ☠ Vertigo, fits, psychosis; megaloblastic anaemia
Ciprofloxacin

Steroids: Oral glucocorticoids used in TB meningitis or CNS tuberculoma; pericardial or pleural effusions
Surgery, e.g. for spinal disease: Osteomyelitis/orchidectomy
Source isolate or face-mask while still has +ve sputum smears (usually within 1 week of starting Rx) + contact-trace + notify CDC

Prophylaxis

BCG:

- **Intramuscular** injection of live, attenuated *Mycobacterium bovis*
- Given in UK only to neonates at risk (e.g. immigrants from high-prevalence areas); health-care workers

Isoniazid in exposed children with +ve Heaf test

MYCOBACTERIA

The following types of mycobacteria occur:

T.A.X. S.L.U.M.

Mycobacterium	**T***uberculosis* (see p. 200)
	A*vium intracellulare/cheloni*
	X*enopi/kansasii*
	S*crofulaceum*
	L*eprae:* Leprosy (see p. 205)
	U*lcerans:* Buruli ulcer
	M*arinum*: Fish-tank granuloma

Atypical Mycobacteria

M. avium intracellulare* (MAI)/*M. cheloni

Epi: Immunocompromised – terminal phase of AIDS (CD4 count <50/mm^3); elderly

M.A.I.

Megaly: Hepatosplenomegaly (ALP ↑), lymphadenopathy
Anaemia: Bone marrow infiltration
Intestine: Chronic diarrhoea, weight loss + systemic – fever, night sweats

Ix: Cultures from urine, stool; blood; bone marrow; liver; lymph node

Rx:

Needs **C.A^2.R^2.E.**

Clofazimine, Ciprofloxacin
Azithromycin (or clarithromycin), **A**mikacin
Rifampicin, **R**ifabutin (also used as prophylaxis in AIDS)
Ethambutol

***M. xenopi/kansasii*/MAI**

Epi: Occurs in pre-existing lung lesions, e.g. bronchiectasis, fibrosis
PC: Lung cavities (but note that sputum cultures may be +ve in healthy people)

***M. scrofulaceum*/MAI**

Epi: Children
PC: Lymphadenitis

M. ulcerans: 'Buruli ulcer'

Epi: Tropics
PC: Indurated, fluctuant nodule that breaks down to form painless ulcer with necrotic base and extensive scarring

M. marinum: 'Fish-tank granuloma'

Epi: Fish collectors, swimming pools
PC: Painless nodular ulcer

LEPROSY

Epi

Inc: 10 million cases worldwide
Age: In endemic areas, acquired in childhood, but not manifest until teens – 30s
Geo: Tropics, Mediterranean, Southern USA
Aet: *M. leprae* spread by nasal aerosol from lepromatous leprosy patients; prolonged contact required, but bacteria may survive for <7 days outside of body

PC

Incubation period 2–15 years, as leprosy has slowest bacterial replication (12 days per cycle!)

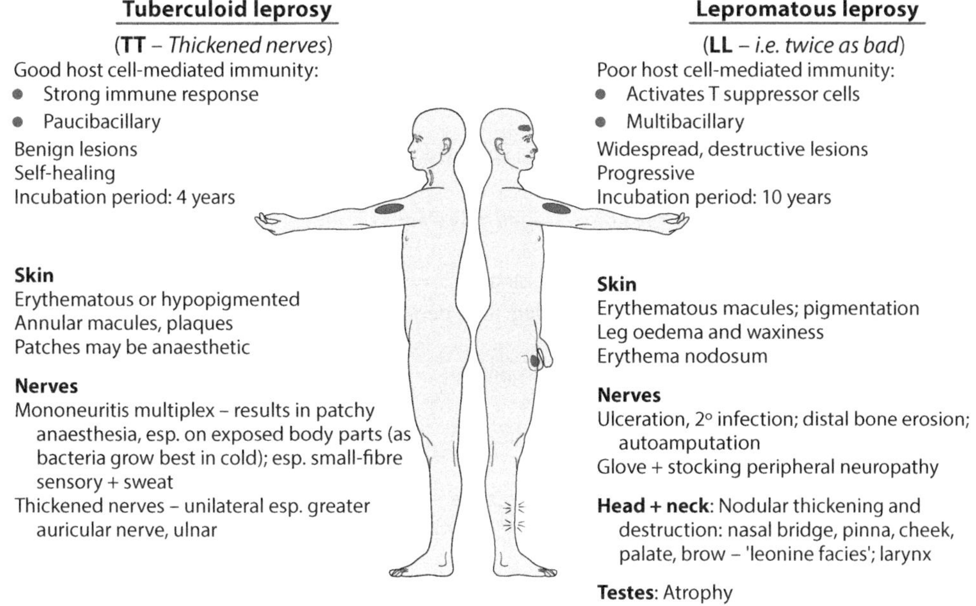

Tuberculoid leprosy
(**TT** – *Thickened nerves*)
Good host cell-mediated immunity:
• Strong immune response
• Paucibacillary
Benign lesions
Self-healing
Incubation period: 4 years
Skin
Erythematous or hypopigmented
Annular macules, plaques
Patches may be anaesthetic
Nerves
Mononeuritis multiplex – results in patchy anaesthesia, esp. on exposed body parts (as bacteria grow best in cold); esp. small-fibre sensory + sweat
Thickened nerves – unilateral esp. greater auricular nerve, ulnar
Lepromatous leprosy
(**LL** – *i.e. twice as bad*)
Poor host cell-mediated immunity:
• Activates T suppressor cells
• Multibacillary
Widespread, destructive lesions
Progressive
Incubation period: 10 years
Skin
Erythematous macules; pigmentation
Leg oedema and waxiness
Erythema nodosum
Nerves
Ulceration, 2° infection; distal bone erosion; autoamputation
Glove + stocking peripheral neuropathy
Head + neck: Nodular thickening and destruction: nasal bridge, pinna, cheek, palate, brow – 'leonine facies'; larynx
Testes: Atrophy

Ix

Bloods: IgM ↑, ESR ↑ ; TPHA, Rh factor, ANA are often +ve
Lepromin tests:

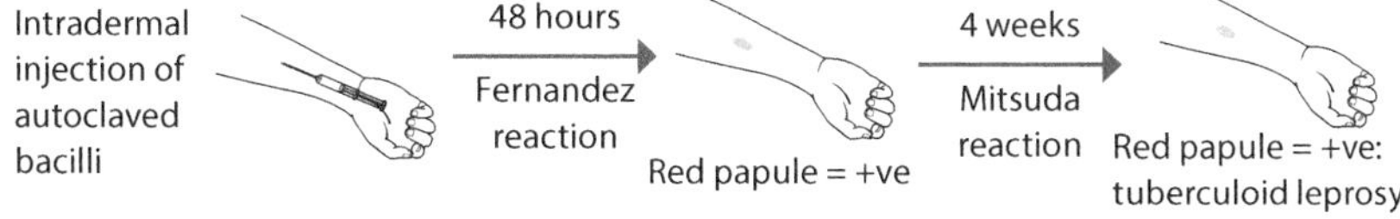

Biopsy: From skin scraping (either type); nerve biopsy (TT only); nasal septum scraping (LL only)
Laboratory:
- Acid-fast bacilli smear for *M. leprae*
- Inoculation: In armadillo or mouse foot pad (can't culture on artificial media!)

Rx

Medical: Dapsone + clofazimine + rifampicin
- Duration: 6 months (tuberculoid leprosy); 2 years or more (lepromatous leprosy)
- Dapsone: Neuropathy, erythema nodosum; N+V; Clofazimine: Blue-black skin lesions, red urine
- Steroids may be needed if lesions worsen acutely on starting Rx ('reversal reaction')

Surgical: Amputation
Prophylaxis: BCG may protect, esp. in children

SYPHILIS

Treponema pallidum

Epi

Transmitted sexually (horizontal) and transplacentally (vertical); rarely via blood products or fomites

C.L.O^2.U^2.D.Y. A.G.A^3.I.N.

Chancre: Painless papule, breaks down to ulcer and erythematous ring on genitals, anus or mouth
Lymphadenopathy (generalized), fever, headache
Oral ulcers: 'Snail-track'
Organomegaly: Hepatomegaly, hepatitis
Uveitis
Urine: Protein-nephrotic syndrome
Dermatological:

- Non-pruritic, maculopapular rash on palms, soles, trunk
- Scarring alopecia

Y: cond**Y**lomata lata = large pink–grey discs around vulva, anus or under breasts (highly infectious)

Arthralgia, nocturnal bone pain (periostitis), meningism
Gumma: Granulomatous swellings in skin (e.g. leg, foot, periorbital), oropharynx (tongue, palate), viscera (testis, liver, lung)
Aortic: **A**scending aortic aneurysm; **A**ortic regurgitation
Immune: Paroxysmal cold haemoglobinuria
Neurological – classified according to onset of signs:

- 2 months–2 years:
  - Meningitis (may occur during secondary stage)
  - Cranial nerve palsies, incl. deafness, vertigo, optic neuritis
- 2–5 years: Strokes (Heubner endarteritis)
- 5–15 years: General paresis of insane = dementia, psychosis, Argyll–Robertson pupils
- 10+ years: Tabes dorsalis = rombergism, Charcot joints, numbness and lightning pains

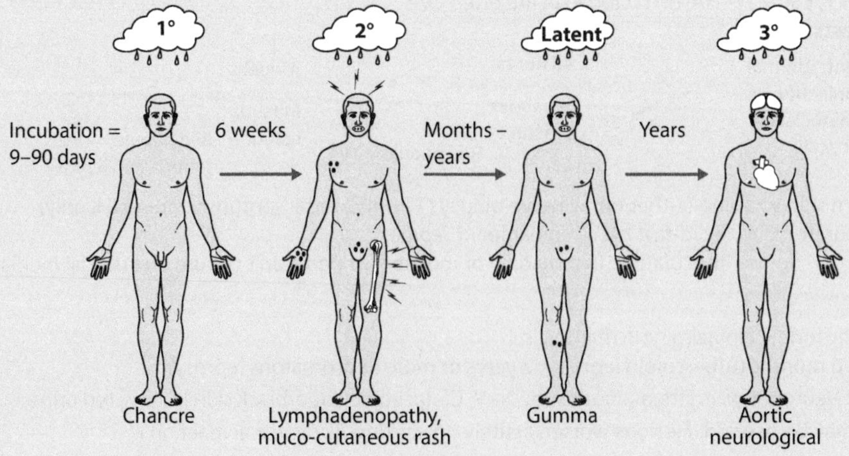

PC

Congenital syphilis

S^2.H.O^2.C^2.K.

Sniffles (watery nasal discharge)
Saddle-shaped nose (also sunken maxillae and frontal bossing)
Hutchinson incisors – notched, widely spaced;
+ Mulberry molars – multiple cusps
+ Linear rhagades – scars around mouth
Optic atrophy, salt + pepper choroidoretinitis; keratitis – blindness
Otitic: Sensorineural deafness
Clutton joints (painless knee effusions); sabre shins
Cold haemoglobinuria, paroxysmal
Kills: 50% babies die pre- or perinatally!

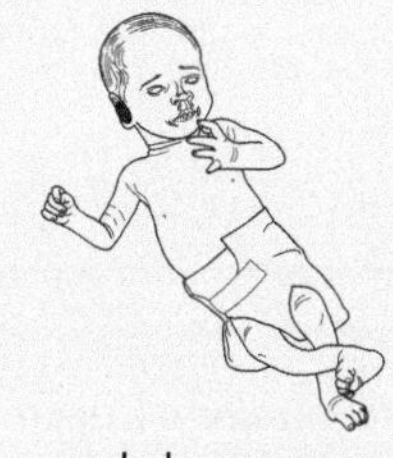

my baby comes as something of a **S.H.O.C.K.**

Ix

Micro: Chancre swab with dark-ground microscopy – characteristic spiral-shaped bacterium
Serology:

- Non-specific: Anti-cardiolipin, e.g. VDRL (Venereal Diseases Research Lab) or RPR (rapid plasma reagin):
  - Advantage: Becomes –ve with Rx
  - False +ve = infections (e.g. herpes, HIV, TB), SLE, pregnancy, elderly (10%)
  - False –ve, esp. in late syphilis, HIV
- Specific: TPHA (*Treponema pallidum* haemagglutination assay), FTA (fluorescent treponemal assay), or TPI (TP immobilisation)
  - Advantage: More specific, but remains +ve even when successfully treated
  - False +ve = non-venereal treponemes, leptospirosis, Lyme
- CSF: Pleocytosis + protein ↑ + antibody tests +ve

Rx

- Procaine penicillin IM 600 mg od × 10 days (2–3 weeks if tertiary disease)
  ☠ Jarisch–Herxheimer reaction = septic shock on initiating Rx, due to endotoxin release, which is most likely in 2° syphilis, but most dangerous in 3° syphilis. Risk can be reduced by administering steroids at same time
- Contact-trace

Non-venereal Treponemes

Def

These diseases are characterized by being:

- Non-venereal: Transmitted skin-to-skin, esp. as children; shared kitchen utensils
- Endemic to Africa, S. and Central America

Types

- Yaws (*T. pallidum* subsp. *pertenue*) – West-Central Africa, S. America, SE. Asia
- Pinta (*T. carateum*) – S. and Central America
- Endemic syphilis (*T. pallidum* subsp. *endemicum*) – Central Africa

PC

1°: Raspberry-like papules ('framboesia')
2°: Lymphadenopathy; periostitis
Latent: Bone gummae – destroy facial bones

BORRELIOSIS

Lyme disease

Borrelia burgdorferi (USA, esp. New England [Lyme, Conneticut]), *B. afzelii*, *B. garinii* (Middle Europe and Asia)

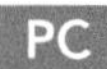

S.N.A.C.K.

Skin

Erythema chronicum migrans in initial phase (days after infection):

- Annular erythema that expands from centre
- Accompanying fever/lymphadenopathy/headache
- Organism can be cultured from rash on Kelly medium

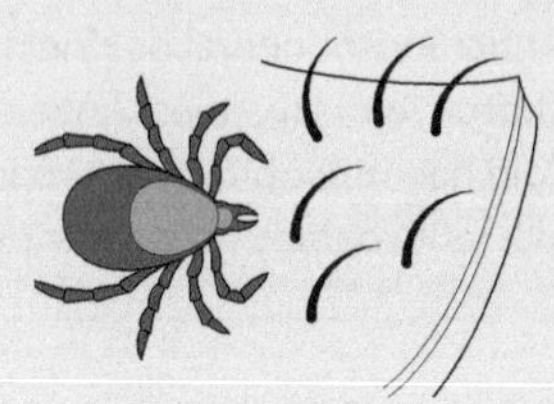

Vector: Deer tick
(Ixodes scapularis)

Neuro

Meningo-encephalitis:

- Cranial neuropathy, esp. VII
- Peripheral neuropathy
- Lymphocytic meningo-radiculitis (Bannwarth syndrome)

Arthritis: Oligoarticular, esp. knees

Cardiac: Heart block, incl. 3° (temporary – does not need pacing)

K: Acrodermatitis chronica atrophicans – only sign of *B. afzelii/B. garinii*

Ix

ELISA

Rx

- Rash: Tetracycline, doxycycline, amoxicillin
- Systemic: Benzylpenicillin, ceftriaxone

Relapsing fever

Louse-borne: *B. recurrentis* – Ethiopia (body lice occur with poor hygiene and overcrowding)
Tick-borne: *B. duttoni* – Sub-Saharan Africa (or *B. hermsii* – NW. USA)

PC: Leptospirosis-like (see p. 209):

- Flu-like symptoms with fluctuating high temperature (>40°C), myalgia–arthralgia, headache
- Injected conjunctivae
- Respiratory (dry cough), neuro. (lymphocytic meningitis), gastro. (abdominal pain, vomiting)

Vincent angina

B. vincenti; PC: Acute gingivitis

LEPTOSPIROSIS

Leptospira interrogans (serotype *icterohaemorrhagie* or *copenhageni* = 'Weil disease')

Epi

Transmitted by contact of rats' urine with skin abrasions or mucous membranes, e.g. sewerage workers

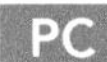

PC

Types:
- Anicteric (90%): Flu-like, aseptic meningitis
- Icteric (10%): Additional liver and renal failure, and DIC = 'Weil disease'

M.O.U.R.N.S.

Myalgia: Severe calf, back, abdominal pain (flu-like with high fever)
Ophthalmic:
- Injected conjunctivae
- Uveitis: Iritis or retinochoroiditis – present several weeks to months later
- Deeply jaundiced due to hepatitis (Weil disease)

Urine:
- Proteinuria, red cells, white cells, granular, hyaline casts – invariable!
- Tubulointersitial nephritis; acute tubular necrosis (2nd week)

Respiratory: Cough, haemoptysis, chest pain
Neurology:
- Aseptic meningitis – CSF: Early neutrophilia, late lymphocytosis; high protein
- Encephalopathy

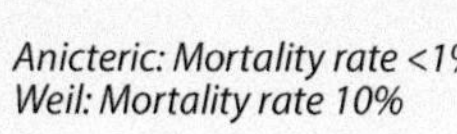

Skin:
- Maculopapular rash
- Purpura, bruising due to vasculitis or DIC
- **S**pleno-/hepatomegaly/lymphadenopathy

Ix

Bloods: CK ↑
U&E – urea ↑, creatinine ↑ – in Weil
LFT – bilirubin ↑, ALP ↑
FBC – neutrophilia, thrombocytopenia, haemolytic anaemia, deranged clotting, CK ↑
(NB: Viral hepatitis: ALT ↑ ↑, leucopenia and normal CK)

Urine: Active urine sediment

Micro: **1st week –** blood/CSF culture; **2nd–4th weeks –** urine culture (EMJH medium)
MAT (microscopic agglutination test) – rise in titre at 2nd week
Hanta virus serology – similar presentation with myalgia and meningism

ECG, **E**CHO: Associated myocarditis, pericarditis

Radiol: CXR – lower-zone air-space shadowing

Rx

Antibiotics:
- Mild: Doxycycline or amoxicillin
- Severe: Benzylpenillicin, ampicillin or erythromycin
  ☠ Jarisch–Herxheimer reaction (fever, myalgia)

Renal dialysis

Prophylaxis: Doxycycline 200 mg × 1/week, or vaccine – in exposed personnel

RICKETTSIA

Q.ua.R.TI.L.E².S.

Q-Fever

Coxiella burnetii

Epi: Acquired from pregnant farm animals or pets, and rarely from other affected humans

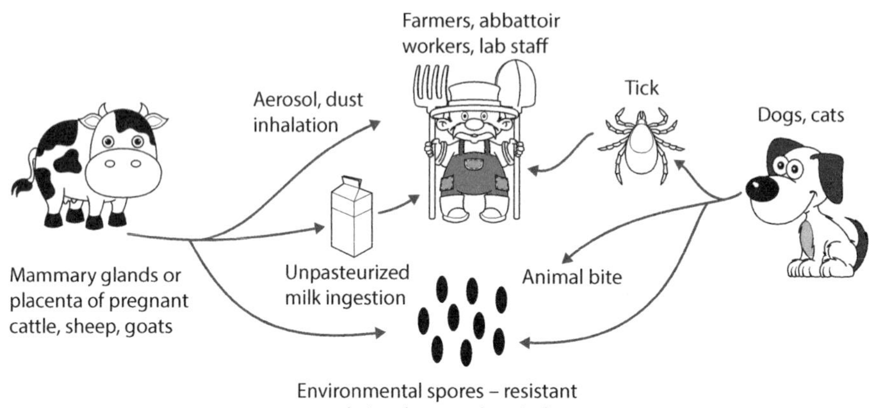

PC

F.R.I.C.T.I.O.N.

Flu -like symptoms: Fever, myalgia
Respiratory: Atypical pneumonia, i.e. mild, dry cough, but CXR shows consolidation or masses
Intestine (1): D+V
Cardiac: Acute phase – myocarditis, pericarditis; chronic – aortic valve endocarditis
Thrombosis: DVT, miscarriage; early, platelets ↑ → later, platelets ↓
Intestine (2): Granulomatous hepatitis
Organomegaly: Hepatosplenomegaly
Neurological: Headache common, meningoencephalitis, optic neuritis, parkinsonism

Ix

Serology: Exists in 2 antigenic forms due to 'phase variation' of lipopolysaccharide:

- Phase I Ag = chronic infection: Highly infectious
- Phase II Ag = acute infection: Avirulent

Rx

Tetracycline ± rifampicin, or ciprofloxacin

Typhus

Rocky mountain spotted fever
- Organism: *Rickettsia rickettsii*
- Vector: Rocky Mountain wood tick, American dog tick
- Geog: SW. USA, Mexico

TIck-borne typhus – other
- Ehrlichiosis
  - Organism: *Ehrlichia chaffeensis* (monocytes), *E. phagocytophilia* (granulocytes)
  - Vector: Deer tick
  - Geog: USA
- Mediterranean spotted fever
- Organism: *Rickettsia conorii*

Louse-borne:

Epidemic and **E**ndemic typhus
- Epidemic typhus
  - Organism: *Rickettsia prowazekii*
  - Vector: Body lice *(Pediculus humanis)*
  - Geog: Poor hygiene, overcrowding, e.g. prisons, famine
- Endemic typhus
  - Organism: *Rickettsia typhi*
  - Vector: Flea; rats, cats, opossums act as reservoir
  - Geog: S. USA

Scrub typhus
- Organism: *Orientia tsutsugamushi*
- Vector: Larval mite
- Geog: SE. Asia, Australia

PC

F.R.I.C.T.I.O.N.

Flu -like symptoms: Fever, myalgia

Rash:
- Eschar of original bite
- Vasculitic: Maculopapular, purpura, haemorrhagic, esp. palms, soles (on 4th day)

Intestine (1): D+V, enterocolitis, GIT bleeding

Cardiac: Arrhythmias

Thrombosis: DVT; limb gangrene – thrombocytopenia

Intestine (2): Transaminitis

Oedema, peripheral and pulmonary: Due to widepread increased vascular permeability, leads to sh**O**ck

Neurological: Headache common, meningoencephalitis, ataxia, deafness

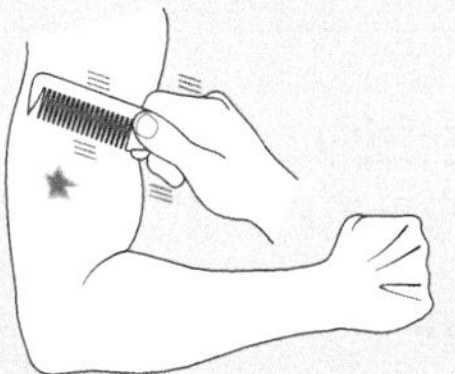
Eschar from tick or larval bite, in tick or scrub typhus

Serology: Indirect IF (the 'Weil–Felix heterophile antibody test' is less sensitive and specific)
PCR, esp. *Rickettsia typhi*
Skin biopsy, esp. Rocky Mountain spotted fever

Tetracycline or chloramphenicol

MALARIA

Plasmodium falciparum

Incubation period 1–2 weeks (but may be up to 1 year)
Duration: 3 weeks, but mortality rate = 20%
Relapses do not occur – if successfully treated

F.A.L.C.I.P.A.R.U.M^2.S.

Flu-like:
- Fever: Continuous, daily or paroxysmal (subtertian – every 36 h, or tertian – every 48 h)
- Other: Myalgia, lymphadenopathy

Anaemia: Intravascular haemolytic anaemia causes haemoglobinuria ('Blackwater fever')
Leucopenia/thrombocytopenia:
- Leucopenia:
  - Although B cells and IgM increased (incl. cryoglobulinaemia)
  - Imunodeficiency → herpes labialis, septicaemia, Burkitt lymphoma (EBV)
- Thrombocytopenia (due to malaria or quinine)/DIC

Cerebral malaria (causes 80% deaths):
- Headache common
- Encephalopathy, cerebral oedema: Drowsiness, seizures, pyramidal signs, psychosis
- Retinal haemorrhages, papilloedema, nystagmus

Intestine: D + V common
Pulmonary oedema: Due to ARDS, uraemia or injudicious rehydration
Acidosis, lactic: Due to hypotension/parasite occlusion of tissue vessels
Renal: Acute tubular necrosis 2° to shock ('algid'), or mesangiocapillary glomerulonephritis
Uraemia
Metabolic:
- Na ↓
- Glucose ↓ due to reduced hepatic gluconeogenesis, or quinine

Miscarriage
Splenomegaly/splenic rupture/hepatosplenomegaly: Repeated infections over long time

Non-falciparum malaria

Incubation period :	*P. vivax* or *ovale*: 2–3 weeks
	P. malariae: 3–6 weeks, although 10% present after 1 year
Duration:	*P. vivax* or *ovale*: 1–2 months
	P. malariae: 1–6 months, with recrudescences over 20 years
Rx:	Oral artesunate or chloroquine

F.A.R.

Fever, paroxysmal:
- *P. vivax/ovale* – tertian (i.e. every 48 h); *P. malariae* – quartan (i.e. every 4th day)
- Due to dormant hypnozoites in liver (*P. ovale/vivax*), or blood (*P. malariae*)
- Fever regularity not seen in early infection

Anaemia, haemolytic: *P. vivax*
Renal – nephrosis: *P. malariae* (esp. in children)

Life-cycle

Alternates between **spores** (products of asexual reproduction) and **gametes** (products of sexual reproduction)

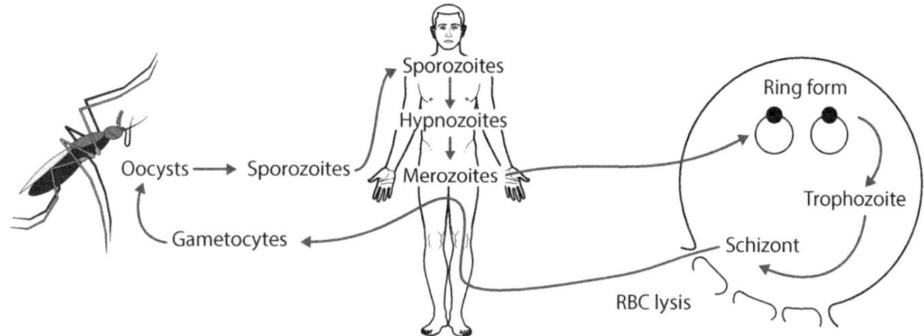

Ix

Thick and thin films ×3:

- Parasitaemia >2% = symptomatic; >10% = exchange transfusion required
- May take several days to rise to true level after becoming symptomatic, so repeat films over 3 days
- Parasites may persist in blood for weeks to months after cure

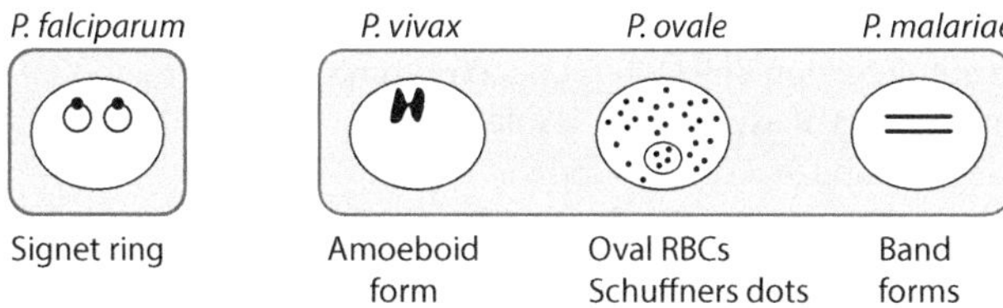

Bone marrow smear: May be needed in partially treated patients, with –ve blood smears

P. falciparum

- Artesunate OR
- Quinine for 7 days (PO or IV) OR
  ☠: Cinchonism: Tinnitus, visual loss, abdominal pain, headache + thrombocytopenia; glucose ↓; renal failure
- Malarone (proguanil + atovaquone)

Prophylaxis

Conservative: Drain swamps; long sleeves; permethrin-impregnated nets; DEET lotion
Chemoprophylaxis: Start 1–3 weeks pre-visit to endemic area; stop 4 weeks post-visit:

- Weekly chloroquine (☠: Visual loss, fits, blood dyscrasia) + daily proguanil
- Weekly mefloquine (☠: Acute psychosis, fits, arrhythmias)
- Daily doxycycline

NEMATODES (ROUNDWORMS)

Intestinal

S.N.A².K.E².

S*trongyloides stercoralis*

Inc: 1 month, and may last for decades due to autoinfection

PC: Worms penetrate skin from soil

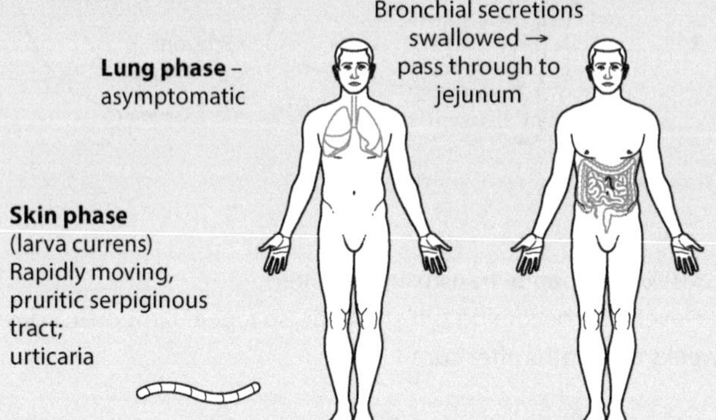

'Hyperinfection': Severe autoinfection due to immunocompromise, e.g. steroids, that may occur after many years of asymptomatic infection

N*ecator americanus/****A****ncylostoma duodenale* ('hookworm')

Inc: 1-3 months, and can last for several years (<8 years for *A. duodenale)*

PC: Skin phase: Worm penetrates toe furrow – pruritus; serpiginous tract (cutaneous larva migrans)

Lung phase: Mild pneumonitis

GIT phase: Fe-deficiency anaemia; hypoalbuminaemia

A*scaris lumbricoides* ('human roundworm' – largest!)

Inc: 2 months, and lasts up to 1 year

PATH: Eggs are ingested → larvae invade jejunal mucosa → enter portal vein and lymphatics → lung phase → swallowed to re-enter jejunum, where mature worm develops

PC: Lung phase: Dry cough, wheeze; CXR shows transient, round infiltrates (Loffler pneumonitis)

GIT phase: Bowel, biliary, pancreas obstruction (esp. heavy infestation in children)

K: Anisa**K**iasis, capillariasis – raw fish; trichostrongyliasis – vegetation; abdominal angiostrongyliasis

E*nterobius vermicularis* ('pinworm' or 'threadworm')

PATH: Larvae colonize appendix and caecum → worms migrate nocturnally to release eggs perianally

PC: Pruritus ani in children; abdominal pain, weight loss; vulvovaginitis; pelvic granulomas

Extra: Rectal prolapse-causing – *Trichuria trichuris* ('whipworm')

Inc: 2–3 months, and may last for 5 years

PATH: Eggs hatch in duodenum → larvae migrate and mature in caecum and colon

PC: Abdominal pain, PR bleeding (colitis); rectal prolapse esp. in children

For all:

Stool samples for ova or larvae

Eosinophilia (during migration phase of hookworm, *Ascaris***,** *Strongyloides)*

ELISA: *Strongyloides*

Albendazole, mebendazole; thiabendazole (*Strongyloides*)

Tissue

FI.G.h.T².S.

FIlariasis – lymphatic nematodes:

- *Onchocerca volvulus* – 'river blindness'
  - Vector: *Simulium* blackfly
  - PC: Keratitis, choroidoretinitis, secondary optic atrophy
    - Rash: Generalized papular, pruritic
    - 'Hanging groin' = inguinocrural lymph node blockage
  - Ix: Skin snip – motile microfilariae
- *Wuchereria bancrofti* – 'elephantiasis'
  - Vector: Mosquitoes – *Aedes aegypti* or *Anopheles* spp.
  - PC: Systemic: Fever, myalgia, photophobia, diffuse lymphangitis, lymphadenopathy
    - Local: Leg lymphoedema, hydrocoele, pleural effusion, ascites
  - Ix: Blood film: Parasites present
- Loa loa
  - Vector: Deerfly – *Chrysops* spp.
  - PC: Calabar swellings of limbs (= evanescent angioedema)
    - Subconjunctival worm
    - Endomyocardial fibrosis
- Brugia malayi
  - Vector: Mosquitoes – *Mansonia* or *Anopheles* spp.
  - Rx for all: Diethylcarbamazine (onchocerciasis: Add suramin, ivermectin)
    - Nodulectomy: Prevents continued production of microfiariae

Guinea worm (*Dracunculus medinensis*)

PATH: Larvae swallowed in drinking water contaminated with vector *Cyclops* spp. (freshwater crustacean) → invade stomach → migrate subcutaneously or to joints → female penetrates skin and release larvae into water

PC: Painful vesicle; subcutaneous nodule; arthritis

***T**oxocara canis/cati* ('visceral larva migrans')

PATH: Eggs in soil contaminated by dog or cat faeces ingested by children → larvae migrate to liver and lungs → systemic spread

PC: Migration: Asthma, fever, dermatitis
Chronic: Choroidoretinitis; hepatosplenomegaly

Ix: Serology

Rx: Albendazole

***T**richinella spiralis*

PATH: Larvae swallowed in infected pork → invade small intestine, portal circulation → systemic spread

PC: Migration: Periorbital oedema, fever, diarrhoea (+ eosinophilia)
Muscles: Myalgia, myopathy, myocarditis
Other: Meningo-encephalitis, gastroenteritis, pneumonia

Ix: Muscle biopsy, serology

Rx: Thiabendazole (intestinal phase) + steroids for systemic infection

Skin: 'Cutaneous larva migrans'

e.g. *Anclyostoma brasiliense, A. caninum, Uncinaria stenocephalia, Bunostomum phlebotomum*

PATH: Animal hookworms that cannot develop further in humans (human hookworms also cause initially)

PC: Serpiginous, erythematous, pruritic, vesicular rash, esp. in children, and on feet; eosinophilia

Ix: Skin biopsy

CESTODES (TAPEWORMS)

There are 2 main types of disease, depending on which stage of the worm's life-cycle is ingested:
Larvae or proglottid segments: Matures to produce adult tapeworm within the intestine
Eggs: Penetrate intestine (as an 'oncosphere') and spread to brain, muscle, liver and lung

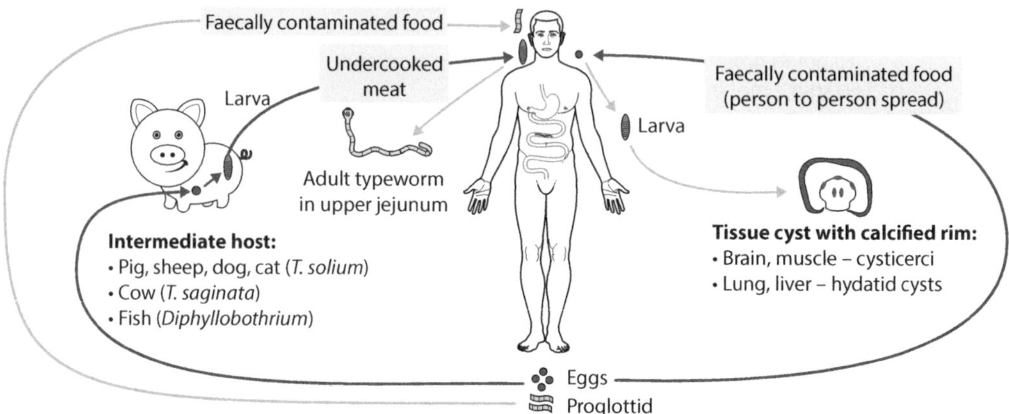

Intestinal tapeworms

P.H.D.

Pork tapeworm – *Taenia solium*
- Epi: *T. solium* – pork: Africa, Latin America, SE. Asia
  T. saginata – beef: Africa, Middle East
- PC: Perianal pain, incl. faecal passage of proglottids
  Epigastric pain, nausea, diarrhoea
  Appetite ↑, weight ↓
- Ix: Stool microscopy: Eggs, proglottids
  Perianal swab with cellophane tape: Detects eggs
  FBC: Eosinophilia; IgE ↑
- Rx: Praziquantel – single dose

***H**ymenolepis nana* (dwarf tapeworm)
- Epi: Commonest cestode infection – endemic in temperate and tropical regions
  Doesn't require intermediate host – auto-infection with eggs common
- PC: Asymptomatic, or anorexia, abdominal pain, diarrhoea

***D**iphyllobothrium latum* (fish tapeworm)
- Epi: Eggs are eaten in raw freshwater fish, e.g. Finland
- PC: Abdominal pain, diarrhoea, bowel obstruction
  Cholangitis, cholecystitis
  Vitamin B12 deficiency – due to consumption by worm

Tissue tapeworms

P.E.T.S.

Pork tapeworm – *Taenia solium*
- PC: Cysticerci form in brain, muscle, subcutaneous:
  - Focal seizures, weakness
  - Obstructive hydrocephalus, meningitis
  - Subretinal: Ocular parasite
- Ix: MRI brain: Ring-enhancing cysts with scolex
  X-ray: 'Cigar-shaped' calcifications in muscle
  ELISA of serum, CSF; tissue biopsy
- Rx: Praziquantel/albendazole; prednisolone + anti-convulsants; CSF shunt

***E**chinococcus granulosus* (dog tapeworm)
- Epi: Dog-handlers, ingesting eggs in vegetables or water
- PC: Hydatid cysts expand:
  - Hepatic: RUQ pain, obstructive jaundice
  - Lung: Chest pain, haemoptysis
  - Other organs: Bone, brain, myocardium
- Ix: Serum ELISA (fluid aspiration risks anaphylaxis!)
- Rx: Cyst excision, with albendazole cover

***T**aenia solium* (pork tapeworm) – see Intestinal

Sparganosis (spirometra tapeworm)
- Epi: Water contains infected crustacean *Cyclops* spp.
- PC: Periorbital – orbital destruction

TREMATODES (FLUKES)

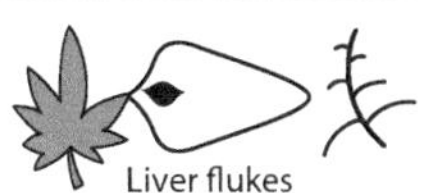

S.C.O.F.F.s H.em.P.

Schistosomiasis (blood fluke = 'bilharzia')

Epi: Fluke (*Schistosoma* sp.) acquired from being bitten by freshwater snails, e.g. in Lake Victoria, S. America

PC: Has acute and chronic manifestations, depending on which part of the life-cycle

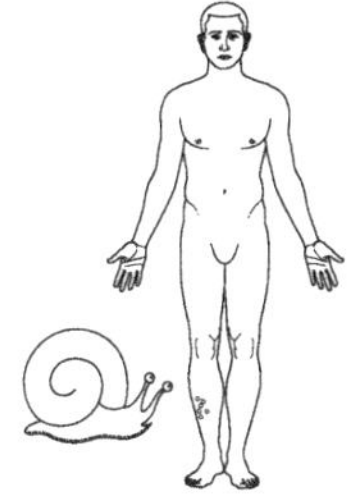

Skin penetration

Freshwater snail eats fluke larvae ('miracidia') and releases cercariae ('freshwater bodies')

Cercariae attach to skin, lose tails, and penetrate to form 'schistosomulae',

PC: 'Swimmers' itch': Dermatitis, papules generalized urticaria

Occurs on day 1, and may persist for 2 weeks

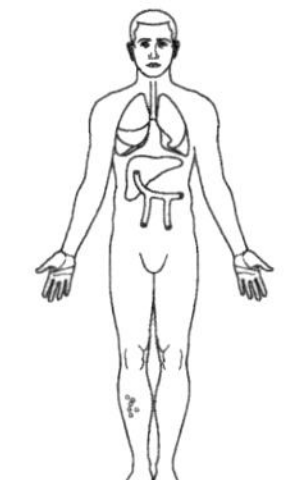

Migration

Skin → lung → portal vein

PC: 'Katayama fever':
- Lymphadenopathy
- Hepatosplenomegaly
- Cough, myalgia
- Headache, diarrhoea
- Encephalopathy, death

Occurs within first month; worst for S. japonicum

Outcome of migration:

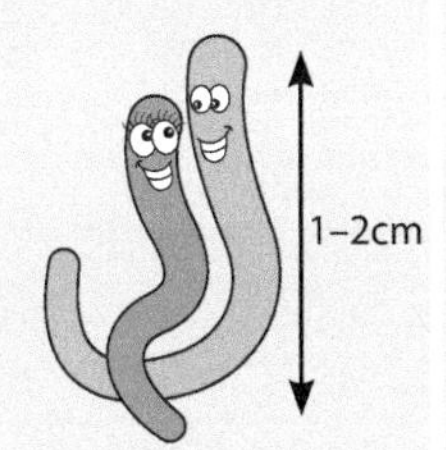

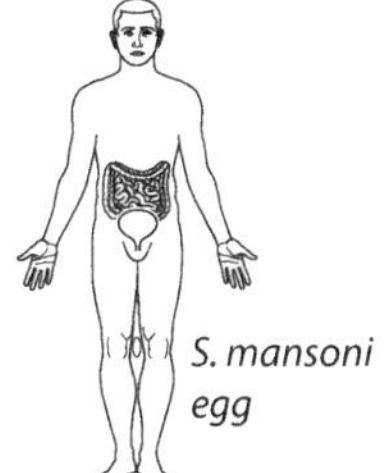

Egg deposition

Schistosomulae settle in portal vein, and mature to form adult male and female pairs, which copulate for many years, and release eggs that are deposited in venules and incite local granulomatous reactions

PC:
- Colon: *S. mansoni* – polyps, bleeding, protein-losing enteropathy; *S. japonicum* – colon carcinoma
- Ileum: *S. japonicum* – colic, malabsorption
- Bladder: *S. haematobium* – haematuria, squamous cell carcinoma

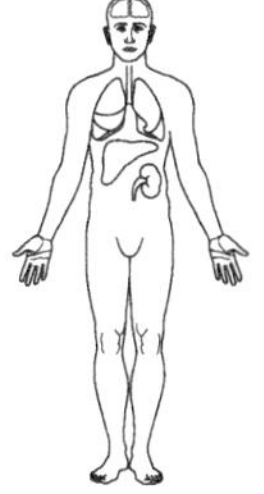

Systemic spread

Liver:
- Hepatosplenomegaly
- Portal hypertension, due to periportal pipestem fibrosis

Lung:
- Fibrosis
- Cor pulmonale

CNS:
- Brain (*S. japonicum*) – focal seizures
- Transverse myelitis/cauda equina syndrome (*S. mansoni/ haematobium*)

Renal:
Glomerulonephritis

***C**lonorchis, **O**pisthorchis, **F**asciola* spp. (liver flukes)

Epi: Raw fish in SE. Asia (*Clonorchis, Opisthorchis*); raw liver or watercress in S. America (*Fasciola*)

PC: RUQ pain; cholangitis with secondary hepatitis or obstructive jaundice; cholangiocarcinoma

***F**asciolopsis, **H**eterophyes* (liver flukes)

Epi: Aquatic plants in SE. Asia (*Fasciolopsis*); raw freshwater fish in Nile, China (*Heterophyes*)

PC: Abdominal pain, mucoid diarrhoea

***P**aragonimus westermani* (lung fluke)

Epi: Crayfish, crab ingestion

PC: Lung – haemoptysis, bronchiectasis, bronchitis; brain – focal seizures, weakness

Rheumatology

OSTEOARTHRITIS – CAUSES

Def

Common final pathological pathway of synovial joints, arising from variety of insults (although commonly refers only to age-related '1° osteoarthritis', with no identifiable insult)

Causes

I.T.'S. A.C.H.I.N.G. M.E^2.

Idiopathic (1°), i.e. age-related – *see pp. 221*
Trauma – old fracture: due to abnormal joint loading after healing, ± articular surface damage
Softened bone, *see p. 221*:
- Developmental – congenital dislocation of hip, Perthes disease, slipped capital femoral epiphysis
- Osteochondritis
- Osteonecrosis (avascular necrosis)

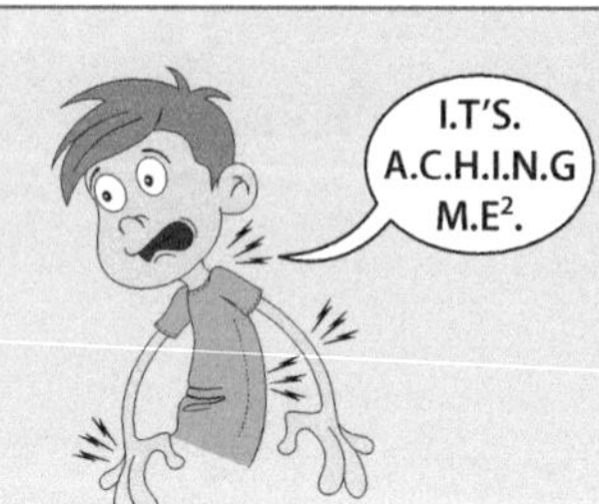

The remainder occur due to weakened cartilage:

Autoimmune: Rheumatoid arthritis; seronegative arthropathies, SLE, polymyalgia rheumatica
Crystal: Gout, pseudogout, hydroxyapatite, hypercholesterolaemia
Haemorrhage: Haemophilia, previous AML
Infection:
- Septic arthritis, incl. viral, gonococcal, TB – Lyme; congenital syphilis (Clutton joints)
- Reactive: Endocarditis, rheumatic fever
- Foreign body arthropathy, e.g. rosethorn → symmetrical polyarthritis

Neuropathic ('Charcot joints' – gross changes of dislocation, disorganisation and debris):
- Cord: Syringomyelia (shoulders), syphilis, vitamin B12 deficiency (hip, knee)
- Neuropathy: Diabetes, leprosy, Charcot–Marie–Tooth disease (ankle, feet)

Genetic:
- Osteogenesis imperfecta, Marfan, homocystinuria, hyperlysinaemia
- Immunodeficiency: Bruton agammaglobulinaemia or common variable

Malignancy:
- Infiltration, incl. leukaemia, amyloid
- Paraneoplastic: Giant-cell arteritis-like syndrome, HPOA (squamous cell carcinoma)

Endocrine – metabolic:
O.W.T.C.H.A. – *see p. 221*
Exogenous:
- Vitamin deficiency: D (rickets), C (scurvy)
- Kashin–Beck disease: Fungal infestation of wheat in China

Idiopathic

Inc: 10% over-60s
Age: Linear increase with age (radiographic progression)
Sex: F > M (esp. knee, hand); M > F (elbow); M = F (hip)
Geo: More common in Caucasians
Aet: Genetic, i.e. family history
Cumulative repetitive movements, i.e. age
Excess loading, i.e. obesity

Softened bone

Developmental

Congenital dysplasia of hip – posterior hip dislocation due to acetabular flattening or joint laxity
PC:

- Neonate: Failure to abduct flexed hips to 90°, and difficulty reducing head (Ortolani test)
- Child: Waddling gait, hyperlordosis (bilateral), asymmetrical skin crease (unilateral)

Perthes disease – avascular necrosis of femoral head secondary to minor trauma
PC: Painful hip in 5–10-year-old, esp. boys
Slipped capital femoral epiphysis – insufficiency fracture of physeal growth plate
PC: Painful hip or knee at puberty, esp. obese, hypogonadal boys

Osteochondritis

Crushing – necrosis of cuboidal bone in hand or feet, esp. during puberty
Types: Hand – lunate or capitulum; feet: metatarsal head or navicular
Splitting (dissecans – osteochondral fracture of convex joint, due to repeated minor trauma
Types: Medial femoral condyle, talus, capitulum (humeral part of elbow joint)
Pulling (traction apophysitis) – bone that receives tendon insertion is pulled off during puberty
Types: Tibial tuberosity (Osgood–Schlatter), calcaneum (Sever)

Osteonecrosis ('avascular necrosis')

F.I.N.A.L.I.T.Y.

Fractured: Neck of femur, carpal (scaphoid, lunate), foot (talus, metatarsal head)
Infection: Septic arthritis or osteomyelitis, TB, endocarditis
Nitrogen: Following rapid decompression N_2 bubbles act as emboli, e.g. in deep-sea divers
Autoimmune: Rheumatoid arthritis, SLE, vasculitis
Lipodystrophy: Gaucher disease
Ischaemic: Sickle cell anaemia, polycythaemia, diabetes, shock (e.g. acute pancreatitis)
Toxins: Steroids (incl. pregnancy, Cushing), alcohol
Young: Perthes – as above

Endocrine – metabolic

O.W.T.C.H.A.!

Ochronosis (homogentisic acid oxidase deficiency – alkaptonuria); PC: Black cartilage
Wilson disease
Thyroid: Graves disease – acropachy, hypothyroidism
Calcium: Hyper- or hypoparathyroidism
Haemochromatosis
Acromegaly

OSTEOARTHRITIS – PC

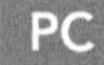

PC

1° OA

Distribution: Localized (1–2 joints) or generalized (≥3 classes of joints)

History:

- Pain ↑ by movement; evening–night; stiffness ↑ after rest
- Slow onset → flares every few months → deformity occurs late

O/E: Crepitus felt on movement, due to osteophytes; locking; effusions

A. Foot/Hand

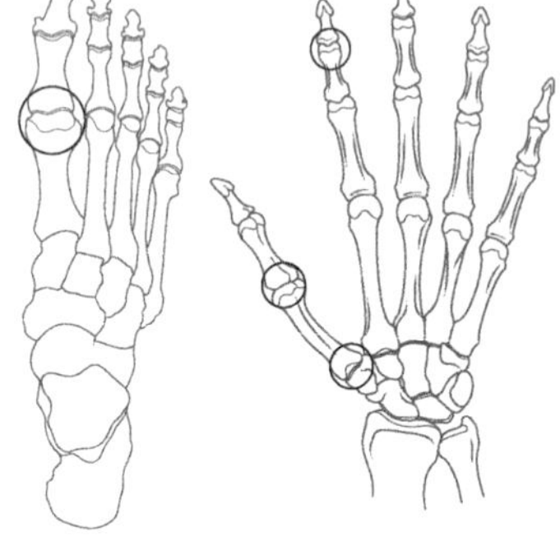

1st MTP joint affected first

DIP and PIP joints (Heberden and Bouchard nodes):

O/E: Binodular (cf. scleroderma – uninodular)

- DIP only: Mild disease; post-menopausal; familial
- PIP: 'Erosive DA' with synovitis
  Associated large-joint DA and cervical spondylosis

Thumb base: 1st MCP and CMC joints:

O/E: Stiffness, subluxation and squaring of thumb base

Familial 'persistent generalized osteoarthropathy' =

- CMC + DIP + knee DA
- Assoc. carpal tunnel syndrome, ulnar neuropathy

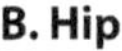

B. Hip

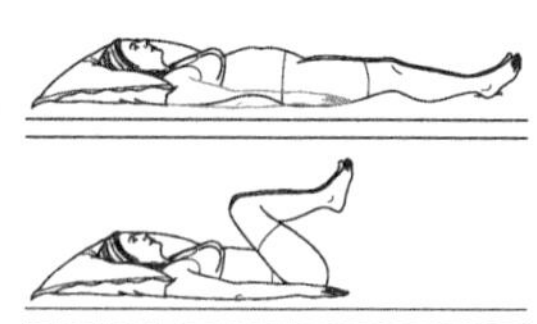

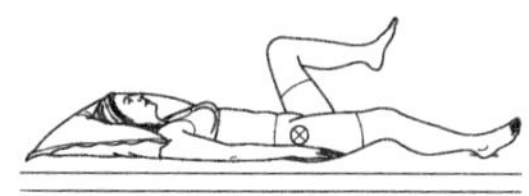

Pain inguinal; buttock; thigh, radiating to knee; limited passive internal rotation (normal: 50° external; 40° internal)

Fixed-flexion deformity: Thomas test (see diagram):

- Legs flat on bed – hyperlordosis apparent
- Flex both hips to straighten back
- Extend one hip, while holding pelvis straight → fixed-flexion deformity
- apparent in hip

True shortening of leg:

- Distance between ASIS and trochanter decreases
- Telescoping may occur with severe instability

C. Knee

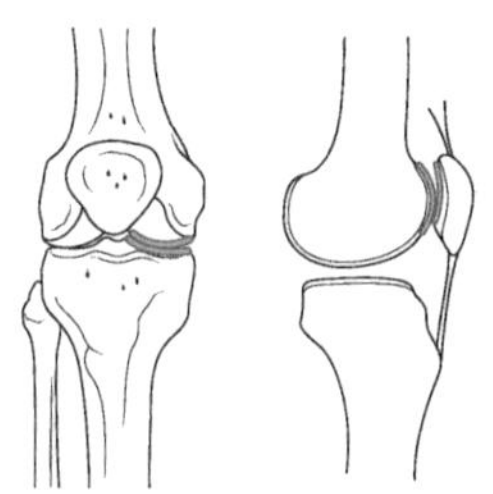

Medial compartment osteoarthritis

- Varus and fixed flexion deformity
- Gait disturbance:
  - Bilateral: waddles
  - Unilateral: Trendelenburg's sign +ve: pelvis sags on diseased side, on standing on one leg

Patella-femoral osteoarthritis

Baker's cyst

D. Spine

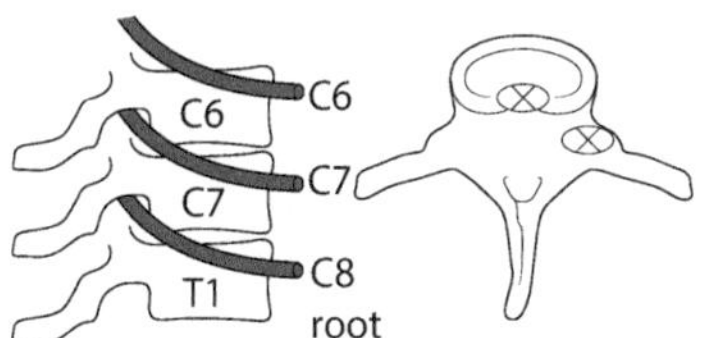

Cervical spondylosis – facet joints: Radiculopathy; myelopathy

Lumbar spondylosis – posterior disc and facet joints: Radiculopathy; cauda equina syndrome, spinal stenosis, spondylolisthesis

Other: Sacro-iliitis, skeletal hyperostosis (ligament ossification)

Other: Shoulder (glenohumeral, acromioclavicular, sternoclavicular), tibio-talar, temporomandibular

OSTEOARTHRITIS – IX AND RX

Ix

Radiol: X-ray

☠ Complications

Soft tissue swelling and effusion → acute pain; locking due to:

- Osteophyte separation
- Synovitis in 'erosive OA'
- Crystal deposition

Bone marrow vascular congestion → chronic pain
Capsular fibrosis, bony ankylosis → stiffness
Osteoporosis, 2° to immobility → fracture

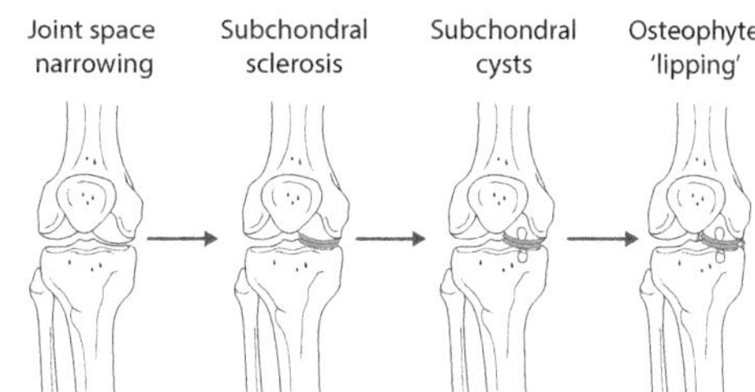

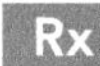

Rx

Conservative

- Physiotherapy:
  - Exercise – pain ↓, function ↑, power ↑
  - Hydrotherapy – joint load ↓, mobility ↑; heat or ice therapy – for acute flares
  - Serial splintage – fixed flexion deformity (e.g. knee), stabilizes joints
- Orthotics and occupational therapy:
  - Stick, frame – joint load ↓, mobility ↑; shoe-raiser for shortened leg
  - Home appliances – stair + bath rail, firm chairs, high toilet-seat ('doughnut')

Medical

- Effusion: Joint aspiration and injection of steroid (e.g. triamcinolone), hyaluronic acid, osmic acid
- Analgesia:
  - Mild: Paracetamol, co-dydramol
  - NSAIDs: Ibuprofen, diclofenac, COX-2 inhibitors (if no arteriopathy) – for acute flares
    ☠: Gastritis, peptic ulceration, renal disease
  - Other: Capsaicin cream, TENS

Surgical

- Arthroscopy:
  - Debride unstable cartilage and osteophytes (but recurrence common)
  - Drilling exposed bone causes cartilage remodelling
- Osteotomy:
  - Genu varum
  - Realign tibial plateau by removing wedge from lateral tibia
  - Divide meduallary veins, which reduces pain
  - 1st MTP joint: Keller osteotomy – excision of proximal MTP and proximal phalanx
- Arthroplasty:
  - Hip, knee, elbow – replacement hemi or total
  - 1st MTP joint – joint excision or insertion of Silastin sponge
- Arthrodesis: Fusion of joint removes pain and can improve resting position, but requires neighbouring joints to be normal to allow compensation

RHEUMATOID ARTHRITIS – PC

Def

Multisystemic cell-mediated immune autoimmune disease, characterized by chronic synovitis

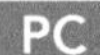

A.N.N.O.Y.I.N.' S.C.A²**.R.S²****.**

Arthritis:

- Small-joints, symmetrical + generalized (≥3 joint areas)
- Pain + stiffness: ↑ with rest, e.g. early morning stiffness
- Subacute onset → periodic + progressive; flare frequency ↓, deformity ↑ → quiescence

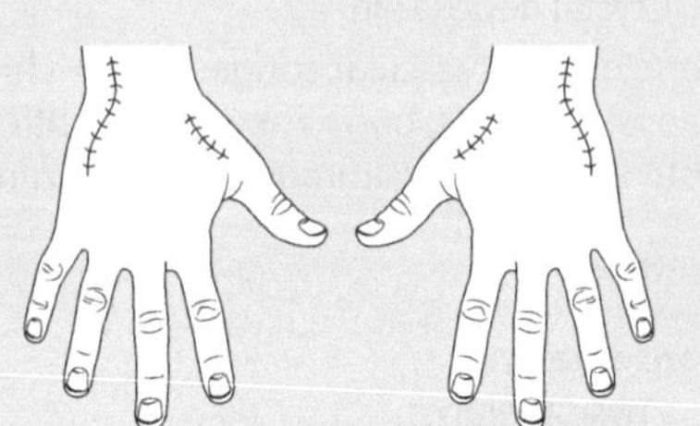

Nodules (25%):

- Elbows, feet, ischial tuberosity; Achilles tendon; periosteal; visceral (e.g. lung, eye, bowel)
- EPI: Elderly men; sero +ve; serositis, e.g. pleural effusions; may ulcerate and become infected

Nails and skin:

- Longitudinal ridges, clubbing (if lung fibrosis), splinter haemorrhages (if vasculitis), palmar erythema
- Vasculitis (10%), incl. dusky cyanotic digits, Raynaud syndrome, cryoglobulinaemia livedo reticularis
- Leg ulcers, incl. pyoderma gangrenosum; ankle oedema

Ophthalmology:

- Keratoconjunctivitis sicca: 2° Sjögren syndrome (40%) – associated lethargy + lymphoma
- Episcleritis (also scleromalacia perforans); scleral nodules
- Vasculitis: Central retinal; anterior ciliary arteries (obliterative endarteritis)

Y: L**Y**mphadenopathy – proximal to affected joints; resembles giant follicular-cell lymphoma on histology

Immunocompromise: Due to disease and immunosuppressive drugs

Neurology:

- Peripheral – entrapment neuropathy, e.g. carpal tunnel syndrome; vasculitic mononuritis multiplex
- CNS: Ischaemic stroke due to medium-vessel vasculitis
- Myositis: Polymyositis or vasculitis (also hand wasting due to disuse atrophy)

Systemic: Fatigue, low-grade fever, anorexia, weight loss, steroid side-effects (e.g. skin thinning)

Cardiac: Pericarditis ± effusion, myo- or endocarditis, mitral regurgitation, coronary arteritis

Anaemia of chronic disease/**A**myloid AA (hepatosplenomegaly, malabsorption; renal failure)

Respiratory:

- Pulmonary fibrosis: Lower zone ± 2° pulmonary hypertension
- Pleurisy, pleural effusions
- Rare: Lung nodules, pneumonitis (esp. with methotrexate), bronchiolitis

Syndrome, Felty (1%) – severe arthritis, splenomegaly, low platelets and neutrophils (leg spots, ulcers)

Still disease ('juvenile chronic arthritis'): PC: Evening rash coincident with fever

Arthritis

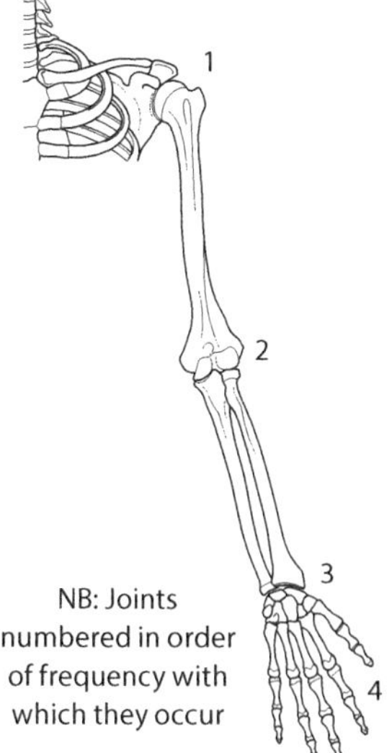

Upper limb

1 Shoulder/clavicle
Shoulder: Unable to abduct; rotator cuff tears, superior subluxation
Acromioclavicular, sternoclavicular arthritis, subacromial bursitis

2 Elbow: Unable to extend, olecranon bursitis

3 Wrist
Extensor tenosynovitis and effusion: Tender, hot, red, boggy swelling
Volar subluxation of wrist joint, dorsal subluxation of distal radio-ulnar joint
Prominent distal radius and ulnar: 'Piano-key deformity' (radius), tendon rupture

4 PIP/MCP joints
PIP: Fusiform or sausage-shaped fingers. effusions, 2° osteoarthritis
MCP: Ulnar deviation of fingers, volar subluxation, Z-shaped thumb
Deformities: Swan-necking, bouttonière (tendon rupture), trigger finger

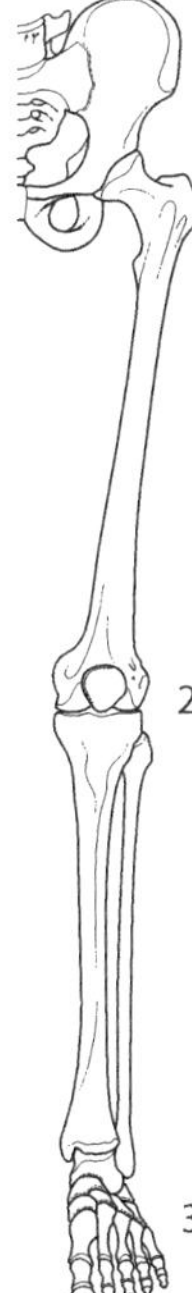

Lower limb

1 Hip
Osteoporosis
Avascular necrosis, incl. due to steroids
Protrusio acetabula
Trochanteric bursitis – anterior thigh pain

2 Knee
Genu valgus
Baker's cyst – popliteal bursitis ruptures to cause acute pain and swelling in calf

3 Foot
Toe clawing and hallux valgus
Metatarsal callosities
Volar subluxation of metatarsal heads – 'walking on pebbles'
Talar, subtalar joint synovitis

Cervical spine/other head–neck

1 Atlanto-axial dislocation
Odontoid peg – atlas synovitis:
when separation ↑ to >2 mm, on flexion:

- Cord compression (limb paraesthesia)
- Paroxysmal medullary dysfunction (e.g. vertigo, dysphagia, LOC) or vertebral artery TIA or stroke
- Head feels like falling forwards on flexing

2 Neurocentral joints of Luschka (C3–7) synovitis
Def: Synovial joints occur at upturned lateral lips of vertebral bodies
PC: Neck + head pain and stiffness, cord compression

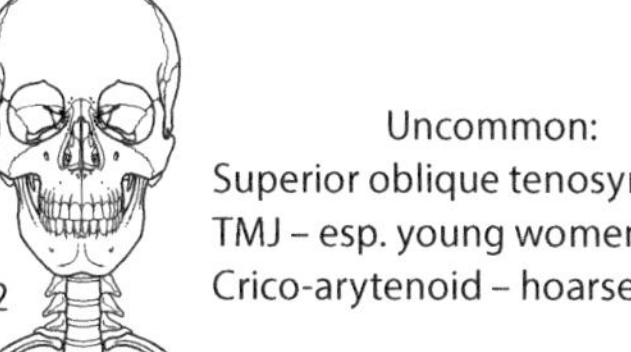

Uncommon:
Superior oblique tenosynovitis
TMJ – esp. young women
Crico-arytenoid – hoarseness

RHEUMATOID ARTHRITIS – EPI, IX AND RX

Epi

Inc: Prevalence 3% (women), 1% (men)
Age: Presents between 40 and 60 y
Sex: F:M = 3:1
Geo: Urban > rural
Aet: Cell-mediated immunity: CD8 + T cells
Pre: Genetic: HLA-DR4 or -DR1 (relative risks of 6 and 2, respectively)
Smoking

Ix

Bloods:

Anti-cyclic citrullinated peptide (anti-CCP) antibody: High specificity, low sensitivity
Rheu**M**atoid factor = Ig**M** (± IgG) directed against Fc of IgG, found in serum and synovial fluid: High sensitivity, low specificity
Other autoantibodies, or markers of inflammation:

- ANA +ve in 30%
- ESR, CRP ↑ (correlates with severity)
- C3, C4, IgG ↑ or normal (unlike SLE)

Routine bloods:
FBC:

- Hb – normochromic, normocytic anaemia (ferritin ↓ if Fe-def.; ↑ if active inflammation)
- WBC – eosinophilia, lymphocytosis in severe RA (except in Felty syndrome – leucopenia)
- Plt – thrombocytosis (except in Felty syndrome – thrombocytopenia)

LFT: ALP ↑, LDH ↑, albumin ↓

Micro – aspirate of synovial or serosal fluid:

Straw-coloured, turbid, low viscosity
Neutrophilia; CD8 + T cells ↑
Complement Ig ↑, glucose ↓

Radiol:

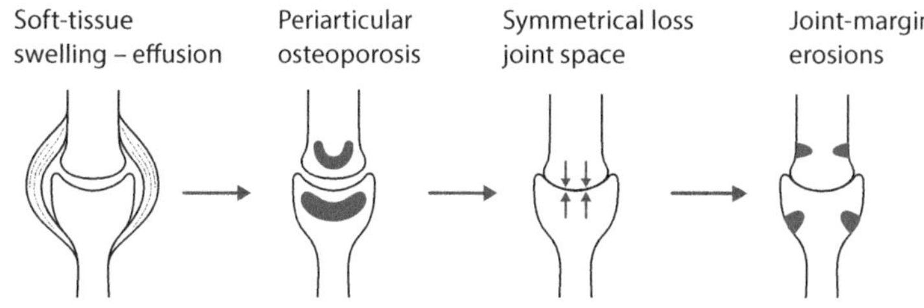

☠ Subluxation + deformity

Arthritis mutilans = telescoped digits

2° OA, e.g. Bouchard nodes

Cervical X-ray: Atlanto-axial distance should be <2 mm on flexion
MRI: Cervical cord compression by synovial hypertrophy
CXR: Lower-zone fibrosis

Surgical – biopsy, e.g. of skin, nerve:

Vasculitis:

- Obliterative endarteritis, e.g. retina, nailbeds
- Necrotising arteritis (large vessel), e.g. ischaemic colitis, CVA, PVD (limb)
- Subacute arteritis (medium and small vessel), e.g. nerves (vasa nervorum), muscles

Rx

Conservative

- Physiotherapy: Stretching (decreases joint contractures); hydrotherapy; heat or ice therapy; orthotics, aids, incl. collar; neck protection during surgery
- Diet: Low-fat, high in omega-3 fatty-acids

Medical

Anti-inflammatories

Ind: Steroids:

- Acute flares: Intra-articular; short oral course; IM or IV pulse
- Maintenance (<7.5 mg prednisolone od): Decreases erosion and systemic disease
  ☠Steroids: Add bisphosphonate and omeprazole; check glucose, ABP
  NSAIDs: Peptic ulcer; hypertension; fluid retention; renal failure; asthma

Disease-modifying anti-rheumatoid drugs (DMARDs)

1. Should always be used; 2. Takes several months to start working; 3. Efficacious for 1–2 years

Synthetic DMARDS

Sulphasalazine:
☠: Oligospermia; headache, nausea, dizziness; rash

Antimalarials – chloroquine, hydroxychloroquine:
☠: Retinopathy (annual fundoscopy and visual fields); rash

Methotrexate (purine antagonist) – weekly PO or IM:
1st choice as quicker onset of action: 1–2 months; and longest-lasting efficacy of approx. 6 years
☠: Liver failure; lung fibrosis, acute pneumonitis; cytopenia; nausea

Azathioprine (purine synthesis inhibitor)
☠: Immunosuppression; cytopenia; lymphoma and haemorrhagic cystitis (cyclophospamide)

Biological DMARDS

Infliximab or etanercept (TNF-α antagonists)
(etane**RCEPT** = receptor antagonist; inflixim**AB** = anti-TNF antibody)
☠: Opportunistic infections – TB, fungal, bacterial septicaemia; autoimmunity – SLE or MS

Surgical: Arthroplasty (hip, knee, elbow); arthrodesis (wrist, atlanto-axial); osteotomy (e.g. radial head, forefoot) + tendon transposition; synovectomy

SERONEGATIVE ARTHROPATHIES – 1

Def

Generalized arthropathy centred on axial skeleton, with systemic features
Negative rheumatoid factor/anti-CCP antibody
Familial component, esp. via association with HLA-B27

Types

R.A.P.p.E.R.S.

Reactive arthritis: Large joint arthritis in response to infection elsewhere
PC: Classic triad = monoarthritis, urethritis, conjunctivitis; may also have banalitis and keratoderma blennorrhagicum

Ankylosing spondylitis:
Assoc: HLA-B27 – strongest association
PC: Spondylosis, chest, arthritis, enthesopathy

Psoriatic arthropathy:
Assoc: Psoriasis, nail pitting
PC: Arthritis – may precede skin problems

Enteropathic:
Assoc: IBD, Whipple or Behçet syndrome
PC: Arthritis – may precede bowel problems

Rheumatic fever:
Assoc: *Streptococcus pyogenes* (not HLA-B27)
PC: Pancarditis, arthritis, subcutaneous nodules, Sydenham chorea, erythema marginatum, streptococcal infection in past

Still disease, adult-onset:
PC: Arthritis, serositis, rash, organomegaly

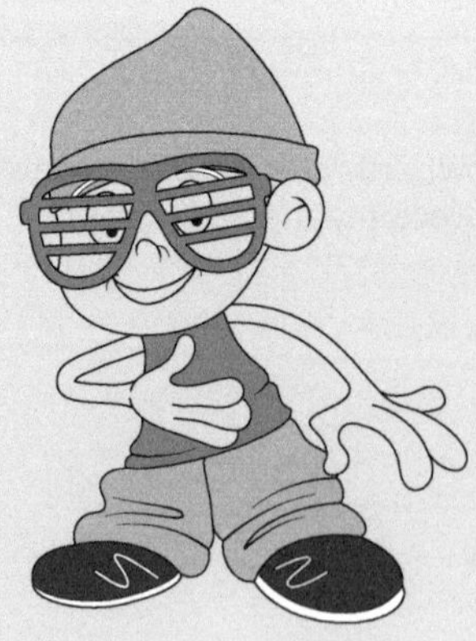

PC

S^2.C.A.R.E.D. S.L.O.U^2.C.H.E.R.S.

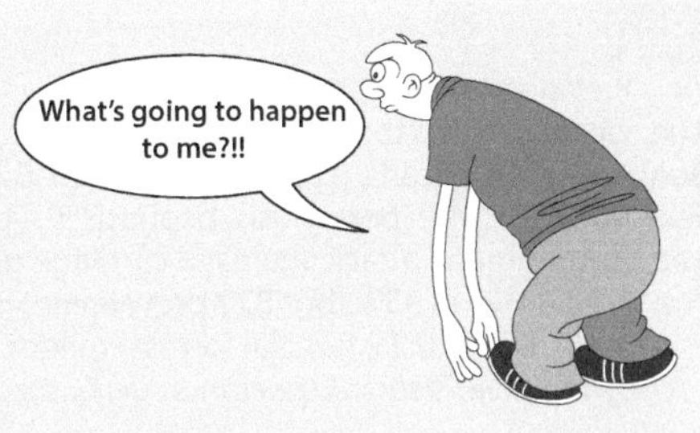
What's going to happen
to me?!!

Sacro-iliitis/**S**pondylosis:

- Sacro-iliitis:
  PC: Painful buttocks, hamstrings; thighs: ↑ in morning or with rest; difficult high-stepping
  O/E: Tender over SI joints – induced by pressure on sacrum centre and both iliac crests
- Spondylosis (fibrous bony ankylosis):
  PC: Stiff, painful back and neck
  O/E: Restricted lateral or anterior flexion; lumbar flattening or lordosis on forward flexion; thoracic kyphosis (wall–tragus distance ↑);
  Schober test: max. excursion of two points, 10 cm apart upwards from L5, is <15 cm

Complications: Spinal fracture (incl. end-plate collapse); cauda equina syndrome; spinal fusion

Costochondritis: Sternocostal and costovertebral enthesitis, resulting in ankylosis; thoracic spondylosis
O/E: Max. inspiratory excursion below breasts <5 cm circumference increase

Arthritis: Asymmetrical, mono- or oligoarthritis, esp. women; knee, ankle, TMJ

Respiratory:

- Chest wall ankylosis – restricted excursion and pain
- Apical fibrosis (*Aspergillus* may infect fibrotic lung)

Enthesopathy (painful inflammation of tendon and ligament insertions): Pelvis (iliac crests, ischial tuberosity, greater trochanter), patella, Achilles, plantar fasciitis

Dactylitis

Systemic: Fatigue, low-grade fever, anorexia – weight loss; ESR, CRP ↑

Liver and GIT:

- Fatty change, chronic active hepatitis, cirrhosis (ALP ↑), sclerosing cholangitis
- Inflammatory bowel disease, incl. silent ileal ulcers

Ophthalmology: Iridocyclitis (anterior uveitis), phlyctenular conjunctivitis, episcleritis

Ulcers/**U**rethritis: Orogenital ulceration, incl. circinate balanitis

Cardiac: Aortic root fibrosis and regurgitation; myocarditis – arrhythmias

Haematology: Anaemia of chronic disease; DVT; Sweet syndrome (purple plaques, fever, neutrophilia)

Extra: Hepatosplenomegaly due to AA amyloid or adult-onset Still disease (also lymphadenopathy)

Renal: IgA nephropathy, plasma IgA ↑

Skin:

- Pyoderma gangrenosum (esp. UC): O/E: Violaceous everted edge
- Erythema nodosum or multiforme
- Vasculitis or Raynaud syndrome

SERONEGATIVE ARTHROPATHIES – SPECIFIC

Ankylosing spondylitis

Epi

Inc: Prevalence = 0.5% population
Age: Onset in teens to 30s
Geo: Native Americans, e.g. Pima (high HLA-B27 occurrence)
Sex: M:F = 3:1; M – spondylosis, psoriasis; F – peripheral arthritis, Crohn disease
Aet: **A**utoimmune attack against a cartilage glycoprotein, e.g. 'aggrecan'
Pre: 1. HLA-B27 in 95% (but B27 prevalence = 10%; so only 5% of people with HLA-B27 have ank. spond.)
2. MZ/DZ = 70:25; familial forms – milder severity
3. Infective: *Klebsiella pneumoniae, Campylobacter* spp. (serology often +ve)

PC

S^2.C.A.R.E.D. S.L.O.U.C.H.ers.

Sacro-iliitis/**S**pondylosis: Back and buttock pain, stiffness
Costochondritis and thoracic ankylosis
Arthritis: Mainly women sufferers – knees, ankles, shoulder
Respiratory: Apical fibrosis; chest wall ankylosis (restricted excursion and pain)
Enthesopathy: Ligament insertion inflammation, e.g. plantars, Achilles, knees (also responsible for spondylosis and sacro-iliitis)
Dactylitis

Systemic: Fatigue (esp. elderly); fever (low-grade); anorexia; weight loss
Liver/GIT: Liver fatty change, ALP ↑, silent ileal ulcers
Ophthalmic: Acute iridocyclitis (commonest complication) – poor prognosis
Urethritis
Cardiac: Aortic regurgitation; heart block
Haematology: Anaemia of chronic disease

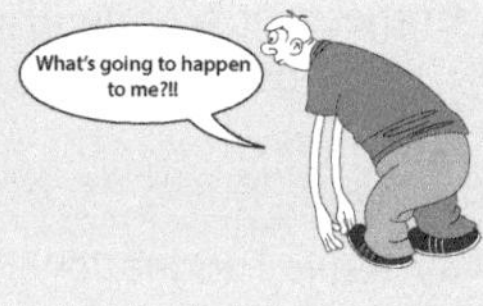
What's going to happen to me?!!

Ix

Bloods: ESR, CRP ↑; IgA ↑; CK; ALP ↑
Radiol: X-ray

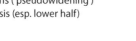

Sacro-iliac joints
Blurred cortical margins
Erosions ('pseudowidening')
Sclerosis (esp. lower half)

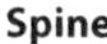

Spine
Initially upper lumber spine
Calcification of annulus fibrosus ends = 'syndesmophytes'

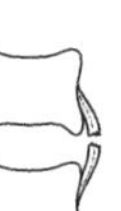

Ossification of annulus and posterior longitudinal ligament ('bamboo spine')
Loss of joint space

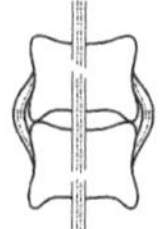

Squared-off bodies
Sclerotic end-plate
Osteoporosis

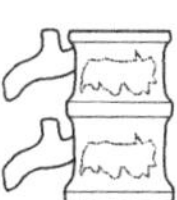

MRI – spinal arachnoid cysts

Rx

Conservative: Physiotherapy; swimming; avoid contact sports
Medical: NSAIDs: Esp. indomethacin, phenylbutazone (most efficacious, but ☠ cytopenias!)
Steroids: Pulsed methylprednisolone, CT-guided sacro-iliac injection, eye-drops for iritis
DMARDs: Sulphasalazine, methotrexate (for peripheral arthritis), infliximab, thalidomide
Surgical: Total hip arthroplasty; spinal osteotomy – in severe cases only

Reactive arthritis

Def

Arthritis following bacterial infection of any kind
May have classical triad of **G.O.A.** – see below (if arthritis alone, then it is called 'reactive arthritis')
Systemic autoimmune reaction, secondary to cross-reactivity with Gram-negative bacteria: gastroenteritis (e.g. *Yersinia, Salmonella spp., E. coli);* STD (*Chlamydia spp.,* gonococcus)

Epi

Occurs in 1–2 % of those with associated infections, esp. in young, with equal sex distribution

PC

A real **G.O.A.**

Genital:
- Urethritis (discharge), prostatitis
- Pelvic inflammatory disease, cervicitis
- Orogenital ulcers, incl. circinate balanitis

Ophthalmic: Conjunctivitis, anterior uveitis
Arthritis:
- Lower limb, mono- or oligoarthritis
- Resolves within 6 months, although 1/3 relapse
- Enthesopathy, incl. Achilles tendonitis, plantar fasciitis

+ Keratoderma blenorrhagica – pustular psoriasis on soles or palms
+ Diarrhoea

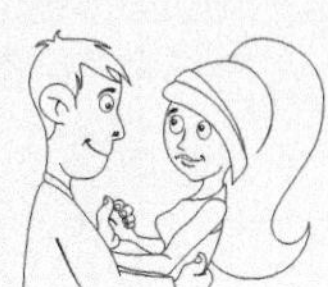

Ix

Micro: Microscopy and culture of blood; stool; urine; urethral, cervical + rectal swabs
Serology: Ligase chain reaction for *Chlamydia spp.,* HIV, syphilis (if STD suspected)
Joint aspirate: Neutrophil or monocyte exudate, but sterile

Rx

Acute: Rest initially, physio, later; aspirate effusions; NSAIDs ± steroids
Chronic: Sulphasalazine, methotrexate or azathioprine (but must exclude HIV first!)

Psoriatic arthropathy

Epi

2% population have psoriasis, of whom 7% develop arthropathy, esp. young men

PC

Arthritis
Small-joint, esp. DIP joints – commonest
Large-joint – symmetrical or asymmetrical
Sacro-iliitis; spondylitis
'Arthritis mutilans' = telescoping of digits

Skin
Psoriasis: Poor correlation with arthritis
Nail pitting; onycholysis; horizontal ridging: esp. on same digits with DIP arthritis

Iritis

Distinction from rheumatoid arthritis
DIP joints (rheumatoid = PIP joints)
Asymmetrical, oligoarthritis (rheumatoid = symmetrical, polyarthritis)
Sacro-iliitis, spondylitis (rheumatoid = atlanto-axial disease)
Dactylitis – uniform-swelling (rheumatoid = spindle-shaped fingers)

Ix

Radiol: X-ray: osteolysis of phalanx ends – 'pencil-in-cup' deformity

Rx

NSAIDs: Avoid steroids (worsen psoriasis on withdrawal)
DMARDs: Sulphasalazine, methotrexate, infliximab, etanercept (avoid antimalarials worsen psoriasis)

SEPTIC ARTHRITIS

Predisposing

All the **I's**

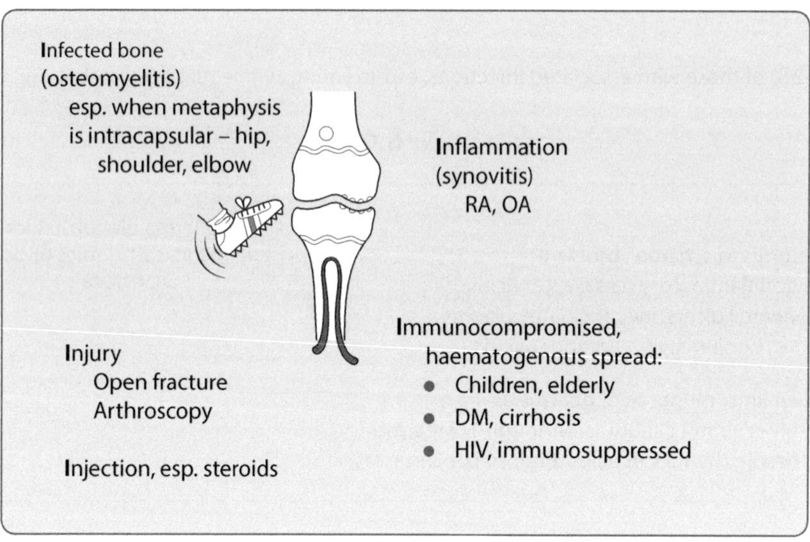

Organisms

 **Gram +ve cocci**

Staphylococcus aureus: 80%
Streptococcus viridans: SBE
Streptococcus pneumoniae: Immunocompromised

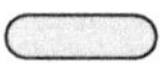 **Gram –ve rods**

Salmonella: Sickle cell, elderly
Brucella: Endemic areas
Haemophilus: Children <5 y

 **Gram –ve cocci**

Neisseria gonorrhoea
Neisseria meningitidis

 **Atypical bacteria**

Mycobacterium tuberculosis:

- Children: Discitis, vertebral body collapse; adults: painful large-joint synovitis
- Poncet disease (reactive non-septic arthritis)

Mycobacterium bovis: Carpal tunnel infection
Lyme disease: Rash followed by recurrent large-joint arthritis

---

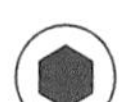 **Viruses**

DNA	RNA
Parvovirus	Rubella
EBV	Mumps
Hep B	Enteroviruses: Coxsackie, hep A

Patterns

Monoarthritis: Pyogenic, TB
Polyarthritis:

- Virus (rubella = rheumatoid-pattern in hands that lasts months)
- Lyme

Migratory: Gonoccoccus – occurs several weeks after acute infection; moves between hand, wrist and knee, before settling in 1 or 2 joints
Vertebral: TB (painless), staphylococal (painful); cause discitis, vertebral body collapse, psoas abscess, radiculopathy

PC

Arthritis
Acute, severe pain; tender, hot effusion; muscle spasm (pseudoparesis)
Secondary osteomyelitis (tender along bone), sinus, abscess
Chronic immobility due to:

- Fibrous-bony ankylosis: Begins within 24 h of infection!
- Secondary wasting and osteoporosis

Systemic
Fever, N+V
Associated: Rash (virus, incl. parvovirus, gonococcus, Lyme), diarrhoea (parvovirus, enterovirus)
Risk groups: Sickle cell anaemia, sexually active (gonorrhoea, HIV)

Ix

Bloods: FBC, ESR, CRP
Uric acid, rheumatoid factor, ANA (acute gout and rheumatoid are differential diagnoses)
Urine: Microscopic haematuria – SBE
Micro: Blood cultures and serology: For suspected viral infections
Synovial aspirate: Urgent Gram stain
Radiol:

X-ray

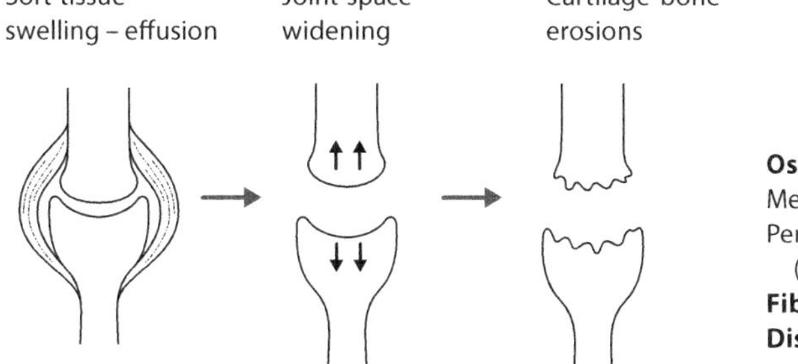

Osteomyelitis:
Metaphyseal mottling
Perisoteal elevation
(involucrum + sequestrum)
Fibrous or bony ankylosis
Dislocation – tense effusion

Radio-isotope scan: Reveals adjacent osteomyelitis, even in absence of X-ray changes

Rx

Medical – Antibiotics:
S. aureus – flucloxacillin, vancomycin, clindamycin (fusidic acid if osteomyelitis)
Coliforms – gentamicin (IV for first 2 weeks, PO for 6 weeks thereafter)
Surgical: Arthroscopy and drainage – indicates whether synovial damage and osteomyelitis
Supportive:
NSAIDs, e.g. indomethacin
Daily aspiration – relieves pain
Physio: 1st – splint or cast in appropriate position (hip: 30° flexion + adduction); rest
2nd – gradual exercise from 1 week after acute stage

CRYSTAL ARTHROPATHIES

Gout

Def

Precipitations of NaH urate (monosodium urate monohydrate) and uric acid crystals, in synovial joints and soft tissue (cf. 'Pseudogout' = calcium pyrophosphate crystals)

Occurs acutely and chronically against a background of hyperuricaemia, that is caused by:

Causes

G.O.U.T.Y².

Genetic: Enzyme defects in purine metabolism

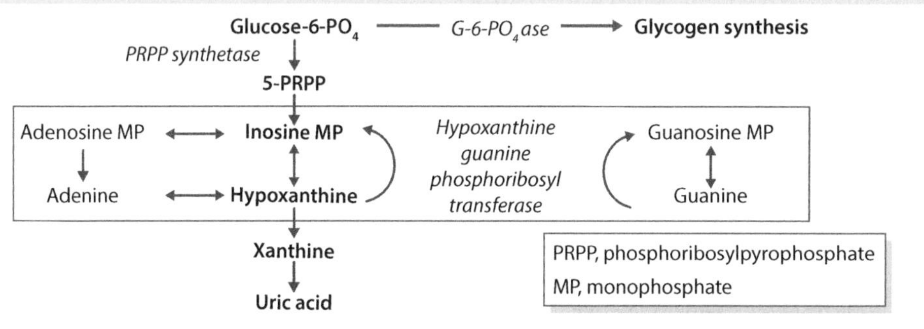

- Lesch–Nyhan syndrome (X-linked) = HGPRT deficiency
  PC: Spasticity, developmental delay, self-mutilation
- PRPP synthetase overactivity
- Glycogen storage disease, type 1: Glucose-6-phosphatase deficiency

Overproduction of uric acid:

- Ingestion of purines – offal, oily fish
- Increased cell turnover:
  - Myeloproliferative disease, leukaemia, myeloma, carcinomatosis – esp. with chemotherapy
  - Chronic haemolytic anaemia
  - Severe psoriasis
- Hypoxia, e.g. cyanotic congenital heart disease, incl. Down syndrome;
  ATP production ↓ → inosine → xanthine production ↑

Underexcretion of uric acid:

- 'Idiopathic' (95% cases) – often have positive family history
- Chronic renal failure – due to decreased glomerular filtration rate, and hence urate clearance:
  - Esp. with hypertension
  - Tubular disease: uric acid may be lost excessively (hypouricaemia)
- Acidosis: urate → uric acid → resorbed in renal tubules, e.g. starvation, alcoholism (lactic acidosis)

Toxins:

- Alcohol
- Diuretics: Thiazide, loop
- TB Rx: Pyrazinamide; ethambutol
- Other: Salicylates (so don't treat pain with aspirin!), cyclosporin, metformin

Y: h**Y**pothyroidism or h**Y**perparathyroidism

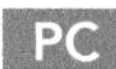

Epi

Inc: 5% hyperuricaemia → of which 15% have gout
Age: Middle-age or elderly – urate levels increase until 30 y (men) or menopause (women)
Sex: Men: 10–20 ×↑
Pre: Alcohol-drinking, meat-eating, obese; hypertensive-IHD

PC

Acute:

Arthritis
Location:
- Small-joint monoarthritis
- 75% = 1st MTP ('podagra')
- 10% = >1 joint

Painful, red, shiny, desquamates
Fever

Triggers of **A.T.T.A.C².K.**

Acute illness: Infection, trauma, dehydration, exertion
Toxin-1: Allopurinol, uricosuric
Toxin-2: Diuretic, chemotherapy
Alcohol: Esp. binge, withdrawal
Cold, **C**onsumption of high-protein meal
Ketoacidosis: DKA, starvation

Chronic:

A.R.T.

Arthritis: Irregular nodules, recurrent flares; tenosynovitis, olecranon bursitis
Renal: Tubulointerstitial nephritis
Tophi: Crystal deposition and calcification in skin (finger tips); pinna; eyes; cartilage, bone, bursae, tendon

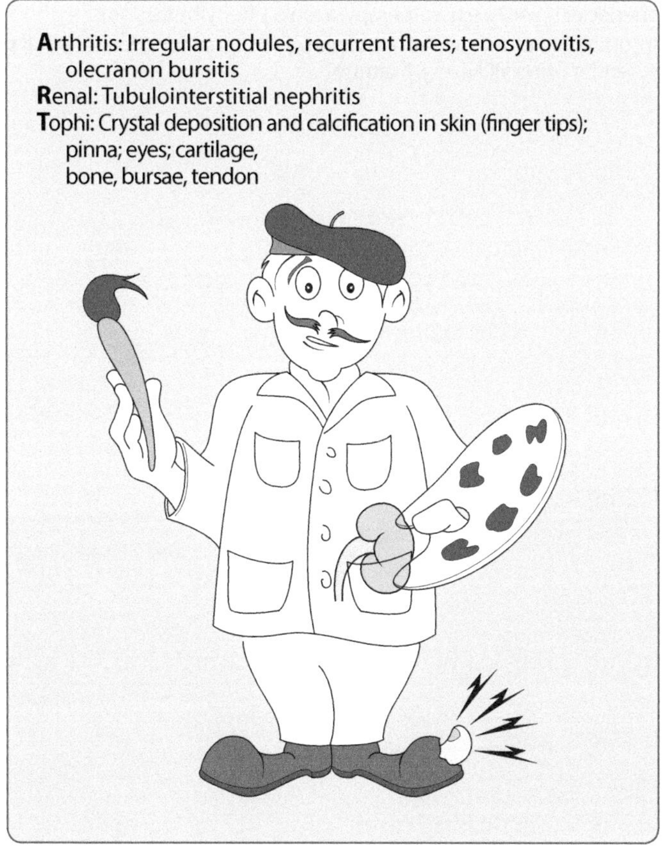

Ix

Bloods: Uric acid (<480 μmol – males; <390 μmol – females); but levels do not correlate with acute attack – an attack may be precipitated by a **reduction** in levels!

Urine: 24-h uric acid, collected after a 70 g protein, purine-free diet; distinguishes 'overproducers' (high urinary uric acid) from 'underexcretors'

Micro: Synovial aspirate microscopy:

- Polarized light: Strongly negative birefringence (cf. pseudogout = weakly positive birefringence)
- Neutrophils contain crystals
- Blood-staining suggests pseudogout,or hydroxyapatite crystals (e.g. Milwaukee shoulder)

Radiol: Bone X-ray: Subcutaneous calcification; 'moth-eaten' phalanges; 'punched-out' erosions
Abdominal X-ray: Calculi – radiolucent, unless mixed with calcium

Rx

Acute:

NSAIDS, high-dose – e.g. indomethacin, diclofenac, azapropazone (but not aspirin!)
Colchicine: Microtubule assembly inhibitor; ☠ Diarrhoea, N+V, neuropathy

Chronic:

Strategy: Wait >1 month after acute attack; cover for 3 months with NSAID or colchicine; continue indefinitely, incl. during attacks

- Allopurinol (xanthine oxidase inhibitor): Indicated in 'overproducers' or severe disease
  ☠: Hypersensitivity reaction or rash – necessitates withdrawal; dyspepsia
- Rasburicase = oxidases uric acid into allantoin
- Uricosuric (probenecid; NSAIDs, e.g. sulphinpyrazone, phenylbutazone):
  - Indicated in 'underexcretors', mild disease, preserved renal function ☠: Renal stones (ensure high fluid intake, render urine alkali, e.g. K citrate)

PYROPHOSPHATE ARTHROPATHY

AKA Calcium pyrophosphate dihydrate crystal deposition disease
AKA Pseudogout

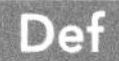

Def

Precipitation of calcium pyrophosphate dehydrates crystal in synovial joints

Causes

Unclear – familial cases are rare

Epi

Mostly elderly patients >80 y, equal M:F

PC

Either:
- Acute large joint monoarthritis (50% knee joint)
- Chronic/insidious polyarthritis

May be associated with carpal tunnel

Ix

Micro: Rhomboid crystals, weakly positively birefringent on polarized light microscopy
Radiol: Evidence of chondrocalcinosis on plain X-ray

Rx

Steroids – oral or intra-articular injection
NSAIDS or colchicine for acute flares

MULTISYSTEMIC AUTOIMMUNE DISEASES

Classification

Rheumatoid arthritis
Sjögren syndrome

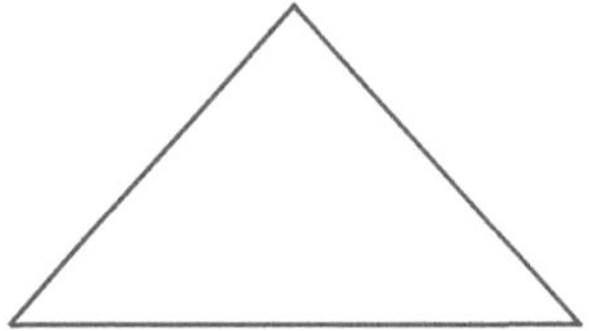

Connective tissue diseases

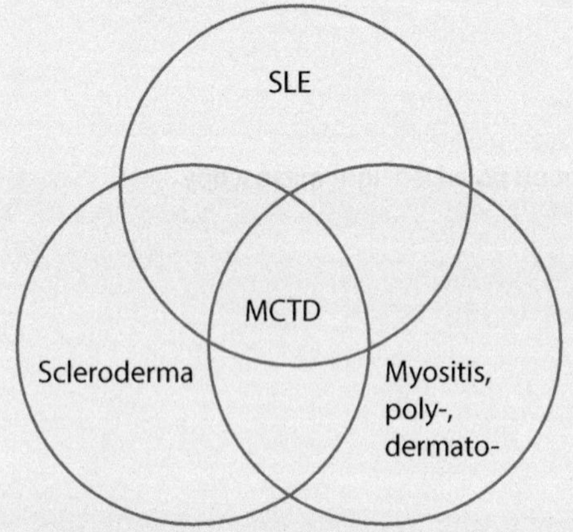

Associations

1. Anti-phospholipid syndrome (recurrent thromboses and miscarriages) – associated with SLE
2. Raynaud disease/cryoglobulinaemia
3. Primary biliary cirrhosis – both 2 and 3 associated with connective tissue diseases, rheumatoid arthritis and Sjögren

Vasculitides

Primary

Large	PMR, GCA, Takayasu arteritis
Medium	Buerger disease, Kawasaki disease, PAN
Small	Granulomatosis with polyangiitis Eosinophilic granulomatosis with polyangiitis HSP Behçet

Autoimmune: connective tissue disease
Infection:
- HBV – PAN
- HCV – 'essential mixed cryoglobulinaemia'
- HIV, parvovirus B19, rickettsia

Neoplasia: Lymphoma, carcinoma – paraneoplastic
Toxins

GCA, giant-cell arteritis
HSP, Henoch–Schönlein purpura
MCTD, mixed connective tissue disease
PAN, polyarteritis nodosa
PMR, polymyalgia rheumatica
SLE, systemic lupus erythematosus

Auto-antibodies

Anti-Cardiolipin IgG: Anti-phospholipid syndrome ± SLE
Anti-RBC, -platelet or -lymphocyte Abs: Respective cytopenia ± SLE

RheuMatoid factor
Def: Ig**M** directed against Fc portion of IgG
Positive: 1. Rheumatoid arthritis, Sjögren, connective tissue disease (in 50%)
2. Malaria, leprosy, rubella
False –ve: Other Ab serotypes, e.g. IgG or IgA

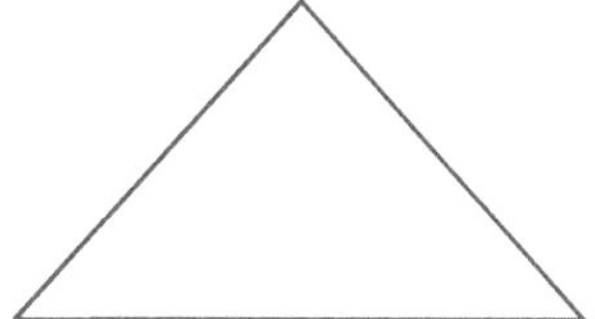

ANA (anti-nuclear abs)

High sensitivity (SLE 95%), but poor specificity:
False +ve: Rheumatoid arthritis, PBC, drugs, elderly
False –ve: Complement deficiency, subacute cutaneous LE
Types: Classified according to:

Indirect immunofluorecence (HEP-2 cells)	**ENA**
Rim = **R**egular SLE	Double-stranded DNA Smith (Sm) antigen: • Small nuclear RNP
Diffuse = **D**rug-induced or regular SLE	Histone
Speckled = **S**ystemic: • Myositis • Raynaud • Cardio-pulmonary	U_1 ribonucleprotein: • MCTD Jo-1 (histidyl tRNA synthetase): • Myositis + pulmo. fibrosis
Speckled = **S**jögren syndrome	SS-A (Ro); SS-8 (La): • Sjogren syndrome • Subacute cutaneous LE, or lupus nephritis (Ro) • Neonatal heart block
Nucleolar = scleroderma	Anti-Scl-70: • Diffuse cutaneous Anti-centromere: • Limited CREST

ANCA (anti-neutrophil cytoplasmic abs)

p-ANCA
Def: Abs against perinuclear antigens – myeloperoxidase, cathepsin, elastase, lactoferrin, lysozyme
Diseases: **P.U.R.G.E**
PAN, micro**PAN** (70% sensitivity) or eosinophilic granulomatosis with polyangiitis (EGPA)
Ulcerative colitis, or:
- Chronic active hepatitis
- Primary biliary cirrhosis
- Primary sclerosing cholangitis

Rheumatoid arthritis with vasculitis
Glomerulonephritis, idiopathic crescentic
Endocarditis, HIV

c-ANCA
Def: Abs against cytoplasmic antigens, esp. proteinase-3 (neutral serine protease)
Diseases:
- Granulomatosis with polyangiitis
- α_1-anti-trypsin deficiency

NB: ANCA titre indicates disease severity better than ESR or CRP

SYSTEMIC LUPUS ERYTHEMATOSUS (SLE)

PC

S.O.S. A.N.A. ...
S.O.S. A.N.A

Skin
- Photosensitivity due to IL-1 secretion from keratinocytes:
  - Malar, 'butterfly', rash: Erythematous maculopapular rash involving chin and ears
  - Discoid LE: Hyperkeratotic, follicular plugs; atrophic scars, raised erythematous rim
  - Subacute cutaneous LE: Extensive papules, annular, hypopigmented rash; fatigue
- Alopecia: Patchy or total
- Vasculitis: Purpura, cryoglobulinaemia, Raynaud, nail fold infarcts, ulcers–nodules
- Other: Urticaria, bullae, erythema multiforme, lichen planus, panniculitis

Oral ulcers, or nasopharyngeal ulcers: aphthous – white base with red surround
Serositis:
- Pleural effusions, pericarditis, peritonitis
- Other respiratory: Basal fibrosis, linear atelectasis, pulmonary hypertension
- Other cardiac: 'Libman-Sacks endocarditis', myocarditis
- Other GIT: Abdominal pain, N+V+D

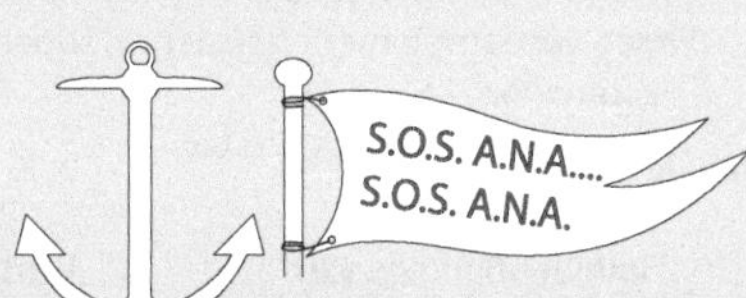

Arthritis:
- Non-erosive arthritis of ± 2 joints: 'Jaccoud arthropathy'
- Joint effusions, contractures, avascular necrosis; tendonitis
- Myalgia, myositis

Neurological:
- Headaches: Common
- Seizures, psychosis, dementia, encephalopathy, cerebellar ataxia
- Transverse myelitis, peripheral neuropathy

Anaemia and other haematological:
- Haemolytic: direct Coombs' test +ve, warm agglutinins
- Lymphopenia – immunosuppressed: Miliary TB; toxoplasmosis; histoplasmosis, candida
- Thrombocytopenia

Splenomegaly, hepatomegaly (fatty change), lymphadenopathy
Ophthalmic: Sicca, conjunctivitis, episcleritis, retinal vasculitis, cytoid bodies
Systemic: Fever, fatigue, LOW

Acute **N**ephritis (or chronic): Proteinuria (3+; >0.5 g/24 h)/cellular casts
Antibodies:
- ANA+ve incl. dsDNA, anti-Sm, false +ve VRDL (or LE cell prep. +ve)
- Anti-cardiolipin (or lupus anticoagulant) → 'anti-phospholipid syndrome' = arterial and venous thromboses (incl. recurrent miscarriages), thrombocytopenia, liveo reticularis, nephritis, cerebral disease, endocarditis

Disease-defined by presence of any 4 of SOS, ANA and ANA

Epi

Inc: Prevalence = 1/10,000
Age: Onset 15–30 y
Sex: F:M = 9:1 (discoid LE = 2:1)
Geo: Black:White = 9:1; SLE also highly prevalent in Chinese
Aet: Inherited: C2, C4 deficiency (5%)
Oestrogen: OCP pregnancy, menses worsen SLE
Drug-induced:

- Fast acetylators: Hydralazine
- **SL**ow acetylators: **SL.I.P^2.P^2.E.D.**
  Isoniazid
  Phenytoin, **P**henothiazine (chlorpromazine)
  Procainamide, **P**enicillin (or tetracycline)
  O**E**strogen (oral contraceptive)
  Diuretic (thiazide)
  PC: Rash, serositis, pulmonary fibrosis (**NOT** neurological or nephritis)

Ix

ANA (anti-nuclear antibodies):

- ENA: Anti-Ro, anti-La, anti-Sm, Anti-scl-70, anti-Jo
- Anti-dsDNA – very specific for SLE
- Anti-histone antibodies – strongly assoc. with drug-induced lupus

Other auto-antibodies:

- Rheumatoid factor +ve in 40%
- Anti-cardiolipin ELISA IgG; or lupus anticoagulant assay (APTT ↑)
- Direct Coombs' test (warm agglutinins); anti-neutrophil, -lymphocyte, -platelet abs

Other:

- ESR ↑ but CRP normal (unless superimposed infection or active serositis)
- Complement: C3, C4 ↓ (C3 normal in C1, C4 deficiency, or drug-induced SLE); CH50 ↓
- Biopsy, e.g. rash, renal, brain: Fibrinoid necrosis; small-medium–vessel vasculitis

Rx

Acute flares:
Steroids
NSAIDS
Opioids
DMARDS:

- Hydroxychloroquine
- Azathioprine
- Methotrexate
- Cyclophosphamide for severe lupus nephritis

Surgical:
Splenectomy, esp. if ITP
Kidney transplant for severe renal disease

Other: Anticoagulation, e.g. warfarin for recurrent thromboembolic disease

SCLERODERMA

Types

Scleroderma – Localized

Morphoea: Plaque of thick, waxy skin
Linear scleroderma: En coup de sabre (linear alopecia), facial hemiatrophy
Eosinophilic fasciitis:

- Acute inflammation, and cobblestone-like induration of all extremities, after exertion
- Flexion contractures, carpal tunnel syndrome, myositis (CK normal)
- Aplastic anaemia, myelodysplasia

Systemic sclerosis – Limited

PC

C.R.E.S.T.

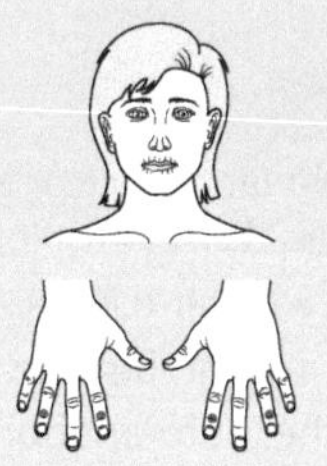

Calcinosis, subcutaneous
Raynaud phenomenon: May precede CREST by several years
O**E**sophageal dysmotility: PC: Dysphagia (present in 50%)
Sclerodactyly: Tight, tense, thick, tender, tanned skin (oedema and fibrosis); ulcers; claw hand
Telangiectasia: No central arteriole, cf. liver disease

NB: Cutaneous disease is confined to forearms and face

Systemic sclerosis – Diffuse

PATH

Organ fibrosis

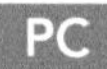
PC

C.R.A.C.K.I.N.G.

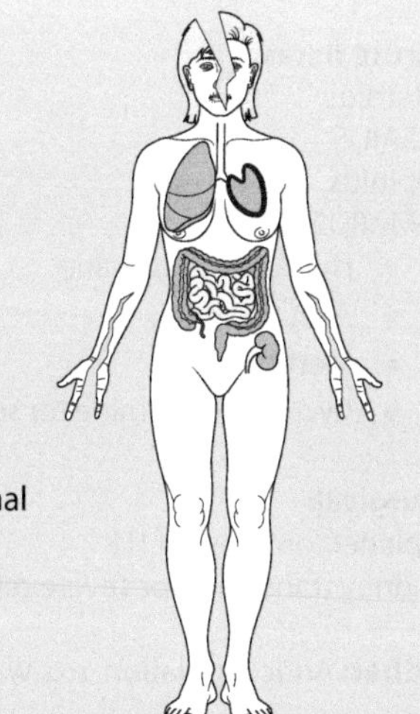

Cutaneous disease spreads to entire body
Respiratory:

- Pulmonary fibrosis
- Pulmonary hypertension

Arthritis:

- Non-erosive arthritis
- Tapered fingers; phalangeal tuft erosion and osteolysis

Cardiac:

- Restrictive cardiomyopathy
- Pericardial effusion

Kidney:

- Rapidly progressive renal failure, or chronic renal failure (PATH: Intimal proliferation + medial fibrinoid necrosis)
- Malignant hypertension, flash pulmonary oedema
- Microangiopathic haemolytic anaemia (MAHA)

Intestine:

- Small bowel: Dysmotility, bacterial overgrowth, malabsorption
- Large bowel: Constipation, diverticulae, pseudo-obstruction, pneumatosis coli

Neurological: Polymyositis
Gastric: Oesophageal dysmotility – peptic oesophagitis

Epi

Inc: Prevalence = 50/100,000
Age: 20–40 y
Sex: F:M = 3:1 (esp. limited systemic sclerosis)
Geo: Choctaw Native Americans (Oklahoma) – highest incidence
Aet: Limited systemic sclerosis: Small-vessel vasculitis
Diffuse systemic sclerosis: Necrosis → overproduction of collagen and ground substance → fibrosis
Pre: Industrial toxins: Vinyl chloride, aromatics, epoxy resins – scleroderma-like disease
Iatrogenic – bleomycin; breast implants – localized scleroderma around silicon implants
Autoimmunity: Sjögren, primary biliary cirrhosis, vitiligo

Ix

Bloods:
Routine:
Hb ↓: Normocytic, due to chronic inflammation or microangiopathic haemolytic anaemia
Macrocytic, due to vitamin B12 deficiency (bacterial overgrowth)
ESR ↑; urea and creatinine ↑
Autoantibodies:
Limited systemic sclerosis: ANA: anti-centromere pattern
ENA: Anti-centromere
Diffuse systemic sclerosis: ANA: anti-nucleolar pattern
ENA: anti-Scl-70 (topoisomerase)
Others: Rheumatoid factor, cryoglobulins
Urine: RBC and WBC casts
ECG, **E**CHO
Radiol:
CXR, high-resolution CT
Barium swallow, meal + follow-through: Abnormal in 90% systemic sclerosis dilated 2nd part of duodenum
Special:
Oesophageal manometry
Wide-angle microscopy (or ophthalmoscopy) of nail fold:

- Limited systemic sclerosis: Capillary enlargement
- Diffuse systemic sclerosis: Capillary enlargement and areas of capillary loss

Rx

Immunosuppressive:
Azathioprine, mycophenolate, methotrexate, cyclophosphamide
Tyrosine kinase inhibitors – imatinib
Autologous bone marrow transplant

Symptomatic:
cR.E.S.t
Raynaud: Nifedipine, IV prostacyclin
O**E**sophageal dysmotility: Metoclopramide, domperidone, proton-pump inhibitor
Sclerodactyly: Emollients (keep skin moist), subcutaneous relaxin (pregnancy hormone)

Diffuse
GIT: Laxatives, cyclical antibiotics (bacterial overgrowth)
Respiratory – pulmonary hypertension: IV prostacyclin
Kidney: ACE inhibitors, beta-blockers

SJÖGREN SYNDROME

Def

Autoimmune destruction of exocrine glands that is either primary, or secondary to:

- Rheumatoid arthritis (30% of RA pts.); SLE, scleroderma, polymyositis; vasculitides
- Organ-based autoimmunity: Chronic active hepatitis, primary biliary cirrhosis, thyroiditis

Epi

Inc: Prevalence = 0.5–1% (primary SS)
Age: Onset commonest in 30s–40s
Sex: F:M = 9:1 (*same as SLE*)
Pre: HLA-B8, -DR3 – associated with extraglandular involvement and auto-antibodies

X.X.X. S.U.R.R.O.U.N.D.I.N.G.S.

Xerophthalmia (dry eyes):
- Grittiness, soreness, photophobia, every day for >3 months
- O/E: Keratitis, conjunctivitis, corneal ulcers (Rose Bengal stain)

Xerostomia (dry mouth):
- Dysphagia: Need to take water to swallow ('cream cracker Sx'); awakes at night to drink water
- Bilateral parotid enlargement (uncommon in secondary Sjögren, massive in HIV)
- Angular stomatitis, dental caries, fissured tongue; atrophic filiform papillae, oral candida

X: Ix: 2 out of 4 must be positive to establish diagnosis, see p. 245

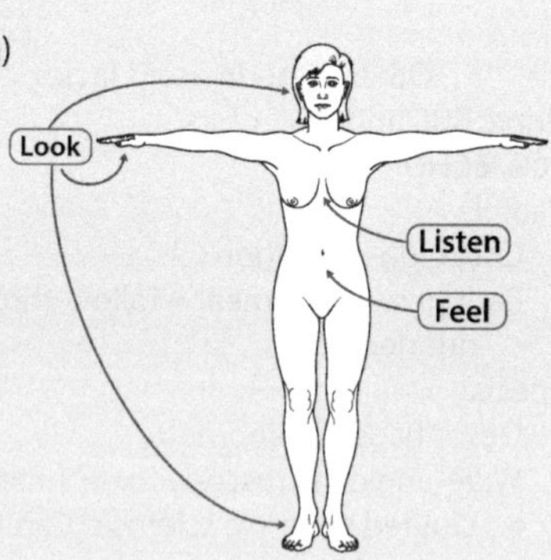

Skin:
- Dry skin + dry hair
- Vasculitis, incl. Raynaud syndrome, ulcers, urticaria, livedo reticularis

Ulcers: Orogenital, corneal, leg ulcers (incl. pyoderma gangrenosum)
Rheum: Reversible deformity, e.g. swan-necking PIP joints (Jaccoud arthropathy)
Respiratory:
- Dry respiratory passages: Xerotrachea, bronchitis (dry cough), sinusitis
- Basal pulmonary fibrosis

Ophthalmic: Xerophthalmia causes keratoconjunctivitis sicca and corneal ulcers
Urine:
- Tubulointerstitial nephritis, renal tubular acidosis – nephrocalcinosis, osteomalacia
- Glomerulonephritis (vasculitis-associated)

Neurology:
- Central nervous system vasculitis: Seizures, multiple sclerosis-like syndrome
- Peripheral neuronopathy: Sensory, painful, facial numbness, Rombergism

Deafness: Sensorineural
Intestine:
- Atrophic oesophagitis–gastritis (due to lack of mucosal barrier), achlorhydria
- Pancreatitis (subclinical)

Neoplasia: Lymphoma or Waldenstrom macroglobulinaemia (5% risk)
Genital: Dyspareunia (dry secretions) – 30% (often presenting complaint)
Systemic: Fatigue, anorexia, loss of weight, low-grade fever, lymphadenopathy

Differential diagnosis

Causes of dry eyes and dry mouth

S.A.L^2.I.V.A.T.E.

Sarcoidosis
Autoimune: Sjögren (primary or secondary)
Lymphoma or **L**eukaemia (CLL) or graft-versus-host disease
Infection: TB
Virus: HIV 'sicca syndrome'
Amyloid
Toxin: Anticholinergics, incL. tricyclic antidepressants
Endocrine: Diabetes mellitus

NB: Glandular enlargement (Mikulicz syndrome) is common with these conditions

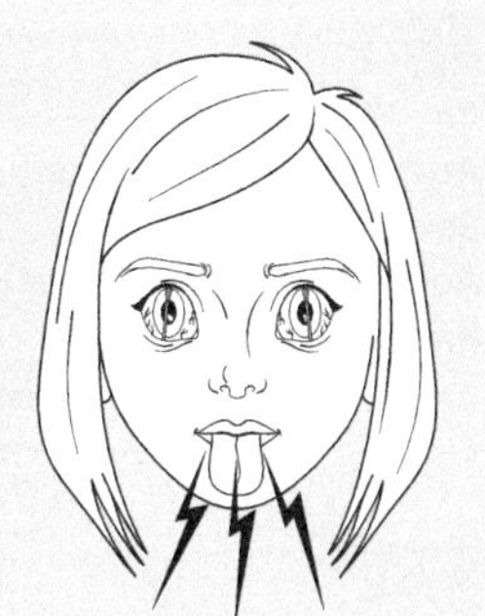

Causes of dry, gritty eyes
Ocular: Blepharitis, conjunctivitis, corneal ulcers, proptosis
Neurological: 5th or 7th cranial nerve palsies, myopathy
Vitamin A deficiency

Causes of bilateral parotid enlargement
Viral: Mumps, EBV, influenza
Gastroenterological: Cirrhosis, chronic pancreatitis, hyperlipoproteinaemia
Bulimia nervosa (painless)

Ix

1. Autoantibodies:
   ENA: SS-A (Anti-Ro), SS-B (Anti-La): Associated with severe disease and extraglandular symptoms
   ANA (immunofluorescent staining = speckled), rheumatoid factor, thyroid auto-antibodies
2. Schirmer test <5 mm in 5 min (usual >15 mm)
3. Salivary function tests: Salivary scintigraphy, parotid sialography, salivary flow test
4. Labial minor salivary gland histology:
   Clusters of CD4+ lymphocytes around salivary acini (↑ 'focus' >50 lymphocytes)
   + gland destruction; duct dilation
   (cf. HIV: CD8+ lymphocytes in glands; sarcoid: granulomas)

Rx

Symptomatic:
Sicca symptoms – artificial tears and saliva; oral pilocarpine; avoid anticholinergics or diuretics
Arthralgia: Hydroxychloroquine

Immunosuppressants:
Steroids, IVIg or cyclophosphamide – used for extraglandular disease, e.g. vasculitis, respiratory

AUTOIMMUNE MYOSITIS

Dermatomyositis

Epi

Inc: 1/100,000 p.a.
Age: Adults and children
Sex: F:M = 3:1
Aet: Primarily a vasculitis of muscle and skin capillaries → ischaemia + CD4 infiltration
Pre: Malignancy:
Present in 10%: Bronchial, breast, ovary, GIT, lymphoma (non-Hodgkin)
May pre-date or post-date malignancy by 2 years

PC

Similar organ involvement as for diffuse systemic sclerosis:

C.R.A.C.k.I.N.G.

Cutaneous
Respiratory:
- Pulmonary fibrosis: Assoc. anti-Jo-1 (tRNA synthetase); anti-KL6 (mucin-like glycoprotein)
- Respiratory muscle weakness

Arthritis: Arthralgia; flexion contractures (children)
Cardiac: AV-conduction block, arrhythmias, myocarditis
Intestine: Visceral myopathy – constipation, dysphagia
Neurological:
- Proximal myopathy develops acutely over days–weeks
- Bulbar and respiratory weakness

Gastro-oesophageal – dysphagia, due to involvement of striated muscle of oropharynx, upper oesophagus

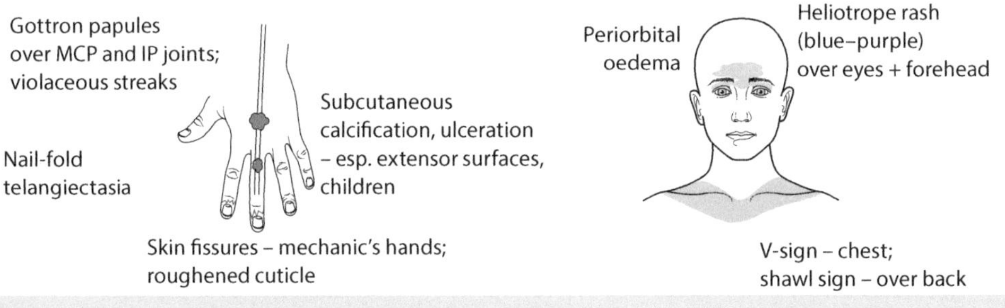

Ix

Bloods: CK ↑↑
Auto-abs: Anti-Jo1 (histidyl tRNA synthetase), anti-SRP (signal recognition particle)
EMG: Small-amplitude, polyphasic potentials; positive sharp-waves; fibrillations
Radiol: Plain X-rays – subcutaneous calcification
CT thorax–abdomen–pelvis, or PET scan – search for occult malignancy
Special – muscle biopsy (site can be guided by prior MRI)

Rx

Steroids: 80 mg od, taper over 10 weeks
Steroid-sparing drugs: Methotrexate (acts faster), azathioprine, mycophenolate, IVIg

Polymyositis

Epi

Inc: 0.5/100,000 p.a.
Age: Adults only
Sex: F:M = 3:1
Aet: Primarily myositis → CD8 infiltration
Pre: Autoimmunity: SLE, Sjögren syndrome, RA
Infection: HIV

PC

As for dermatomyositis, except:

- No cutaneous features
- Myopathy develops sub-acutely over weeks–months (cf. acutely for dermatomyositis)

As for dermatomyositis, except no need to hunt for neoplasia, but do HIV test

As for dermatomyositis

Inclusion body myositis

Epi

Inc: Commonest myopathy of 50+s
Age: Elderly
Sex: F:M = 1:3
Geo: Caucasians
Aet: Myositis + degenerative components:
Myositis: Similar to polymyositis
Degenerative: Vacuolated fibres, amyloid-positive inclusions, mitochondrial DNA deletions
Pre: Autoimmunity
Family history

PC

Myopathy:

- Distal (foot extensors, wrist extensors, finger flexors), or quadriceps weaknesss
- Dysphagia in 60%
- Sub-acute onset over weeks–months
- Unresponsive to steroids

Bloods: CK normal or slightly ↑
EMG: As for dermatomyositis
Special – muscle biopsy: Distinguished from DM and PM due to rimmed vaculoes, amyloid-positive inclusions and abnormal mitochondria (ragged-red fibres and cytochrome oxidase-negative fibres)

Rx

Immunosuppressants (steroids, azathioprine, IVIg) can be tried, but no or little response is often found – in contrast to other inflammatory myopathies

VASCULITIS

Types

P.A.I.N.T.

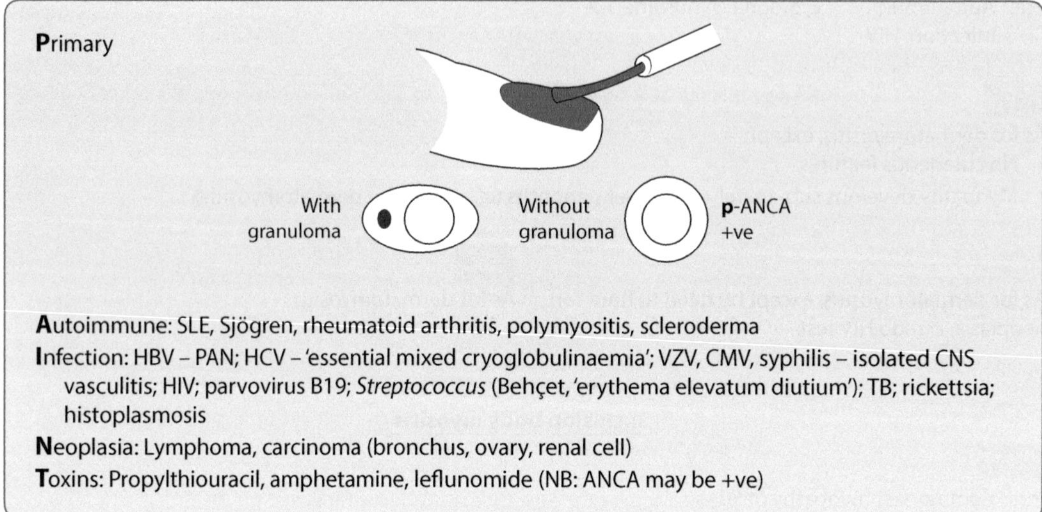

Autoimmune: SLE, Sjögren, rheumatoid arthritis, polymyositis, scleroderma

Infection: HBV – PAN; HCV – 'essential mixed cryoglobulinaemia'; VZV, CMV, syphilis – isolated CNS vasculitis; HIV; parvovirus B19; *Streptococcus* (Behçet, 'erythema elevatum diutium'); TB; rickettsia; histoplasmosis

Neoplasia: Lymphoma, carcinoma (bronchus, ovary, renal cell)

Toxins: Propylthiouracil, amphetamine, leflunomide (NB: ANCA may be +ve)

Typical presentations of primary vasculitides

GCA:
- Epi: Elderly (>60), women (2:1)
- PC: Headache, proximal weakness, optic neuropathy

Takayasu disease
- Epi: Young, Asian women
- PC: CVA, PVD, renal failure

Buerger disease
- Epi: Middle-aged, Mediterranean men; smoking, HLA-B5 (B51)
- PC: CVA, PVD, Raynaud

Eosinophilic granulomatosis with polyangiitis (EGPA - formerly Churg–Strauss syndrome)
- Epi: Any age, M:F = 1.3:1
- PC: Asthma, mononeuritis multiplex, eosinophilia

Granulomatosis with polyangiitis (GPA – formerly Wegener's granulomatosis/Wegener disease)
- Epi: Caucasian, any age, M:F = 1:1
- PC: ENT, pulmonary infiltration, renal failure

Kawasaki disease
- Epi: **C**hildren
- PC: **C**ervical lymph nodes, **C**onjunctivitis, **C**utaneous (rash), **C**oronary microaneurysms

Polyarteritis nodosa (PAN)
- Epi: HBV-infection PC: see p. 249

MicroPAN: As for PAN

Henoch–Schönlein purpura
- Epi: Children (4–11), boys, post-URTI; IgA ↑
- PC: Maculopapular rash on extensor surfaces
  - Haematuria (IgA nephropathy)
  - PR bleeding (ischaemic bowel, intussusception)

PC

Examine the **S.U.R.R.O.U.N.D.I.N.G.S.**

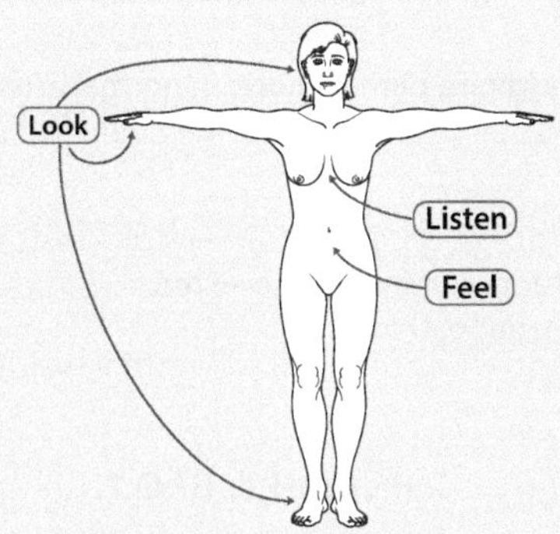

Skin: PAN, GPA: Purpura, nodules, Raynaud syndrome, infarcts, livedo reticularis
Ulcers: Orogenital ulcers, esp. Behçet
Rheumatology: Arthralgia or myalgia (esp. PMR – morning stiffness); arthritis
Respiratory and Cardiac
Respiratory: PAN, microPAN: Pulmonary infarction, haemorrhage
GPA: Haemoptysis; pulmonary infiltrates, atelectasis, nodules, cavitation
EGPA: Asthma, fleeting eosinophilic infiltrates
Cardiac: Takayasu, PAN: MI, CCF, pericarditis, aortic regurgitation, aortic dissection, aneurysm
Ophthalmic: Retinal infarcts ('cotton-wool spots'), uveitis, scleritis, conjunctivitis
GPA: Orbital pseudotumour with proptosis
Urine: Glomerulonephritis: Proliferative or crescentic
Neurological: CNS: Headache, stroke (both infarction and haemorrhage), fits, dementia, psychosis
PNS: Neuropathy, mononeuritis multiplex (esp. EGPA, GPA, PAN), myopathy (GCA)
Deaf (ENT) GPA: Deafness due to otitis media (conductive) or sensorineural; nasopharynx necrosis (epistaxis, sunken nasal bridge); sinusitis; subglottic stenosis (hoarseness, stridor); dacrocystitis
Intestine PAN, HSP: Mesenteric ischaemia (pain, perforation, PR bleeding, intussusception)
PAN: Cholecystitis; pancreatitis; hepatic infarction
Neoplasia: Cyclophosphamide side-effect
Genito-urinary: PAN: Ovarian, testicular–epididymal pain; Behçet: ulcers
Systemic Fever, weight-loss and anorexia, depression-fatigue
Hypertension (suggests glomerulonephritis)
Bloods: Normocytic anaemia, CRP ↑, ESR ↑; polyclonal Ig ↑; complement normal

Ix

ANCA: p-ANCA +ve in PAN, microPAN, HSP, EGPA
c-ANCA +ve in GPA (level indicates severity)
Angiogram (e.g. renal, cerebral, retinal): Aneurysms, stenosis, beading, corkscrew collaterals
Biopsy: Skin, renal, liver, nerve, muscle, brain: Immunofluorescence for immune complexes, IgA
Superficial temporal artery (may be negative due to skip lesions)

Rx

Immunosuppression: Steroids, cyclophosphamide, methotrexate, plasma exchange, IVIg
Anti-platelet/anti-coagulation: Kawasaki, giant-cell arteritis if ischaemia, optic neuropathy
Surgical: Angioplasty (Takayasu), renal transplant (GPA, PAN)

Prog

Poor: PAN, microPAN, EGPA: 5-y SR = 50% treated; 10% untreated
Intermediate: GPA – 75% achieve remission, of whom 50% relapse: Takayasu (variable)
Good: HSP (self-remitting usually), GCA (if steroids given promptly), Kawasaki

RAYNAUD PHENOMENON

Def

Episodic vasospasm of extremities (digits, pinnae, nose) in normal arterioles (idiopathic form)

PC

Pain
Characteristic pattern of colour change: white → blue → red
Chronic: Ulcers and necrosis (not in idiopathic form)

Causes

P^2.A.I.N.T. P^2.O.T.

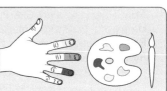

Primary ('Raynaud disease')/**P**ulmonary hypertension:
Epi: Accounts for 50% of Raynaud phenomenon
Women in 20–40s. Assoc: Primary pulmonary hypertension
PC: Triggered by cold, emotion, smoking

Autoimmune:
- Scleroderma (90% pts. have Raynaud – due to digital vessel calcification)
- SLE, RA, poly- or dermatomyositis

Injury:
- Repetitive injury: Pneumatic drills, chainsaws, drums, piano
- Frostbite

Neurological: Reflex sympathetic dystrophy, following trauma ('Volkmann ischaemia')

Toxins:
- Migraine Rx: Beta-blockers (β_2-mediated), ergotamine; methysergide
- Bromocriptine (ergot derivative)
- Chemo Rx: Bleomycin, cisplastin
- Heavy metals/vinyl chloride

Paraproteinaemia; **P**olycythaemia; cold agglutinins – hyperviscosity
- Paraproteinaemia (myeloma, Waldenstrom), esp. cryoglobulinaemia
- Cold agglutinins (e.g. mycoplasma, EBV, lymphoma), typhoid

Outlet obstruction, thoracic:
- Cervical rib; fascial band behind scalenus anterior; prominent transverse process C7
- Fractured 1st rib or clavicle; sleep-related

O/E: Symptoms ↑ and radial pulse ↓ with shoulder abduction to 90°, and external rotation
Supraclavicular fossa bruit

Thromboembolism:
- Atherosclerosis
- Buerger disease (thromboangiitis obliterans)

Rx

- Conservative: Avoid cold; mittens and coats (cold induces generalized vasospasm); stop smoking
- PO meds: Ca antagonists (nifedipine), α_1-blockers (prazosin), losartan, fluoxetine (via platelet 5-HT effect)
- IV prostacyclin
- Surgical: Sympathectomy

CRYOGLOBULINAEMIA

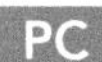

Def

Immunoglobulins that precipitate at 4°C

PC

S.A.U.N.A.

Skin:
- Palpable purpura (leucocytoclastic vasculitis)
- Raynaud, with digital ulcers
- Cold urticaria

Arthralgia: Rheumatoid arthritis-like
Urine: Mesangiocapillary glomerulonephritis
Neurology: Mononeuritis multiplex, cranial nerve palsies
Additional: Pericarditis, thyroiditis

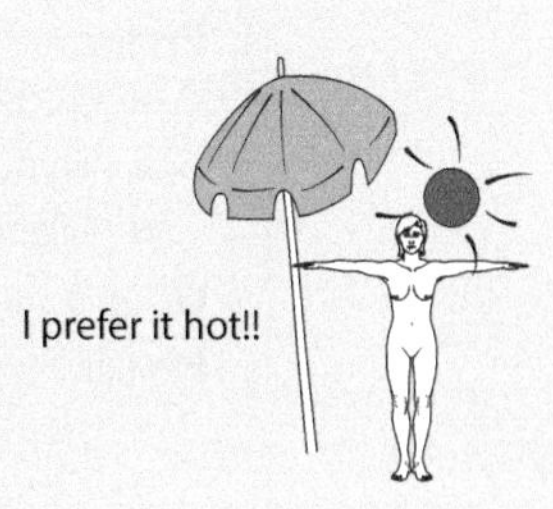

The full syndrome is typical of mixed essential cryoglobulinaemia; other causes result predominantly in rash

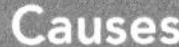

Causes

P.A.I.N.

Primary – 'mixed essential cryoglobulinaemia': Most cases have chronic hepatitis C
Autoimmune:
- SLE, RA, systemic sclerosis
- Primary biliary cirrhosis

Infection:
- Hepatitis C, B virus: 5% chronic hepatitis C patients develop cryoglobulinaemia
- Herpes (EBV, CMV)
- Bacteria:
  - Endocarditis
  - *Streptococcus* (esp. post-acute glomerulonephritis)
  - Leprosy, kala-azar, malaria (hyper-reactive form with splenomegaly)

Neoplasia:
- Myeloma, granulomatosis with polyangiitis, amyloid
- CLL, Hodgkin lymphoma

Ix

Type 1: Monoclonal Ig – myeloma
Type 2: Polyclonal IgG (e.g. specific to hep C) + monoclonal rheumatoid factor
Type 3: Polyclonal IgG (e.g. to herpes, bacteria) + polyclonal rheumatoid factor

Differential diagnosis

Acrocyanosis:
PC: Cyanotic digits irrespective of ambient temperature
Epi: Women in 20s

Erythromelalgia:
PC: Burning, erythematous extremities; feet > hands; worse in warmth and dependency; normal pulses
Epi: Middle-aged men; myeloproliferative disease, nifedipine, bromocriptine
Rx: Aspirin

CARPAL TUNNEL SYNDROME

P.O.M.E.G.R.A.N.A.T.E.

Pregnancy
OCP (oral contraceptive pill)
Menopause, pre-menstrual
Endocrine:
- Acromegaly
- Hypothyroidism
- Diabetes mellitus

Gout
Renal:
- Nephrotic syndrome (fluid overload)
- Chronic renal failure or congestive cardiac failure (fluid overload) (and, as in CCF, symptoms worsen at night)
- Haemodialysis: Accumulation of β_2-microglobulin
- AV – fistula: Steals blood from median nerve vasa nervorum

Amyloid, multiple myeloma
Neuropathy: Hereditary neuropathy with liability to pressure palsies (autosomal dominant)
Arthritis:
- Rheumatoid arthritis with associated wrist tenosynovitis
- Osteoarthritis, esp. familial 'persistent generalized osteoarthropathy'

Trauma: Carpal fracture or anterior dislocation of lunate
Extra: TB, sarcoid

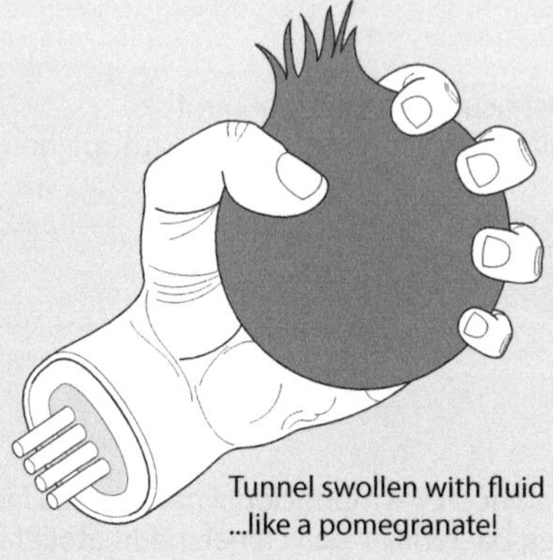
Tunnel swollen with fluid
...like a pomegranate!

PATH

Swelling of flexor synovial sheaths beneath flexor retinaculum, due to generalized fluid accumulation, or synovitis

PC

Pain and paraesthesia in hand – often more extensive than just lateral 3½ fingers!

- Radiates up medial forearm and towards shoulder (thus mimicking a cervical root lesion)
- Worse at night; relieved by shaking hand

Clumsy hand or weak grip

O/E

Motor: Wasting and weakness of hand muscles supplied by the median nerve:

L.O.A.F.

Lumbricals 1 + 2
Opponens pollicis
Abductor pollicis brevis (most sensitive)
Flexor pollicis brevis

Sensory: Sensory loss over palmar aspect, and tips, of lateral 3½ fingers, and adjacent palm (but not over thenar eminence, which is supplied by superficial palmar branch that traverses over the transverse ligament!)

Special: **T**inel test = **T**apping gently over carpal tunnel reproduces paraesthesia
Phalen test = **F**lexing wrist maximally for 1 min reproduces symptoms

Distinguish this pattern from diffuse wasting of hand muscles, whose causes are:

- Upper motor–neuron: CVA, Parkinson (disuse atrophy)
- Cervical cord: Syringomyelia
- Anterior horns: Motor neurone disease, polio
- Roots: Cervical spondylosis
- Brachial plexus: 'Klumpke's palsy'
- Neuropathy:
  - Brachial neuritis (viral)
  - Mononeuritis multiplex (e.g. vasculitis)
  - Generalized neuropathy (CIDP, multifocal motor neuropathy)
- Joints, e.g. rheumatoid arthritis
- Constitutional, e.g. carcinoma, malnutrition

Ix

EMG: Slowing of median nerve across wrist

Rx

S.I.D.S.

Splint wrist
Injection of hydrocortisone
Diuretics
Surgical decompression

COLLAGEN AND ELASTIC-TISSUE DISEASES

Defects in collagen

Genetics: All are **autosomal dominant**, except severe forms of osteogenesis imperfecta and severe epidermolysis bullosa (autosomal recessive), and Alport disease (X-linked)

Type I: Osteogenesis imperfecta

O.S.T.E.OC.L.A.S.T.

Osteopenia: Frequent fractures; kyphoscoliosis; *in utero* fractures – short stature; perinatal death
Skin: Thin
Teeth: Dentinogenesis imperfecta
Eyes: Blue sclera – also seen as familial trait, Ehlers–Danlos, Marfan; PXE, pseudohypo-PTHism
Otos**C**lerosis, and sensorineural deafness >20 y
Ligament laxity: Joint dislocations
Aortic regurgitation; mitral regurgitation
Systemic hyperthermia
Thyroid, hyper

Type II: Achondroplasia

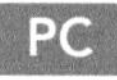

C.H.O.N.D.R.O.

Craniofacial: Frontal bossing, midface hypoplasia
Height: Short – due to short thighs (rhizomelic), but normal trunk size
Orthopaedic: Hip, pelvic abnormalities due to metaphyseal flaring
Neurological: Spinal stenosis, cervicomedullary compression, hydrocephalus
Deafness: Recurrent otitis media, partly due to cleft palate
Respiratory: Restrictive defect; obstructive sleep apnoea, incl. central apnoea
Ophthalmic: Cataracts, vitreal degeneration, retinal detachment

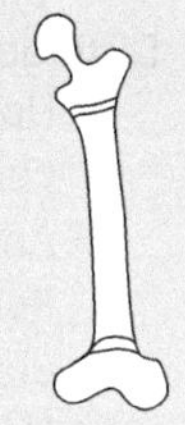

Type III: Ehlers–Danlos syndrome

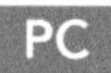

E.L.A².S.T.I.c.

Eyes: Keratoconus; ocular rupture (lysyl hydroxylase def. variant – AR)
Ligament laxity: Hypermobile joints, osteoarthritis
Aortic regurgitation; **A**ortic dissection–aneurysm; mitral valve prolapse
Skin: Hyperextensible (cutis laxis), fragile (cigarette paper), purpura
Thoracic: Kyphoscoliosis
Intestine: Bowel or uterine perforation

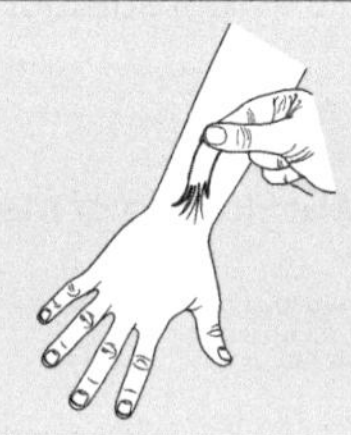

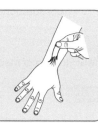

Type IV: Alport disease

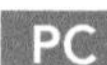

Glomerular and interstitial nephritis (recurrent haematuria), sensorineural deafness, lenticonus

Type VII: Epidermolysis bullosa

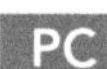

Epithelial blisters and breaks following minor trauma:
Mild: Epidermal keratin
Severe: Dermal collagen VII, or junctional laminin

Defects in elastic tissue

Fibrillin: Marfan syndrome

PATH

Fibrillin mutation in epidermal growth factor-like regions of gene (chromosome 15)
Fibrillin is a constituent of **elastic** tissue and microfibrils, incl. suspensory ligaments of lens
Autosomal dominant (as opposed to phenotypically-similar homocystinuria: AR)

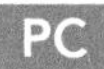

$E^2.L^2.A^2.S^2.T^2$.I.C.

Eyes: Ectopia lentis (upward displacement, cf. homocystinuria – downwards)
Elevated (high-arch) palate
Limbs: Long arms, fingers (arachnodactyly) and toes
Long trunk, i.e. upper:lower segment ratio increased
Ligament laxity: Hypermobile joints (thumb sign, Walker–Murdoch's wrist sign)
Aortic regurgitation; mitral regurgitation or mitral valve prolapse
Aortic: Aneurysm–dissection (esp. ascending aorta)
Skin: Striae
Skin: Purpura on buttocks, shoulders
Thorax: Pectus excavatum or carinatum, kyphoscoliosis; dural sac dilatation
Thorax: Pneumothorax
Intestine: Herniae
Circulation: Varicose veins

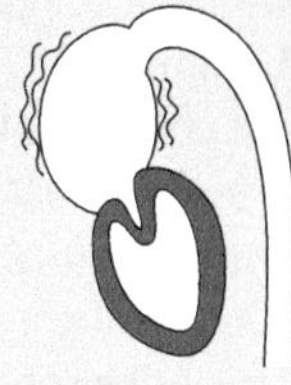
Aortic aneurysm

Elastin (1): Pseudoxanthoma elasticum

PATH

Calcium deposition in elastic fibres of skin; arteries and retina–choroid Bruch membrane
Autosomal recessive/dominant, or as an effect of penicillamine; worsened by steroids!

E.L.A.S.T.I.C.

Eyes: Angioid streaks (also seen in Paget, sickle cell disease, Ehlers–Danlos) – blindness
Ligament laxity: Hypermobile joints; osteoarthritis
Aortic regurgitation; mitral regurgitation
Skin: 'Plucked-chicken' = coalesced yellow maculopapules; spares follicles
Hanging, lax skin folds, esp. neck, axillae, antecubital fossae
Purpura on buttocks, shoulders
Thorax: Scoliosis, pneumothorax
Intestine: Haematemesis
Circulation: Hypertension, ischaemic heart disease, peripheral vascular disease; and haemorrhage – subarachnoid, GIT, genito-urinary; haemoptysis

Angioid streaks

Elastin (2): Williams syndrome

PATH

Sporadic large deletion on chromosome 7, incorporating elastin and actin-regulator *LIMK* genes

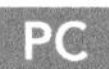

WI.L.L.I.A.M.

WIde mouth, short, upturned nose. **L**ow growth. **L**ow **I**ntelligence but gregarious (opposite of autism)
Aortic stenosis – supravalular. **M**etabolic – hypercalcaemia

BACK PAIN

Epi

Commonest cause of chronic disability in under-50s
1% of general population are chronically disabled by back pain
2nd most common primary care consultation (after viral URTIs)

Causes

M.A.D.D.E.N.I.N.G^3. P.A.I.N.

Mechanical: Injury-related – ligament strain; also fracture
Autoimmune:
- Seronegative arthropathies – ankylosing spondylitis, enteropathic, etc.
- Rheumatoid arthritis

Disc prolapse/**D**egenerative – other:
- Adults: Spondylosis, canal stensosis
- Adolescents: Kyphosis, spondylolisthesis, spondylolysis

Endocrine–metabolic: Osteoporosis (microfractures, verterbral compression), osteomalacia, Paget
Neoplasia – vertebral or cord
Infection: Discitis, epidural spinal abscess, osteomyelitis – pyogenic, TB
Neurological: Guillain–Barré syndrome, meningoradiculitis, haematomyelia (e.g. subarachnoid haemorrhage, AVM), spina bifida occulta
Gastroenterological or **G**ynaecological or **G**enito-urinary:
- Gastroenterological: Duodenal ulcer, pancreatitis
- Gynaecological: Endometriosis, pelvic inflammatory disease, ovarian cyst
- Genito-urinary: Prostatitis, pyelonephritis

Psychological
Aortic aneurysm or retroperitoneal haematoma
Ischaemic – sickle crisis
Neurofibromatosis

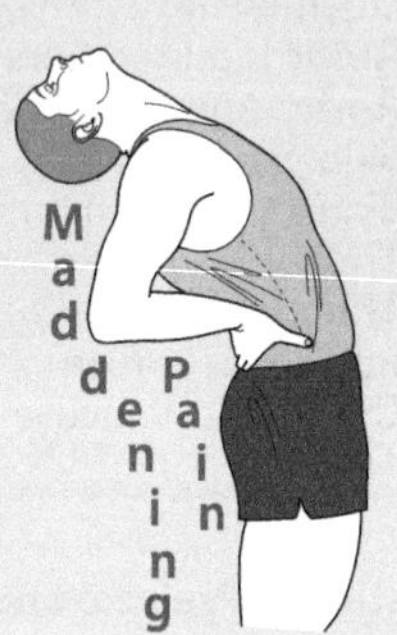

Mechanical

Cause: Minor injury, e.g. lifting heavy object or sudden deceleration in car accident
PC: Pain confined to lower back or neck, but no radiation to buttocks or legs
O/E: Paraspinal muscle spasm – if unilateral, causes scoliosis to that side

Autoimmune

Ankylosing spondylitis
PC: Lower back and buttock pain and stiffness, worse at night or morning; better with exercise
O/E: Loss of lumbar lordosis and exaggeration of thoracic kyphosis; reduced chest expansion

Rheumatoid arthritis
PC: Painful limitation of movement due to facet joint involvement

Disc prolapse

PATH:

- Disc prolapse most common at L4–5 or L5–S1, although may occur at any level
- Affected nerve root lies lower than affected disc space, e.g. L4–5 causes either L5 or S1 radiculopathy
- Lateral disc prolapse causes radicular pain; central disc prolapse causes cauda equina syndrome

PC:

- Lower back and leg pain, with variable sensory symptoms in leg; worsened by cough or sitting
- Bilateral leg pain, saddle anaesthesia, or sphincter–erectile dysfunction suggest cauda equina syndrome

O/E:

- Ipsilateral scoliosis; hip and knee kept in flexed position
- Straight leg raising reduced (often to $<30°$); Lasegue manoeuvre (pain on extending knee with hip flexed)
- Radicular signs, e.g. absent ankle jerk or numbness of 5th toe (both suggest S1 root lesion)

Degenerative – other

Spondylosis
PATH: Osteoarthritis-like changes in lumbar or cervical spine, e.g. flaval or facet joint hypertrophy
PC: Radiculopathy, myelopathy or headache (esp. cervical spondylosis)

Lumbar spinal stenosis (neurogenic claudication)
PC: Back, buttock or leg pain in elderly (rarely congenital); triggered by standing (unlike ischaemic claudication) or walking; relieved by sitting (unlike disc prolapse)
O/E: Radiculopathy may be present; normal peripheral pulses (to exclude ischaemic claudication)

Neoplasm

Vertebral

B^2.O.N.E.1. M. (Boney M!)

> **B**reast, **B**ronchus, **O**varian, **N**ephro (renal, prostate, testes), **E**ndocrine (thyroid) – metastatic carcinoma **1**° bone tumour – Ewing, osteosarcoma, **M**yeloma/lymphoma

Cord

1 Extradural: All causes of vertebral tumours (**B^2.O.N.E.1. M.**)
2 Extramedullary: Neurofibroma, meningioma, leptomeningeal metastases
3 Intramedullary: Glioma, ependymoma, medulloblastoma 'drop' metastases

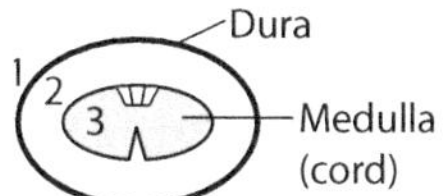

BONE CYSTS

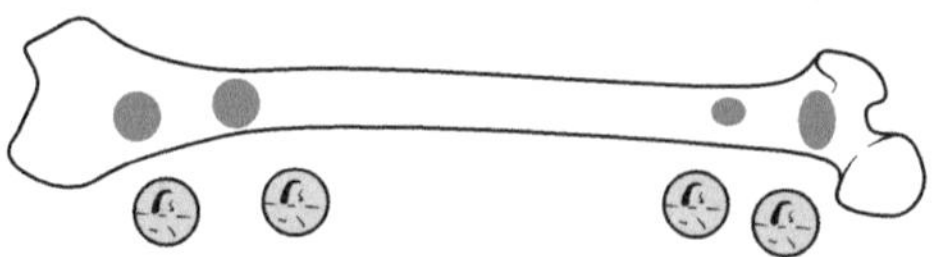

P.E.N.N.I.E.S.

Primary

S.A.F.E. *(all benign)*

Simple bone cyst:
Epi: Pre-pubertal
PC: Pain or pathological fracture
Rx: • Intracystic steroid injection
• Curettage; pack with bone chips

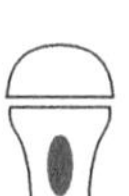

- Central, metaphyseal
- Knee, proximal humerus, skull ('congenital cranial lacunae')

Aneurysmal cyst or AVM:
Epi: Young adults

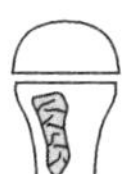

- Expanding, eccentric
- Blood-filled, trabeculated
- Long bone, spine, skull AVM

Fibrous cortical defect:
Epi: Children

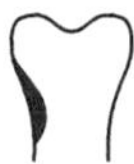

- Cystic centre, sclerosed edge
- Long bones

Enchondroma:
Ollier syndrome (multiple enchondroma)

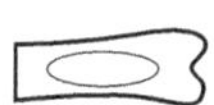

- Tubular bones
- Specks of calcification

Endocrine: Primary hyperparathyroidism

'Pepper-pot skull'

Neoplasia – primary – giant-cell tumour:
Epi: 20–40 (epiphyses must have fused)
PATH: Multinucleate giant cells; stromal proliferation
PC: Pain and swelling near joint; pathological fracture
Prog: 1/3 benign; 1/3 local invasion; 1/3 metastasize

Soap-bubble/ ballooned cortex in sub-articular site , e.g. knee, distal radius, proximal humerus

Neoplasia – secondaries: **B^2.O.N.E.1. M.**
Breast, **B**ronchus
Ovary
Nephrology: Renal, prostate
Endocrine: Tumour
1 °– primary
Myeloma/Langerhans cell histiocytosis; also pseudotumour of haemophilia

Infection: Osteomyelitis – 'Brodie abscess'

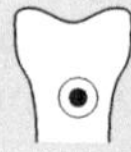

- Metaphyseal
- Round, cystic centre
- Sclerosed edge

Electrolytes: Gout
Sarcoid: Dactylitis (enlarged phalanges)

SCLEROSIS

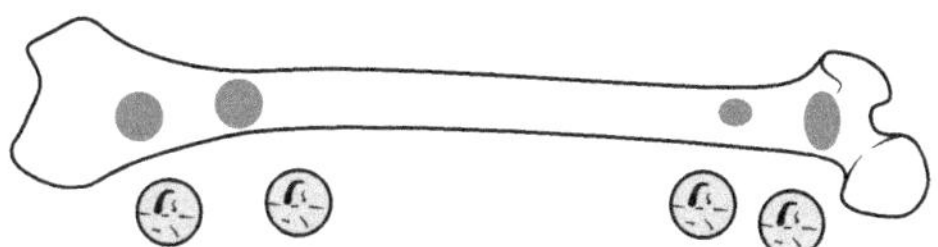

P.E.N^2.N.I.E.s

Paget disease
Endocrine: Secondary hyperparathyroidism – renal osteodystrophy
Neoplasia – primary – benign
- Osteoid osteoma – appears similar to Brodie abscess
- Osteochondroma = cartilage-capped exostosis

Neoplasia – primary – malignant:

Osteosarcoma (50%):
Epi: Bimodal 10–20%: and >50% (Paget); M:F=2:1
PC: Painful, swollen, warm limb; worse at night
Lung metastases – early
X-ray: Mixed rarefaction and sclerosis
'Codman triangle' (periosteum lifts off shaft)
Sunray spicules – soft-tissue calcification

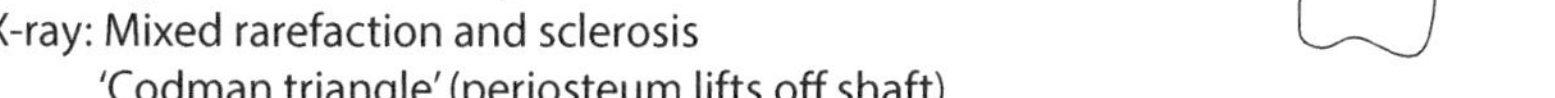

Knee, proximal humerous

Chondrosarcoma (25%):
Epi: Age >40 y
PC: Enchondroma – indolent pain, swelling, pathological fracture
Ecchondroma – early swelling, except pelvic basin exostosis
X-ray: ENC: Medullary rarefaction, calcified specks
ECC: Large exostosis, calcified specks in cartilage cap

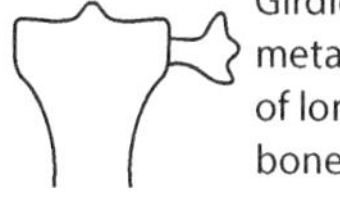

Ewing or reticular cell sarcoma (15%):
Epi: Age 10–20 y; associated with adrenal neuroblastoma
PC: Pain, worsened by walking/limp
Swelling: Warm, firm, rubbery, tender
PUO from liver, lung, bone metastases (like osteomyelitis)
X-ray: Medullary rarefaction
Periosteal onion-skinning (reactive new layers)

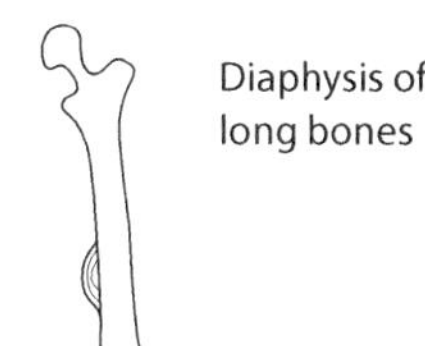

Neoplasia – secondary:
- Metastatic carcinoma: Breast, prostate, colorectal
- Myeloma (incl. POEMS syndrome); Hodgkin lymphoma

Inflammation:
- Osteoarthritis
- Osteopetrosis

Exogenous:
- Lead ('pica'), radium, bismuth, phosphorus (match heads)
- Fluorosis, esp. Persian Gulf, India, China
- Vitamin A toxicity; X-ray – epiphyseal thickening; irregular opacification of lower ribs

Neurology

HEADACHE – ACUTE

Causes

V.I.C.I.O.U.S.

Vascular: Thunderclap onset (i.e. immediate):
- Haemorrhage: Aneurysmal subarachnoid; intracerebral
- Thrombosis: Venous sinus thrombosis; ischaemic stroke (in conjunction with acute hemiparesis)
- Reversible cerebral vasoconstriction syndrome (RCVS):
  - PC: Recurrent thunderclap headaches over 1–4 weeks, mimics subarachnoid haemorrhage
  - Ix: CT angiogram shows vasoconstrictions that reverse by 6 weeks; but no aneurysms; CT may show infarcts or cerebral convexity subarachnoid haemorrhage
- Other: Dissection, vasculitis

Infection/**I**nflammation: Acute or subacute onset (i.e. over hours or days):
- Meningitis:
  - Neutrophilic CSF: Meningococal, pneumococcal, listeriosis, fungal; OR early viral or TB
  - Lymphocytic CSF: Viral (enterovirus, HIV), TB, Lyme, syphilis; OR partially treated bacterial; autoimmune vasculitis, SLE, Behçet syndrome; sarcoidosis
- Brain abscess
- Encephalitis: Infective (e.g. herpes simplex virus) or post-infective (acute demyelinating encephalomyelitis)

Compression: Recurrent paroxysmal, or thunderclap:
- Intraventricular or periventricular tumour, causing transient obstructive hydrocephalus, (e.g. colloid cyst of 3rd ventricle)
  - PC: Drop attacks, acute bilateral visual loss
- Posterior fossa lesion: Tumour, Arnold–Chiari malformation
- Pituitary enlargement: Apoplexy, due to infarction of pituitary macroadenoma; post-partum hypophysitis

Intracranial pressure ↑ or ↓:
- Primary intracranial hypertension:
  - PC: Headache worse on stooping or lying flat; visual disturbance (obscurations; 6th cranial nerve palsy); tinnitus, triggered by weight gain
- Spontaneous intracranial hypotension, due to spinal CSF dural leak
  - PC: Headache worse on standing initially, but may become posture-independent later. May be triggered by exertional event, e.g. lifting

Ophthalmic – acute glaucoma: Unilateral but not necessarily ocular

U: co**U**gh or other 'situational' cause, e.g. exertion, coital cephalgia:
- Commoner in people who suffer with migraines
- Recurrent paroxysmal thunderclap headache

Systemic:
- Hypertensive crisis (e.g. pre-eclampsia, phaeochromocytoma) causing PRES (posterior reversible encephalopathy syndrome) with characteristic MRI cerebral white matter lesions; vasculitis
- Infection, e.g. sinusitis, tonsillitis, dental abscess, UTI, atypical pneumonia (e.g. mycoplasma) – may all cause meningism and encephalopathy, esp. in children and elderly
- Toxins: Carbon monoxide

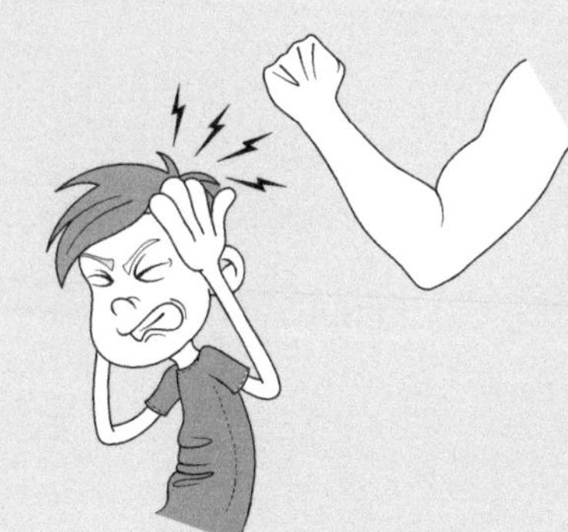

Ix

1st-line: **CT head**: Subarachnoid haemorrhage: Blood in sulci, cisterns – sensitivity = 90% in first 24 h
Mass lesions/midline shift: Intracerebral haemorrhage, abscess, tumour

Bloods:
WBC: Neutrophils – bacterial meningitis, abscess, **LiS**teria (**L**ymphocytes in **S**erum)
Lymphocytes: **LyM**e disease (**L**ymphocytes in **M**eninges)
Monocytes: TB
ESR, CRP: Meningitis

Urine:
MSU, glucose, protein

Micro:
Blood cultures
Serology: Bacterial meningitides, enterovirus, HIV, syphilis,
Fungal antigens: Cryptococcal (serum CRAG), galactomannin
TB 'EliSpot'

Radiol:
CT angiogram (more sensitive than MR angiogram):

- Detects aneurysm, RCVS, AVM, dissection, vasculitis; sensitivity for aneurysms >5 mm = 90%
- CT venogram if patient at risk of cerebral venous thrombosis

Catheter angiogram if aneurysm or AVM suspected, sensitivity = 95% (but risk of stroke due to procedure = 0.5%)

MRI:

- MRI: Posterior fossa lesion, ADEM, CSF dural leak (brain and spine MRI with contrast)
- MRA: Aneurysm, AVM, dissection, vasculitis; sensitivity for aneurysm >5 mm = 90%
- MRV: Cerebral venous thrombosis

Special: CSF: Always do brain scan before performing lumbar puncture to exclude mass-lesion or cerebral oedema

Opening pressure:

- Normal = 5–20 cmH_2O
- Raised: Subarachnoid haemorrhage, primary intracranial hypertension, meningitis
- Depressed: Spontaneous intracranial hypotension (avoid LP if history is suggestive!)

Appearance:

- Normal = clear
- Xanthochromic (yellow): Traumatic tap, subarachnoid haemorrhage, high protein
- Bloody: Traumatic tap, subarachnoid haemorrhage, so if subarachnoid haemorrhage is a possibility, send for immediate centrifugation and spectrophotometry on supernatant for bilirubin (+ve between 12 hours and 2 weeks) and CSF ferritin (+ve in SAH)

Microscopy, culture and sensitivity:

- Normal: RBC count raised if traumatic tap, but should see decrease from bottles 1 to 3
  WBC count 0–4 (lymphocytes); deduct 1 WBC for every 700 RBCs
- Neutrophilia: Meningococal, pneumococcal, listeriosis, fungal; OR early viral or TB
- Lymphocytosis: Viral (enteroviruses, HIV), TB, Lyme, syphilis; OR partially treated bacterial autoimmune vaculitis, SLE, Behçet syndrome; sarcoidosis
- Stains: Gram – bacteria, some fungal; Ziehl–Nielsen – TB; Indian Ink – *Cryptococcus*

Chemistry:

- Normal: Protein 0–0.45 g/l; deduct 0.01 g/l for every 1000 RBCs; glucose 2.8–4.2 mmol/l, or >50% serum glucose
- Protein >1 g/l: Bacterial, TB or fungal meningitis, or subarachnoid haemorrhage
- Glucose <40%: Bacterial, TB, fungal or mumps meningitis

Other: Cryptococcal antigen (CSF CRAG), herpes class PCR, ACE, oligoclonal bands, cytology

HEADACHE – CHRONIC

Causes

M.A.D.D.E.N.I.N²·G². *noise*

Migraine – episodic, severe lasting hours to days, or continuous mild-moderate ('transformed')
Autonomic (trigeminal autonomic cephalgias or TACs):
Cluster headaches: Strictly unilateral, severe pain, min to hours, unilateral tearing, red eye, ptosis, rhinorrhea
SUNCT: Like cluster headaches but lasting seconds
Paroxysmal hemicrania/hemicrania continua: Like cluster headaches but continuous
Depression/Tension headaches
Degenerative disease – cervical spondylosis: Causes unilateral fronto-occipital pain worsened by neck movements
Exogenous:
Drugs:
- Medication-overuse headache syndrome: Migraine commonly becomes continuous and bilateral due to 'medication overuse headache syndrome', i.e. consuming any analgesic (paracetamol, NSAID, triptan, codeine, more than once a week)
- Hormonal: Oestrogen contraceptive pill – worsens migraine
- Direct effect: Vasodilators, e.g. nitrate, calcium-antagonists; lamotrigine; sulphasalazine; antibiotics
- Traumatic brain injury: Causes chronic tension headache, depression, and cognitive impairment
- Extracranial structures: Sinuses, neck, eyes, ears, TMJ (PC: preauricular, temple pain; associated crepitus), teeth

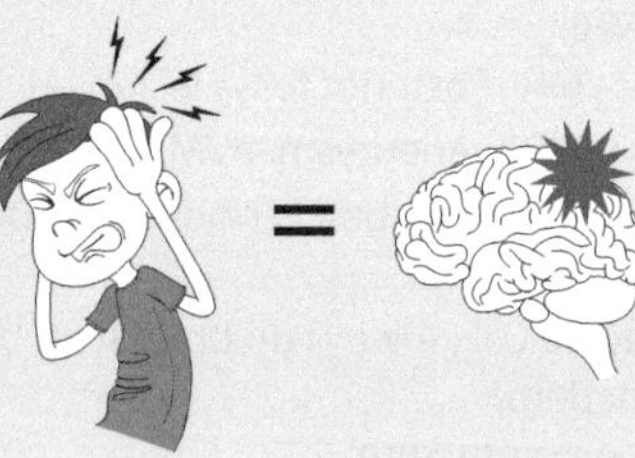

Neuralgia:
Trigeminal: Commonest in V3, or V2 territories; lancinating pain triggered by trivial stimuli or movement
Occipital: Pain over unilateral occipital-parietal area, triggered by pressure over greater occipital nerve
Intracranial pressure ↑ or ↓:
ICP raised: Primary intracranial hypertension – assoc. with obesity, young females; thrombosed or narrow cerebral venous sinuses; serious because causes progressive visual loss
ICP low: Spontaneous intracranial hypotension (due to CSF dural leak)
- Inflammatory disorders, e.g. SLE, Behçet, sarcoid, vasculitis due to systemic inflammation, or less commonly, direct CNS inflammation

Neoplasia: Brain tumour or meningeal infiltration; aneurysm or AVM; structural causes such as these account for ~1/100,000 chronic headache presentations
Nocturnal headaches ('hypnic headaches'): Variant of migraine
Giant-cell, temporal arteritis; or**G**an failure or other systemic impairment
Hypercapnia (e.g. obstructive sleep apnoea, causing morning headaches), hypoxia (e.g. mountain sickness)
Uraemia, hepatic failure, hypoxia, e.g. mountain sickness
Anaemia or hyperviscosity
Severe hypertension
Endocrine, e.g. cortisol ↑ or ↓; thyroxine ↑ or ↓
APUDoma: Phaeochromocytoma, carcinoid, mastocytosis – episodic headaches, with flushing; recurrent hypoglycaemia
Seizures: Headaces occur post-ictally, e.g. morning headaches indicative of nocturnal epilepsy

PC

Migraine

Temporal: Attack duration = 4–72 h; may also develop background continuous headache ('transformed migraine')

Character: Throbbing, unilateral but may cross midline, severe; worse with movement; patient lies down

Assoc: N+V, photophobia, phonophobia, osmophobia:

- Premonitory symptoms in 50% (e.g. change in appetite, arousal, mood)
- Aura in 20% (preceding focal neurological Sx, esp. visual)

Epi:

- Age: Begins in childhood (as cyclical abdominal pain or motion sickness) or teens
- Sex: Females > males; family history common
- Triggers: Carbohydrates (cola, citrus, chocolate, alcohol); premenstrual; exertion; lying-in

Autonomic: trigeminal autonomic cephalgias (TACs)

Cluster headaches

Site: Orbital or temporal

Timing: Attack duration = 5–120 min

Onset: Typically same time every night/day. Cluster length = 2–12 weeks; remission length = 3 months–3 years

Character: Non-throbbing; strictly unilateral peri- or retro-orbital pain; patient paces room and is agitated

Assoc: Ipsilateral Horner syndrome, lacrimation, nasal congestion or rhinorrhoea, sweating

SUNCT = Short-lasting unilateral neuralgiform headache with conjunctival injection and tearing

Usually men in their 50s

Severe pain lasting seconds of minutes (much shorter than cluster headache)

Non-responsive to triptans, opioids, oxygen

Require AEDs for long-term prophylaxis

Hemicrania continua/paroxysmal hemicrania

Temporal: Continuous symptoms of cluster headache-like symptoms

Female preponderance

Completely responsive to indomethacin

Depression/tension headaches

Temporal: Attack duration = 30 min – continuous ('chronic daily headache' >15 days/month)

Character: Tightness, pressure, heaviness, ice-pick pains, vertex-bitemporal; mild (patient works through)

Assoc: Mild photophobia, nausea, depression; dizziness (due to hyperventilation)

Neuralgia, trigeminal

Temporal: Attack duration = sudden, momentary pain, repeated in bursts:

- Triggered by touching trigger zone or action, e.g. chewing, swallowing, talking

Character: Lancinating (stabbing) pain, in distribution of V2 or V3 dermatome typically

Intracranial

Raised: Worse with stooping; visual obscurations; obese women (primary intracranial hypertension)

Low: Worsens on sitting or standing; associated with previous trauma, often minor

Giant-cell, temporal arteritis

Character: Unilateral temple pain and tenderness; worse at night; anorexia and weight loss; myalgia; jaw claudication

Assoc: 'Law of 60' = >60 years; ESR >60; responds within days to prednisolone 60 mg OD

Complications: Anterior ischaemic optic neuropathy (blindness); ophthalmoplegia, ischaemic stroke; aortitis, aortic regurgitation

ACUTE CONFUSIONAL STATE

Def

Impairment in the **level** of consciousness (GCS), with a secondary global impairment in the **content** of consciousness (i.e. cognition) over hours, days or weeks (cf. dementia, which refers to primary impairment in cognition, with preserved alertness

O/E

Glasgow Coma Scale: Fluctuates – worse in evenings ('sundowning')
Physical examination: Sympathetic overactivity – tachycardia, hypertension, diaphoresis
Mental state examination

Appearance: Agitated, aggressive, but purposeless
Affect: Labile
Thought:

- Speech incoherent, rapid or slow
- Delusions: Paranoid, but poorly systematized and poorly sustained
- Hallucinations: Visual; illusions-distortions

Cognition: Globally impaired
Insight: Impaired

Causes

Intracranial: Primary disturbance in structures subserving consciousness
Extracranial:

- Interruption of energy substrate delivery: Glucose ↓, O_2 ↓, Hb ↓, blood supply ↓
- Alteration of neuronal membrane physiology: Toxaemia, electrolyte disturbance

I.N.V.I.T.E./P.A.S.S. I.S. F.R.E.E.

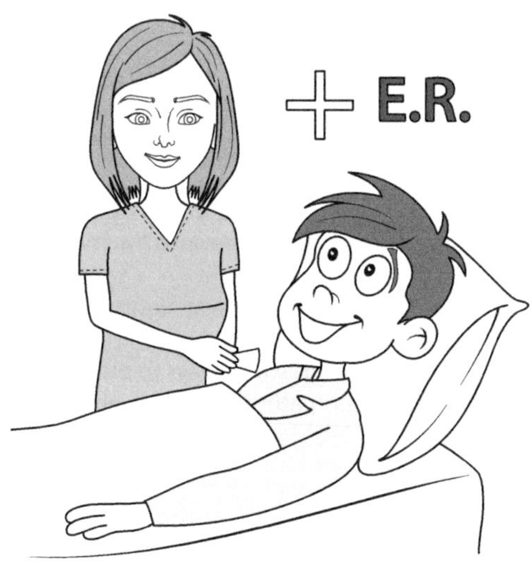

ACUTE CONFUSIONAL STATE – CAUSES

Intracranial

I.N.V.I.T.E. /P.A.S.S. I.S. F.R.E.E.

Infection:
- Meningitis: Bacterial, TB, fungal, syphilis
- Encephalitis: HSV, VZV, flavivirus (Western Nile/Japanese encephalitis virus)
- Other: Abscess, HIV-dementia, malaria

Neoplasia:
- Brain tumour: 1° or 2°
- Meningeal: Carcinoma, melanoma, lymphoma; paraneoplastic syndrome, e.g. anti-neuronal antibodies from lung carcinoma

Vascular:
- Infarction: Non-dominant temporoparietal region; thalamic, upper brainstem
- Haemorrhage: Subarachnoid haemorrhage
- Migraine: Vertebrobasilar

Injury: Trauma – diffuse brain injury; extradural or subdural haemorrhage

Toxins/nutritional:
- Prescribed:
  - β-blockers, anticholinergics, dopaminergics, steroids, NSAIDs
  - Overdose: Anticonvulsants, paracetamol, aspirin, digoxin
- Abused:
  - Alcohol: Intoxication, withdrawal ('delirium tremens'), Wernicke syndrome
  - Recreational: Opioids, cannabis, amphetamines, LSD
- Nutritional: Vitamin B12 deficiency

Epilepsy:
- Postictal
- Non-convulsive status epilepticus – often complex partial seizures (temporal lobe)

Psychiatric: Mania or catatonia

Autoimmune:
- Autoimmune limbic encephalitis, e.g. anti-K^+ voltage-gated channel antibodies, anti-NMDA receptors antibodies (associated with ovarian teratoma)
- ADEM: Post-viral, vaccination; multiple sclerosis
- Cerebral vasculitis, SLE, antiphospholipid syndrome

Sarcoid

'**S**enile': Degenerative dementia, esp. Lewy body; end-stage Alzheimer; prion disease

Extracranial

Infection:
- Pneumonia, esp. mycoplasma, legionella/endocarditis/tonsillitis
- Gastroenteritis, esp. campylobacter/leptospirosis/UTI/cellulitis/septic arthritis
  - NB: Infection presenting solely with confusion is most common in elderly or children

Systemic:
- Haematological: Anaemia, hyperviscosity, acute intermittent porphyria
- Autoimmune: SLE, vasculitis, Hashimoto encephalopathy (anti-thyroid abs)
- Hypothermia, hyperthermia

Failure, organ:
- Respiratory/cardiac, due to ↓ O_2 or ↑ CO_2
- Renal/liver: Due to toxins uraemia, plasma NH_4^+↑, CSF glutamine

Retention: Acute urinary/faecal impaction

Electrolytes:
- Na^+ or Ca^{2+} ↑/↓; NH_4^+ ↑ (esp. valproate)

Endocrine:
- Glucose ↑/↓ (esp. HHS, insulinoma)
- Thyroxine ↑/↓
- Steroid hormones ↑/↓ (Addison, hypopituitarism, Cushing)

COMA – CAUSES

Def

Persistent unconsciousness, i.e. inability to arouse the patient by painful stimuli

PATH

Consciousness requires normal functioning of three 'systems':

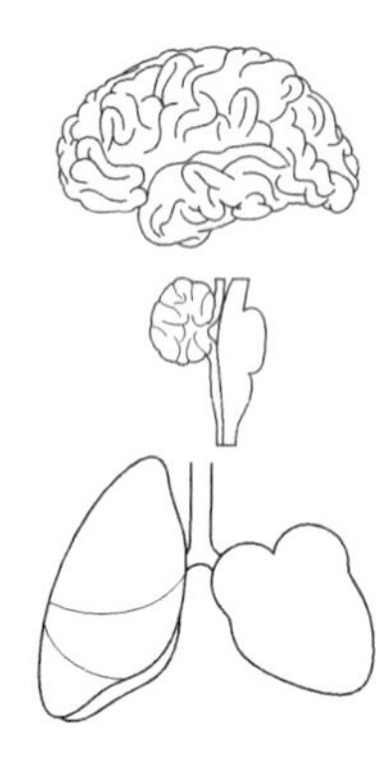

Cerebral cortex
An extensive area of cortex needs to be deranged before consciousness is impaired, i.e. diffuse process, e.g. encephalitis, trauma, epilepsy

Ascending reticular activation system (ARAS)
A limited set of areas need to be deranged for consciousness to be impaired, viz thalamus, upper brainstem, e.g. CVA, tumour, MS

Systemic
Metabolic factors may depress all brain regions, e.g. anoxia, toxins, septicaemia

Causes

I.N.V.I.T.E. /P.A.S.S. I.S. F.R.E.E.

Intracranial

Infection: **Focal**: abscess; **diffuse**: meningo-encephalitis – HSV, bacterial, TB, malarias
Neoplasia: **Focal**: tumour; **diffuse**: meningeal carcinoma; lymphoma; paraneoplastic limbic encephalitis
Vascular: **Focal**: large cerebral stroke with mass effect; or paramedian thalamic stroke, or basilar artery thrombosis with upper brainstem infarction
Diffuse: subarachnoid haemorrhage; cerebral venous thrombosis, cerebral anoxia
Injury: **Focal**: sub-, extradural, intracerebral bleed, contusion; **diffuse**: axonal injury, oedema
Toxins: Opioids, alcohol (central pontine myelinolysis, Wernicke syndrome), sedative overdose
Epilepsy: Non-convulsive status epilepticus, post-ictal, anti-convulsant overdose

Psychiatric: Catatonia
Autoimmune: Autoimmune encephalitis, ADEM, vasculitis, antiphospholipid syndrome
Sarcoid
Special: Degenerative dementia, prion

Extracranial

Infection: Endocarditis, septicaemia
Systemic: SLE, vasculitis, Hashimoto encephalopathy, hypo- or hyperthermia

Failure, respiratory/cardiac: ↑ CO_2, ↓ O_2
Renal/liver failure: Toxin accumulation
Electrolytes: Na^+ ↑/↓, Ca^{2+} ↑/↓, NH_4^+ ↑
Endocrine: Glucose ↑/↓, thyroid ↑/↓, cortisol ↓

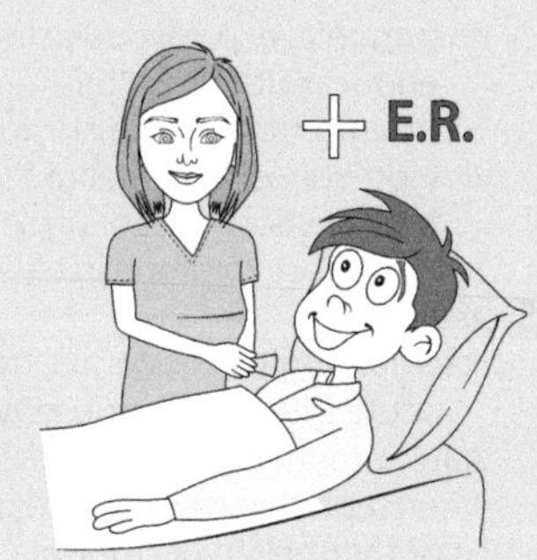

COMA – MANAGEMENT

ITU transfer, if ventilation required

Neurosurgeons if abscess, tumour, bleed or ICP bolt-monitor needed

B. Breathing

Oxygen: 60%

Ventilation if GCS <9

Hyperventilation may be needed to treat raised ICP

C. Hydration

Dextrose 50%, 50 ml IV

- If hypoglycaemic

Normal saline

Caution if:

- Severe hypertension
- Pulmonary oedema
- Alcoholic or hyponatraemia, as at risk of central pontine myelinolysis

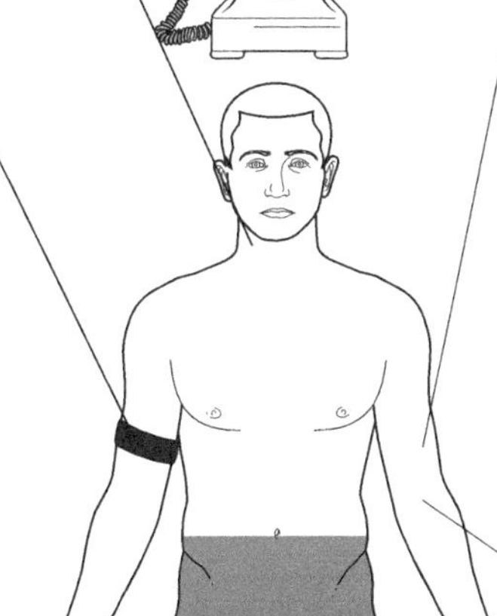

A. Assessment

A.B.C.Disability

GCS:

- Eyes: **S.S.P.S.**
  Spontaneous, Spoken, Pain, Shut
- Motor: **O.L. W.F.EN.**
  Obeys, Localizes Withdraws. Flex, Ext, None
- Vocal: **O.C.I.I.N.**
  Orientated, Confused, Inappropriate, Incoherent, None

Brainstem tests:

- Pupils
- Ocular movements
- Corneal/gag
- Respiration pattern

C.O.A.T.

Cardiac monitor; **O_2** sats; **A**BP, CVP line; **T**PR

Investigations

Bloods:

- Glucose
- Arterial blood gases
- FBC, U&E, LFT
- Ca, PO_4, Mg, NH_4
- Vitamin B12, drug levels, autoAbs, anti-neuronals, ACE

Urine:

- Toxicology/porphyrins

Micro

- Blood cultures; serology
- CSU
- LP (post-imaging)
- Culture, spectrophotometry

Monitor: GCS

EEG, ECHO

Radiol:

- CT brain (urgent)
- MRI, A, V

D. Drugs

Vitamin B complex IV

(esp. thiamine – vitamin B1)

Antimicrobials:

- Cefotaxime IV
- Aciclovir IV 10 mg/kg tds
- Also consider
  - HIV/immuno-suppressed: ? TB, fungal or toxoplasmosis
  - Foreign travel: ? malaria, W. Nile virus

+

Drug overdose:

- Naloxone 400 μg IV
- Flumazenil 200 μg IV

Anticonvulsants:

- Lorazepam, phenytoin,
- Phenobarbitone IV

Dexamethasone:

Indicated in

- Vasculitis
- Tumour

Nursing, bedsore avoidance, catheterize

Physio, flexion contracture avoidance

DEMENTIA

Def

Chronically impaired content of consciousness (i.e. cognition) that affects multiple cognitive domains, e.g. memory, attention, language (cf. amnesia or aphasia) and is acquired and progressive (cf. learning disability, e.g. due to cerebral palsy)

Causes

D².I.V.I.N.I.T.Y⁴.

Degenerative/**D**evelopmental

Degenerative: Classed by clinical syndrome and abnormal protein inclusion

Alzheimer: Spatial disorientation, word-finding impairment, beta-amyloid

Frontotemporal:

- Behavioural variant: Ubiquitin (TDP-43-A) or phosphorylated tau
- Aphasia: Fluent ('semantic dementia'): TDP-43-C
  Non-fluent: Phosphorylated tau
- Other neurological syndomes: Motor neurone disease (weakness, wasting) – TDP-43-A; Parkinsonism – tau

Parkinion-plus dementias:

- Cortical Lewy body disease: Visual hallucinations, neuroleptic sensitivity
- Corticobasal ganglionic degeneration: Alien limb, aphasia, apraxia, neglect; or PSP – supranuclear gaze palsy
- Genetic: Huntington disease, Wilson disease

Rarer: Prion – seizures, cerebellar signs, myoclonus, cortical blindness

Developmental **F.A.M.I.L.I.A³.L.**

Fragile X
Aneuploidy (Down)
Mitochondrial
Ictal (myoclonic epilepsy syndrome)
Lipoidoses
Intermediary metabolism (glycogen storage disease)
Acidaemia, organic or **A**mmonaemia, or **A**taxia spinocerebellar
Leucodystrophy

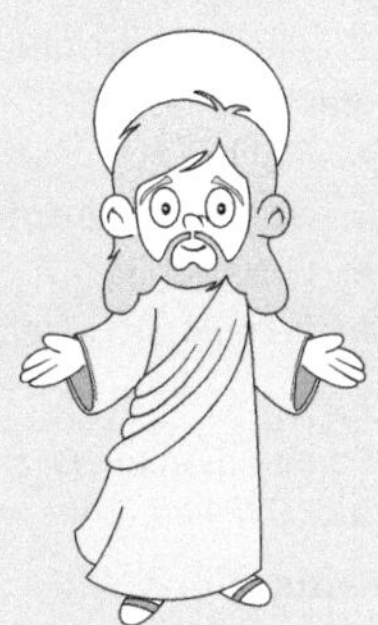

Infection:

Viruses: HSV; HIV, PML (JC virus)
Bacterial: Syphilis (tertiary), Whipple disease, TB (all cause low-grade, chronic meningitis)
Other: Fungal; prion – CJD (classical, new-variant)

Vascular:

Vascular dementia – cortical (multi-infarcts), subcortical (hypertensive arteriosclerosis, CADASIL)
Subdural haematoma, chronic (also presents with fluctuating confusion, SIADH)
Cerebral anoxia, e.g. after cardiac arrest

Inflammation:

Autoimmune limbic encephalitis, e.g. anti-voltage gated K^+-channel autoantibodies (assoc. seizures, low Na)
Vasculitis incl. SLE, antiphospholipid syndrome, Behçet syndrome
Sarcoidosis; multiple sclerosis (late)

Neoplasia:

Brain tumour, especially frontal, callosal or temporal location
Meningeal carcinoma, melanoma, lymphoma
Paraneoplastic syndrome, esp. small-cell lung cancer (anti-Hu limbic encephalitis), lymphoma (PML)

Injury/Epilepsy: Single or repetitive head trauma (dementia pugilistica); non-convulsive status

Toxin/Nutritional:

Toxins: Alcohol; anti-convulsants, long-term use, esp. phenytoin; lead; aluminium
Nutrition: Vitamin B12, folate, or niacin deficiency; malabsorption syndrome, e.g. coeliac

Y: h**Y**pothyroidism, h**Y**poadrenalism (Addison or hypopituitarism)

h**Y**drocephalus, normal-pressure – PC: dementia, gait apraxia and urinary incontinence
ps**Y**chiatric - depression ('pseudodementia')

Alzheimer disease

PATH: Intracellular: Neurofibrillary tangles (paired helical filaments)
Extracellular: Senile plaques; amyloid angiopathy (β-amyloid)

PC Memory loss, esp. spatial
Language: Empty speech, anomia
Other cognitive: Apraxia, attention, executive, mood (depression, aggression, psychosis)
Other neurology: Incontinence; primitive reflexes, myoclonus, epilepsy

Ix: MRI – medial temporal lobe atrophy occurs early
EEG – loss of normal posterior alpha rhythm
CSF – low amyloid beta 1-42: tau ratio
PET – amyloid scan (Amyvid or Florbetapir)

Rx: Cholinesterase inhibitor, e.g. donepezil, rivastigmine
Glutamate receptor antagonist, e.g. memantine

Frontotemporal dementia

PATH: Numerous genetic associations, e.g. microtubule-associated protein tau (MAPT) (40%), progranulin (10%)
Pick bodies (argyrophilic tau cell inclusions) + Pick cells (swollen chromatolytic neurones)

PC: Behavioural variant:

- Overactive: Disinhibition, distractibility, stereotypy, ritualism, predilection for sweet food
- Underactive: Apathy, withdrawal, emotion lack

Primary progressive aphasia variants:

- Non-fluent (frontal)
- Fluent (left anterior temporal) = 'semantic dementia'

Other neurological syndromes: Motor neurone disease (fasciculations deltoids, weakness); parkinsonism:

Ix: MRI: Frontal or temporal atrophy

Rx: None

Lewy body disease

PATH: Lewy bodies (eosinophilic inclusion bodies containing ubiquitin and neurofilament), predominantly within occipito-parietal cortex (cf. Parkinson disease – occur predominantly within substantia nigra)

PC: Fluctuating cognitive dysfunction (esp. attention, visuospatial), and fluctuating consciousness
Visual hallucinations, paranoid delusions
Parkinsonism, incl. falls, sensitivity to neuroleptics, due to nigral Lewy bodies

Ix: MRI; EEG – normal initially

Rx: Cholinesterase inhibitor, avoid dopamine agonists

Vascular dementia

PATH: Cortical: Multiple and/or large infarcts – deficits determined by regions and size of infarcts
Subcortical ('lacunar state'): Hypertensive arteriosclerosis

PC Pattern: Abrupt onset, fluctuating course, stepwise deterioration, nocturnal confusion
Patchy deficits; personality and insight preserved/Psychiatric: depression/emotional lability
Pyramidal signs, 'marche à petit pas'
PMH of hypertension, arteriopathy, atrial fibrillation, diabetes mellitus

Ix: MRI – extensive infarcts or small-vessel disease, with secondary atrophy

Rx: Treat predisposing factors – hypertension, diabetes; aspirin; statin

PARKINSONISM

Def

Parkinsonism refers to the constellation of signs listed (tremor, rigidity, akinesia, etc.)
Parkinson disease refers to the commonest cause of parkinsonism, viz primary neurodegeneration

Causes

D².I.V.I.N.I.T.Y.

Degenerative/**D**evelopmental

Degenerative

Idiopathic Parkinson disease:

Epi: Prevalence: 0.5% over 50 years old

PATH:
- Degeneration of >80% substantia nigra pars compacta dopaminergic neurones and other neuromodulatory systems of brainstem (e.g. locus coeruleus) and basal forebrain
- Lewy bodies (eosinophilic inclusions) occur in areas of cell loss and in cerebral cortex

Parkinson-plus, i.e. Parkinsonism PLUS other neurological syndrome:
- Multiple systems atrophy: Parkinsonism symmetrical, poorly responsive to L-DOPA, +/– autonomic (postural hypotension, urinary frequency), +/– cerebellar and/or pyramidal signs
- Progressive supranuclear palsy – **P.S.P.**
  Postural instability; **S**peech disturbance (+ dementia); **P**alsy, supranuclear down-gaze
- Corticobasal degeneration:
  - Cortical: Aphasia, dysarthria, stimulus-sensitive myoclonus, apraxia (alien-hand), neglect
  - Basal-ganglia: Parkinsonism asymmetrical, intention or kinetic tremor

Dementia-associations: Cortical Lewy body disease, Alzheimer, frontotemporal dementia,

Developmental: Young- or late-onset PD

Genetic:
- Autosomal dominant, e.g. LRRK2 mutation (pronounced 'Lark 2'): Commonest genetic cause of sporadic, late-onset PD; Huntington disease, esp. juvenile form
- Autosomal recessive: Parkin mutation (commonest cause of young-onset PD), PKAN (pantothenate kinase-associated neurodegeneration [iron accumulation]; Wilson disease (copper accumulation)

Perinatal: Cerebral palsy (anoxia, kernicterus)

Infection:

Streptococcus, group A: Post-infective encephalitis lethargicum – anti-basal ganglia antibodies
Structural: Syphilis, toxoplasmosis, cysticercosis, CJD

Vascular:

Hypertensive arteriosclerosis; PC: Lower-body parkinsonism
Cerebral anoxia: Opiate overdose, cardiac arrest, CO poisoning

Inflammation: Vasculitis

Neoplasia: Brain tumour affecting basal ganglia

Injury: 'Dementia pujilistica' – boxers

Toxin:

Dopamine-receptor-2 antagonists: Haloperidol, metoclopramide
Toxins: MPTP (heroin contaminant), manganese, cycad (endemic in Guam)

Y: h**Y**drocephalus, normal-pressure; PC: Lower-body parkinsonism

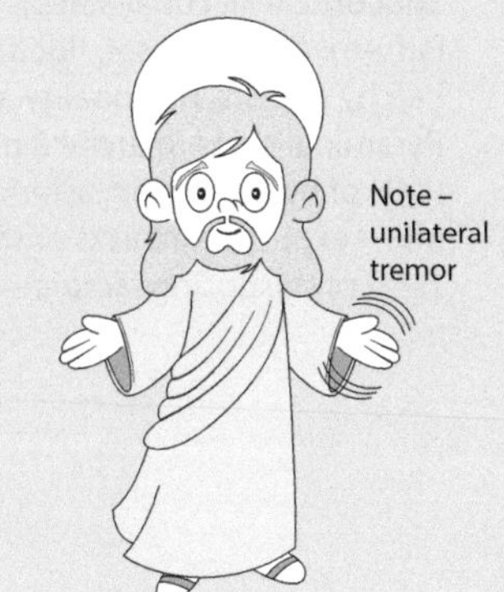

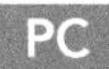

The Parkinson patient is **T.R.A.P.P².E².D².**

Tremor:
- Resting, 4–6 Hertz, pill-rolling (less commonly, intention or postural 6–8 Hz tremor)
- Initially unilateral
- Worsened by stress, walking; reduced by relaxation, sleep

Rigidity:
- Lead-pipe, cog-wheeling (= rigidity + tremor)
- May present subtly with pain or numbness in limb, or writer's cramp
- When advanced, may cause foot dystonia, hand or swan-neck deformities, scoliosis

Akinesia (decreased frequency and decreased speed of movements):
- Difficulty with repetitive movements, e.g. opposing finger + thumb
- External cues and emotional input promote movement

Postural instability: Stooped gait with festination and shuffling; retropulsion

Prose: Monotone, quiet dysarthria, micrographia, drooling (due to reduced swallowing)

Perseveration: When asked to clap 3 times, will clap more; palilalia; doesn't inhibit blinking with glabellar tap

Expression/**E**yes: Mask-like face, stare (widening of palpebral fissures), blinking ↓ (5–10/min)

Depression/**D**ementia: Thought slowing/**D**epressed autonomics: constipation, detrusor instability

Rx

Pro-dopaminergic

L-DOPA:
- Given with dopa-decarboxylase inhibitor (carbidopa, benserazide) to minimize peripheral conversion
- Side-effects: **D.O².P.A.M.I.N.E.**
  - **D**yskinesia, e.g. chorea – occurs >5 years of therapy with peak dose, or end of dose
  - **O**n-**O**ff phenomenon, i.e. fluctuations, occur >5 years from starting therapy
  - **P**sychosis, insomnia
  - **A**BP ↓ (postural hypotension)
  - **M**ental: Addiction, e.g. gambling, OCD (more problem with dopamine agonists)
  - **I**ntestinal (diarrhoea)
  - **N**+V; pre-treat with domperidone if this occurs
  - **E**xcretions – red urine

Dopamine agonist:
- Oral: Ropinirole, pramipexole; transdermal: rotigotine patch
- Delays time to requirement of L-DOPA, but not as effective and causes confusion in elderly
- Subcutaneous: Apomorphine – indicated in pts with severe fluctuations due to L-DOPA

MAO-B inhibitor (selegeline, rasagaline, safinamide) – can increase time before L-DOPA needed; helps reduce fluctuations; safinamide is also a calcium-channel blocker and may be neuroprotective

COMT inhibitor (entacapone, tolcapone; combined with levodopa = 'Stalevo') – given with L-DOPA to increase its bioavailability

Other oral

Anticholinergics: Benzhexol (trihexyphenidyl) – good for tremor and drug-induced parkinsonism, but causes confusion in elderly

Amantadine (indirect dopamine agonist + anticholinergic) – good for dyskinesias, but causes livedo reticularis, ankle oedema and confusion

Non-oral

Deep brain stimulation of subthalamic nucleus or internal pallidum

Duodopa: Levodopa + carbidopa gel, administered as continuous jejunal infusion via PEG tube and external pump – for severe cases with dyskinesias and fluctuations

Subcutaneous exenatide: Glucagon-like peptide receptor agonist used in diabetes; research drug – may be neuroprotective

CHOREA

Def

C.H.O.R.E.A.

Continuous (brief jerks, e.g. forearm pronation-supination, tongue poking)
High-speed and brief
Odd or bizarre movements
Random (flit over body), irregular
Exacerbated by movement
Actions intruded upon by chorea, or chorea incorporated into normal activity, e.g. lurching gait

Causes

H.I.T.T.I.N.G. M.E^2.

Hereditary:
- Dominant: Huntington disease:
  - Epi: 35–50 y, onset inversely proportional to length of CAG trinucleotide repeat
  - PATH: PolyGlutamine (CAG) repeat causes mutated Huntingtin (IT) gene, on chromosome 4p; MRI brain: caudate atrophy
  - PC: Chorea or parkinsonism in young; apraxia; dementia, violence, depression
  - Rx: ?anti-sense interfering RNA – under trial; where genetic risk known – pre-implantation diagnosis
  - Benign, hereditary chorea
- Recessive: Wilson disease
- Complex: Acanthocytosis – 'neuroacanthocytosis' or McLeod syndrome (abnormal Kell blood group)

Infection/**I**nflammation:
- *Streptococcus pyogenes*: Sydenham chorea in childhood (cross-reactivity with basal ganglia)
- AIDS
- SLE, antiphospholipid syndrome

Toxins:
- L-DOPA
- Neuroleptics (dopamine antagonists) – immediate or tardive, esp. orofacial or akathisia (legs)
- Phenytoin

Toxins: Alcohol withdrawal or thiamine deficiency, pellagra

Ischaemic:
- Cerebral palsy
- Small-vessel disease ('senile chorea' = vascular + degenerative damage to basal ganglia)
- Traumatic or anoxic brain injury; carbon monoxide poisoning

Neoplasia, in basal ganglia; or other mass-lesion – abscess, CVA, subdural haemorrhage – violent, flinging movements suggest hemiballismus due to subthalamic lesion

Gynaecological: Chorea gravidarum (pregnancy)/oral contraceptive pill users

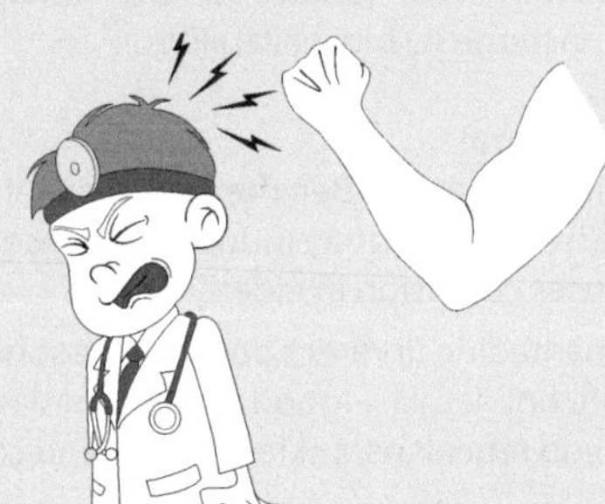

Myeloproliferative: Polycythaemia rubra vera
Endocrine: Thyroxine ↑ or ↓, glucose ↓ or ↑
Electrolytes: Na^+ ↑ or ↓, Ca^{2+} ↓, Mg^{2+} ↓

DYSTONIA

Def

'Abnormal tone': Continuous co-contraction of agonist–antagonist pair with joint in unusual posture, e.g. flexed and pronated wrist with flexed digits, or inverted foot, or retrocollis with neck tremor

Types:

- Idiopathic focal dystonia – this is the commonest form of dystonia:
  - Spasmodic torticollis
  - Hemifacial or blepharospasm
  - Oromandibular dystonia or spasmodic dysphonia
  - Writer's, musician's or sportsman's cramp
- Secondary focal or generalized

Causes

H.I.T.T.I.N.G. M.E.

Hereditary:
Dominant: Huntington disease
DOPA-responsive dystonia (GTP cyclohydrolase mutation)
Recessive: Wilson disease
Pantothenate kinase-associated neurodegeneration (PKAN): Associated parkinsonism, dementia, retinitis pigmentosa – caused by brain iron accumulation
Complex: Primary generalized dystonia (DYT1 mutation)

Infection/**I**nflammation :
AIDS
SLE, antiphospholipid syndrome

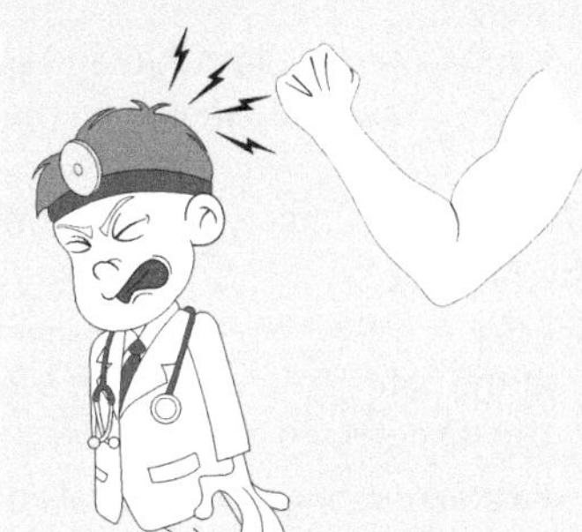

Toxins:
L-DOPA (or Parkinson disease itself, esp. young onset)
Neuroleptics (dopamine antagonists) – immediate or tardive
Phenytoin, flunarizine (calcium antagonist)

Toxins: Alcoholic liver disease; methanol

Ischaemic:
Cerebral palsy
Small-vessel disease ('senile chorea' = vascular + degenerative damage to basal ganglia)
Traumatic or anoxic brain injury; carbon monoxide poisoning

Neoplasia, in basal ganglia; or other mass-lesion – abscess, CVA, subdural haemorrhage; paraneoplastic

Groan! Depression/post-traumatic

Multiple sclerosis – with cord lesion

Electrolytes $Ca^{2+}\downarrow$ or idiopathic striatal calcification (Fahr disease)

TREMOR

Def

Regular, rhythmic oscillation, that needs to be distinguished from:

- Myoclonus: Irregular, discontinuous jerks (however, asterixis = rhythmic myoclonus)
- Epilepsia partialis continua: Abrupt onset, striking asymmetry

Types

R.A.P.I.D. TA.P.S.

Resting
Cause: Parkinsonism
O/E: 4–6 Hz, 'pill-rolling' tremor of thumb-index finger; jaw tremor; ↑ with distraction; postural or action tremor may also occur

Action/**P**ostural
Cause: *see opposite*
O/E: 6–12 Hz (slows with age), worse with outstretched hand or movement, equally bad at all stages of movement (i.e. 'kinetic tremor', as compared with intention tremor)

Intention
Cause: Cerebellar outflow – dentate nucleus, superior cerebellar peduncle, red nucleus
O/E: >6 Hz, terminal tremor, past-pointing and ataxia on reaching or pointing; severe, 'wing-flapping' tremor, incl. at rest and posture, suggests midbrain ('rubral tremor')

Dystonic
Cause: Mostly idiopathic, and as for dystonia
O/E: Varies depending on precise position of joint; associated cervical dystonia

TAsk-specific: Primary writing tremor

Psychogenic

Special:

Orthostatic – comes on after a few seconds of standing; patient prefers to walk than stand still; can be detected by palpating ankle dorsiflexor tendons or auscultating thighs

Palatal tremor (previously called 'palatal myoclonus')

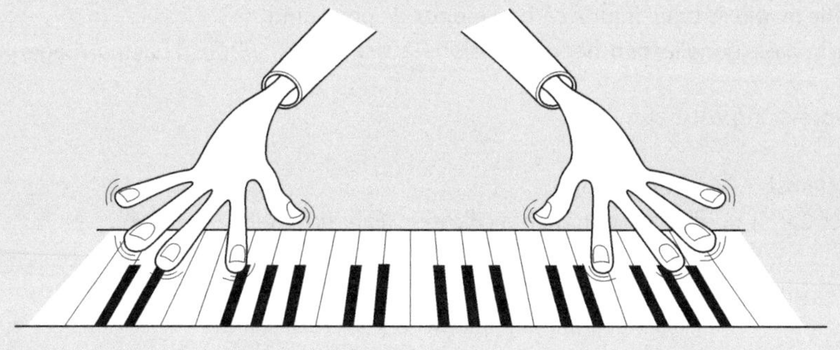

Causes

The following are causes of an action or postural tremor:

B.E.A.T.I^2.N.G.S.

Benign essential tremor
  Epi: Autosomal dominant
  PC: Action > rest; arms, neck, voice tremor (discriminates from Parkinson disease)
Endocrine: Thyrotoxicosis, phaeochromocytoma, hypoglycaemia
Alcohol withdrawal ('delerium tremens'); or caffeine, or opioid, withdrawal
Toxins:
  Prescribed: Lithium, tricyclic antidepressants; salbutamol, theophylline; phenytoin, valproate
  Drugs of abuse
  Lead, arsenic, mercury ('hatter's shakes')
Infection/**I**nflammation:
  Infection: Syphilis
  Inflammation: Multiple sclerosis, SLE
Neuropathy, peripheral: IgM paraproteinaemia, Charcot–Marie–Tooth disease (Roussy–Levy syndrome)
Genetic: Autosomal recessive – Wilson disease
Sympathetic – enhanced physiological tremor: Physiological tremor is present in everybody at 8–12 Hz but is usually too small to be apparent. It may be enhanced by factors that increase sympathetic output: endocrine, toxins, fatigue, anxiety, hypothermia

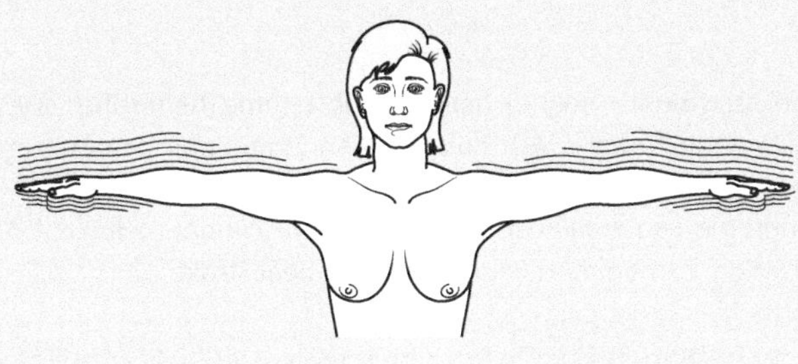

Rx

Alcohol in moderation – improves essential tremor
Propranolol, primidone, topiramate
Botulinum toxin (Botox) injections
Surgery: ViM nucleus thalamus stimulation/lesion/MR-guided focal ultrasound therapy

CEREBELLAR DISEASE – CAUSES

D².I.V.I.N.I.T.Y.

Developmental/**D**egenerative

Developmental

Structural: Arnold–Chiari or Dandy–Walker malformations

Spinocerebellar ataxias:

- Autosomal recessive: Friederich ataxia
- Autosomal dominant: SCA 1-14

Other genetic: Ataxia telangiectasia, Refsum disease, progressive myoclonic epilepsy

Degenerative

Parkinson-plus syndrome: Multiple-systems atrophy (MSA)

Prion: Gerstmann–Straussler–Schenker syndrome

Inflammation:

Multiple sclerosis

Coeliac disease (or other malabsorption, e.g. Whipple disease)

Vascular:

Infarction: PICA, AICA, superior cerebellar artery

Haemorrhage

Infection:

Virus: VZV, EBV, HIV

Bacteria: *Mycoplasma*, *Legionella*, abscess

Neoplasia:

1°:

- Children: Medulloblastoma (midline), haemangioblastoma (hemispheric), astrocytoma
- Cerebellopontine-angle tumour: Vestibular schwannoma, cholesteatoma, meningioma

2°: Bronchus, breast, bowel

Paraneoplastic syndrome, esp. small-cell lung cancer (anti-Purkinje cell = anti-Yo)

Injury: Oxygen deprivation, carbon monoxide poisoning, heat stroke

Toxin/Nutritional:

Alcohol (commonest cause): Causes anterior vermis degeneration or Wernicke syndrome

Anticonvulsants, in overdose or long-term use, esp. phenytoin

Nutrition:

- Vitamin B12, folate or vitamin E deficiency
- Lead poisoning

Y: h**Y**pothyroidism

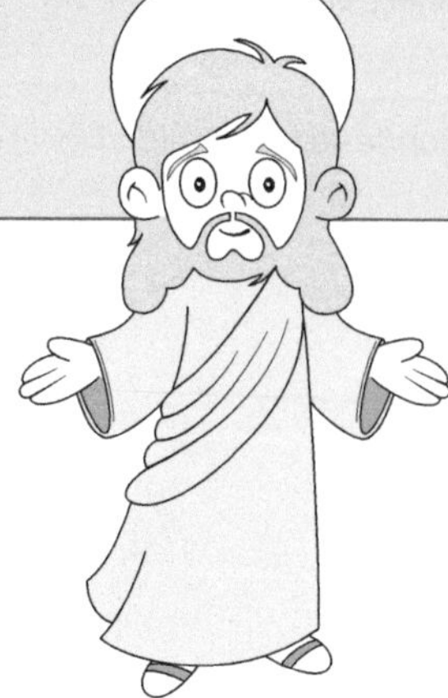

CEREBELLAR DISEASE – PC

D.A.N.I.S^4.H. PAST.R.Y^2.

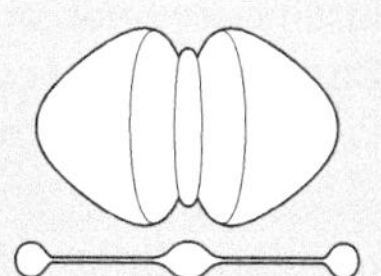

Dysdiadochokinesia: Failure of rapidly alternating movements

Ataxia:
- Limb, incl. gait
- Trunk, titubation (neck tremor)
- Gait: Due to anterior vermis degeneration

Nystagmus:
- Horizontal: Ipsilateral hemisphere
- Downbeat: Inferior cerebellum, e.g. Arnold–Chiari malformation, SCA

Intention tremor:
- Tested by finger-to-nose, and heel-to-shin test
- Severe 'bat's wing' tremor suggests lesions of superior cerebellar peduncle or nuclei

Speech – **S**lurred, **S**taccato and **S**canning dysarthria; writing enlarges

Hypotonia

PAST-pointing (hypermetria): Also seen with saccadic eye movements that overshoot and then correct themselves

Rebound: Overcompensatory response to passive disturbance of position:
- Reflexes: Reduced (due to hypotonia) but pendular (due to overshoot)
- Riddoch's sign: Hyperpronation and elevation of outstretched hand

Y: **WI**de-based gait
- awr**Y** head: Head tilts to side of lesion, due to imbalance of postural tone, dural irritation or 4th cranial nerve palsy

Additional notes

Ipsilesional due to crossing of connections from motor to cerebellar cortex

Acute: Nausea + severe vomiting; occipital headache

Chronic: Signs may improve with time, due to compensatory mechanisms

BLACKOUTS

Causes

Causes of blackouts can be broken down logically into:

Insufficient cerebral flow (syncope)
Disorder of blood composition or metabolites (systemic)
Primary neurological

C.R.A.S. H.

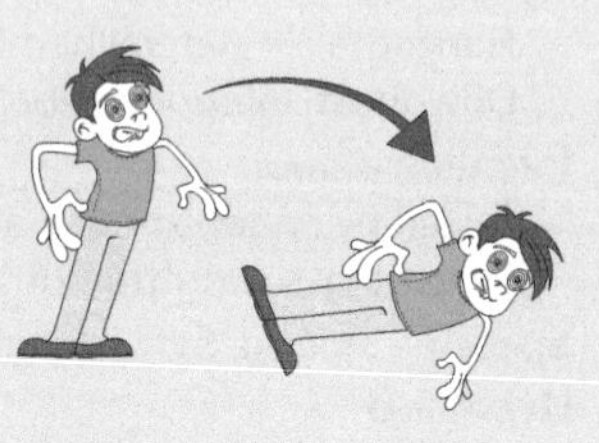

Cardiac:

Bradycardia: Heart block, sick sinus syndrome, tachy–brady syndrome

Tachycardia: SVT (atrial fibrillation, Wolff–Parkinson–White syndrome), VT

Structural:

- Weak heart: LVF, pericardial tamponade
- Blockage: Aortic stenosis, HOCM, myxoma, pulmonary embolism, SVCO

Cardiac, reflex and arterial causes give rise to syncope, i.e. cerebral hypoperfusion

Reflexes

1. Vagal overactivity (venodilation + cardioinhibition)

Vasovagal syncope: Constitutional or situational – cough, micturition, exercise, pain
POTS (postural orthostatic tachycardia syndrome)
Carotid sinus hypersensitivity; glossopharyngeal neuralgia

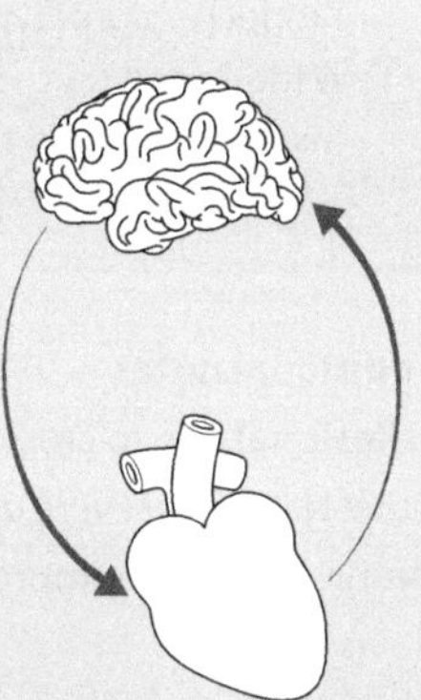

2. Sympathetic underactivity (postural hypotension)

S.T.A.N.D. U.P.

Salt deficiency: Hypovolaemia, Addison disease

Toxins:

- Cardiac: Diuretics, ACE inhibitors, α_1-antagonists, nitrates
- Neuro: L-DOPA, antipsychotics, TCAs, benzodiazepines

Autonomic **N**europathy: Guillain–Barré syndrome, diabetes (both peripheral); Parkinson, MSA (central)

Dialysis

Unwell: Chronic bedrest

Pooling, venous: Varicose veins, prolonged standing

Arterial/venous insufficiency

Vertebrobasilar or bilateral carotid insufficiency, i.e. severe stenosis or occlusion
Systemic hypotension ('shock'): See p. 28
Venous obstruction: Cerebral venous sinus thrombosis

Systemic

Metabolic: Hypoglycaemia or hypothyroidism
Respiratory: Hypoxia or hypercapnia
Blood: Anaemia or hypervicosity

Head (i.e. primary neurological)

Epileptic seizure: Generalized tonic-clonic, atonic, absence, or complex, partial
Non-epileptic attacks (dissociative states)
Structural lesion affecting consciousness pathways: Hydrocephalus, colloid cyst of 3rd ventricle, brainstem tumour (drop attacks)

PC, Ix

Cardiogenic syncope

Trigger: Exertion – esp. sinus bradycardia, SVT, outflow obstruction; drug
Before: Palpitations, chest pain, dyspnoea or no warning
During: As for vasovagal; brady- or tachycardic, ABP ↓
(*if prolonged* – cyanosed, apnoeic, brainstem signs or extensor plantars)
After: Rapid recovery (*if prolonged* – confusion, focal neurological signs)
Ix: ECG, 24-h tape; ECHO; event recorder; intracardiac electrophysiological recording

Reflex – vasovagal

Trigger: Prolonged standing, heat, fatigue, stress
Before:

- Gradual onset over minutes
- Faint, nausea, anxiety, blurred or tunnel vision, visual spots or fading, tinnitus

During: Pale grey, clammy, eyes closed; limp; bradycardic; ABP ↓; quiet respiration
After: Rapid recovery (may feel cold, nausea)
Ix: Tilt-table testing – blood-pressure initially maintained → HR ↑ → HR ↓, ABP ↓

Reflex – postural hypotension

Trigger: Standing for short or long delay
Before, During, After: As for vasovagal
Ix: Tilt-table testing – blood-pressure drops immediately (esp. with autonomic failure)

Arterial

Trigger: Arm elevation (subclavian steal)
Before, During, After: As for vasovagal ± brainstem Sx (diplopia, nausea, dysarthria)
Ix: MRA or duplex vertebrobasilar circulation

Systemic

Before, During, After: As for vasovagal

Head – epileptic attacks

Trigger: Flashing lights, fatigue, fasting
Before: Complex partial seizure – 'strange feeling'; epigastric rising; olfactory hallucinations; déjà vu; automatism, grimacing frontal seizures – sudden onset; 'heralding cry'; occurs in frequent clusters
During: Tongue-biting; urinary and faecal incontinence; stiffness (tonic phase); eyes open
O/E: Sympathetic activation – pupillary dilation; tachycardic; ABP ↑; cyanosed; reduced oxygen sats; pyrexia; brainstem signs
After: Headache, sleeps, confused, Todd paresis
Ix: EEG; videotelemetry; serum prolactin at 10–20 min elevated

Head – non-epileptic attacks

Trigger: Emotional stress; presence of other people; psychiatric history; sexual abuse
During: Eyes closed firmly; head turns side-to-side; pelvic thrusts; flailing limbs; persists for >10 min with no cyanosis and normal oxygen saturation

Dizziness – Causes

With impaired consciousness e.g. blackout or light-headedness

Blackout causes: **C.R.A.SH**

Without impaired consciousness

Vertigo: Spinning sensation – vestibular
Imbalance – unsteady on feet: Vestibular, cerebellar, extrapyramidal

EPILEPSY

Causes

D^2. I. V. I. N. I. T. Y^3.

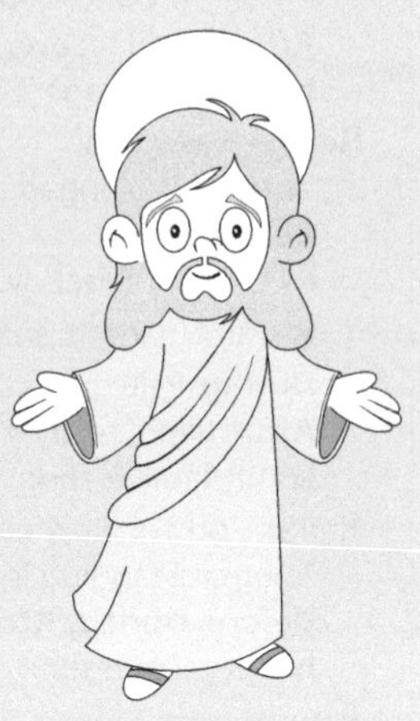

Degenerative/**D**evelopmental
- **D**egenerative: Alzheimer, prion disease
- **D**evelopmental
  - Primary:
    - Generalized: Generalized tonic–clonic seizures on awakening ± absences ± myoclonus
    - Focal: Benign rolandic, occipital
    - Complex: Lennox–Gastaut syndrome
  - Secondary:
    - Structural: Mesial temporal sclerosis, cortical heterotopia, dysplasia
    - Neurocutaneous: Neurofibromatoses, tuberous sclerosis/PKU
    - Progressive myoclonic epilepsy, e.g. mitochondrial

Infection:
- Viral encephalitis, esp. herpes simplex
- Bacterial abscess
- HIV, syphilis, Whipple (or coeliac disease)

Vascular:
- Large stroke, multi-infarcts, hyperviscosity syndrome, TTP
- Cortical venous thrombosis
- Cerebral AVM, angioma

Inflammation:
- Autoimmune limbic encephalitis: Anti-voltage gated K^+-channel antibodies – faciobrachial dystonic seizures; anti-NMDA receptor antibodies; Rassmussen encephalitis (anti-glutamate receptor)
- Multiple sclerosis
- SLE, antiphospholipid syndrome, vasculitis, sarcoidosis

Neoplasia:
- Brain tumour: Primitive neuroectodermal tumour (PNET), glioma
- Meningeal carcinoma, melanoma, lymphoma
- Paraneoplastic syndrome, esp. small-cell lung cancer (anti-neuronal Hu limbic encephalitis)

Injury:
- Head injury: Early or late
- Cerebral anoxia

Toxins:
- Withdrawal from alcohol; sedatives
- Drugs: Penicillin, ciprofloxacin, opioids

Y: h**Y**poglycaemia, h**Y**pocalcaemia (or Mg ↓ or Na ↓), h**Y**perthermia

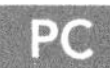

Complex partial seizures

A.A.A.A.A.

Aura: Rising epigastric sensation; déjà vu; olfactory or auditory hallucinations
Autonomic: Change in skin colour, temperature, palpitations
Absence: Motor arrest, motionless stare lasts longer than typical absences of childhood
Automatism: Lip-smacking, chewing, swallowing; fumbling, walking
Amnesia: Amnesia of entire attack usual

Cause:
- Usually arise from mesial temporal lobe, esp. 'mesial temporal sclerosis'
- Associated with febrile convulsions in childhood, but the complex partial seizures may not begin until middle-age

Absences

AB.S.E.N.C.E.

ABrupt onset + offset
Short – usually <10 seconds
Eyes: Glazed, blank stare; slight blinking, eye-rolling
Normal, i.e. normal intelligence, examination, brain scan
Clonus, or automatism – may occur, esp. as duration of attack increases
EEG: 3 Hz spike-and-wave, with photosensitivity

Cause:
- Typical absences (as described) are one of the 'primary generalized epilepsies', due to thalamic dysregulation
- Atypical absences (e.g. last longer; focal signs common) may form part of temporal or frontal-lobe seizures, or complexes, e.g. Lennox–Gastaut syndrome

Ix

Bloods: Prolactin 10 min after fit may be increased relative to baseline
Urine: e.g. toxicology
Micro: CSF PCR for HSV; HIV serology
EEG: Resting or with provocation (hyperventilation, photosensitivity); sleep-deprived; telemetry
Radiol: MRI brain with fine temporal lobe cuts
Surgical: Depth or subdural strip electrodes (pre-operative work-up)

Rx

Conservative: No need to treat if a 'one-off'

Counsel:
- Can't drive for 1 year; careful in bath, ladders etc.
- Pregnancy (folate) and pill (interactions)

Medical:
- Generalized: Lamotrigine or valproate are 1st-line; valproate is more effective, and can be increased in dose more rapidly, but cannot be used in women who may become pregnant
- Partial: As for generalized plus levetiracetam, lacoamide or oxcarbazepine adjunct

Surgical:
- Temporal lobectomy
- Callosotomy
- Vagal nerve stimulator

Underlying cause: e.g. alcohol abuse counselling; antiviral for encephalitis

STROKE – ISCHAEMIC

Causes

Ischaemic stroke occurs due to focal arterial ischaemia, i.e. inadequate blood flow to a *part* of the brain (as opposed to the whole brain, as occurs with syncope when temporary, or anoxic injury when sustained)

Focal ischaemia is due to arterial or venous thrombus, the causes of which are given by Virchow triad of thrombosis (p. 484)

Arterial wall (endothelial) injury
Arterial ischaemia

A.D.V.I.S.E.

Atherosclerosis: Hypertension, DM, cholesterol, smoking
Dissection: Hypertension, Ehlers–Danlos, Marfan; dysplasia, fibromuscular
Vasculitis: Autoimmune (PAN, giant-cell arteritis); infection (TB, syphilis)
Injury: Trauma, catheterisation (angioplasty), indwelling central line, radiation
Spasm: Migraine
Embolism, cardiac: AF, endocarditis, myxoma

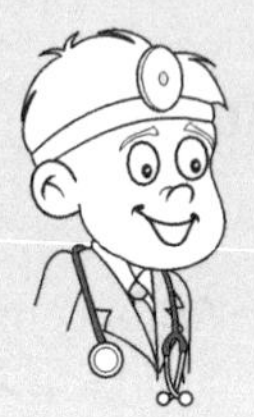

Stasis
Venous, ± arterial, ischaemia

A.nd

Atrial fibrillation

Hypercoagulability
Venous, ± arterial, ischaemia

H.E.P^3.A.R.I.N.I.S^2.E.

Hereditary: Prothrombin, factor V Leiden genes, protein S, C deficiency, homocystinuria, mitochondrial (MELAS – stroke due to metabolic not vascular defect)
Endocrine: Oestrogens – pregnancy, OCP, HRT; androgens; diabetic HHS
Polycythaemia; **P**araproteinaemia; **P**NH
Autoimmune: Antiphospholipid syndrome, SLE, Behçet
Renal: Nephrosis, dehydration
Injury
Neoplasia: Adenocarcinoma, acute leukaemia
Infection: Septicaemic; local – cellulitis; otitis media, sinusitis
Smoking; **S**enility (increasing age)
Exogenous: Chemotherapy, steroids; COX-2 inhibitors

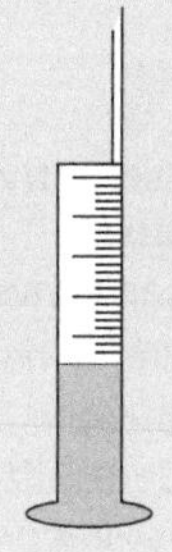

CT head +/– CT angiogram carotids and intracranial are 1st-line

Bloods: FBC, U&E, cholesterol, ESR, CRP, autoAbs, thrombophilia screen
Urine: Glucose, blood
Micro: VDRL, HIV serology, blood cultures
Monitor: ABP, neuro. obs., glucose
ECG, **E**CHO
Radiol:

- CXR
- Brain: MRI, MRA; catheter angiogram
- Carotid Doppler USS

Rx

5 Rs

Resuscitation:
O_2, nasogastric tube, fluids, temperature, glucose, ICP
Blood pressure should be 110–180 mmHg systolic; use IV labetalol or GTN (for acute hypertension); or IV saline (for hypotension)

Revascularisation: Performed immediately after arrival in A&E and subsequent CT head +/– CT carotid+cerebral angiogram

- IV thrombolysis: Must be given in 4.5 hour window, improves disability but not survival; +/–
- Thrombectomy for proximal occlusion of middle cerebral artery, or basilar artery: Must be performed within 6 hours (unless MRI/CT perfusion imaging shows perfusion deficit, but no infarct, for up to 24 hours)
- Anticoagulation – doesn't dissolve thrombus but stops thrombus propagation: May be used if arterial thrombus present but no large infarction, and if thrombolysis not given; 1st-line treatment for venous thrombosis

Rest of medical therapy – secondary prevention:

- Antiplatelet (aspirin or clopidogrel) – started day after thrombolysis, statin
- Anti-hypertensives
- Anticoagulant (if AF or persistent large vessel thrombus), antihypertensives

Removal of cranium (hemicraniectomy) or removal of plaque (carotid endarterectomy)
Other surgical, e.g. VP shunt if hydrocephalus occurs after cerebellar stroke

Rehabilitation:
Patient should be cared for in a Hyperacute stroke unit, then a step-down stroke early swallow assesment – NGT, PEG?

- TED stockings
- Physiotherapy, OT, speech therapist, psychologist

STROKE – HAEMORRHAGIC

Causes

H.A.E.M.A.T.O.M.A^2.

Hypertension: Causes Charcot–Bouchard microaneurysm: putaminal/thalamic/brainstem bleed

Aneurysm :

- Berry aneuysms occur at arterial bifurcations and usually cause subarachnoid haemorrhage, but can bleed intracerebrally
- Assoc. with hypertension, family history, APKD

Elderly: Amyloid angiopathy causing lobar haemorrhages

Malformations: AVM, dural fistula, cavernous angioma, moya-moya syndrome

Autoimmune/infection: Vasculitis, TB, endocarditis

Trauma

Occlusive venous or arterial disease:

- Cerebral venous thrombosis
- Haemorrhagic transformation of infarct
- Reversible vasoconstriction syndrome (RCVS) – typically non-aneurysmal subarachnoid hemorrhage

Metastases/primary brain tumour:

- Mets: Bronchial, melanoma, choriocarcinoma (pregnancy, testes), thyroid, renal
- Glioma

Amphetamine, cocaine; **A**nticoagulation

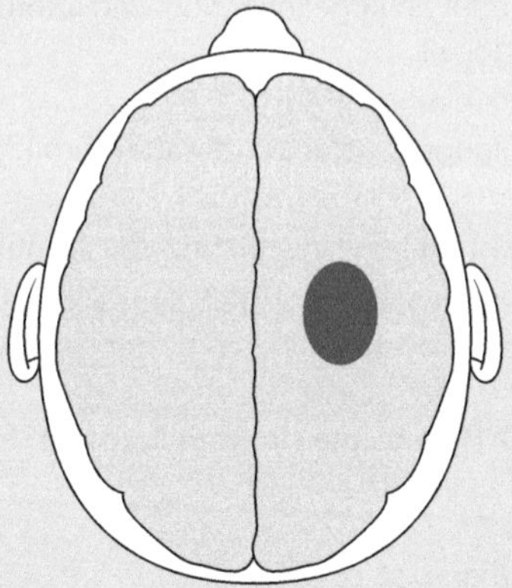

Ix

Bloods: FBC, clotting, G&S, autoAbs
Urine: Glucose (subarachnoid bleed); toxicology
Micro: Blood cultures
Monitor: ABP, neuro. obs., glucose
ECG: Ischaemic changes in SAH
Radiol:

- CXR (pulmonary oedema in SAH)
- Brain: CT, MRI, MRA
- Cerebral angiogram

Special: LP for xanthochromia if SAH suspected

Rx

Resuscitation

O_2, IV fluids, nasogastric tube, BP/ECG monitor, ITU if drowsy

+

A.B.C.D.

Anticoagulant reversal: If patient on anticoagulant, give activated coagulation factors, vitamin K (if on warfarin), specific monoclonal antibodies for direct oral anticoagulants (e.g. for dabigatran)

Blood pressure control:

- Acute: IV labetalol, GTN
- Chronic: ACE inhibitor, calcium-channel blocker, etc.

Craniectomy/Coiling

+

D: Drugs, e.g. lactulose (decrease intracranial pressure with defaecation), levetiracetam (for seizures)

ACUTE WEAKNESS

Cerebrum/Brainstem
Vascular: Infarction, haemorrhage
Infection: Encephalitis, abscess
Inflammation, e.g. ADEM

Cord
Vascular: Anterior spinal artery infarction, AVM
Inflammation: Transverse myelitis
Injury

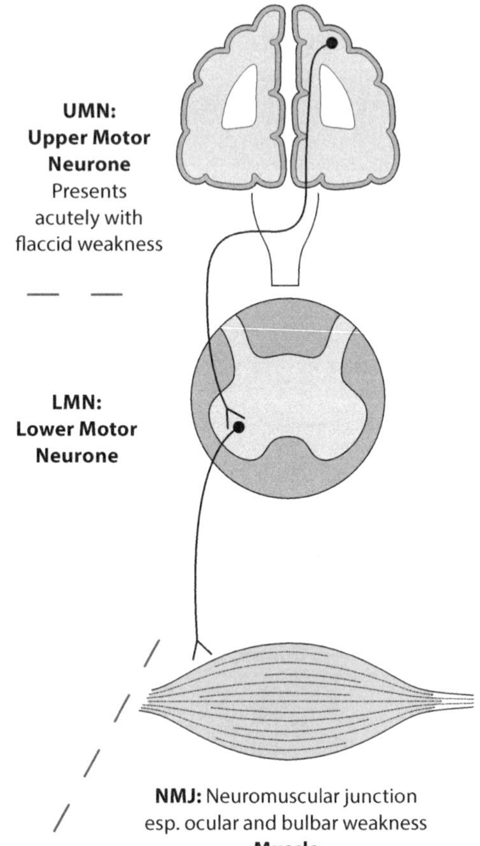

Anterior horn cells
Infection: Polio, West Nile virus
Paraneoplastic

Roots/Plexus
Proximal nerve inflammation: Brachial neuritis
Plexitis: Carcinoma, radiotherapy

Motor nerves (p. 296)
Demyelinating
- **I**nflammatory: GBS
- **T**oxin: Diphtheria, buckthorn, seafood (ciguatoxin), suramin
- **S**ystemic – uraemia

Axonal
- **P**orphyria, acute intermittent
- **A**utoimmune: Vasculitis
- **I**nfection: Lyme disease/ITU neuropathy
- **N**eoplastic: Paraneoplastic, lymphoma

NMJ
Autoimmune: Myasthenia gravis
Toxin: Botulism
Neoplasia: Lambert–Eaton myasthenic syndrome
Calcium ↑ or ↓

Muscle
Toxins: Steroids, statins, ITU, cocaine, alcohol
Hereditary: Periodic paralysis, malignant hyperthermia
Inflammation: Myositis, trichinosis, HIV
Neoplastic: Paraneoplastic
Electrolytes: K^+ ↓, PO_4 ↓
Rhabdomyolysis: Due to any of above

GUILLIAN–BARRÉ SYNDROME

Types

- GBS = AIDP (acute inflammatory demyelinating polyneuropathy) 90% – various antibodies
- AMAN (acute motor (± sensory) axonal neuropathy) 5% – anti-GD1a antibodies
- Miller–Fisher syndrome (ophthalmoplegia + ataxia + areflexia) 5% – anti-GQ1b antibodies
- Acute sensory/autonomic neuropathy 1%
- NB: AMAN constitutes 30–50% cases in China and South America

Causes

Cross-reacting antibodies to gangliosides (glycosphingolipids on myelin sheath or axolemma), with clinical syndrome beginning 1–4 weeks, following exposure to:

- Bacteria: *Campylobacter jejuni* (30%, esp. AMAN), *Mycoplasma*
- Viruses: CMV, EBV, HIV, unidentified virus, e.g. flu (majority of cases)
- Vaccines, esp. rabies

PC, Ix

G.B^3.S. = A.I.D.P.

Growing weakness:
Typically, proximal weakness that ascends from legs to trunk, arms, head; nadir <4 weeks
Variants include brachiocephalgic (bifacial palsies) or paraparesis (mimic cord lesion)
Areflexia very common; fasciculations may occur
Breathing and **B**ulbar problems/**B**ack pain
Respiratory support required in 25% due to bulbar and respiratory muscle weakness
Back pain common due to inflammation of proximal nerve roots
Sensory disturbance
Paraesthesia in extremities is often first symptom
Sensory ataxia common, esp. in Miller–Fisher syndrome

Autonomic neuropathy: Arrhythmias, labile blood pressure, urinary retention, constipation
Immune: Serology for anti-gangliosides; *Campylobacter,* HIV, etc.; stool sample
Demyelinating nerve conduction studies: Motor conduction velocities – slow; central motor conduction times (F-wave) – delayed
Protein in CSF:
Protein usually>1 g/l by second week; white cells <4 × 10^9/l (i.e. 'albuminocytological dissociation')
High CSF protein can cause papilloedema and optic neuropathies (check visual acuity)

Rx

Immunuosuppression: IVIg or plasma exchange – the earlier, the better
Supportive
Airway/ventilation support: transfer to ITU if FVC<1.0 l (15 ml/kg)
Analgesia (NSAIDs, gabapentin, antidepressants)
Autonomic: Cardiac monitor; labetalol or noradrenaline etc.; laxatives; urinary catheter
Antithrombotic: TED stockings, low-molecular-weight heparin
Physiotherapy: Prevent flexion contractures

Prog

Death 5%; permanent disability 20%
Bad prognosis – rapid onset; *Campylobacter*-positive
Good prognosis – Miller–Fisher variant

HAND WASTING – CAUSES

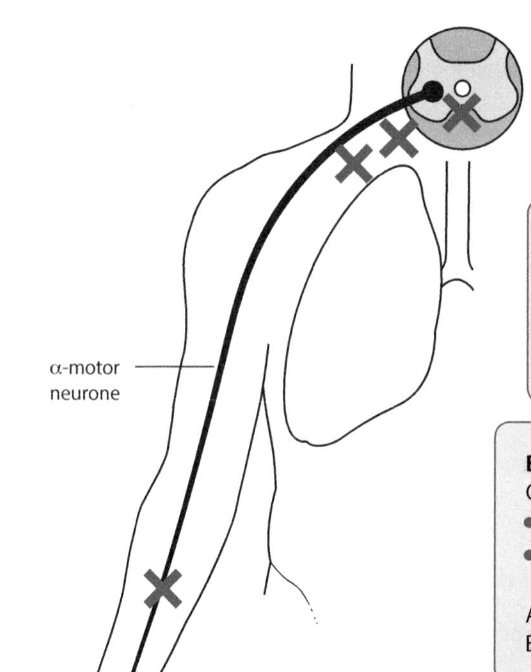

Cord
Syringomyelia
Anterior horn cell disease:
- Motor neurone disease
- Polio, syphilis, paraneoplastic

Roots (C8, T1)
Compression:
- Spondylosis
- Neurofibroma

Meningeal infiltration

Brachial plexus (lower)
Compression:
- Cervical rib, fibrous band
- Tumour: Pancoast tumour (apical lung ca.); breast ca. or lymphoma; radiotherapy

Avulsion (Kiumpke's palsy)
Brachial neuritis (usually proximal wasting)

Neuropathy
Generalized:
- Chronic inflammatory demyelinating polyneuropathy (CIDP)
- Multifocal motor neuropathy with conduction block (MMN)
- Charcot–Marie–Tooth disease (CMT)

Mononeuritis multiplex: Diabetes, vasculitis
Mononeuropathy – compressive:
- Median (wasting of thenar eminence; numb lateral 3½ digits): Carpal tunnel syndrome
- Ulnar:
  - At axilla (sensory loss over medial arm, forearm, palm)
  - At elbow (sensory loss over palm): repetitive injury, old supracondylar fracture of humerus
  - At wrist (no sensory changes): trauma, ganglion in Guyon canal

Other
Compartment syndrome – Volkmann ischaemic contracture: Fibrosis of wrist and finger flexors
Disuse atrophy:
- Rheumatoid arthritis (also causes carpal tunnel syndrome, ulnar neuropathy and mononeuritis)
- Long-standing neurodisability: Parkinson, stroke, multiple sclerosis

Cachexia

WALKING DISTURBANCE – CAUSES

Apraxic (frontal lobes)
O/E: Wide-based, short steps,
out-turned toes,
+ dementia, incontinence,
primitive reflexes
Lacunar state: Marche à petit pas
Normal-pressure hydrocephalus

UMN Bilateral
O/E: Spastic, scissoring
+ brisk jaw jerk,
pseudobulbar speech,
emotional incontinence,
sphincter dysfunction
Bihemispheric disease:
Cerebral palsy, ALS
parasagittal meningioma
Cord lesion (myelopathy):
Cervical spondylosis,
hereditary spastic
paraparesis

UMN Unilateral
O/E: Circumducting, spastic gait
Cerebral hemisphere lesion:
CVA, MS, tumour
Hemicord (Brown-Sequard syn.):
MS, tumour

Functional
O/E: Distractible,
bizarre

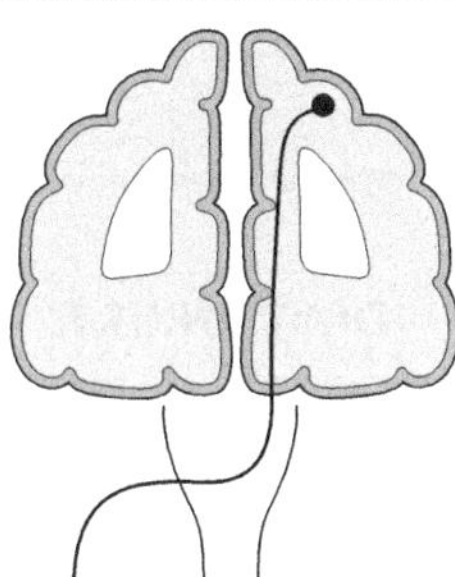

UMN:
Upper motor
neurone

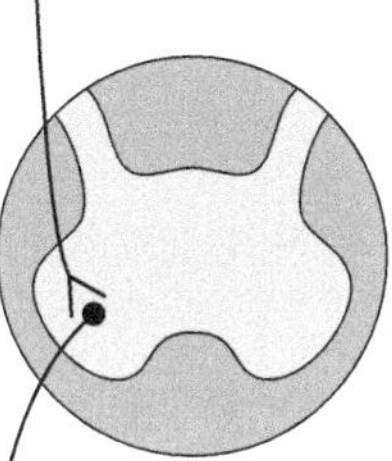

Vestibular
O/E: Veering (ipsilateral),
Romberg +ve, nystagmus,
drop attacks (paroxysmal)

Cerebellar
O/E: Wide-based, ataxic,
nystagmus

Basal ganglia (extrapyramidal)
Parkinsonism
O/E: Short-step, shuffling,
flexed, loss of arm
swing, festinant
Choreiform
O/E: Lurching
Dystonia
O/E: Hand or foot held in odd
fixed position; torticollis
Myoclonus
O/E: Knees give way

LMN Bilateral
O/E: Bilateral foot drop,
flaccid paraparesis, areflexia
Peripheral neuropathy:
CMT, Guillain-Barré syn., CIDP
Cauda equina:
Lumbar disc prolapse
(also sphincter dysfunction,
saddle anaesthesia)

LMN Unilateral
O/E: Foot-drop: high-steppage
gait
Radicular lesion, e.g. L5
Sciatic or lateral popliteal nerve:
Trauma, diabetes, vasculitis

Mixed UMN + LMN
Conus medullaris lesion
Vitamin B12 deficiency
Motor neurone disease

LMN:
Lower motor
neurone

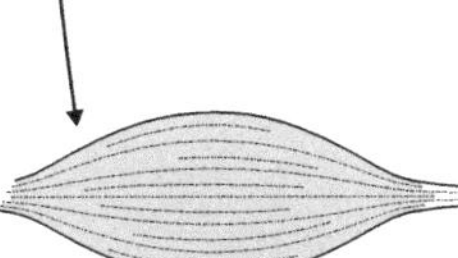

Myopathy
Myasthenia
O/E: Waddling gait

Proprioceptive loss
O/E: Romberg +ve
Dorsal column disease:
- Vitamin B12 deficiency
- Syphilis, HIV (mixed UMN + LMN disease)

Large-fibre peripheral
neuropathy, or dorsal-root
ganglionopathy

Visual loss

Other medical
Vascular:
- Postural hypotension
- Intermittent claudication

Cardiac: Stokes-Adams attacks
Arthritis

MYELOPATHY

Spastic paraplegia or quadriplegia (i.e. upper motor neuron syndrome) is nearly always caused by spinal cord injury, due to 1) extrinsic cord compression, or 2) intrinsic cord disease

Cord compression

Pain
Radicular symptoms

Causes

D².I.V.I.N.I.T.Y.

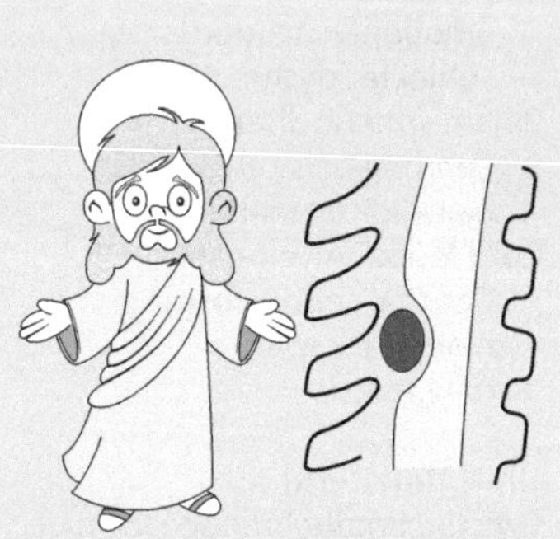

Degenerative/**D**evelopmental
- **D**egenerative
  - Cervical disc prolapse/cervical spondylosis
  - Osteoporosis
  - Paget disease
- **D**evelopmental
  - Spina bifida (cauda equina syndrome/lipoma, haemangiomas)
  - Klippel–Feil syndrome

Infection
- TB
- Pyogenic:
  - Epidural abscess
  - Infected intradural dermoid

Vascular: Extradural haematoma

Inflammation
- Rheumatoid arthritis of atlanto-axial joint
- Ankylosing spondylitis: Increased risk of vertebral fracture

Neoplasia
- Extradural: Vertebral – **B².O.N.E.1. M.** (see p. 257)
- Intradural, extramedullary:
  - Neurofibroma – 'dumb-bell'
  - Meningioma (esp. in thoracic cord, in middle-aged women)
  - Lipoma (assoc. with spina bifida)
  - Dermoid
- Arachnoid cyst

Injury
- Fracture
- Spondylolisthesis

Toxin/Nutritional: Nutritional – rickets/osteomalacia

Y: k**Y**phoscoliosis

Intrinsic cord disease

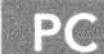

Painless
Early sphincter/erectile dysfunction

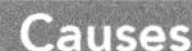

D^2.I.V.I.N.I.T.Y.

Degenerative/**D**evelopmental
Degenerative: Amyotrophic lateral sclerosis/primary lateral sclerosis
Developmental:
- Friedreich ataxia and other spinocerebellar ataxias
- Hereditary spastic paraplegia

Infection
Virus: HIV (selective dorsal column disease), HTLV-I, VZV
Syphilis – 'tabes dorsalis' (selective dorsal column disease)

Vascular
Infarction:
- Thromboembolism, atheroma, diabetes mellitus
- Dissection of aorta
- Vasculitis, esp. polyarteritis nodosa (anterior spinal artery infarction causes spinothalamic loss)

Haemorrhage, intramedullary, incl. AVM (spinal haemangioma)

Inflammation
Demyelination:
- Multiple sclerosis, ADEM
- Post-infective transverse myelitis
- Devic disease (transverse myelitis + optic neuritis)

SLE, vasculitis
Sarcoid

Neoplasia – intradural, intramedullary (rare)
Glioma (esp. in cervical cord, in young adult)
Ependymoma; haemangioblastoma (assoc. Von Hippel–Lindau syndrome)

Injury
Trauma: Contusion, syrinx, myelomalacia secondary to compression
Radiation myelitis

Toxin/Nutritional
Toxin: Lathyrism (chick-pea ingestion in India)
Nutritional: Vitamin B12 deficiency (selective dorsal column disease)

Y: s**Y**ringomyelia

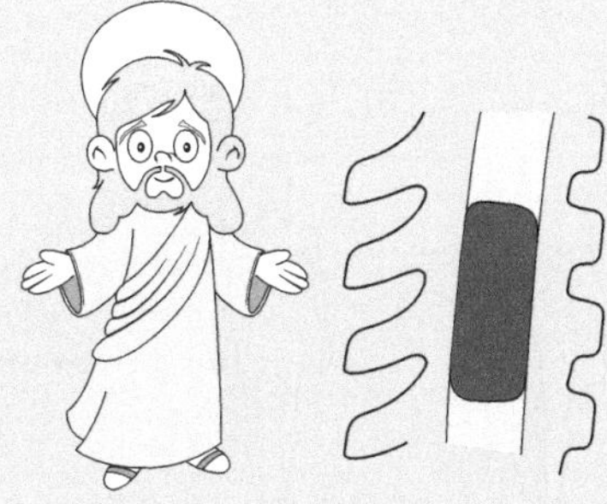

ANTERIOR-HORN CELL DISEASES

The following are causes of a pure lower motor neurone syndrome (wasting, fasciculations, weakness), with or without upper motor neurone signs

A. S.K.I.N.N^2.Y. MA.N.

Amyotrophic lateral sclerosis (ALS)/other motor neurone disease

- **I**nc: 1/100,000 p.a.; prevalence 5/100,000
- **A**ge: >60 years
- **S**ex: M:F = 1.5:1
- **G**eo: Guam, West New Guinea, Japanese Kii Peninsula: Associated with ALS-dementia–Parkinson complex
- **A**et: Neurotoxin: Glutamate excess, e.g. higher in leather workers
  Genetic: 10% are familial, of which 40% are due to C9ORF72 (chromosome 9 open reading frame 72) mutation, and 20% are due to Cu-Zn SOD1 mutation (free-radical clearance enzyme) – that are also cause of frontotemporal lobar degeneration
- **M**icro: Degeneration of both LMN (anterior horns) and UMN (corticospinal tract)
  Ubiquitin positive Bunina inclusion bodies are found within anterior horn cells

Spinal muscular atrophy (SMA)

- PATH: Autosomal recessive disorders linked to 5q
- PC: Infantile and childhood forms are severe and fatal within a few years
  Adult-onset form causes mild proximal limb wasting

Kennedy disease (bulbospinal muscular atrophy)

- PATH: Due to androgen receptor mutation, comprising CAG repeat on X chromosome
- PC: Head: Facial fasciculations, bulbar palsy, dysarthria
  Limbs: Proximal wasting, postural tremor, sensory involvement
  Endocrine: Gynaecomastia, infertility, type 2 diabetes, prostate carcinoma

Infection

- Acute: Polio or West Nile virus; Lyme disease
- Chronic: Post-polio syndrome; syphilis (meningeal)

Neoplasia – 1: Direct motor nerve or meningeal infiltration

Neoplasia – 2: Paraneoplastic (esp. lymphoma) or radiotherapy to pelvis

Neoplasia – 3: Cervicomedullary tumour (or syringomyelia, or cervical spondylosis) may mimic ALS

Y: Ta**Y**–Sachs disease, adult-equivalent – GM2 gangliosidoses due to hexosaminidase deficiency

Monomelic **A**myotrophy: Non-progressive wasting of one distal limb in young adult (i.e. 'benign')

Neuropathies, motor

- Multifocal motor neuropathy with conduction block: Anti-GM1 anti-ganglioside; important not to miss, as this can be treated successfully with IVIg!
- Toxins, e.g. vincristine, lead

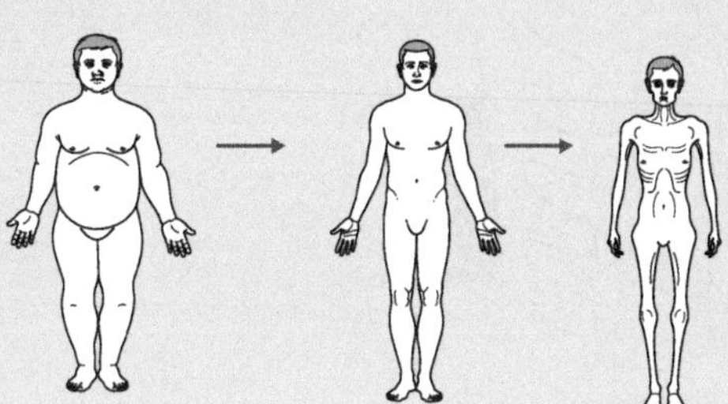

ALS typically causes marked weight loss as well as distal wasting

ALS/MOTOR NEURONE DISEASE

Types/PC

A.P.P.L.E.

Amyotrophic lateral sclerosis (80%)
LMN: Bulbar palsy, distal limb wasting, fasciculations, cramps
UMN: Pseudobulbar palsy, spastic paraparesis, extensor plantars
Spares: Ocular movements (III, IV, VI nuclei)
Bladder, anus control
Sensory signs (although symptoms may occur)
Cerebellum

Progressive bulbar palsy (10%)
LMN: Tongue atrophy and fasciculations, dysarthria, nasal regurgitation
UMN: Pseudobulbar speech, brisk jaw jerk

Progressive muscular atrophy (10%)
LMN: Fasciculations, distal limb wasting, claw hand
Respiratory – poor cough, tachypnoea

Lateral sclerosis, primary (1%): UMN signs only

Extra features (1%): Frontal dementia, parkinsonism – usually hereditary forms
C9ORF72, or SOD1 mutations, and other genetic forms of ALS
Younger onset, more severe course

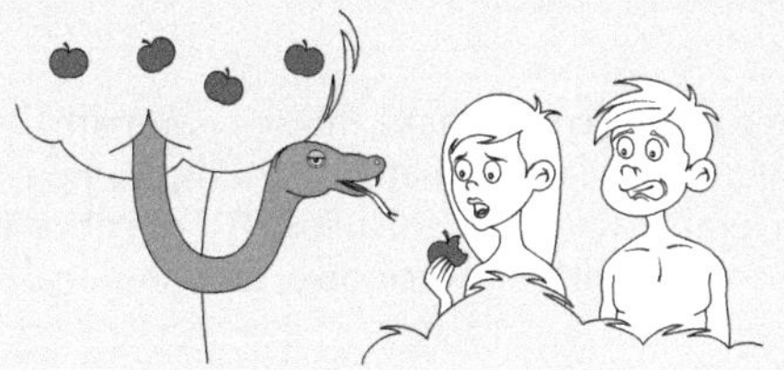
Don't pick that or
we'll be cursed!

Ix

Bloods: CK: Due to spasticity and cramps
Alternative diagnoses: Anti-GM1 (anti-ganglioside Abs), VDRL, hexosaminidase
EMG: MND: Fasciculations, fibrillation potentials; ↓ no. of spikes on maximum contraction
MMN: Conduction block
Radiol: CXR
MRI brain and cervical cord
Special: CSF: VDRL, cytology

Rx

Riluzole: Inhibits glutamate release – prolongs life by 3 months
Supportive: Quinine (cramps); baclofen (spasticity); propantheline (drooling)
Other: Nerve growth factors, IVIg, pyridostigmine (improves weakness in early MND)

PERIPHERAL NEUROPATHY – CAUSES

Demyelination

I.T.'S. T.H.I.N.

Acute

Inflammatory: Guillain–Barré syndrome
Toxin: Diphtheria; arsenic, buckthorn berry
Syndrome: Refsum disease; **S**ystemic: acute uraemic

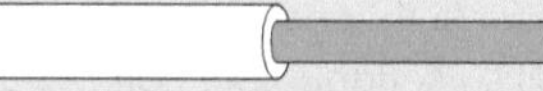

Loss of myelin sheath around axon causes slowing of conduction (cf. axonal – reduced action potential)

Chronic

Toxins: Amiodarone, suramin, industrial solvents
Hereditary: Charcot–Marie–Tooth disease – type 1A (*PMP22* duplication); 1B (protein 0)
Hereditary neuropathy with liability to pressure palsies (*PMP22* deletion)
Metabolic: Refsum disease, abetalipoproteinaemia, leucodystrophies
Inflammatory: Chronic inflammatory demyelinating polyneuropathy, multifocal motor neuropathy
Neoplasia: Myeloma, anti-myelin-associated glycoprotein IgM, POEMS syndrome

Axonal

P.A.I.N. E.N.D.I.N.G.S. H.U.R.T.

Acute

Porphyria, acute intermittent: Recurrent acute attacks, motor neuropathy
Autoimmune: Vasculitis, cryoglobulinaemia, rheumatoid arthritis, Sjögren syndrome, SLE
Infection: Lyme disease (painful lumbosacral polyradiculitis)/ITU or critical illness
Neoplasia: Paraneoplastic (assoc. small-cell lung carcinoma; anti-neuronal Abs), lymphoma

Chronic

Endocrine: Diabetes, hypothyroidism, acromegaly (compression neuropathies, e.g. carpal tunnel)
Nutritional: Vitamin B12 deficiency (+ myelopathy + dementia), thiamine deficiency (alcohol), coeliac
Drugs: Chemotherapy (cisplatin, taxanes), antibiotics (isoniazid), nucleoside analogs (ddI)
Infection: HIV, leprosy
Neoplasia: Infiltration (e.g. lymphoma, carcinoma), amyloidosis
Granulomatous: Sarcoidosis
Systemic: Amyloidosis

Hereditary: CMT disease type 2, HSAN, familial amyloid polyneuropathies, Fabry disease
Uraemia/**R**espiratory failure (COPD): Cirrhosis
Toxins: Thallium (cockroach poison, causes hair loss, may be acute), lead (motor neuropathy)

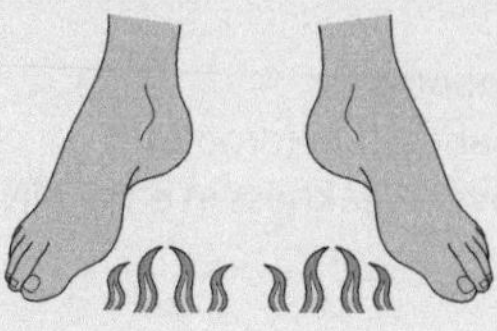

Predominantly sensory symptoms, e.g. burning paraesthesia (cf. demyelinating – motor symptoms)

PERIPHERAL NEUROPATHY – PATTERNS

Mononeuropathy multiplex

Def

Dysfunction of non-contiguous peripheral nerves, e.g. median and peroneal nerve

H.E.A.T.I.N.G. (*some are painful***)**

Causes

Hereditary neuropathy with liability to pressure palsies
Endocrine: Diabetes, hypothyroidism, acromegaly
Autoimmune: Vasculitis, cryoglobulinaemia
Toxin: Lead (radial nerve, peroneal nerve palsies)
Infection: HIV, Lyme, leprosy/**I**nflammatory: CIDP variant (MADSAM, MMN)
Neoplastic: Amyloid, direct infiltration with lymphoma or leukaemia
Granulomatous: Sarcoid

Small-fibre neuropathies

H.E.A.T.I.N.g. (*most are painful***)**

Causes

Hereditary: HSAN, familial amyloid polyneuropathies
Endocrine: Diabetes
Autoimmune: Sjögren syndrome
Toxins: Alcohol (large and small fibres, but painful)
Infection: HIV
Neoplastic: Amyloid

Dorsal-root ganglionopathy

Sensory **A.T.A.X.I.C.**

Causes

Acute: Guillain–Barré syndrome, esp. Miller–Fisher type
Toxins: Cisplatin
Autoimmune: Sjögren syndrome
Xs: Excess vitamin B6
Infectious, post
Carcinoma: Paraneoplastic; also paraproteinaemia with anti-MAG

Palpable nerves

L.A.R.G.E.

Causes

Leprosy
Amyloidosis
Refsum disease
Genetic, other: Charcot–Marie–Tooth types 1, 3; neurofibromatosis
Endocrine: Acromegaly

Autonomic involvement

Causes

Acute: Guillain–Barré syndrome, toxin (vincristine), paraneoplastic, porphyria
Chronic: Diabetes, hereditary (HSAN, FAP), amyloid, HIV

NEUROMUSCULAR JUNCTION DISEASE

Causes

A.C.T.I.O.N.

Autoimmune – myasthenia gravis

PATH: Antibodies to skeletal muscle nicotinic-ACh receptors (nAchR), or muscle-specific kinase (MuSK) causing receptor endocytosis, receptor block and complement fixation

Types:

Thymic hyperplasia (60%, esp. young women): High Ig level; good response to thymectomy

Thymic atrophy (20%, esp. old men): Low Ig level; poor response to thymectomy

Thymoma (10%, middle aged): High Ig level; poor response to thymectomy

Neonatal: Due to placental transfer of IgG in 10% of myasthenic mothers (PC: arthrogryposis)

Assoc: HLA-B8, DR3; thyrotoxicosis, type 1 diabetes mellitus, rheumatoid arthritis, SLE

Congenital myasthenia

PATH: Genetic defect in ACh receptor subunits, or presynaptic ACh synthesis or vesicle packaging

Toxins

PATH: Penicillamine: generates Ach-receptor Abs, and causes myasthenia gravis-like syndrome

Other drugs may exacerbate primary causes of NMJ defects, e.g.

- Pre-synaptic:
  - Ca-channel antagonists: Verapamil, magnesium, aminoglycosides
  - Na-channel blockers: Anti-arrhythmics (Ia, e.g. procainimide), β-blockers
  - Black widow spider venom: Depletes ACh from motor terminals
- Post-synaptic: Anaesthetics; AChR blockers – atracurium, vecuronium, suxamethonium
- Pre- and post-synaptic: Ciprofloxacin

Infection – botulism

PATH: *Clostridium botulinum* toxin acquired from:

- Food-poisoning, esp. home-preserved food, cans
- Food colonisation, esp. infants, raw honey
- Wound contamination, esp. intravenous drug users ('skin popping')

Botulinum toxin (Botox) prevents docking of ACh vesicles with presynaptic cell membrane

Organophosphates, nerve gas

PATH: Act as irreversible acetylcholinesterase inhibitors, causing cholinergic excess and depolarising block

Neoplasia – Lambert–Eaton myasthenic syndrome

PATH: Antibodies to presynaptic voltage-gated calcium channel

Types: 2/3 of cases are paraneoplastic (esp. small-cell lung cancer); 1/3 are primary autoimmune

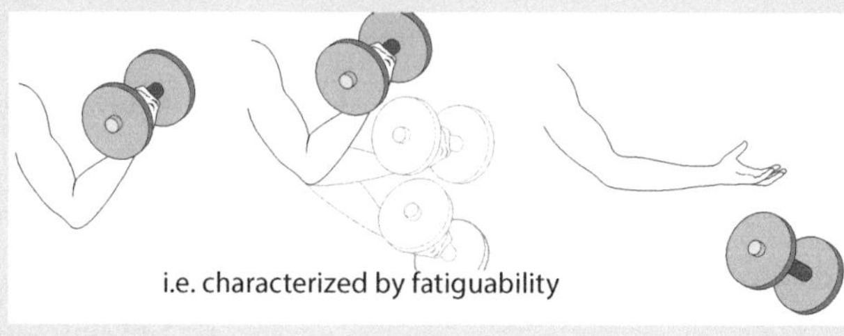
i.e. characterized by fatiguability

Myasthenia gravis

Fluctuating weakness – fatiguable (worsens during day, with infection, drugs, dysthroidism)

Eyes: Ptosis, worse with sustained up-gaze; Cogan lid twitch
Ophthalmoplegia, diplopia (if ptosis not complete)
Face: Weak, snarling-smile, jaw-droop
Bulbar: Nasal dysarthria; nasal regurgitation; aspiration
Neck: Marked weakness, head droop
Limbs: Proximal weakness, asymmetric, brisk reflexes
Ventilation: ↓ FVC (worse on lying) – usually late

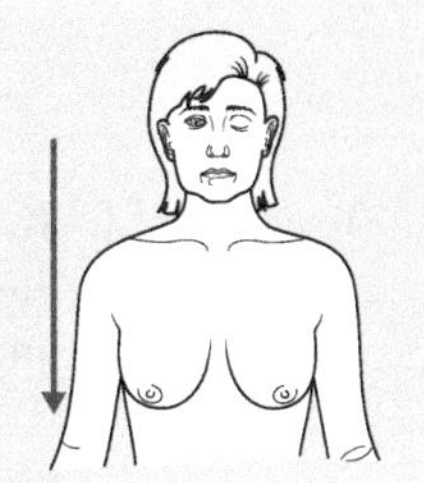

LEMS

As for myasthenia gravis, except **L.E.M.S.**

Leg weakness early, **E**xtra (areflexia, autonomic), **M**ovement improves, **S**ensory symptoms

Botulism

As for myasthenia gravis, plus prominent anticholinergic effects:

Eyes: Iridoplegia, mydriasis, cycloplegia (blurred vision and diplopia are always early symptoms)
Abdominal: Nausea and vomiting (and vertigo); constipation; urinary retention
Systemic: Bradycardia, constipation

Bloods: AutoAbs: nAChR, MuSK, striated muscle (assoc. with thymoma), VG-Ca channel (LEMS)
TFT: Dysthyroidism may precipitate myasthenic crisis
Associated autoimmunity: Glucose, vitamin B12, U&E (Addison), rheumatoid factor, ANA

EMG: Repetitive stimulation: ↓ in compound action potential in myasthenia (↑ with LEMS; botulinum toxin)
Single-fibre studies: Jitter and block – represents delay between two fibres within one motor unit

Radiol: CT thorax – exclude thymoma

Special:

'Tensilon' test: Patient injected with IV 'Tensilon' (edrophonium), which acts as short-acting cholinesterase inhibitor. Becoming less popular due to risk of cholinergic crisis

Ice pack test: An ice pack held on the eyes of the patient improves the symptoms of ptosis in 2 minutes, due to a reduction in the activity of anticholinesterases

Myasthenia gravis

Anticholinesterase inhibitors: Pyridostigmine

☠: N+V, colic, diarrhoea; bradycardia; cholinergic crisis (weakness)

Thymectomy (via mediastinectomy): 85% improve; 50% develop remission by 10 years

Immunosuppression:

- Steroids (start at low dose to avoid initial 'steroid dip')
- Azathioprine (check TPMT level), mycophenolate mofetil
- IVIg, plasma exchange (myasthenic crises)

LEMS

3, 4-Diaminopyridine, steroids, IVIg, plasma exchange

Botulism

Benzylpenicillin, intravenous for active infection with *C. botulinum*

Antiserum, trivalent (anti A, B, E) within 24 hours

MYOPATHY

Causes

T.H.I.N.N.E.R.

Toxins **S³.I³.C⁴.K.**

Prescribed: **S**teroids, **S**tatins, **S**kin
Immune – penicillamine, colchicine; **I**nfection – zidovudine, amphotericin
ITU (anaesthetics)
Chemotherapy: Vincristine; **C**hloroquine, **C**arbimazole, **C**ardiology (amiodarone)
K$^+$-losing diuretics, e.g. thiazides, carbenoloxone, liqourice

Drugs of abuse: Alcohol, amphetamines, opioids, cocaine, barbiturates

Hereditary

Muscular dystrophy:
XL: Duchenne, Becker, Emery–Dreifuss; AR: limb-girdle; AD: facioscapulohumeral, oculopharyngeal
Congenital myopathy
Myotonic dystrophy, myotonia congenita
Channelopathy: Periodic paralysis (K^+), paramyotonia congenita, neuromyotonia
Metabolic: Glycogen-storage, fatty-acid metabolism, mitochondrial disease

Inflammatory

Myositis: Dermatomyositis; polymyositis; inclusion-body myositis (primarily a degenerative disease)
Infective: *Trichinella,* cysticercosis, HIV
Sarcoidosis
(Polymyalgia rheumatica – causes proximal muscle pain, although power and CK usually normal)

Neoplasia

Carcinoma: Advanced or paraneoplastic (incl. dermatomyositis)
Haematological: Eosinophilia (e.g. tryptophan), amyloid, graft-versus-host disease

Nutritional

Ca^{2+} (or Mg^{2+}) ↕ : Osteomalacia, due to poor intake, malabsorption, chronic renal failure
K^+ ↕
Malnutrition, malabsorption: Vitamin E deficiency

Endocrine

Corticosteroids ↕ :

- Cushing syndrome: Due to catabolic effects on muscle; acute or chronic
- Hyperaldosteronism – due to ↓ K^+, hypoaldosteronism (Addison) – mainly muscle fatigue

Thyroid ↕
Other: Acromegaly, diabetes – ischaemic infarction of thigh

Rhabdomyolysis

Toxins: Prescribed (e.g. statin + clofibrate, cyclosporin), neuroleptic malignant syndrome, drugs of abuse
Hereditary: Metabolic – McArdle disease; CPT or acyl CoA deficiency; mitochondrial; malignant hyperthermia (ryanodine receptor gene)
Injury: Trauma, epilepsy

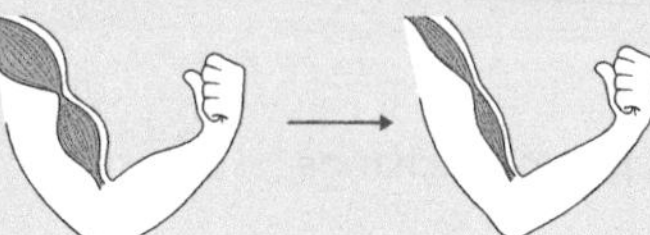

PC

Weak

Proximal pattern usually:

- Girdles, e.g. rising from chair, combing hair
- Ocular–lids, facial, bulbar, neck weakness (esp. myotonic dystrophy and myositis)
- Respiratory (nemaline, McArdle myopathy, myositis)

Distal pattern: Myotonic dystrophy, Emery–Dreifuss or FSH dystrophy, inclusion body myositis

Pain

Toxins (alcohol, heroin), hereditary (McArdle), inflammatory (polymyositis), neoplasia, nutrition (Ca^{2+} ↓), stiffness or cramps: if better with movement – myotonia; worse with movement – paramyotonia

Associated

Arrhythmias: Muscular dystrophy, myotonic dystrophy, mitochondrial myopathy
Infertility: Myotonic dystrophy

O/E

Inspection: Wasting, proximal, symmetrical; ptosis; jaw droop; scapula winging; pseudohypertrophy calves
Tone: Normal; test for hand-grip release and percussion myotonia (thenar eminence, tongue) in myotonia
Reflexes: Relatively spared (except muscular dystrophy or myotonia, in which areflexia occurs)
Gait: Waddle
Other:

Myotonia: Frontal balding, cataracts, dilated cardiomyopathy
Mitochondrial myopathy: Salt and pepper retinitis pigmentosa, deafness, dementia, ataxia
Myositis: Periorbital oedema, rash, lower-zone pulmonary fibrosis

Ix

Bloods: CK ↑ , but normal in PMR, IBM, myotonia, mitochondrial myopathies, chronic steroids
AutoAbs – ANA, ENA, incl. anti Jo-1 (polymyositis), ESR ↑, AChR Abs (myasthenia mimics)
Genetics: Dystrophin, FSH (facioscapulohumeral dystrophy); lactate ↑ in mitochondrial myopathy
Urine: Myoglobin: rhabdomyolysis
Micro: ELISA
Monitor: FVC if dyspnoeic
ECG: Muscular dystrophy, myotonic dystrophy, mitochondrial myopathy
EMG: Small, brief, polyphasic potential (due to recruitment of ↑ no. of weaker motor units)
Insertional activity, fibrillation potentials, positive sharp waves in polymyositis
Myotonia: Waxing and waning amplitude and frequency: 'dive-bomber/motor bike' revving sound
Radiol: CXR (polymyositis, sarcoid, carcinoma)
MRI – directs muscle biopsy location
Surgical – biopsy:
Lymphocytic infiltrate –myositis, sarcoidosis, dysferlinopathy
Mitochondrial myopathy – COX-staining, genetics and respiratory chain assay

Rx

Hereditary: Myotonia – phenytoin, mexiletine (Na^+ channel blockers); dystrophy – myostatin inhibitors?
Inflammatory: Steroids, IVIg

Distinction with steroid-induced myopathy can be made on basis of pain, CK, EMG, MRI and biopsy

ACUTE VISUAL LOSS – CAUSES

Aqueous

Closed-angle glaucoma

Epi
- **I**nc: 10% glaucoma
- **A**ge: Elderly
- **S**ex: F:M = 3:1 (Caucasions)
- **G**eo: Asians
- **A**et: 2 types:
  - Apposition of back of iris to lens blocks aqueous flow → iris pushed forwards, blocking drainage
  - Uveitis → iris adhesions
- **Pre**: Hypermetropes (short eye)
- **Macro**: Corneal oedema

PC:
- Pain: eye, head; severe
  - ↑ in evening (semidilated pupil)
  - ↓ in sleep (pupil constricts)
- N+V, photophobia
- Vision: blurry, haloes

O/E:
- Inspection: red eye, hazy cornea, pupil fixed, semidilated
- Palpation: tender, hard
- Visual acuity ↓
- Fundi: papilloedema
- Late: anterior synechiae, grey atrophy of iris, lens flecks

Ix: Intraocular pressure >21 mmHg (often 40–80 mmHg)

Rx: Acetazolamide (top/IV)
- Mannitol (IV)
- Urgent iridotomy: laser/surgical

Vitreous

Vitreal haemorrhage

Epi:
- Diabetes mellitus
- High myope

PC:
- Floaters
- Blurred vision

O/E:
- Visual acuity ↓
- Red reflex ↓

Retinal detachment/tear

PC:
- Floaters
- Flashing lights (retinal traction)

Retina

Central retinal artery or vein (or branch) occlusion

Epi:
- Artery: thromboembolism, e.g. diabetes, AF, aortic stenosis
- Vein: hypertension, diabetes, hyperviscosity

PC:
- Visual loss:
  - Sudden onset ± offset
  - Curtain descending ± rising

O/E:
- Altitudinal scotoma
- Fundoscopy:
  - Arterial: pale retina, embolus at bifurcation, macular cherry-red spot
  - Vein: flame haemorrhages, papilloedema (sausage-strings – hyperviscosity)
- Late: rubeosis iridis, glaucoma

Macular degeneration

Epi:
- Disciform type >60 years old
- Central serous chorioretinopathy = leakage of fluid into subretinal space: side-effect of steroids

PC:
- Metamorphosia, micropsia,
- Positive central scotoma
- Photo-stress test +ve

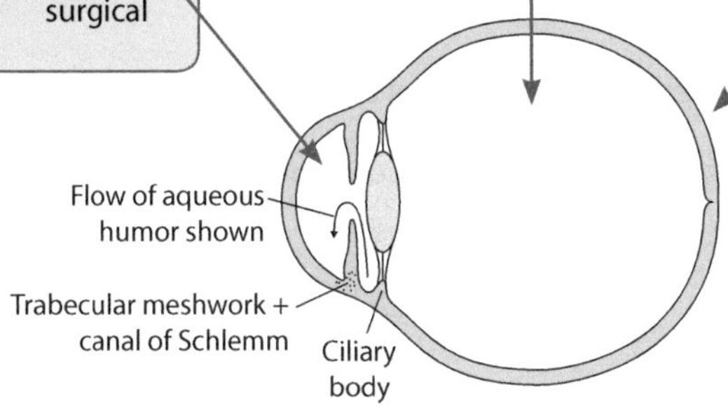

Flow of aqueous humor shown

Trabecular meshwork + canal of Schlemm

Ciliary body

Examination

Characteristic eye or retinal appearance

Usually unilateral

Optic nerve

V.I.S.I.O.N. & O.P.T.I.C.

Vascular: anterior ischaemic optic neuropathy (AION)
- Thromboembolic
- Vasculitis: giant-cell arteritis, SLE, antiphospholipid syn.

Inflammatory – 'optic neuritis'
- Multiple sclerosis
- NMO (neuromyelitis optica)
- ADEM

Sarcoid/other granulomatous
- CRION (chronic relapsing inflammatory optic neuropathy)

Infection:
- Virus, e.g. VZV
- TB, syphilis
- Sinus infection (contiguous)

Other: GBS

Neoplasia: Lymphoma, leukaemia

Ocular

Papillitis/papilloedema

Toxin: Sildenafil, methanol, tobacco/alcohol

Inherited: Leber's hereditary optic atrophy (mitochondrial disease)

Compression: Tumour, trauma, carotid aneurysm

CSF/Chiasm

Intracranial pressure ↑

Epi:
- Mass lesion, e.g. tumour
- Cerebral venous thrombosis
- Primary intracranial hypertension

PC: Visual obscurations

O/E: Papilloedema

Obstructive hydrocephalus

Pituitary apoplexy

Cortical

Vascular

Epi: Causes of vertebrobasilar insufficiency:
- Thromboembolic, incl. AF, cardiac catheterisation, hyperviscosity
- Hypoperfusion, incl. vasovagal, arrhythmia, post-cardiac arrest
- Migraine – usually hemifield loss
- Trauma

Occipital epilepsy

Functional

O/E:

Optokinetic nystagmus present with rolling striped drum

Tunnel vision that does not widen with distance

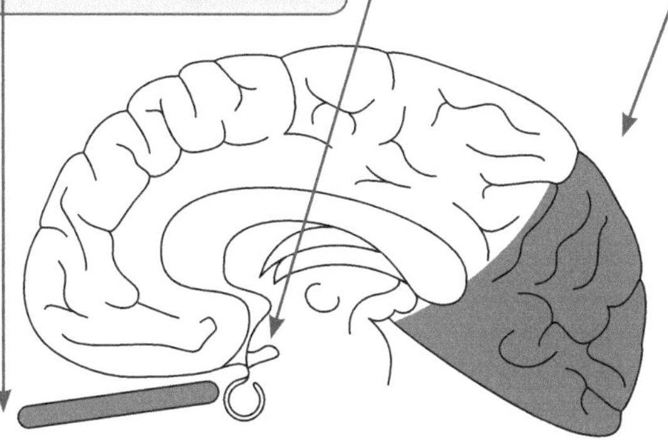

Examination

Optic disc abnormal (optic neuritis, AION, papilloedema) or normal (retrobulbar neuritis; cortical)

Unilateral (optic nerve), sequential (optic nerve or chiasm), bilateral (cortex or chiasm)

OPTIC ATROPHY – CAUSES

O.P.T.I.C.

Papillitis/Papilloedema

Papillitis or retrobulbar neuritis = inflammation of optic nerve head or behind nerve head

V.I.S.I.O.N.

Vascular: 'AION' or 'PION' (anterior or posterior ischaemic optic neuropathy)
- Thromboembolic
- Vasculitis: giant-cell arteritis, SLE, antiphospholipid syn.

Inflammatory: 'Optic neuritis':
- Multiple sclerosis
- NMO (neuromyelitis optica)
- ADEM

Sarcoid/other granulomatous: CRION (chronic relapsing inflammatory optic neuropathy)

Infection:
- Virus
- TB, syphilis
- Sinus infection – contiguous

Other: GBS, vaccination

Neoplasia: Lymphoma, leukaemia

Chronic papilloedema may also cause optic atrophy, e.g. due to primary intracranial hypertension

Toxins/Nutritional

Toxins

Chloroquine
Isoniazid, ethambutol
Lead, thallium

Nutritional

Vitamin B12 deficiency
Vitamin B1 deficiency' – 'tobacco/alcohol amblyopia'
- Due to combination of cyanide in tobacco and thiamine (vitamin B1) deficiency
- Strachan syndrome is association of this with peripheral neuropathy, ataxia and dermatitis

Inherited

Leber's hereditary optic atrophy (LHOA)

Epi:
- Mitochondrial disease
- Men are more symptomatic
- Onset in 20–30s

PC:
- Attacks of acute visual loss, sequentially in each eye
- Ataxia, cardiac defects

O/E: Initially papilloedema, circumpapillary telangiectasia

Neuropathy-associated
- Charcot-Marie-Tooth disease
- Refsum disease

Ataxia-associated
- Friedreich ataxia
- Leukodystrophies

D.I.D.M.O.A.D.
= Diabetes insipidus
Diabetes mellitus
Optic atrophy
Deafness
(autosomal recessive)

NB: Hereditary causes are often associated with **retinitis pigmentosa**, which presents as nyctalopia (night-blindness)

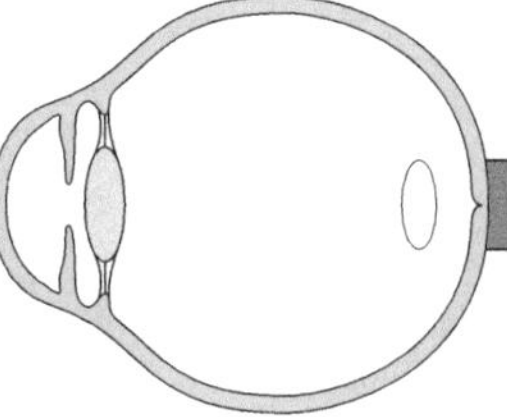

Ocular

Glaucoma
Chronic open-angle: presents with visual loss due to arcuate scotomas and tunnel vision
Graves disease
High myopia

Compression

Neoplasia
- Optic nerve tumour: glioma, sheath meningioma
- Pituitary tumour
- Meningeal ca., leukaemia

Carotid aneurysm
Paget disease

PAPILLOEDEMA – CAUSES

ICP ↑

D.I.V.I.N.I.T.Y[3].

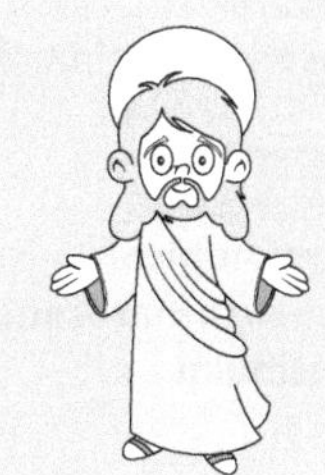

Developmental: Hydrocephalus – esp. obstructive
Infection: Meningo-encephalitis
Vascular:
- Large cerebral infarct or bleed with oedema
- Subarachnoid haemorrhage

Inflammation: Vasculitis, sarcoid
Neoplasia:
- Brain tumour, or spinal cord tumour (high CSF protein)
- Meningeal

Injury: Trauma
Toxin/Nutritional
- Drug overdose, alcohol, lead poisoning; oestrogens (OCP, pregnancy), vitamin A excess
- Vitamin B12 deficiency

Y:
- h**Y**pertension, idiopathic intracranial (assoc. obesity)
- h**Y**ponatraemia (esp. rapid), h**Y**pocalcaemia (esp. hereditary)

Pseudopapilloedema

Hypermetropes
Drusen on disc
Medullated nerve fibres

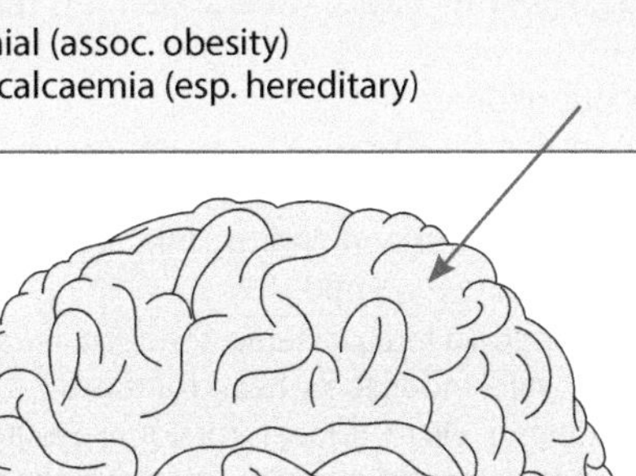

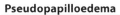

Papillitis

V.I.S.I.O.N.

Vascular – 'AION' (anterior ischaemic optic neuropathy)
- Thromboembolic
- Vasculitis: giant-cell arteritis

Inflammatory: 'Optic neuritis': multiple sclerosis/ADEM
Sarcoid/CRION
Infection
- Virus, TB, syphilis
- Sinus infection – contiguous

Other: Guillain-Barré syndrome, due to high CSF protein
Neoplasia: Lymphoma, leukaemia

Vascular

Arterial flow ↑
- Malignant hypertension
- CO_2 retention
- Haematological
  - Chronic anaemia (high-output state)
  - Polycythaemia
  - Coagulopathy, e.g. DIC

Venous flow ↓
- Venous occlusion
  - Central retinal vein occlusion
  - Cavernous sinus thrombosis, carotico-cavernous fistula
  - SVCO
- Compression of optic nerve
  - Optic glioma/meningioma
  - Orbital cellulitis
  - Thyroid eye disease

VERTIGO

Def

Illusory sensation of movement, especially rotation

Causes

Physiological e.g. post-rotation, caloric testing
Visual/somatosensory e.g. refractive error, extraocular muscle palsy, peripheral neuropathy
Vestibular

I².M. B.A.L.A.N.C².E².d.

Peripheral

Infection/**I**njury – labyrinthitis
PATH: Virus (associated with URTI), ischaemia (internal auditory artery), head injury
PC: Severe vertigo, N+V for days to weeks; deafness may also occur if cochlea involved

Ménière disease
PATH: Endolymphatic oedema
PC: Paroxysmal vertigo for 20 min–3 h, severe; associated N+V, aural fullness – may also present as paroxysmal drop attacks or ataxia with past-pointing
Low-frequency deafness and tinnitus: Initially paroxysmal, later continuous

Benign Paroxysmal Positional Vertigo (BPPV)
PATH: Utricle sheds otoconia into posterior semicircular canal; often follows labyrinthitis
PC: Vertigo for sec–min, induced by head rotation
O/E: Hallpike manoeuvre elicits upbeat–torsional nystagmus that exhibits:
Latency; adaptation; fatiguability; position-changing with return of position

Aminoglycosides (e.g. gentamicin)/furosemide

Lymph, peri-, fistula
PATH: Trauma, congenital deformity, or superior-canal dehiscence
PC: Paroxysmal vertigo, high-frequency deafness, esp. when lying on ear
O/E: Nystagmus evoked by loud sound (Tullio phenomenon) or pressure in external meatus

Arterial
Migraine, vertebrobasilar
PC: Headache, N+V may accompany, or occur at other times; focal numbness; dysarthria
Posterior circulation TIA/stroke (e.g.in arteriopathy, atrial fibrillation)
PC: Attacks usually shorter than migraine

Nerve, vestibulocochlear lesion
PATH: Acoustic neuroma, meningitis, sarcoidosis, base of skull fracture

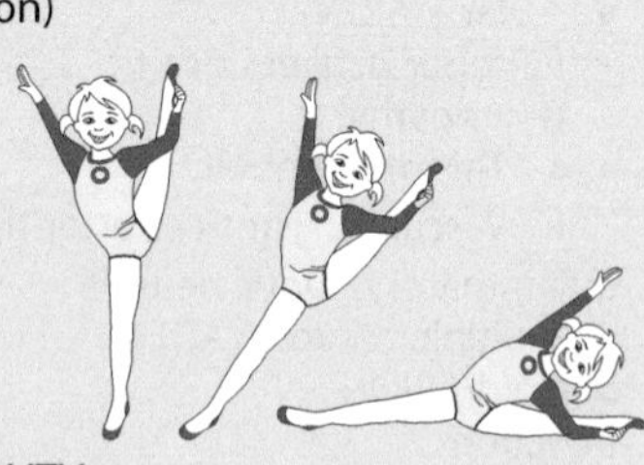

Central

Central lesions – brainstem, cervico-medullary lesion
PATH: Stroke, demyelination (multiple sclerosis, ADEM), tumour, VZV

Channelopathy (episodic ataxia)

Excitement: Anxiety, panic attacks, psychogenic
PPPD – persistent postural-perceptual dizziness: chronic sense of motion or imbalance triggered by prior episode or peripheral vertigo, or primary psychogenic

Epilepsy, complex partial

DEAFNESS

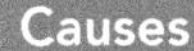

Causes

Conductive

W.I.D.E.N.In.G.

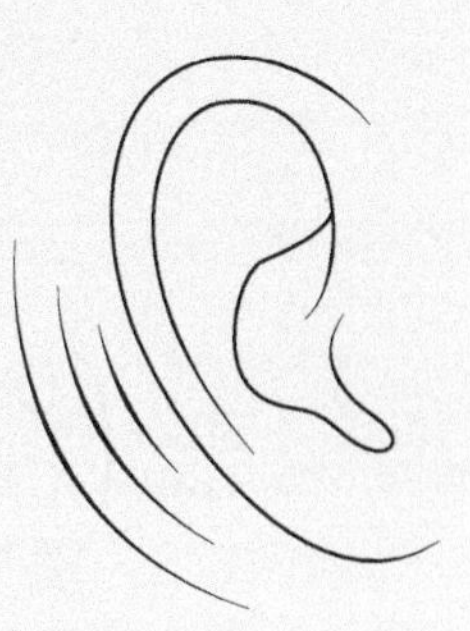

Wax in external auditory meatus
Infection – otitis media
PATH:
- Acute: *Streptococcus pyogenes, Haemophilus influenzae*
- Chronic ('glue ear'): Assoc. large adenoids, cleft palate, Down syn., TB

O/E: Effusion on otoscopy
Drum perforation: Noise injury; barotrauma (e.g. pilots, divers)
Extra: Ossicle discontinuity – otosclerosis, trauma (NB: Normal otoscopy)
Neoplasia: Glomus jugulare, carcinoma
Injury
Granulomatous: Granulomatosis with polyangiitis/sarcoid

Sensorineural

D².I.V.I.N.I.T.Y².

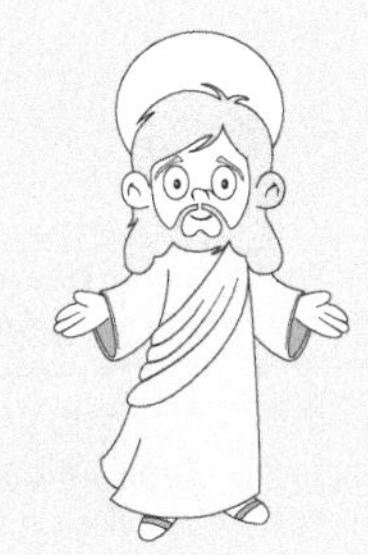

Developmental/**D**egenerative
Developmental:
Genetic: Connexin mutation, Refsum disease, Waardenburg syndrome
Congenital: TORCH infections, esp. syphilis (late-onset), rubella
Perinatal: Anoxia (cerebral palsy)
Degenerative: Presbyacusis – high-tone deafness
Infection
VZV (O/E: Vesicles on eardrum!), measles, mumps, influenza
Meningitis: *Haemophilus influenzae*
Vascular
Ischaemia: Internal auditory artery 'AICA' – sudden hearing loss and vertigo
Haemorrhage: Superficial siderosis (slow haemorrhage following old brain op.)
Inflammation: Vasculitis, sarcoid
Neoplasia
Cerebellopontine angle tumour, e.g. acoustic neuroma – commonest cause of unilateral sensorineural deafness
Meningeal carcinoma, leukaemia, melanoma
Injury
Noise: 4 kHz notch in audiogram, later high-frequency
Trauma: Including trivial head injury
Toxins: Gentamicin, furosemide, quinine, aspirin
Y: l**Y**mph
Endol**Y**mph h**Y**drops = Ménière disease – low-tone deafness
Peril**Y**mph fistula (ruptured oval or round window)

FACIAL NERVE PALSY

Anatomy

The facial nerve (cranial nerve VII) has a long course, with branches at different points

The location of the lesion can be ascertained by testing the several functions that it serves, as well as by testing functions of adjacent structures

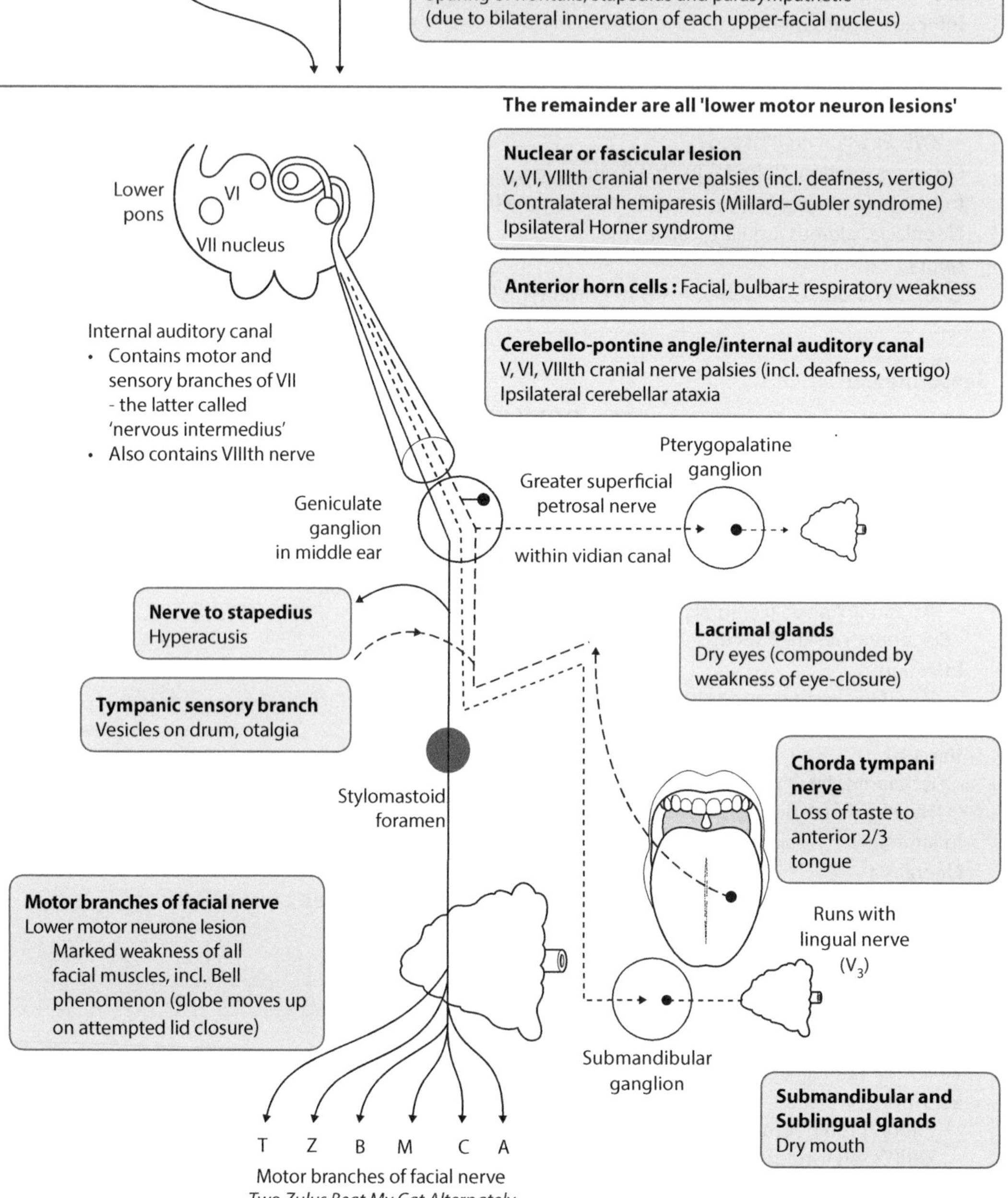

Motor branches of facial nerve
Two Zulus Beat My Cat Alternately

Causes

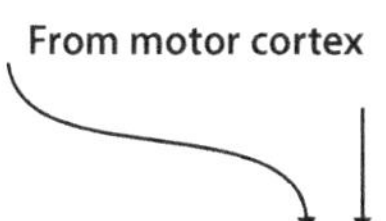

Upper motor neurone lesion
Cerebral infarct or tumour, multiple sclerosis

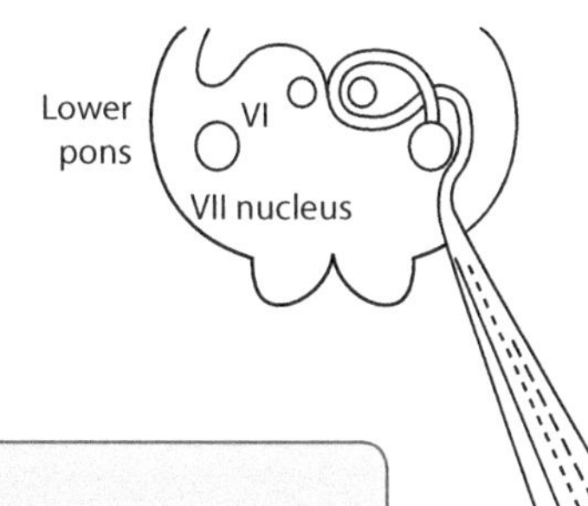

Nuclear or fascicular lesion
Developmental: Möbius syndrome, syringobulbia
Vascular: Pontine infarct, basilar artery aneurysm
Inflammatory: Multiple sclerosis, sarcoid, vasculitis

Anterior horn cells: Motor neurone disease, polio, tetanus

Cerebello-pontine angle/internal auditory canal
Structural:
- Tumour: Acoustic neuroma, meningioma, met.
- Trauma: Basal fracture

Meningeal: Carcinoma, lymphoma, sarcoid, TB

Middle ear
Infection:
- HSV-1: Commonest cause of 'idiopathic Bell's palsy'
- VZV (Ramsay-Hunt syn.): May cause cranial polyneuritis or CNS vasculitis
- Acute otitis media

Neoplasia: Glomus jugulare, cholesteatoma
Injury: Petrous fracture

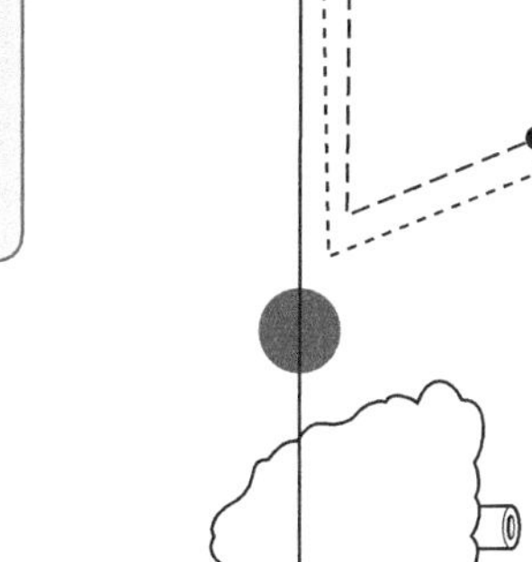

Idiopathic Bell's palsy

Path
HSV-1

PC
Onset at night, worst at 2 days
Retroauricular pain, facial numbness
Recovery-phase: Aberrant reinnervation causes synkinesia (hemifacial spasm), crocodile tears

Rx
Prednisolone 60–80 mg od for 1 week, starting within 3 days
Famciclovir 750 mg tds
Hypromellose eye drops
± surgical decompression if EMG shows >90% denervation within 1st week

Parotid/stylomastoid foramen
Neoplasia:
Injury: Trauma, surgery

Peripheral neuropathy
Demyelinating: Guillain-Barré syndrome
Axonal:
- Diabetes mellitus
- Lyme disease, leprosy, HIV, EBV
- Sarcoid (uveoparotid fever)
- Hereditary: Melkersson syn. (recurrent facial oedema, furrowed tongue)

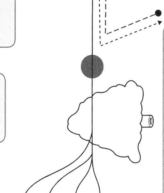

NMJ/muscle
Myasthenia gravis/botulism
Myopathy: Dystrophy, myesitis

NEUROFIBROMATOSIS

Type 1

Epi

Prevalence = 1/3000 (30% sporadic mutations)
Gene: Chromosome 17
Autosomal dominant tumour suppressor gene (as for all neurocutaneous syndromes)
Neurofibromin gene normally inhibits Ras-GTPase mitogenic signalling

PC

C.A.F.É. N.O.I.R^2.

Café-au-lait spots: >5 spots of >1.5 cm diameter (or >5 mm, prepuberty)
Axillary freckling, also inguinal
Fibromas, neuro-:
Subcutaneous: Soft, firm, lobulated, mobile at right-angles to nerve only
Plexiform: Overgrowth of nerve trunk and overlying tissues, esp. temporal scalp
PC: Cutaneous masses
Compression:
- Spine/nerve roots: Myelopathy, radicular pain, muscle atrophy
- Cranial nerves: Trigeminal neuralgia, cerebellopontine angle tumour
- GIT: Bowel obstruction, bleeding

Sarcomatous transformation in 10%
Eye Lisch nodules (iris hamartomas); retinal astrocytoma; optic nerve glioma

Neoplasia
CNS: Meningioma, ependymoma, astrocytoma; complicating obstructive hydrocephalus
Chronic or acute myeloid leukaemia
MEN2b syndrome = medullary carcinoma, thyroid, phaeochromocytoma, marfanoid
Orthopaedic
Spine – canal stenosis, spina bifida, kyphoscoliosis, short stature
Sphenoid dysplasia
IQ ↓/epilepsy
Renal: Wilms tumour, renal artery stenosis/**R**espiratory: pulmonary fibrosis, pneumothorax

Type 2

Epi

Prevalence = 1/50,000
Gene: Chromosome 22 (MERLIN gene = cytoskeletal proteins: Moesin, Ezrin, Radizin)

PC

Think of diseases in **2**s

Bilateral acoustic neuromas; also meningiomas, ependymomas
Bilateral posterior subcapsular cataracts (café-au-lait spots and peripheral neurofibromas occur rarely)

NEUROCUTANEOUS DISEASES – OTHER

S.O.N.S. *of neurofibromatosis*

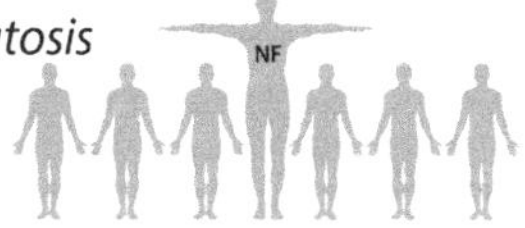

Tuberous sclerosis

Epi Gene: Chromosome 11 (80% sporadic mutations); autosomal dominant

PC

Skin
- Adenoma sebaceum (angiofibromata): Papular rash around nose, worsens after puberty
- Shagreen patch (lumpy plaque), ash leaf macule (depigmentation seen with Wood lamp)
- Periungual or intraoral fibromas

Ocular: Retinal phakomas (50%; appear yellow), retinal pigmentation, optic disc drusen

Neurology
- Epilepsy (75%); IQ ↓ (50%)
- Brain tumours: Subependymal tubers (hamartomas), lateral ventricle gliomas

Systemic
- Renal: Adult polycystic kidney disease, angiomyolipomata (66%; cause loin pain, haematuria)
- Respiratory: Pulmonary cysts, pneumothorax, pulmonary fibrosis
- Cardiac: Rhabdomyosarcomas that cause arrhythmias and CCF

Sturge–Weber syndrome

PC

Skin
- Port-wine stain (capillary haemangioma) on face – although most port-wine stains are not associated with the syndrome
- Associated with ipsilateral intracranial calcified haemangioma whose location depends on dermatome involved by stain: Vi – occipital; Vii – frontal or parietal

Ocular: Strabismus, congenital glaucoma (appears as buphthalmos or 'ox-eye'), optic atrophy

Neurology
- Epilepsy (due to 'tramline' calcification of cortical vessels); IQ ↓
- Infantile hemiplegia–hemiatrophy

Von Hippel–Lindau disease

Epi Gene: VHL tumour suppressor gene (chromosome 3)

PC

Skin: Polycythaemia, secondary to renal cysts or cerebellar haemangioblastoma

Ocular: Retinal angioma

Neurology: Cerebellar or spinal cord haemangioma (-blastoma)

Systemic
- Polycystic kidney disease, renal cell carcinoma
- Adrenal phaeochromocytoma
- Other: Epididymis, liver, pancreas cysts

Endocrinology

DIABETES MELLITUS – CAUSES

P.E.P.S.I. & C.O.K.E. – *make sure it's diet!*

Primary

Type 1: Autoimmune destruction of β-cells of pancreatic islets of Langerhans; always leads to insulin dependency.

Epi: **I**nc: Prevalence = 1–2% population, and rising

Age: Children to 30 y

Aet: Genetic: DR3, 4 increases risk, but MZ concordance = 50%

Infection: CMV, EBV, Coxsackie, congenital rubella (seasonal onset of diabetes)

PATH: Anti-islet-cell Abs (esp. glutamic acid dehydrogenase) and/or anti-insulin Abs

Type 2: Peripheral insulin resistance ± insulin ↓ ± hepatic glucose efflux ↑

Epi: **I**nc: Prevalence = 5%

Age: Increases with age, but inherited types occur in children

Geo: Indian, African

Aet: Genetic: MZ concordance = 90%

Syndrome X = DM + central obesity + ↑ABP + ↑lipids, due to ↑ liver fat synthesis

Amylin deposition in islets (= hypoglycaemic hormone secreted by islet cells)

Hereditary: Insulin hyposecretion: MODY (maturity-onset diabetes of young) – like type 2 DM

Aet: Glucokinase deficiency (rare)

Insulin resistance: Donohue syndrome; lipodystrophy

Endocrine

Stress hormone excess: *in temporal order of release:*

Adrenaline → glucagon → glucocorticoid → growth Hormone → T4

(phaeochromocytoma) (glucagonoma) (Cushing) (acromegaly) (thyrotoxicosis)

Stress response: Sepsis, surgery, trauma → hypercortisolaemia → insulin resistance

Oestrogen: Gestational diabetes; polycystic ovaries syn.; oral contraceptive pill

Pancreatic disease: Chronic pancreatitis, (alcohol, cystic fibrosis, malnutrition); haemochromatosis; pancreas ca. (late)

Steroids

Inherited:

Neurological: Myotonic dystrophy; Friedreich ataxia; ataxia telangiectasia; Huntington chorea

Glycogen storage disease

Other: Lawrence–Moon–Biedl syn; DIDMOAD (**D**iabetes **I**nsipidus, **DM**, **O**ptic **A**trophy, **D**eafness) syn.

Chromosomal: Down, Turner, Kleinfelter syndrome

Organ failure: Liver/congestive cardiac failure

Kidney failure: Due to insulin resistance; insulin hyposecretion; peritoneal dialysis (glucose in dialysate)

Exogenous: Diuretics (thiazides, loop), adrenergic stimulants (salbutamol, amphetamines), pancreatic toxins (pentamidine), chemo Rx (e.g. alloxan)

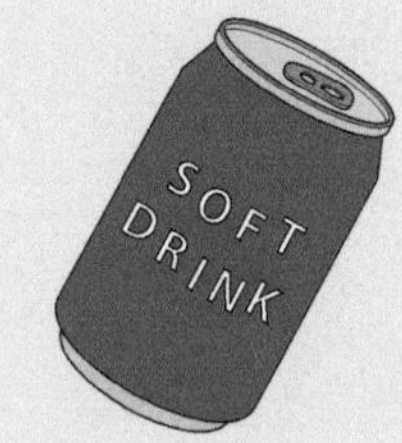

INSULIN – PHYSIOLOGY

The causes, complications and treatment of diabetes are most easily understood by appreciating the normal regulation and actions of insulin:

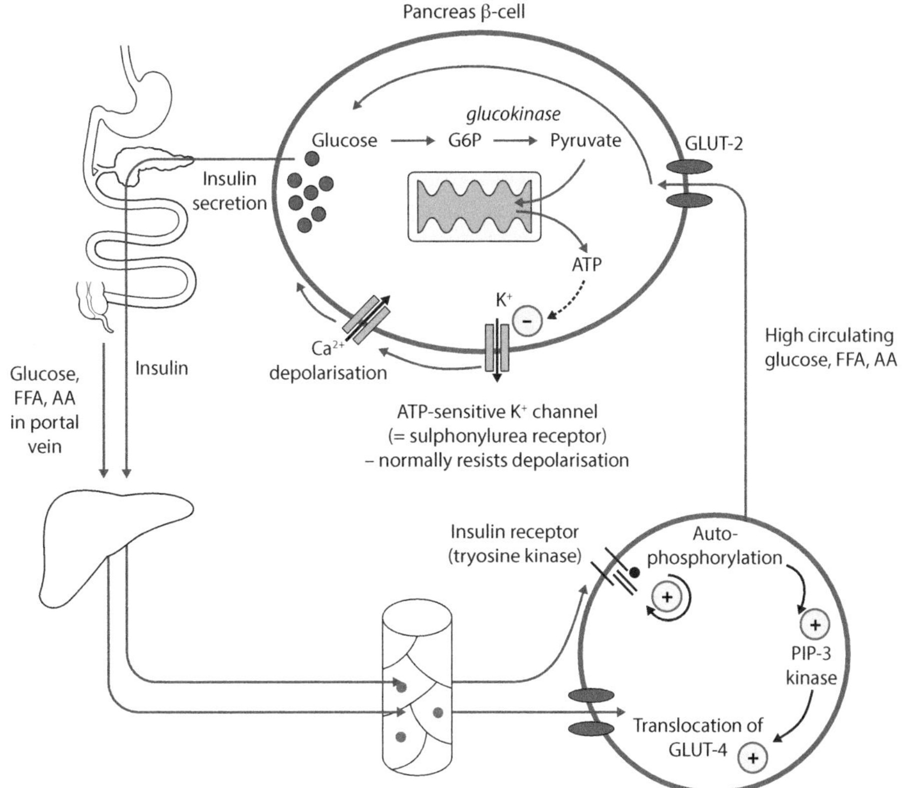

Liver	Endothelium	Periphery
Glycogen synthesis ↑ Gluconeogenesis ↓ ⊕ glucokinase ⊕ glycogen synthase ⊕ phosphofructokinase		Glucose uptake ↑
FFA and TAG synthesis ↑ VLDL release ↑ ⊕ pyruvate dehydrogenase	VLDL, chylomicrons processing ↑ → FFA +m DAG update ↑ ⊕ lipoprotein lipase	FFA and TAG synthesis ↑ ⊕ pyruvate dehydrogenase ⊖ lipase, via PKA
Protein synthesis ↑ ⊕ AA uptake, Kreb cycle		Protein synthesis and growth ↑ ⊕ AA uptake, translation

Key: ⊕ insulin activates; ⊖ insulin inhibits; AA, amino acids; ATP, adenosine triphosphate; DAG, diacylglyceride; FFA, free fatty acids; G6P, glucose-6-phosphate; GLUT, glucose transporter; PIP, phosphatidylinositol phosphate; PKA; protein kinase A; TAG, triacylglyceride; VLDL, very-low density lipoprotein

DIABETIC KETOACIDOSIS

PATH

Combination of **insulin deficiency** (e.g. first presentation, forgot insulin, inadequate dosage) and **sympathetic stimulation** (e.g. sepsis, MI, volume depleted, cocaine), results in:

- Glucose uptake ↓ and glucose release ↑ → hyperglycaemia
- Osmotic diuresis → hypovolaemia → tissue ischaemia and renal failure → lactic acidosis
- Compensation for lack of intracellular glucose by lipolysis (with resultant ketosis) and proteolysis (with resultant amino-acid release) → metabolic acidosis

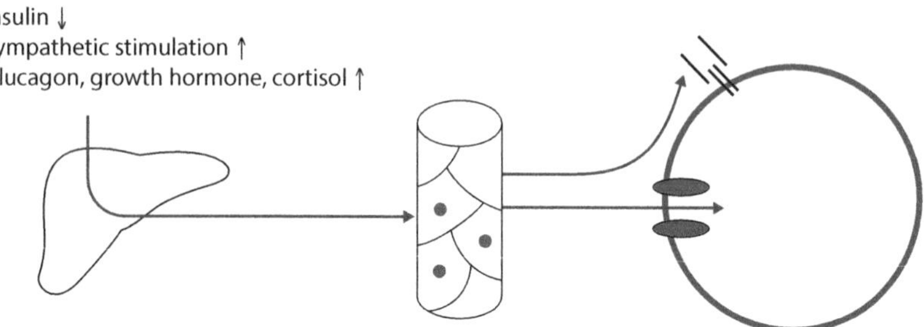

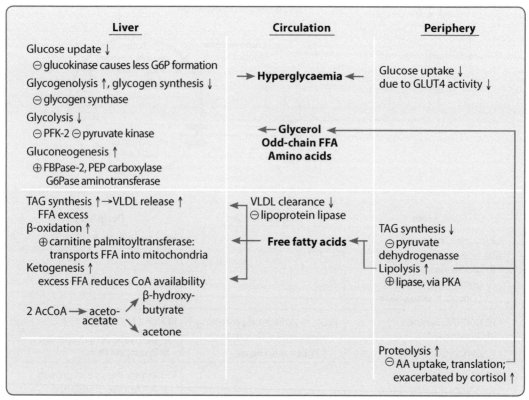

Liver	**Circulation**	**Periphery**
Glucose update ↓ ⊖ glucokinase causes less G6P formation Glycogenolysis ↑, glycogen synthesis ↓ ⊖ glycogen synthase Glycolysis ↓ ⊖ PFK-2 ⊖ pyruvate kinase Gluconeogenesis ↑ ⊕ FBPase-2, PEP carboxylase G6Pase aminotransferase	→ **Hyperglycaemia** ← ← **Glycerol** **Odd-chain FFA** **Amino acids**	Glucose uptake ↓ due to GLUT4 activity ↓
TAG synthesis ↑→VLDL release ↑ FFA excess β-oxidation ↑ ⊕ carnitine palmitoyltransferase: transports FFA into mitochondria Ketogenesis ↑ excess FFA reduces CoA availability 2 AcCoA → aceto-acetate ↗ β-hydroxy-butyrate ↘ acetone	← VLDL clearance ↓ ⊖ lipoprotein lipase ← **Free fatty acids** ←	TAG synthesis ↓ ⊖ pyruvate dehydrogenasse Lipolysis ↑ ⊕ lipase, via PKA
		Proteolysis ↑ ⊖ AA uptake, translation; exacerbated by cortisol ↑

Key: ⊕ activation; ⊖ inhibition; AA, amino acids; AcCoA, acetyl coenzyme A; FBPase, fructose-1, 2-biphosphatase; FFA, free fatty acids; G6P, glucose-6-phosphate; GLUT, glucose transporter; PEP, phosphoenolpyruvate; PFK, phosphofructokinase; PKA, protein kinase A; TAG, triacylglyceride; VLDL, very-low density lipoprotein

PC

D^2.K^3.A.

Diuresis, osmotic/**D**ehydration
- PC: Polyuria, polydipsia, blurred vision (refractive error due to hyperglycaemic osmotic shift)
- O/E: Fast, thready pulse; hypotensive; collapsed veins; dry skin, tongue; skin turgor ↓; temp. ↓
- Comp: Cerebral oedema (confusion, coma); acute renal failure; deep-vein thrombosis

Kussmaul breathing (deep sighs; also air hunger)/**K**etotic breath

K$^+$: Initially hyperkalaemic but becomes hypokalaemic with insulin Rx; risk of cardiac arrest

Abdominal
- Abdominal pain ('acute abdomen') – consider acute pancreatitis due to hyperlipidaemia
- N+V – consider acute gastric dilatation, but appetite ↑ (due to hypothalamic uptake ↓)

Ix

Bloods:
- U&E:
  - Urea: ↑↑ due to dehydration, proteolysis; creatinine ↑ (incl. false +ve due to ketone bodies)
  - Na^+: ↓ (peripheral osmotic activity, and hyperlipidaemia causing pseudohyponatraemia)
  - K^+: initially ↑ → ↓ with insulin Rx; HCO_3^- ↓ (weakness; SOB), and Cl^- ↑: both occur on Rx anion gap ($Na^+ + K^+$) – ($Cl^- + HCO_3^-$) >18 mmol/l, due to ketone bodies, lactate
- ABGs: Metabolic acidosis: PO_4 <24 mmol/l, base excess >2 mmol/l
- Glucose: Typically 15–33 mmol/l; triglycerides ↑ (VLDL or chylomicrons)
- Ketone bodies; ratio of β-hydroxybutyrate: acetoacetate ↑ with hypoxia, due to shock
- FBC: Neutrophilia (leukaemoid reaction); AST ↑ due to shock

Urine
- Glucose + + +
- Ketones +, but may be falsely negative if shocked or hypoxic, due to high BHB:AcAc ratio.

Micro: MSU, blood cultures

Monitor 2-hourly blood glucose, K^+

ECG: Myocardial infarction (cause or effect); effects of hyper- or hypokalaemia

Radiol: CXR – infection; PAXR – gastric dilatation; ground-glass appearance

Rx

Ventilatory support
- O_2
- Ventilation, if persistent acidosis

ITU:
- $NaHCO_3$: If pH <7.1, and SBP <90 mmHg
- Dexamethasone: If cerebral oedema

Assessment — **C.O.A.T.I.N'**
- **C**ardiac monitor
- **O**$_2$
- **A**BP
- **T**PR → space blanket?
- **I**nput + output chart (incl. nasogastric tube, urine catheter)
- **N**eurological observations

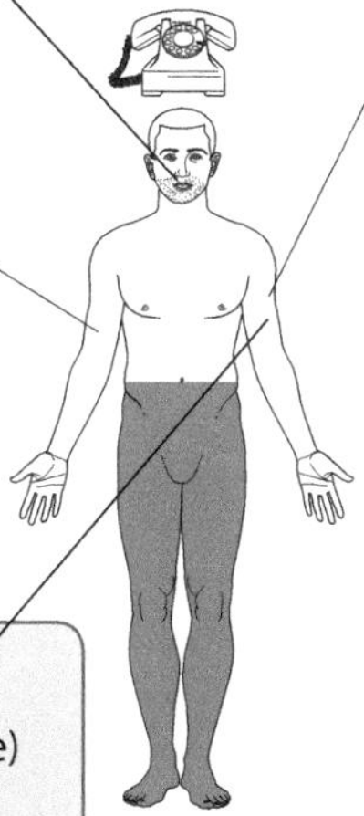

Hydration

Type:
- Colloid 500 ml: If SBP <90 mmHg
- N. saline: 2 l in 2 h° → 2 l in 4 h° → 4 l in 24 h°
- 5% dextrose when glucose <15 mmol/l
- 10% dextrose if persisting acidosis and ketosis

KCL
- Add 20 mmol to each litre after 1st litre
- Titrate: [K^+] of 3 mmol/l = 300 mmol deficit
- Caution if oliguric

Phosphate: IV or PO as K^+ or Na^+ acid salt

Medication

IV soluble insulin (50 units in 50 ml N. saline)
- 10 units stat → 6–10 units/h
- Sliding scale (e.g. 3 units/h, while BM >15)

Treat precipitant, e.g. antibiotics, thrombolysis
LMW heparin

DIABETES – HHS

Def

Hyperosmolar hyperglycaemic state

PATH

Sustained, **partial** insulin deficiency, leads to hyperglycaemia (via ↓ glucose uptake and glucose release), but **not** β-oxidation of lipids or ketogenesis. Consequently, **acidosis does not occur initially**, and the condition presents later than DKA with very high glucose levels and extreme dehydration

Predisposing: Type 2 or type 1 with inadequate insulin dose, plus supervening stress, e.g. sepsis, myocardial infarction, stroke, or initiation of diabetogenic drug (e.g. steroid, thiazide)

PC

HHS presents similarly to DKA, except for the following features:

H.H.S

Hyperosmolar
Hyperglycaemia

Both are more extreme than in DKA

PC:

- Polyuria, polydipsia
- Fatigue
- Blurred vision (refractive error due to hyperglycaemic osmotic shift)

O/E: Fast, thready pulse; hypotensive; collapsed veins; dry skin, tongue; skin turgor↓

Comp: Cerebral oedema (confusion, coma); acute renal failure; deep-vein thrombosis

Ix: Typical values:

- Osmolality, serum >350 mOsm/kg
- Na^+ >150 mmol/l
- Glucose >35 mmol/l

Sticky blood – thrombosis occurs due to hyperviscous blood

Rx

HHS is treated similarly to DKA, except for:

- Fluid: Hyperosmolarity and hyperglycaemia usually respond to fluid infusions alone
- Insulin: Only indicated if fluid fails to correct hyperglycaemia or if ketones present
- Potassium replacement

DIABETES – LACTIC ACIDOSIS

PATH

Lactic acidosis is more likely to occur in diabetics, due to:

Inhibition of gluconeogenesis:

- Metformin therapy (type 2 DM) causes type B lactic acidosis
- Liver or renal failure

Hypoxia secondary to pneumonia or CCF
Shock, e.g. pancreatitis

PC

Hyperventilation
Fatigue, confusion, coma

Ix

Bloods: Lactate >2 mmol/l (also apparent as a wide anion gap, where anion gap = $(Na^+ + K^+) - (Cl^- + HCO_3^-) > 18$ mmol/l)
ABGs: Metabolic acidosis
Renal: May demonstrate renal impairment as a cause of lactic acidosis
Glucose: Normal – slightly elevated
Urine: Ketone –ve
Micro: Blood, urine, CSF cultures
ECG
Radiol: CXR – pneumonia

Rx

Underlying cause
O_2 (± ventilation)
IV $NaHCO_3^-$ ☠ = paradoxical intracellular acidosis!
Haemodialysis, to clear lactic acid, and to clear sodium when $NaHCO_3$ given

DIABETES MELLITUS – CHRONIC COMPLICATIONS

PC

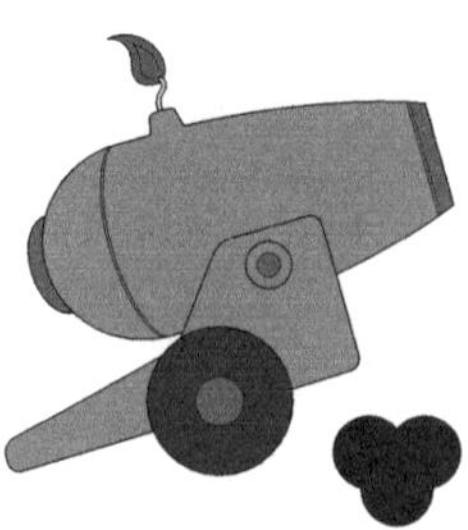

Macrovascular

C.A.N.N.O.N.I.C.A.L².

Cardiology – ischaemic heart disease
PC: Myocardial infarction/acute coronary syndromes:
- Classically 'silent' due to coexisting autonomic neuropathy
- More often complicated by cardiac failure and shock

Rx involves intensive insulin regime, usually with IV 'sliding scale'
Cardiomyopathy – left-ventricular failure in presence of normal CXR and angiogram
Arterial insufficiency – peripheral vascular disease
PC: Intermittent claudication → rest pain, due to tibial or iliofemoral artery insufficiency
Ulcer, gangrene (*see opposite*)
Neurological – large-vessel or lacunar stroke/TIA

Microvascular

Neurological – peripheral and autonomic neuropathy
Peripheral:
- 'Glove and stocking' sensory neuropathy; amyotrophy (painful, wasted quadriceps); cranial neuropathies
- Mononeuritis multiplex
- Entrapment (carpal tunnel or ulnar neuropathies); ulcers (see opposite)

Autonomic: Impotence, frequency, gustatory sweating, gastroparesis, postural hypotension
Ophthalmopathy: Lens/glaucoma/retinopathy (*see opposite*)
Nephropathy, incl. **N**ephrotic syndrome
Microalbuminuria (albumin excretion rate: 30–300 mg/day) → nephrotic syn. (>3 g/day)
Chronic renal failure
Renal tubular acidosis type 4: Hyporeninaemic hypoaldosteronism
Immunocompromise
Bacteria: Boils, UTI, pneumonia, osteomyelitis
Other: Candida (pruritus vulvae, balanitis), mucormycosis (proptosis), TB
Cutaneous
Pigmentation: Acanthosis nigricans, diabetic dermopathy (pigmented scars on shins)
Necrobiosisis lipoidica diabeticorum (erythematous plaque, sunken, yellow atrophic skin)
Other: Vitiligo (association with type 1 DM), scleroderma-like skin, granuloma annulare
Arthritis
Cheirarthropathy – limited joint mobility and contractures; 'prayer sign': can't appose palms
Pseudogout
Charcot joints (neuropathic)
Lethargy/**L**oss of weight

Foot ulcers

May be due either to arterial insufficiency or to neuropathy

Ischaemic ulcer

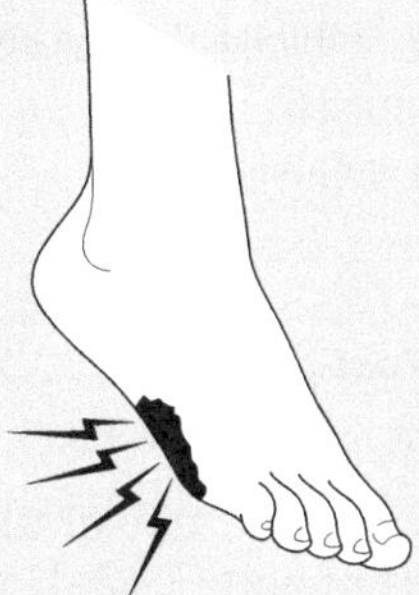

PC:
- Painful ulcer (sensation preserved)
- Colour: white on lying — red on standing

O/E:
- Site: Foot margin
- Edge: ragged
- Skin:
  - Pale, cold, thin, hairless
  - Absent-weak pulses; bruits

Associations: Infection – pus, crepitus, foul odour (also with neuropathic ulcer)

Neuropathic ulcer

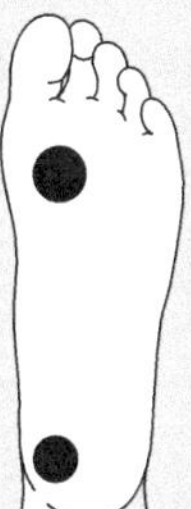

PC: Painless and numb – pt. ignores repetitive trauma

O/E:
- Site: Metatarsal heads, calcaneum
- Edges: Cleanly punched-out ulcer
- Skin:
  - Surrounding callus
  - Dry, fissured skin (sweat loss)
  - Warm, erythema, oedema, distended veins (sympathetic loss)

Associations
- Pes cavus, claw toes, Charcot joints
- Lisfranc deformity: Neuropathic subluxation of tarsal and metatarsals → convex sole

Ophthalmopathy (50%)

Lens:
- Acute blurred vision, due to osmotic-induced swelling of the lens (DKA)
- Cataracts: Senile or juvenile 'snowflake'

Glaucoma – open-angle, or closed-angle due to rubeosis iridis
Retinopathy:

Background	Pre-proliferative	Pro-liferative
Fluorescein angiogram: Leakiness ↑ Haemorrhages: • Dot = microaneurysm • Blot = deep retina • Flame = superficial Hard exudates: Lipoprotein precipitates	Cotton-wool spots: Retinal infarction Venule dilatation; looping; beading Intraretinal microvascular abnormalities (IRMA) Avascular; featureless periphery	New vessels leashes and fronds on disc or vein bifurcations Haemorrhages: Vitreous; pre-retinal Rubeosis iridis: Anterior extension of angiogenesis Advanced: Retinal fibrosis and tear

± Maculopathy: May occur at any stage, due to hard exudates; oedema; ischaemia involving fovea
± Other: Retinal vein or artery thrombosis; ischaemic papillitis; lipaemia retinalis (if chylomicrons ↑)

DIABETES MELLITUS – DIAGNOSIS

Plasma glucose

Method:

- Capillary blood glucose or venous sample (use fluoride oxalate tube – inhibits RBC glycolysis)
- Two samples, on different occasions required (unless plainly symptomatic)
- Post-prandial glucose should not be taken <2 h, due to normal high variability

Fasting (8 h)		**Post-prandial** (2 h post 75 g glucose load)	
Normal	<6 mmol/l	Normal	<7.8 mmol/l
Impaired fasting glycaemia	6–7 mmol/l	Impaired glucose tolerance	7.8–11 mmol/l
Diabetes mellitus	>7 mmol/l	Diabetes mellitus	>11 mmol/l

Urinalysis

Method: Glucose oxidase or reducing-substance reagent
Sensitivity = 30%
False –ve: Elderly, due to higher renal threshold;
(normal threshold for glycosuria >7–13 mmol/l blood glucose)
Specificity = 99%
False +ve:

- Glomerular filtration ↑, e.g. pregnancy
- Tubular resorption ↓, e.g. renal tubular acidosis
- Reducing substances (only, if using reducing-substance reagent), e.g.:
    - Drugs, incl. salicylates, isoniazid, L-DOPA, tetracycline, vitamin C
    - Galactosaemia, fructosaemia, homogentisic acid (alkaptonuria)

Oral glucose tolerance test (OGTT)

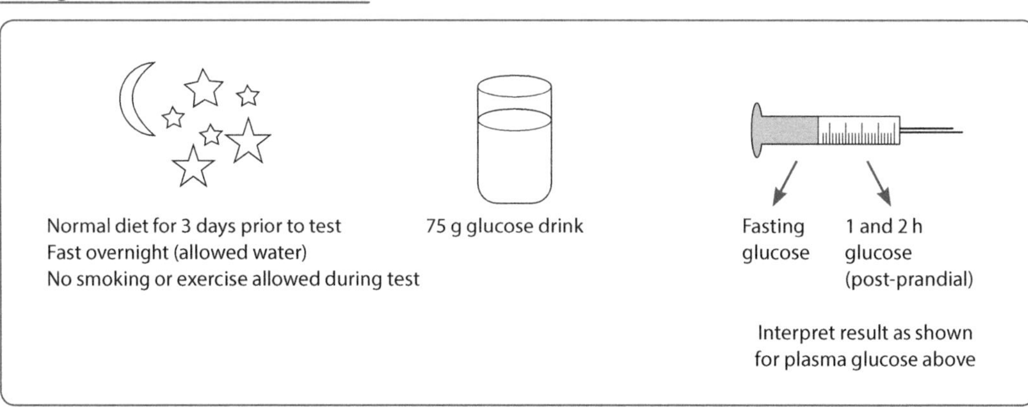
Normal diet for 3 days prior to test
Fast overnight (allowed water)
No smoking or exercise allowed during test
75 g glucose drink
Fasting glucose
1 and 2 h glucose (post-prandial)
Interpret result as shown for plasma glucose above

DIABETES MELLITUS – MONITORING

The **5 Cs**

Control, glycaemic

Record of acute complications: DKA, hypoglycaemic episodes

Self-monitoring:

- Urine dipstick:
  - Indications:
    - Children during infection (ketone sticks), or unwilling to prick finger
    - Elderly or type 2 DM: Tight glycaemic control unnecessary (but higher renal threshold)
  - ☠ Can't detect hypoglycaemia, and reflects mean glycaemia since bladder last emptied
- Capillary-blood glucose ('BM stick'):
  - Mechanism: Glucose oxidase reagent + glucose → hydrogen peroxide → redox potential change
  - Target: Aim for 4.4–6.7 mmol/l (fasting) or 4.4–9 mmol/l (2-hour post-prandial)

Fasting (8 h)		**Post-prandial** (2-h post 75 g glucose load)	
Desirable	4.5–7.0 mmol/l	Desirable	4.5–9.0 mmol/l
Acceptable	<7.8 mmol/l	Acceptable	<10.0 mmol/l

Adjust insulin dose only after several days of abnormal pattern; do not adjust with every measurement (i.e. the 'sliding-scale approach')

- Glycated haemoglobin (HbA1c):
  - Mechanism:
    - HbA-valine + glucose → irreversible non-enzymatic glycation → HbA1
    - Electrophoresis separates HbA1 into more stable component HbA1c
  - Indication: Reflects total glucose exposure over previous 6–8 weeks (RBC half-life):
    - Detects poor compliance with Rx
    - Prognostic indicator for retinopathy
  - Target:
    - Normal 31–64 mmol/mol
    - Acceptable 64–76 mmol/mol

False –ve: Haemolysis: ↑ RBC turnover

False +ve: Abnormally migrating Hb variants

Complications

Peripheral pulses, ABP, cardiac and carotid auscultation

Retinal screening, sensory testing; feet inspection (incl. nails)

Urine albumin:creatinine ratio; U&Es

Competency with insulin administration, 'CBG' monitoring; check insulin injection sites

Career/**C**ontraception etc: Psychosocial, domestic, occupation

DIABETES – CONSERVATIVE RX

D.E.L.A.Y.S³. *complications!*

Diet

Carbohydrate counting, and altering insulin doses accordingly with meals

Low-fat

- High polyunsaturates, e.g. vegetable oil; low eggs; milk-cheese; fried food
- Drugs: Orlistat (gut lipase inhibition), sibutramine (SNRI)
- Surgery: Gastric banding, gastric bypass (roux-en-Y) – ↓ mortality in type 2 patients with body mass index >40 kg/m^2

High-fibre: High-soluble fibre ↓ glucose absorption from gut → overcomes requirement for phase 1 insulin release in type 2 diabetes

Exercise improves glycaemic control; ↓ CVS complications, ↓ weight

Lipids:

Monitor LDL:HDL cholesterol ratio and fasting triglycerides

Start statin in type 1 diabetes if patient:

- Is >45 y
- Has had diabetes for >10 y
- Has established nephropathy

Start statin in type 2 diabetes if patient:

- Has >10% 10-year risk of cardiovascular disease (using QRISK2 assessment tool)
- Has established nephropathy

ABP ↑ (hypertension):

Reduce salt intake, alcohol

Drugs:

- ACE inhibitors or A-II antagonists are best due to their reno-protective effects
- β-blockers discouraged as they mask hypoglycaemia
- Thiazides: Cause hyperglycaemia

Yearly check-up

Ophthalmological assessment: Snellen chart, dilated fundoscopy

Renal function: Albumin:creatinine ratio or 24-hour urine albumin

Smoking, **S**pirits and **S**ex

Smoking: Increases risk of all complications

Spirits (alcohol): Avoid alcohol binges (hypoglycaemia) or heavy consumption (hidden calories, hypertension)

Sex:

- Contraception: Use progestogen-only pill, as oestrogen ↑ glucose
- Pregnancy: Will need more intensive monitoring

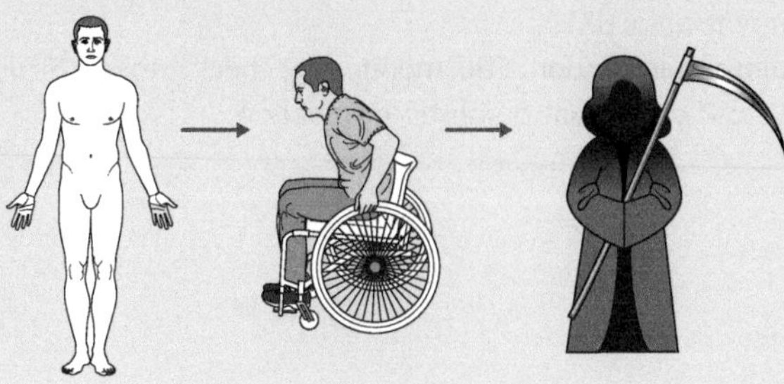

DIABETES – RX OF COMPLICATIONS

Macrovascular

Relationship with glycaemia occurs at *low* HbA1c (so difficult to reduce risk with glucose control)
Cardiac: Ischaemic heart disease – aspirin, anti-anginals, angioplasty, CABG
Arteriopathy: Peripheral vascular disease – aspirin, angioplasty, bypass
Neurological: Carotid disease – aspirin, endarterectomy

Microvascular

Relationship with glycaemia occurs at *high* HbA1c (glycaemic control improves outcome)
Neurological:

Peripheral neuropathy:

- Intensive insulin or continuous insulin infusion
- Duloxetine, amitriptyline or gabapentin for neuropathic pain
- Prosthetics, e.g. foot calipers

Autonomic, e.g. impotence: Sildenafil; intracavernosal or intra-urethral alprostadil (PGE_1); vacuum postural hypotension: increase salt and water intake – fludrocortisone

Ophthalmopathy:

Cataract replacement: ☠ = worsening maculopathy (so perform laser Rx beforehand)
Argon laser photocoagulation:

- Indication: Early proliferative changes; perimaculopathy – laser applied in 'macular grid'
- Mechanism:
  - Focal Rx: Reduces haemorrhage
  - Panretinal (1000–8000 burns): Reduces release of vascular endothelial growth factor → decreases blindness by 60% – ☠ = visual field loss

Vitrectomy: Indication: persistent vitreal haemorrhage, retinal detachment, severe proliferation

Nephropathy:

ACE inhibitors or A-II antagonists:

- Indication: Microalbuminuria
- Mechanism: Delays progression of nephropathy and treats hypertension
  ☠ = acute renal failure (if renal artery stenosis); hyperkalaemia (if hyporeninaemic hypoaldosteronism)

Protein restriction (< 50 g/day for 70 kg man) – reserved for established nephropathy

Feet

Hygiene: Wash, dry and use moisturising cream daily; correctly fitting shoes; avoid ingrowing nails; avoid bare feet; meticulously inspect, and refer early for corns, calluses, etc.
Ulcer care: Remove callus; swab; dressing; cast for pressure relief; antibiotics (e.g. co-amoxiclav, clindamycin)
Surgical: Debridement + lavage; osteotomy for neuropathy or osteomyelitis; arterial bypass; amputation

DIABETES MELLITUS – INSULIN

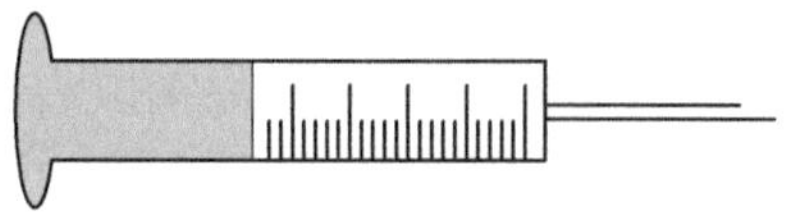

Types

Origin
- Porcine or bovine insulin has problem of antigenicity → allergy, resistance
- Recombinant human form has higher risk of hypoglycaemia, due to faster absorption and shorter effect

Preparation
- Soluble:
  - IV: Peak 5–10 min; duration 30 min – used in DKA, HHS, perioperative or in-patient fasting
  - SC: Peak 2 h; duration 6 h – used as maintenance therapy
- Suspension (S/C): complex of insulin with zinc crystals (lente) or protamine (isophane)
  - Onset 1–2 h; peak: 4–12 h; duration: <24 h
- Biphasic: Soluble + suspension, e.g. 30% soluble + 70% Humulin M3:
  - Pens allow easy delivery of combination
- Recombinant insulin analogue, e.g. insulin glargine or insulin detemir:
  - Allows once-daily delivery

Regimens

Initiation:

Type 1 DM: Start at presentation, e.g. DKA; but may need to ↓ dose or stop over weeks–months, due to 'honeymoon period' = temporary partial islet-cell recovery

Type 2 DM: Used if poor control in spite of oral hypoglycaemics; give metformin at same time (to ↓ weight)
- Benefits: Microvascular complications ↓ by 25%; post-MI mortality ↓ by 50% at 1-year

Maintenance:

'Split-mixed' programme: Morning + evening biphasic insulin doses, given half-hour before breakfast + supper:
- Only 2 injections per day so easier for elderly or patients with cognitive impairments
- Less effective glycaemic control overall

'Basal-bolus' programme: Bedtime long-acting + short-acting half-hour before every meal (adjust dose according to meal size):
- Multiple injections per day
- Allows excellent glycemic control and variation in bolus doses in accordance with carbohydrate counting

Temporary adjustments:

Illness: Fever, vomiting, perioperative, pregnancy:
- Dose must ↑ to counter sympathetic activation even if not eating, but check BMs 2–4-hourly
- Continuous infusion (SC or IV) may be required

Exercise:
- Decrease dose before and 24 h post-exercise; as blood flow ↑ and glucose utilisation
- Avoid injecting exercised limb: ↑ absorption; carry chocolate bar

Side-effects ☠

G.L.A.R.G.IN.E.

Glucose – low (hypoglycaemia): risk factors:
Elderly (can tolerate higher BMs because of less concern of chronic complications)
β-blockers (mask symptoms), alcohol binge
Local:
Lipohypertrophy (due to lipogenic and growth effect) – Rx: Rotate sites; lipoatrophy (allergy); bruising
Inadvertent IM injection, or limb injection (→ more rapid + unpredictable effect) – Rx: If IM then pinch skin
Atherogenesis – in high concentrations
Resistance, insulin >200 units/day:
Associations: Animal insulin (Ab formation), acanthosis nigricans, congenital receptor deficiency
Gain of weight in type 2 DM so give with metformin
INstability – 'dawn phenomenon' or 'Somogyi effect': Insulin given too early in evening → hypoglycaemia through night → rebound hyperglycaemia by morning due to sympathetic activation, and growth hormone, cortisol release
Electrolyte – hypokalaemia – in DKA Rx

DIABETES MELLITUS – ORAL HYPOGLYCAEMICS

Acarbose

Mechanism: Inhibits intestinal α-glucosidase, thereby decreasing starch and sucrose hydrolysis, and so decreasing absorption of glucose

☠ Diarrhoea, flatulence, abnormal LFTs

Sulphonylureas: Glibenclamide, gliclazide

Mechanism: Inhibits ATP-dep. K^+ channel in islet β-cell → ↑ basal secretion of insulin and ↑ phase 1, glucose-mediated stored-insulin secretion

Types:		Metabolism:
Long-acting	(48-h): chloRpropamide	Renal
Intermediate:	(24-h): glibenclamide, glimepRide	Renal
	(12-h): gLiquazone; gLiclazide; gLipizide	Liver
Short-acting	ToLbutamide	Liver

☠ Appetite ↑, weight gain; hypoglycaemia (if long-acting or organ failure); resistance (β-cell dysfunction, receptor downregulation)

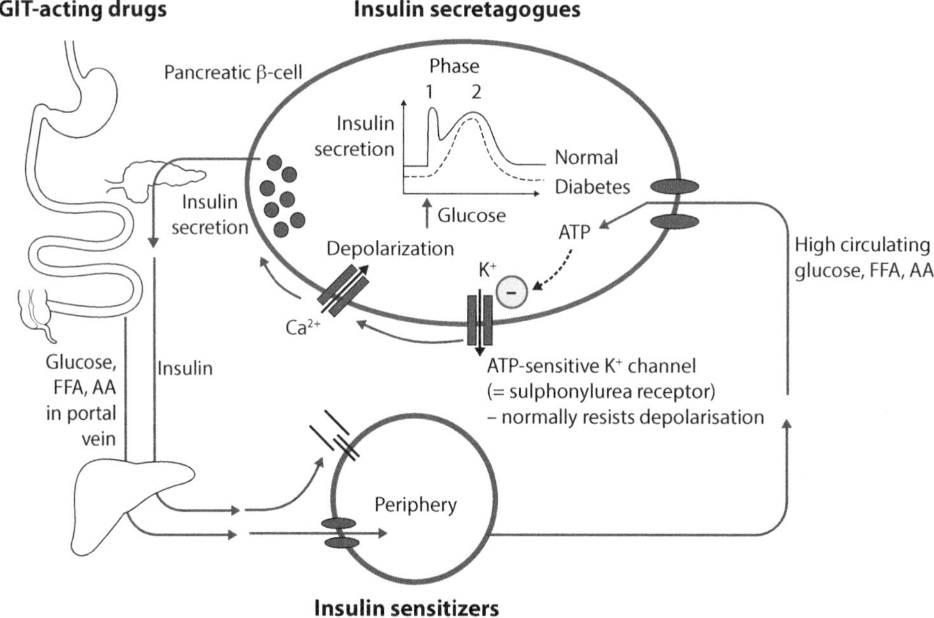

AA, amino acids;
ATP, adenosine triphosphate;
FFA, free fatty acids

Biguanides: Metformin
Mechanism:

- ↑ glucose uptake in presence of background insulin, and BM <14 mmol/l
- Gluconeogenesis in liver, from lactic acid
- LDL+VLDL ↓ and do *not* increase appetite:
  - so used 1st line in **overweight** people

☠ GIT Sx, e.g. diarrhoea, dyspepsia, anorexia
Lactic acidosis, esp. if organ failure
Megaloblastic anaemia – vitamin B12 absorption ↓

Thiazolinediones: Rosiglitazone, pioglitazone
Mechanism: Nuclear PPr receptor y-subunit → tissue responsiveness to insulin
☠ Now mostly withdrawn due to risk of heart failure

Glucagon-like peptide-1 (GLP-1) agonists: Liraglutide, exenatide
Mechanism: GLP-1 is an incretin – a pancreatic hormone that stimulates insulin secretion; GLP-1 agonists are therefore 'secretogogues' (like sulphonylureas)
Benefits:

- Much reduced risk of hypos compared to sulphonylureas
- Associated with significant weight loss, therefore useful in obesity
- However: Only SC preparations exist, requiring twice daily injections

☠ Theoretical risk of pancreatitis and pancreatic cancer (clinically unproven)

Dipeptidyl peptidase-4 (DPP-4) **inhibitors**: Sitagliptin, linagliptin
Mechanism: DPP-4 is an enzyme that degrades pancreatic incretins; DPP-4 inhibitors therefore potentiate the action of incretins and therefore stimulate insulin secretion
Benefits:

- Much reduced risk of hypos compared to sulphonylureas
- Weight neutral
- Oral preparation

Sodium-glucose transport protein-2 (SGLT-2) inhibitors
Mechanism: Act on the nephron to induce glucosuria by blocking SGLT-2 at the proximal tubule
Benefits:

- No risk of hypos
- Improves the cardiovascular risk factors of diabetes
- Associated with weight loss

☠ Chronic glucosuria increases risk of candida and UTI

HYPOGLYCAEMIA

Causes

Divided into: Reactive (occurs after drug or 2–5 h post-prandially)
Fasting (occurs > 5 h post-prandially)

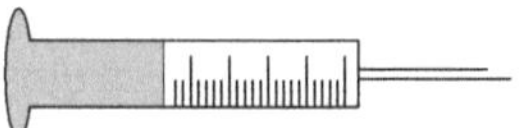

I.A.T.R.O.G².**E.N.I.C.**

Insulin (i.e. in diabetics)
Insulin excess: Distinguished from endogenous insulin by plasma C-peptide absence
Sulphonylureas, esp. chlorpropamide, glibenclamide, esp. in elderly and renal impairment
β-blockers: β2 → gluconeogenesis ↓, glucagon secretion ↓; β1 → masks sympathetic response (although sweating may still occur, being mediated via muscarinic receptor M3)

Alcohol
Acute: Alcohol dehydrogenase → NADH ↑ → hepatic gluconeogenesis ↓
Chronic: ACTH deficiency, malnutrition

Toxins
Aspirin overdose (esp. in children), paracetamol overdose (hepatic necrosis)
Quinine, pentamidine
Ackee (hypoglycine) – Jamaican vomiting sickness

Reactive – 'post-prandial hypoglycaemia'
Idiopathic: Symptoms occur 1–2 h after heavy carbohydrate meal
Secondary: Mild type 2 diabetes, post-gastrectomy (= 'dumping syndrome') TPN (following sudden cessation of IV hypertonic dextrose)

Organ failure – renal/liver
Causes: Gluconeogenesis ↓
Insulin metabolism ↓
Glycogen reserve ↓: Liver failure only
Renal dialysis: Glucose-rich dialysate causes reactive hypoglycaemia

Glycogen storage disease/**G**alactosaemia
Glycogen storage disease 1 (von Gierke): Glucose-6-phosphatase or translocase deficiency
PC: Stunted growth, hepatomegaly, hepatic adenoma
Ix: **G.L.U.T.**: **G**lucose ↓, **L**actic acidosis, **U**ric acid, **T**riglycerides ↑
Galactosaemia and fructose intolerance – both cause reactive hypoglycaemia in infants

Endocrine
Hypoadrenalism: Addison, due to hypocortisolism (adrenaline deficiency does **not** cause)
Hypothyroidism, esp. myxoedema coma
Hypopituitarism (due to TSH and ACTH deficiency; isolated GH deficiency does **not** cause)

Neoplasia
Insulin-secreting (commonest cause of fasting hypoglycaemia):
- Insulinoma: 70% solitary adenoma, 10% multiple (MeN-1), 10% ectopic, 10% malignant – commonest in women in 50s
- Nesidioblastosis, esp. children
- Carcinoid

Insulin-like growth factors/insulin-receptor autoantibodies:
- Adrenal or hepatocellular carcinoma
- Mesothelioma, large retroperitoneal fibrosarcoma; haemangiopericytoma
- Hodgkin lymphoma (insulin receptor autoAbs – may also occur without neoplasia)

Infection: Malaria

Catabolic states: Starvation, esp. neonates, due to ↓ glycogen reserve, sepsis, maternal diabetes

PC

F⁴.A.S².T².i.N.G.

Fatigue/**F**ierce (aggressive)/**F**unny turn/**F**ocal neurological signs, i.e. 'neuroglycopenic symptoms':
- Worse in morning, pre-prandially,or post-exercise; relieved by meal
- Also headache
- Focal neurological signs: Transient hemiplegia, diplopia, dysarthria, ataxia, perioral paraesthesia

Appetite ↑
Sympathetic – pallor (α1 receptor)/**S**weating (M3 receptor)
Tachycardia, palpitations (β1 receptor)/**T**remor (β2 receptor)
Neurological:
- Seizures, confused, coma
- Chronic: Amnesia, dementia, psychosis (may also occur 2° to frequent diabetic asymptomatic 'hypos')

Gain, weight: Chronic hypoglycaemia, esp. with insulinoma

(Whipple triad of insulinoma: wt gain + hypoglycaemia Sx + blood glucose ↓)

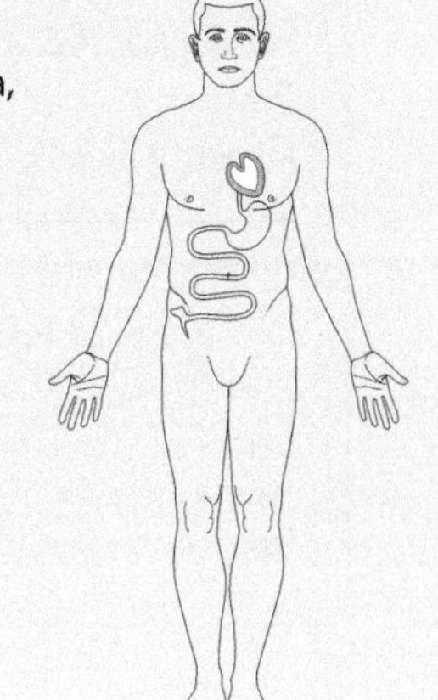

Ix

Bloods: Capillary blood glucose <2.5 mmol/l (normal = 3.5–5.5 mmol/l)
Insulin + C-peptide levels:
- Elevated insulin and low C-peptide = exogenous insulin
- Elevated insulin and normal–high C-peptide = endogenous insulin secretion

Urine: Sulphonylurea assay (is the patient secretly taking sulphonylureas?)
Radiol: MRI pancreas

Rx

Acute:
20 g glucose PO, or 50 ml dextrose 50% w/v IV ± dextrose infusion drip: Use large vein, and leave needle in vein for a while, to reduce risk of thrombophlebitis

Glucagon (1 mg IM): onset = 15 min; offset = 30 min; contraindicated in liver failure or insulinoma

Chronic:
Dumping syndrome:
- Frequent small snacks of complex carbohydrate
- Dietary fibre, guar gum, acarbose

Diabetics: Review medication/education regarding eating, exercise/MedicAlert bracelet

Insulinoma:
Diazoxide or thiazide: Inhibits insulin release (used pre-operatively)
Streptozotocin: Inhibits β-cell growth (used in malignant disease)
Adenoma resection, subtotal pancreatectomy

HYPOPITUITARISM – CAUSES

Anatomy

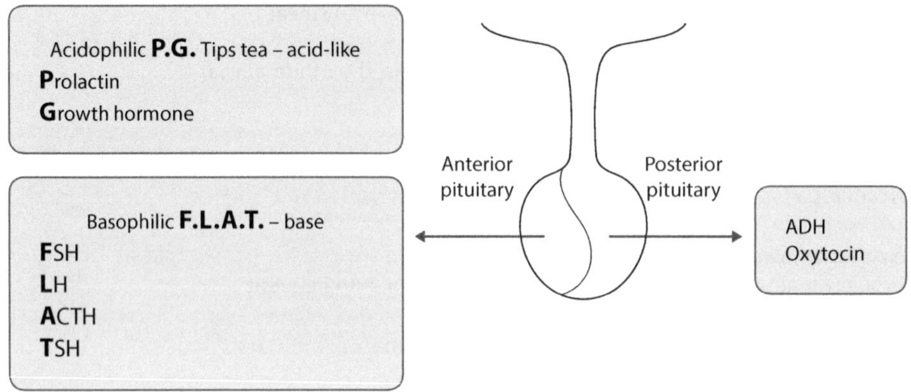

Causes

D.I.V.I.N.I.T.Y.

Developmental:
- Hypothalamic: Kallman syndrome – gonadotrophin deficiency and anosmia
- Pituitary: Genetic panhypopituitarism (*Pit* 1 or *Propl* mutations), isolated GHRH deficiency
- 'Empty sella syndrome':
  - Congenital: Usually a rim of pituitary tissue exists to allow normal pituitary function
  - Acquired: Pituitary mass may silently infarct with CSF replacement

Infection: TB, toxoplasmosis, fungi (PCP, histoplasmosis)

Vascular
- Infarct: Diabetes, vasculitis, Sheehan syn. (post-partum haemorrhage – delayed presentation)
- Haemorrhage or compression by internal carotid aneurysm

Inflammation/**I**nfiltrative:
- Autoimmune: Lymphocytic hypophysitis
- Sarcoidosis, granulomatous hypophysitis
- Haemochromatosis, histiocytosis X

Neoplasia:
- Pituitary: Macroadenoma (commonest):

  in order of frequency ↓
  - Gonadotrope: Silent or non-functioning, i.e. no secretion or secretion of uncombined α(constant) or β subunits
  - Acidophils: Prolactinoma (hyperprolactinaemia), growth hormone (acromegaly)
  - Basophils: ACTH (Cushing – usually microadenoma), TSH (hyperthyroidism – rare)
- Hypothalamic: craniopharyngioma (Rathke's pouch); pineal germinoma, chordoma
- Other: Brain metastasis, glioma, meningioma, arachnoid cyst

Injury: Surgery, trauma, birth injury (2nd commonest)

Toxin: Radiotherapy – for brain tumour

Y: ps**Y**chosocial deprivation: GHRH deficiency

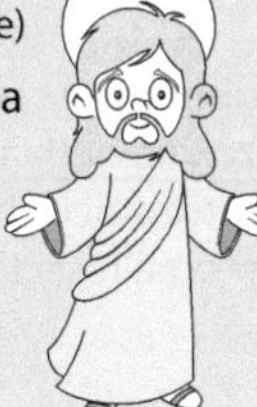

HYPOPITUITARISM – PC

Endocrine dysfunction

If the cause of hypopituitarism is a functioning pituitary macroadenoma, the clinical syndrome will be dominated by the effects of excess secreted hormone:

- Prolactin (infertility, galactorrhoea)
- GH (acromegaly)
- Uncommon: ACTH (Cushing); TSH (thyrotoxicosis)

Hypopituitarism due to any cause results in the following order of endocrine deficiencies:

SEX G.u.I.T.A.R.

SEX hormone-releasers – gonadotrophins: FSH, LH
Menopause-like symptoms: Amenorrhoea, infertility, hot-flushes loss of pubic/axillary hair, dyspareunia, breast atrophy
Loss of libido; impotence; infertility (azoospermia); regression of secondary sex characteristics (soft testicles, fine facial wrinkles)
Adolescent: Delayed puberty
Anaemia: Normochromic, normocytic

Growth hormone:
Children: Failure to grow
Weakness, muscle atrophy, fatigue, depression
Abdominal obesity, cholesterol ↑, HDL ↓ → atherosclerosis
Increased prolactin (due to loss of tonic dopamine inhibition): galactorrheoa, amenorrhea or impotence, infertility
TSH: Hypothyroidism
ACTH: Hypocortisolism → hypomineralocorticoidism
Renal (ADH): Diabetes insipidus

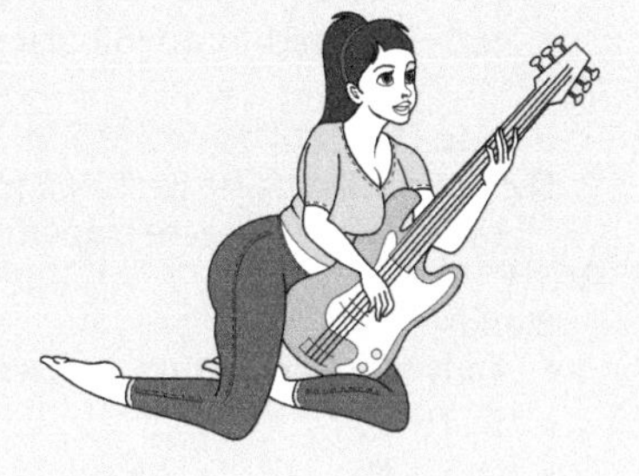

Tumour growth

Cerebral
Personality change
Focal epilepsy or hemiparesis – either direct compression or via carotid artery occlusion in cavernous sinus
Obstructive hydrocephalus

Ophthalmological
Visual-field deficit (70%) – superior-outer quadrantanopia or bitemporal hemianopia
Bilateral central visual acuity or red-vision loss (esp. pituitary apoplexy)
Cranial nerve palsies III, IV, Va, VI via cavernous sinus occlusion

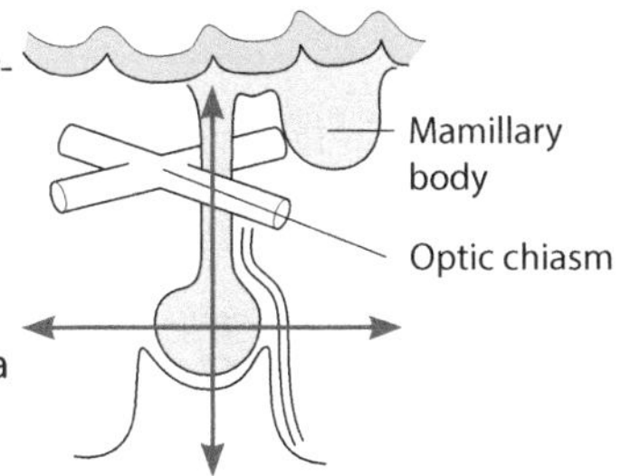

CSF rhinorrhoea

Hypothalamic
Temperature, sleep, appetite dysregulation

Dura stretching
Chronic headache in 40%
- Also due to endocrine effects

Acute headache: Pituitary apoplexy
- Also meningism, drowsiness, bilateral central visual field loss
- Due to haemorrhagic infarction of pituitary tumour

HYPOPITUITARISM – IX

Pituitary function tests

In order of hormone deficiency: **SEX G.u.I.T.A.R.**

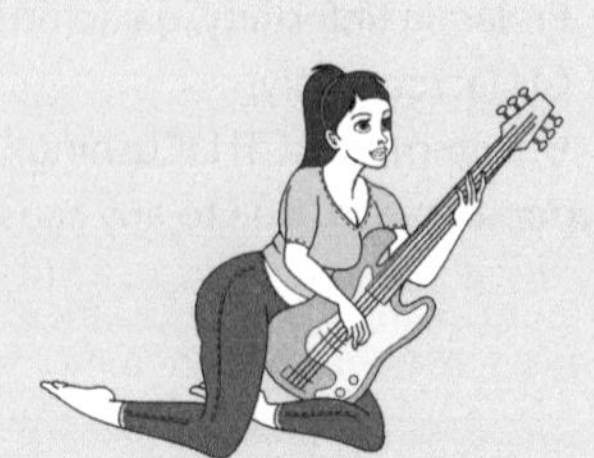

SEX hormone-releasers – gonadotrophins: FSH, LH
Bloods:
- Testosterone ↓ (men) or oestradiol ↓ (women)
- FSH and LH ↓
- Anaemia: Normochromic, normocytic

Dynamic: LHRH challenge: Basal LH normally ↑ x2

Growth hormone
Bloods:
- IGF-1 ↓ or ↑ if GH-macroadenoma is cause of hypopituitarism
- Cholesterol ↑

Dynamic:
- Insulin tolerance test: GH normally ↑ to> 20 IU/l (glucose must ↓ to <2.2 mmol/l)
- GHRH challenge (or L-arginine or L-DOPA): GH should ↑ to >20 IU/l

Increased prolactin
Bloods:
- Prolactin >3600 mIU/l – prolactinoma (commonest functioning macroadenoma)
- 500–3600 mIU/l: Infundibular disconnection, e.g. other type pituitary tumour

TSH
Bloods: TSH↓; fT4 ↓
Dynamic: TRH challenge: TSH normally ↑ to 5–20 IU/l at 20 min; <5 IU/l: hypopituitarism; >20 IU/l: hypothalamic disease (supersensitivity)

ACTH
Bloods:
- Early-morning cortisol ↓ (often normal in early adrenal insufficiency)
- ACTH ↓
- Other: Na^+ ↓, K^+ ↑; glucose ↓; eosinophils ↑, lymphocytes ↑

Dynamic:
- Synacthen test: Should be normal in pituitary insufficiency
- Insulin tolerance test: Cortisol normally >600 mmol/l, or ↑ ×2 from baseline
- CRH challenge: Basal ACTH ↑ 2–4-fold

Cushing syndrome (rarely): 24-hour urine free cortisol; overnight dexamethasone suppression test

Renal (ADH): Diabetes insipidus
Bloods: Serum osmolality and Na^+ ↓
Urine: Urine osmolality ↑
Dynamic:
- Water-deprivation test (for 8 h) – diabetes insipidus is diagnosed if:
  - Serum osmolality >300 mosm/kg
  - Urine osmolality <300 mosm/kg
- Since cortisol deficiency may give false –ve, give dexamethasone before test
- Correctable by prior administration of intranasal desmopressin ('cranial diabetes')

Dynamic tests are performed together as part of **'triple stimulation test'**, i.e. LHRH (IV) + TRH (IV) + insulin tolerance test
Insulin tolerance test is seldomly performed, due to danger of hypoglycaemia in adrenal deficiency

Anatomical localisation

Skull X-ray: Enlarged pituitary fossa, erosion of clinoid processes (historical test)
MRI/CT brain
Goldman's perimetry: Bilateral upper outer quadrantanopia; later, bitemporal hemianopia

HYPOPITUITARISM – RX

Tumour

Medical:

Prolactinoma: Dopamine agonists (bromocriptine, quinagolide, cabergoline):

- Shrink prolactinomas
- Shrink 10% of other pituitary macroadenomas, incl. non-functioning

Acromegaly: Somatostatin analogues (octreotide, lanreotide): Inhibit secretion of GH-secreting adenomas, but only cause shrinkage in 10%

Surgical: Trans-sphenoidal/trans-frontal hypophysectomy

Ind: First-line Rx in non-functioning adenomas; acromegaly; Cushing

- Improves visual acuity/field in 70% pts

☠: Recurrence in 20% (reduced by radiotherapy)

Radiotherapy (external/yttrium implant):

Ind: Used as an adjuvant to surgery, or where surgery inappropriate

Hormone replacement

Sex hormone-releasers – gonadotrophins: FSH, LH

- ♀: EthinylE2 or conjugated E2 for 1st–3rd weeks + medroxyprogesterone in 3rd week (if uterus) with withdrawal bleed on 4th week
- ♂ Testosterone for low libido: Testosterone enanthate (IM every 2 weeks)/decanoate (PO)/ transdermal or implant

Fertility:

- Human menopausal gonadotrophins
- Human chorionic gonadotrophins (LH analogue)
- Recombinant GnRH:
  - Simulates normal pulsatile release of GnRH via pump
  - Less risk of ovarian hyperstimulation and multiple gestation

Growth hormone

- Human recombinant, subcutaneous GH
- GHRH – experimental: Simulates normal pulsatile release of GH

Increased prolactin: Only need to treat if prolactinoma – see under Tumour (above)

TSH

- T4: 75–150 μg/day

  ☠ AF, angina, osteoporosis

  Addisonian crisis: Must replace cortisol first, if deficiency exists

ACTH

- Hydrocortisone: 10 mg mane + 5 mg noon + 5 mg evening
- MedicAlert bracelet
- Need to ↑ in event of illness or operation, e.g. 20 mg tds–qds

NB: Fludrocortisone unnecessary, as ACTH is not a significant releaser of aldosterone

Renal (ADH)

- Desmopressin: DDAVP (PO/intranasal)

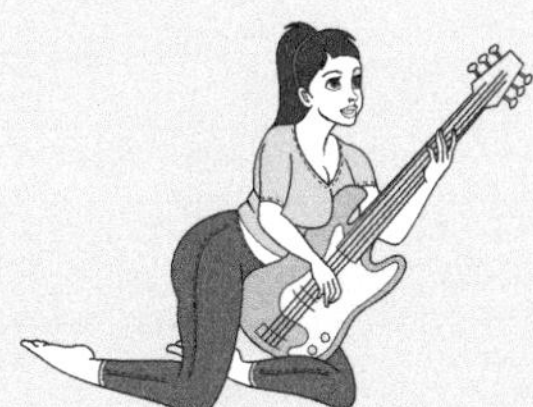

HYPERPROLACTINAEMIA

Causes

Higher brain centres

Stress: Pain (incl. venepuncture), infection, organ failure, esp. renal
Sleep: Pre-awakening
Seizures: 10–20 min postictal or syncope
Sex: Orgasm

Hypothalamus

Dopamine ⊖ ⊕ TRH Estrogen

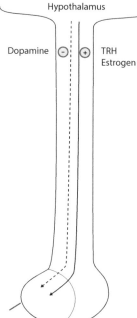

Loss of dopamine inhibition

Hypothalamo-infundibular disconnection:

- Pituitary tumour (any type) or craniopharyngioma
- Pituitary surgery (with damage to stalk)
- Pituitary radiotherapy
- Sarcoid, TB, histiocytosis X

Dopamine antagonists:

- Neuroleptics, TCAs, SSRLs or opioids
- Metoclopramide
- Verapamil

Endocrine stimulation

Hypothyroidism:
T4 ↓ → TRH ↑ → PRL ↑

Oestrogen:

- Pregnancy
  - ↑ size of pre-existing prolactinoma
  - <12 weeks postpartum
- Polycystic ovaries
- Pill (OCP)

Prolactin

Autonomous secretion

Pituitary tumour: Commonest (40%)

- Prolactinoma
  - Microadenoma: women – present early
  - Macroadenoma: men – present later!
- Acromegaly

Ectopic prolactin secretion: Small-cell lung, renal cell carcinoma

Sensory afferents to hypo-thalamus

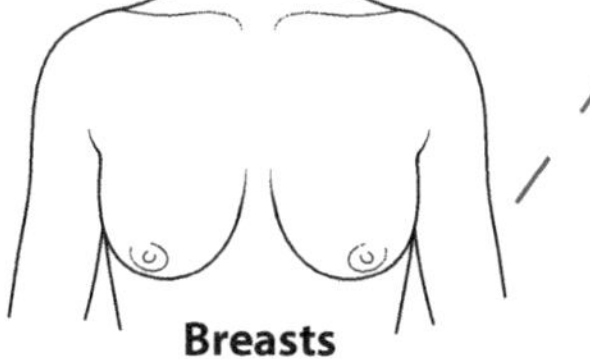

Chest wall stimulation

Breast-feeding; self-examination
Trauma
VZV of thoracic dermatome

PC

Galactorrhoea: Women (rare in men)

Hypogonadotrophic hypogonadism (**GnRH** ↓, gonadotrophins ↓, sex steroids ↓)
♀: Amenorrhoea, infertility
♂: Loss of libido, impotence, infertility (azoospermia)
Osteoporosis

Panhypopituitarism (if due to prolactinoma)
Endocrine deficiencies (**Sex G.u.I.T.A.R.**): Mass effect – headache, hemianopia

Ix

Prolactin (daytime levels)

mIU/l	Cause
<500	Normal
500–3600	Any cause, except prolactin macroadenoma *so if MRI shows pituitary macroadenoma, then cause is infundibular disconnection and the treatment is surgery*
>3600	Prolactin macroadenoma or pregnancy *so if MRI shows pituitary macroadenoma, treat with dopamine agonist*

Dynamic tests
Prolactin: Give domperidone or metoclopramide
Hypopituitarism: Triple stimulation test – LHRH, TRH, insulin tolerance test

MRI pituitary ± visual fields

Rx

Dopamine agonists: Bromocriptine, quinagolide, cabergoline (fewer side-effects)
Ind: Secreting prolactinomas: First-line therapy; 90% respond:

- Within hours, prolactin level normalizes
- Within days–weeks, tumour shrinks
- Can attempt withdrawal after 2 years, as tumour fibroses

Non-secreting prolactinoma + pregnancy:

- Give prophylactically for 6 months pre-conception to ↓ risk of tumour expansion
- Bromocriptine also used for symptomatic expansion during pregnancy

☠: N+V, postural hypotension, Raynaud syn., nasal stuffiness, constipation

Trans-sphenoidal microadenectomy
Ind: Intolerant or resisant to dopamine agonists
Non-secreting tumour/disconnection: 90% cure, but may relapse

Radiotherapy: Ind: Adjunct to surgery

ACROMEGALY

Growth hormone – Normal physiology

Growth hormone is required for both growth and the catabolic response in stressful situations

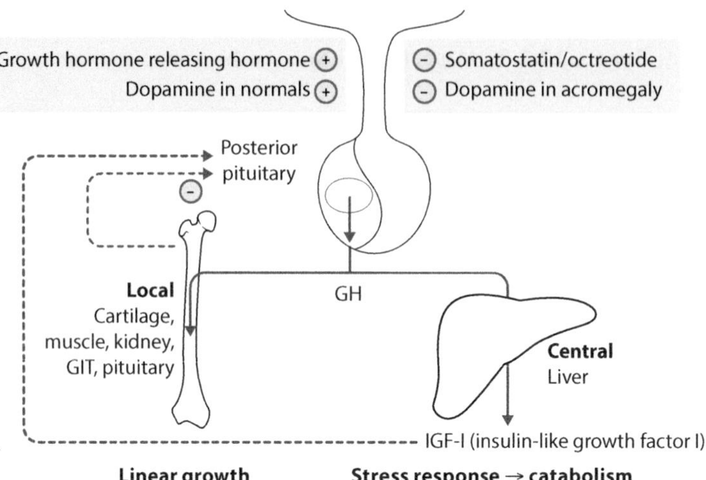

Causes

Pituitary

Epi: Prevalence 5/100,000; age 30–50 years (uncommonly children)

Types:

Adenoma (90%):

- G-Protein Gsα activating mutation → autonomous growth hormone ± prolactin secretion
- Acidophilic adenomas → acromegaly

Genetic syndrome with pituitary adenoma (9%):

- Multiple endocrine neoplasia 1 (MEN-1):
  - Pituitary adenoma, parathyroidism, hyper-, pancreatic insulinoma or gastrinoma
- McCune–Albright syndrome = polyostotic fibrous dysplasia + pigmented patches, due to Gsα activating mutation in mosaic of tissues
- Carney's complex: Spotty pigmentation + myxomas + endocrine tumours
- Familial acromegaly and gigantism: Loss of heterozygosity in tumour cells

Carcinoma (1%)

Extrapituitary

Types:

GHRH secretion: APUDoma (e.g. bronchial carcinoid), small-cell carcinoma, hypothalamic hamartoma

GH secretion: Pancreatic islet cell

PC

G.I.A.N.T. C.O.N.K.

Growth '*acromegaly*' = extremity enlargement:
- Nose: Broad; enlarged sinuses; supraorbital ridge prominence
- Mouth: Prognathism; teeth parting; loss; deep voice; macroglossia
- Skull: Frontal bossing; hat size ↑
- Hands: Spade-like (e.g. ring size ↑); hyperhidrosis
- Feet: Shoe size ↑ ; heel pad thickening (on X-ray)
- Gigantism: If onset occurs before epiphyseal fusion (children)

Insulin resistance or diabetes mellitus (25%):
- Diabetes mellitus; acanthosis nigricans; skin tags
- Hypertriglyceridaemia (due to ↓ lipoprotein lipase activity)

Arthritis: Hips, knees; spine (kyphosis, spinal stensosis, cauda equina syn.)

Neurology: Headache; carpal or tarsal tunnel syndromes; proximal myopathy

Tumour effects:
- Homonymous hemianopia
- Panhypopituitarism, incl. hypogonadism
- Hyperprolactinoma: Galactorrhoea, hirsutism, amenorrhoea

Cardiac:
- Hypertension
- Ischaemic heart disease; CVA: mortality rate = 2×↑
- Dilated cardiomyopathy; cardiac failure

Obstructive sleep apnoea in 60%, due to macroglossia

Neoplasia: Colonic polyps, adenocarcinoma

Kidney stones/hypercalciuria: Normocalcaemic, but PO_4↑ and vitamin D↑

Ix

Insulin-like growth factor I (IGF-I): Does not fluctuate over course of day (unlike GH)
Oral glucose tolerance test (OGTT): GH normally become undetectable following glucose challenge

Rx

Surgical: Trans-sphenoidal or transfrontal hypophysectomy:
- Curative for 90% microadenomas (i.e. <1 cm); less successful for macroadenomas
- ☠ : Panhypopituitarism in 10%; meningitis; haemorrhage

Medical:

Somatostatin analogue: Octreotide or lanreotide (inhibits GH and PRL secretion) – rapid relief of headache, perspiration, obstructive sleep apnoea and carpal tunnel in >90% pts

Dopamine agonists: Bromocriptine, cabergoline – effective in only 10%, but have additive effect with octreotide

GH-receptor antagonists: Pegrisomant

Radiotherapy: GH levels decrease slowly over 10 years

HYPOTHYROIDISM – CAUSES

H.A³.T.R.E.D.

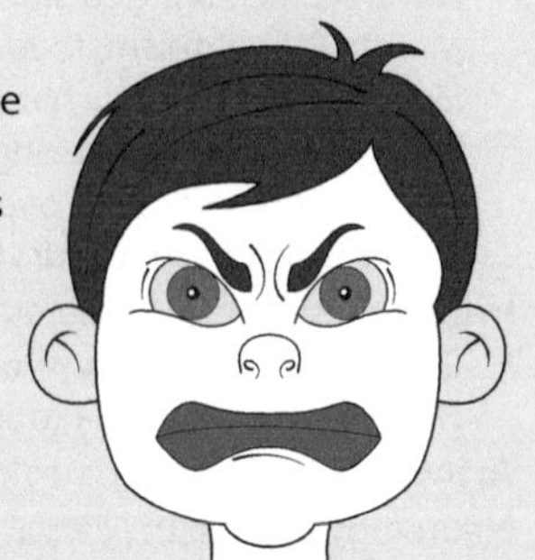

Hashimoto's thyroiditis
- Epi: Middle-aged women; assoc. with other organ-based autoimmune disease, e.g. DM
- PATH: Lymphocytic and macrophage infiltrate with lymphoid follicles
- Course: T4 ↓ → euthyroidism in 40%; a few pts begin/become temporarily hyperthyroid
- Ix: Anti-thyroglobulin (TG) and anti-myeloperoxidase (MPO)

Atrophic/**A**utoimmune, other/**A**myloid and other infiltrative
- Atrophic thyroiditis:
  - PATH: Fibrosis (limited to capsule) and deposition of hydrophilic glycosaminoglycans
  - Course: May represent end-stage Hashimoto or carbimazole-treated Graves
  - Ix: Anti-TSH receptor-blocking Abs (cf. Graves = anti-TSH receptor-stimulatory Abs)
- Autoimmune, other:
  - Graves disease: Late, or following radioiodine therapy or surgery
  - Riedel's thyroiditis (part of multifocal fibrosclerosis, e.g. alveolitis, mediastinitis)
  - Scleroderma
- Amyloidosis, sarcoidosis, haemochromatosis

Toxins/Nutritional
- Anti-thyroid treatment: Carbimazole, radioiodine (^{131}I), surgery
- Other toxin:
  - Lithium, tolbutamide, aminosalicylic acid
  - Cassava excess: Thiocyanate inhibits iodide uptake in thyroid ('trapping')
- Nutritional (iodine excess or deficiency):
  - Excess: Amiodarone (blocks iodination and coupling reactions), or nuclear fallout (^{131}I)
  - Deficiency: Endemic cretinism in Andes, Himalayas, New Guinea (>10% population)
    - Epi: Associated with high $CaCO_3$ in water; pregnancy (high demand)
    - PC: Massive goitre; often euthyroid due to compensation

Resistance to thyroid hormone:
- Autosomal dominant condition, resulting from thyroid receptor β mutation
- Cases are often clinically euthyroid, but have abnormal TFTs – ↑ TSH, ↑ fT4 and ↑ fT3
  - PC: Learning disability, delayed skeletal maturation, goitre; occasionally thyrotoxic!

Endocrine:
- Hypopituitarism, e.g. pituitary tumour; order of endocrine deficiency = (**Sex G.u.I.T.A.R.** = sex hormones GH → TSH → ACTH →ADH: *p. 333*)
- Addison disease: Due to cortisol ↓ or polyglandular autoimmunity (PGAS-2)
  - Ix : Anti-adrenal, anti-MPO

Developmental:
- Thyroid aplasia; ectopic thyroid (e.g. lingual, trachea) – commonest congenital cause
- Dyshormonogenesis: Peroxidase or iodine transferase deficiency:
  - PC: Deaf mutism, learning disability = Pendred syndrome
  - Ix: Perchlorate discharge test: $KClO_4$ leaches out unincorporated ^{131}I
- Down or Turner syndromes

HYPOTHYROIDISM – PC

S.H⁴.O.W.I.N.G. O.F.F. *(their signs)*

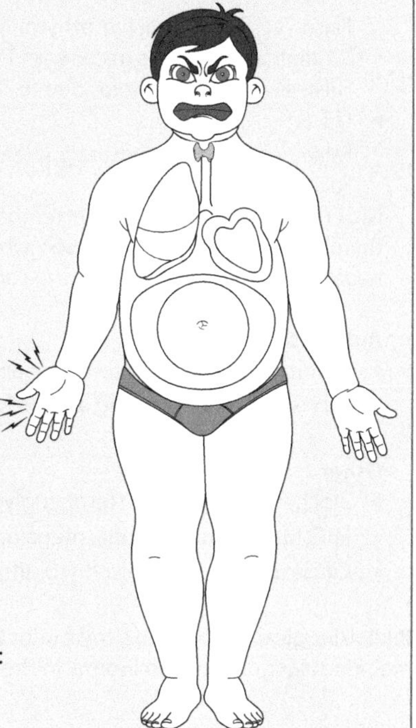

Skin
- 'Myxoedema' = non-pitting, doughy oedema due to impaired hyaluronidase, leading to mucopolysaccharide accumulation:
  - Facies: Puffy, toad-like, apathetic; malar flush; peaches and cream (β-caroteinaemia)
  - Tongue: Macroglossia, glossitis (pernicious anaemia)
  - Voice: Hoarse, gruff (myxoedmatous larynx)
- Other: Erythema ab igne (patient is always cold), pruritus
- Hair: Alopecia; loss of outer 1/3 eyebrow

Hypometabolism/**H**eart disease
- Cold intolerance; hypothermic (myxoedema coma)
- Cardiac:
  - Bradycardia (worsened with digoxin!)
  - Dilated cardiomyopathy (glycosaminoglycan infiltrate)
  - Ischaemic heart disease: Direct effect and via hypercholesterolaemia

Hypoglycaemia/**H**ypercholesterol and triglyceridaemia

Ophthalmic
- Xanthelasma (and tendinous xanthoma) due to hypercholesterolaemia
- Bitemporal hemianopia due to pituitary enlargement from thyrotroph hyperplasia
- Graves disease ophthalmopathy

Weight gain, anorexia

Intestinal: Constipation, abdominal distension (incl. ascites)

Neuropsychiatric
- Dementia (esp. amnesia)/depression (and paradoxical mania):
  - Congenital T4 ↓: Mental retardatation – 'cretinism'; assoc. posterior fontanelle enlargement
  - Juvenile-onset T4 ↓: Mental-slowing only
- Cerebellar ataxia, dizziness, drop-attacks
- Muscle: Proximal myopathy (CK, AST, LDH ↑), slowly relaxing reflexes, myotonia
- Carpal tunnel syndrome
- Deafness (otitis media or Pendred syndrome)

Goitre
- Firm, irregular: Hashimoto's thyroiditis
- Firm, regular: Graves disease ('burnt-out' or treated)
- Woody, hard: Riedel's thyroiditis
- No goitre: Atrophic thyroiditis

Oedema/effusions: Pericardial, pleural, ascites, joint

Females: Menorrhagia or amenorrhoea

Fertility: Infertility delayed or premature puberty; galactorrhoea – all due to secondary hyperprolactinaemia

HYPOTHYROIDISM – IX AND RX

Ix

Bloods: **TFT**

- TSH ↑: Most sensitive test
  False –ve: Secondary hypothyroidism due to hypopituitarism (TSH ↓)
  False +ve:
  - 'Sick euthyroid', e.g. recovery phase of severe systemic illness
  - Generalized thyroid resistance (patients will have high T4 and T3)
- fT4 ↓:
  False –ve: Subclinical hypothyroidism (still requires Rx due to higher risk of ischaemic heart disease; clinical symptoms occur with TSH >5 × upper-limit normal)
  False +ve: 'Sick euthyroid', due to T4 degradation ↑ and rT3 formation ↑
- fT3 ↓:
  False –ve: common, because ↓ TSH causes preferential release of T3 rather than T4
  False +ve: 'Sick euthyroid'

NB: **Free** T4 and **free** T3 are better than total amounts, as they are not influenced by changes in thyroxine-binding globulin (TBG), which may decrease in severe illness, and increase with states such as hepatitis, pregnancy or taking the contraceptive pill

AutoAbs

- Anti-myeloperoxidase (MPO) or anti-thyroglobulin (TG): Graves; Hashimoto
- TSH receptor-stimulating antibody (Graves)

Other

- Biochem: Na^+ ↓; cholesterol, triglycerides ↑; CK, AST, LDH ↑ (sarcolemma damage)
- FBC: Macrocytic anaemia; megaloblastosis suggests coexistent pernicious anaemia
- Cause: ESR ↑↑ – Riedel's thyroiditis; Synacthen test – Addison; FSH, LH – pituitary failure

Radiol/**S**urgical: Hashimoto's thyroiditis may present with asymmetric goitre, which can be confused with multinodular goitre or carcinoma. In these cases, USS and FNA help to distinguish

Rx

Thyroxine, lifelong: Dose 25–200 μg/day

☠: Angina or myocardial infarction in elderly, so introduce dose gradually (by 25 μg every 3 months)
Addison – due to unmasking of hypoadrenalism or hypopituitarism:

- Prior Synacthen test if hypoadrenal features; or, if in doubt
- Cover with hydrocortisone

Acute psychosis

HYPOTHYROIDISM RX – COMPLICATIONS

Myxoedematous coma

Precipitants

Sedatives
MI, CVA
Infection

Ventilatory support

Ventilate: pts often develop type 2 respiratory failure

Assessment

A.B.C.D.
C.O.A.T.
- **C**ardiac monitor:
  - Bradycardia, heart block, long QT interval
- **O**$_2$
- **A**BP
- **T**PR: Hypothermic

Warming

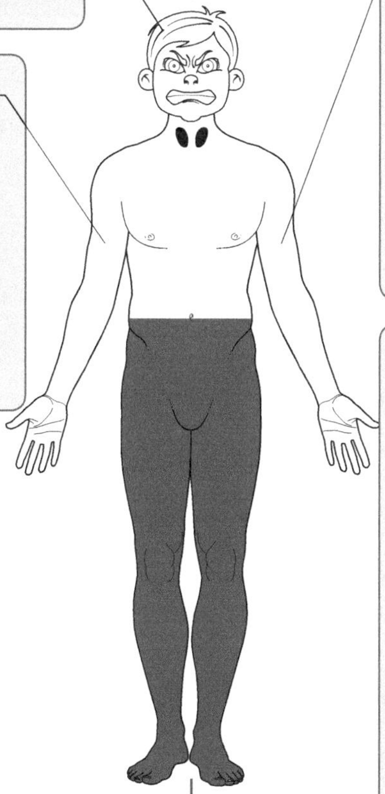

Hydration

CVP line
IV fluids
- Often hypertensive due to compensatory catecholamines, but hypovolaemic
- Hypotension is a poor prognostic sign
- Give 5–50% dextrose, as often hypoglycaemic
- Inotropes are ineffective

Medication

Hydrocortisone: Pre-treat
Thyroxine
- Liothyronine (IV T3):
  - 5–20 μg od for 3 days
  - Rapid onset and offset
  - Overcomes need to convert peripherally, which is suppressed in coma and infection

  ☠: Labile concentrations – angina (give prophylaxis GTN)
- T4 PO or nasogastric, 25–50 μg od

Antibiotics, broad-spectrum

Complications

Hypoglycaemia: 50% dextrose, 50 ml
Seizures (25%): Anticonvulsants
Psychosis: Antipsychotics
ICP ↑: ITU, hyperventilation, inotropes

HYPERTHYROIDISM – CAUSES

G.A.I.N. of F.U.N.C.T.io.N.

Hyperstimulation

Graves disease

- Epi: Prevalence: 1–2%; F:M = 10:1, esp. post-partum; age: 20–40 y
- PATH: Lymphocytic infiltrate with follicles; follicle cell hyperplasia, columnar metaplasia; scalloping of colloid adjacent to follicle cells due to active endocytosis
- Course: T4 ↑ → 40% euthyroidism → 20 % T4 ↓ (may present as hypoT4ism)
  - Neonatal thyrotoxicosis due to maternal LATS (IgG) crossing placenta in 3rd trimester
- Ix: Anti-TSH receptor stimulatory Abs ('long-acting thyroid stimulator')

Follicle destruction

Autoimmune, other

- Hashimoto's thyroiditis: Early
- Post-partum lymphocytic thyroiditis
  - PC: Painless goitre
  - Course: Temporary T4 ↑ or ↓ → 10% develop permanent hypoT4ism
  - Ix: Anti-TSH receptor blocking Abs

Infection: de Quervain's thyroiditis (viral, granulomatous)

- Epi: Women, 20–40 y, assoc. with HLA-B35
- PATH: Coxsackie, influenza or EBV
- PC: Subacute; painful goitre or dysphagia; fever
- Course: Transient ↑ T4 → mild ↓ T4 (exhaustion) → recovery over 2–4 months

Autonomous secretion

Nodular goitre (toxic multinodular goitre or Plummer disease)

- Epi: Age >50 y
- Cause: Long-standing non-toxic goitre, or iodine deficiency

Follicular adenoma (>2.5 cm)/**F**ollicular thyroid carcinoma (esp. metastatic)

U: McC**U**ne–Albright syndrome: GTP activating mutation

Neoplasia: Ovarian teratoma (benign struma ovarii): T4 secretion

Choriocarcinoma: Hydatidiform mole; TSH-related peptide secretion

Toxins

- Iodide, incl. amiodarone (Jod–Basedow disease)
- Thyroid tissue ingestion, e.g. hamburgers; epidemic (T4-toxicosis, with normal T3)
- T4 over-replacement

Neoplasia: Pituitary adenoma – TSH-secreting (rare)

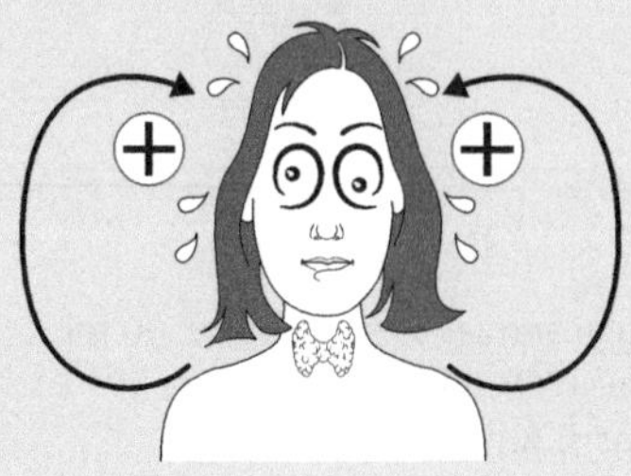

HYPERTHYROIDISM – PC

S.H^3.O.W.I.N.G. O.F.F. *(their signs)*

Skin
- Sweaty, erythematous palms; smooth, salmon-pink face
- Graves disease-associated
  - Pretibial myxoedema:
    - Thickened skin over legs, feet; clearly demarcated; erythema; pruritic
    - Accentuated hair follicles (peau d'orange)
  - Acropachyderma: Clubbing; onycholysis, thick skin, hypertrophic periosteum
- Autoimmune-associated: vitiligo, alopecia

Hypermetabolism/**H**yperdynamic circulation
- Fever, esp. with thyrotoxic storm, or viral infection
- Hyperdynamic circulation:
  - Rapid, bounding pulse or AF
  - Hypertension
  - High-output cardiac failure, dilated cardiomyopathy

Hyperglycaemia

Ophthalmic
- Upper lid retraction (sympathetic stimulation of levator palpebrae superioris)
  - O/E: Staring; infrequent blinking; lid lag on rapid descent
- Graves disease ophthalmopathy:
  - PATH: Due to deposition of hydrophilic glycosaminoglycans in retro-orbital fat pad; lymphocyte infiltrate; muscular fibrosis
  - O/E:
    - Exophthalmos: Superior limbic keratitis (grittiness), chemosis (discomfort, worse in morning)
    - Ophthalmoplegia, esp. upward and outward
    - Retro-orbital compression: Optic nerve atrophy (↓ visual acuity), papilloedema, glaucoma

Weight loss, hyperphagia

Intestinal
- Diarrhoea, malabsorption, abdominal pain, N+V (severe in 'thyrotoxic storm')
- Cholestasis (periportal fibrosis)
- Hyposplenism

Neuropsychiatric
- Emotionally labile, psychosis, depression, anxiety, fatigue
- Tremor (fine, positional), chorea
- Proximal myopathy (rarely ptosis), or hypokalaemic periodic paralysis (esp. in oriental men)

Goitre
- PC: Dysphagia, stridor, dysphonia (due to recurrent laryngeal nerve palsy (esp. if carcinoma)
- O/E: Palpation:
  - Diffuse and smooth – Graves; diffuse and multinodular – toxic multinodular or Hashimoto
  - Focal and mobile – cyst or adenoma; focal and immobile – carcinoma or lymphoma
  - Tender – viral thyroiditis

  Auscultation: Bruit in Graves, carcinoma

  SVCO, esp. on raising arms (Pemberton's sign)

  Lymphadenopathy: Graves, carcinoma, lymphoma

Osteoporosis/hypercalcaemia

Females: Oligomenorrhoea (less commonly menorrhagia, due to ↑ PRL), gynaecomastia

Fertility: Infertility

HYPERTHYROIDISM – IX AND RX

Ix

Bloods: **TFT**

- TSH ↓ or unrecordable (unless cause is TSH-secreting tumour, e.g. pituitary adenoma)
- Free T4 ↑
- Free T3 ↑: If T4 is normal, 5% of patients present with T3 thyrotoxicosis

AutoAbs

- Anti-TSH receptors: 100% specific; 90% sensitive for Graves
- Anti-myeloperoxidase (MPO), anti-thyroglobulin (TG): Graves, Hashimoto, viral, post-partum

Other

- Biochem: Ca ↑, Mg ↓, bilirubin ↑, ALP ↑, glucose ↑, ferritin ↑
- FBC: Normochromic normocytic anaemia, lymphocytosis
- Cause: ESR ↑ (viral thyroiditis), ß-HCG ↑ (choriocarcinoma)

Radiol: ^{99m}Tc – **pertechnate scan**

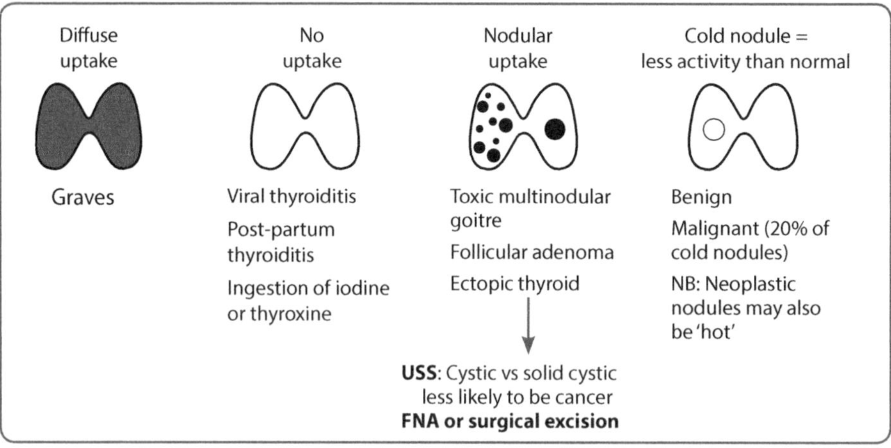

Rx

be **S.T.RI.C.T.** *with them!*

Symptomatic: Propranolol (anxiety, palpitations, tachycardia)

Thiourea: Carbimazole or propylthiouracil (PTU)

Mechanism: ↓ thyroid peroxidase, ↓ oxidative coupling, ↓ T4 → T3, immunomodulation

Indication: Graves or toxic multinodular goitre: Rx for 18 months; 50% relapse

☠: Hypersensitivity (rash, arthralgia, hepatitis – within 6 weeks), agranulocytosis

Radio-**I**odine (^{131}I)

Mechanism: Iodine is only taken up by 'hot' nodules: the rest of the gland is atrophic

Indication: Toxic multinodular goitre or adenoma in over-40s

☠: HypoT4ism (esp. in Graves), malignancy, teratogenic (avoid in women), hypoPTHism

Cause-specific:

- Viral – NSAIDS, steroids
- Gynae – surgery
- Iodide ingestion – Na perchlorate

Thyroidectomy, partial

Indication: Treatment-resistant Graves; large goitre or adenoma

Method: Pre-treat with thioureas for 3 months (avoids thyrotoxic storm), KI for 1 week

☠: Recurrent laryngeal nerve palsy (ENT exam before), hypoPTHism (usually transient)

HYPERTHYROIDISM RX – COMPLICATIONS

Thyrotoxic storm

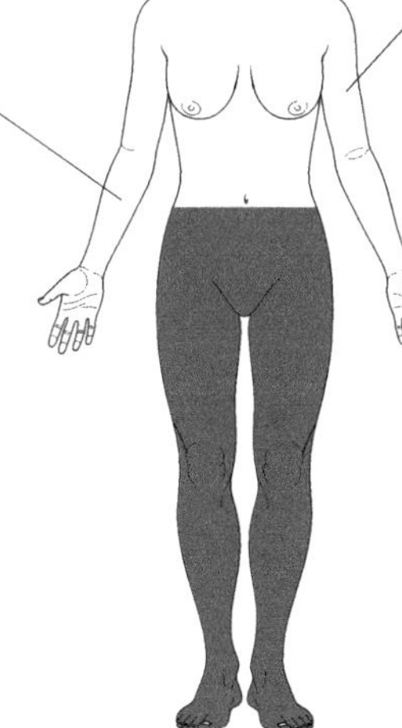

Ventilatory support

Oxygen: 100% – esp. if in CCF

Assessment

A.B.C.D.
C.O.A.T.
Cardiac Monitor: SVT
O_2
ABP
TPR: Hyperpyrexia (>40°C)

Cooling
- Paracetamol
- Blanket
- Do not use aspirin, due to displacement of T4 from TBG

Hydration

N. saline – unless in CCF

Medication

Anti-thyroid
PTU 250 mg 4 hrly:
- Blocks iodine peroxidation

Lugol iodine (I_2/I^-):
- Give 1 h after PTU
- Blocks T4 release

Na ipodate (X-ray contrast):
- Alternative to Lugol iodine
- Blocks T4 release and T3 → T4

Dexamethasone (2 mg qds)
Inhibits T4 release and T3 → T 4
Provides adrenal support
β-Blocker/digoxin
Use β-blocker even if in CCF!
If asthmatic, use guanethidine or reserpine
Vitamin B complex

Complications

Anti-psychotics
Anti-arrhythmics/heart failure treatment
Anti-diarrhoeals/analgesics for abdominal pain

Graves disease ophthalmopathy

Rx

Conservative: Sleep propped up, lubricant eye drops
Medical: Diuretics, steroids (e.g. prednisolone 60 mg od)
Radiotherapy
Surgical: Lateral tarsorraphy, medial orbital wall decompression

Neonatal thyrotoxicosis

PATH

Transplacental transfer of maternal TSH receptor Abs (LATS) to neonate
Check neonatal TFTs at birth and 1 week – maternal antithyroid drugs may initially mask

Rx

Pregnancy:
- Symptomatic: Allows sparing or avoidance of thiourea, esp. at 3rd trimester
- Thiourea (low-dose, as Graves goes into partial remission, and risk of causing neonatal hypothyroidism and goitre, with stridor)

Neonate: β-blockers and carbimazole
Breast-feeding mother: Propylthiouracil

GOITRE

PC

'Lump in the neck'
Dysphagia
Stridor; dyspnoea

O/E

Inspection: Signs of Graves or myxoedema; scar; lingual thyroid (look at back of tongue)
Palpation: Method: palpate from behind; get patient to swallow:

- Diffuse (smooth or irregular) vs nodular
- Other masses:
  - Thyroglossal cyst (elevates on tongue protrusion)
  - Cervical lymphadenopathy (Graves, papillary carcinoma)
  - Delphian node: midline above isthmus (papillary carcinoma)

Auscultation: Bruit in Graves or carcinoma
Manoeuvres: Transillumination: Cystic vs solid nodules
Pemberton's sign: Arm elevation causes SVCO with retrosternal goitre

Causes

Euthyroid
Simple goitre, assoc. women, smoking
Nodules: Non-toxic (i.e. euthyroid), assoc. ionising radiation
Iodine deficiency, compensated

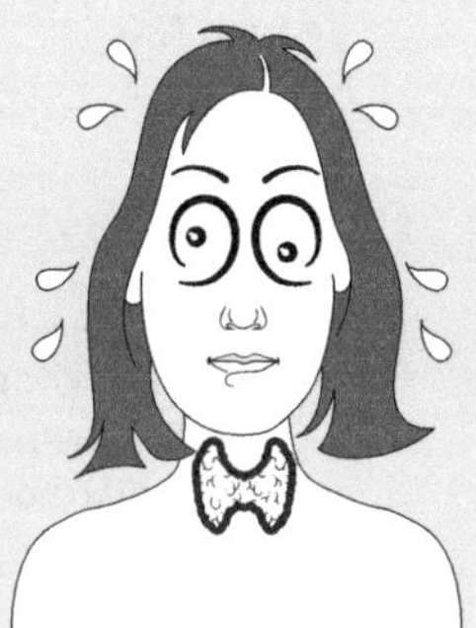

8% population have palpable goitres! (4 × more common in women)

T4 ↑ G.A.I.N. of F.u.N.c.T.ion.
Graves disease: Diffuse enlargement
Autoimmune, other: Post-partum thyroiditis
Infection: de Quervain's thyroiditis (painful, fever, systemic upset)
Nodular: Toxic multinodular goitre – multiple nodules (irregular)
Follicular adenoma: Single nodule
Neoplastic: Metastatic follicular carcinoma
Toxin: Amiodarone

T4 ↓ H.A.T.R.e.D.
Hashimoto: Firm and irregular (may be mistaken for neoplasm)
Autoimmune, other: Riedel – woody hard
Toxin/Nutritional: Iodine deficiency:
Endemic mountainous regions – often massive goitre!
Pregnancy – increased demand
Resistance to thyroid hormone (hereditary, often euthyroid)
Developmental: Ectopic thyroid may be observed, e.g. back of tongue, above thyroid cartilage

Ix

Bloods: TFTs (and associated bloods, e.g. glucose, if autoimmune disease suspected)
Thyroglobulin ↑ in most thyroid diseases and benign adenomas, but especially high in neoplasia
AutoAbs: Anti-TSH R; anti-myeloperoxidase (MPO) or anti-thyroglobulin (TG)
Radiol: Neck X-ray: Calcification – papillary ca. (stippled – psammoma bodies); medullary ca. (dense calcification)
Pertechnetate scan → if single nodule → USS ± FNA (as for thyrotoxicosis – *see p. 345*)

THYROID TUMOURS

PC

Thyroid nodule

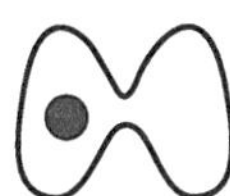

Epi: 50% population have nodules *of any size*
5% population have nodules that are *palpable*:
- 10% of those palpable nodules removed surgically are neoplastic
- 5% of multinodular goitres are neoplastic

Local infiltration

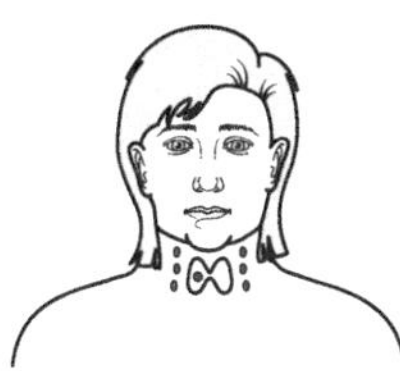

Dysphagia (oesophagus)
Haemoptysis (trachea); hoarseness, dysphonia (recurrent laryngeal nerve)
Neck pain: Radiates to jaw and ear

Endocrine (rare)

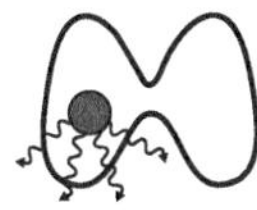

Follicular carcinoma (metastatic): Thyrotoxicosis
Medullary carcinoma:
- Cushing (ACTH)
- MEN-2a (associated phaeochromocytoma, hyperPTHism)

Types

PAP.a.'s. F.A.M.i.LY.

PAPillary (80%) – young adults (20–30s), esp. females
Aet: Radiation, iodine deficiency (TSH overstimulation), *ptc* oncogene
PATH: Psammoma bodies: Stippled calcification (radio-opaque on CXR)
PC: Fixed multifocal neck mass + lateral cervical lymphadenopathy + lung invasion
Rx: T4 – decreases TSH stimulation; surgery or ^{131}I in elderly
Prog: Good: 5-y survival 95% (best prognosis young, women); but 10% relapse after 10 y
Follicular (15%) – middle-aged
PC: Metastasizes early (lung –snowstorm appearance on CXR; bone)
Thyrotoxicosis
Prog: 5-y survival 50% (poor prognosis: Hurthle-cell variety)
Anaplastic (2%) – elderly, esp. females
PATH: Spindle and giant cells
Prog: 5-y survival 10%
Medullary (2%) – young
PATH: Parafollicular C cells (APUDoma derived from neural crest cells)
Secrete calcitonin: Forms amyloid and raises plasma calcitonin
PC: Cervical lymphadenopathy
Diarrhoea (secretion of prostaglandin, 5-HT, polypeptide)
Endocrine: MEN-2a or 2b (assoc. phaeochromocytoma, hyperPTHism), ACTH
Ix: Basal calcitonin; ^{131}I-MIBG scan
LYmphoma: 1% – elderly
Aet: Assoc. Hashimoto's thyroiditis, chronic lymphocytic thyroiditis
PATH: Immunoblastic (large-cell histiocytic)

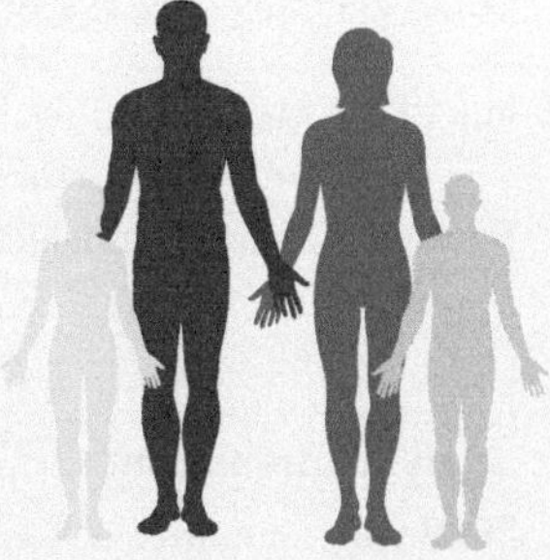

ADRENAL INSUFFICIENCY

Causes

A.D.D.I.S.O.N.'S.

1° Hypoadrenalism ('Addison disease')

PC: Pigmentation
Ix: ACTH ↑

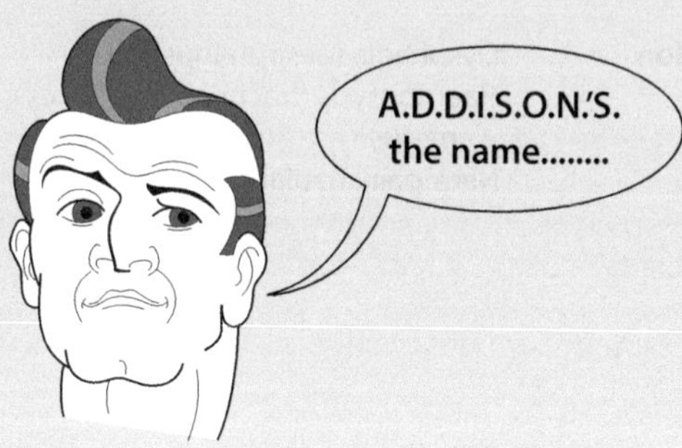

Autoimmune (90%)
F:M = 3:1
Assoc: PGAS-1; 2
Ix: Anti-adrenal Abs (in 50%; may be transient)
Steroid receptor-blocking Abs

Deficiency, enzyme – 1
Congenital adrenal hyperplasia: 21-hydroxylase deficiency (defect in 90%)
PC: Masculinisation of female; male infertility (not all become Addisonian)

Deficiency, enzyme – 2
Adrenoleucodystrophy (X-linked, usually)
PC: Epilepsy, mental retardation, spasticity

Infection: TB
AIDS-related: CMV, histoplasmosis
Meningococcaemia (Waterhouse–Friedrichsen syn.) – adrenal haemorrhagic infarction

Sarcoidosis

Other infiltrative disease: Amyloidosis
Haemochromatosis

Neoplasia: Metastases, esp. from breast
Adrenal vein thrombosis, e.g. from renal cell carcinoma

Surgery: Bilateral adrenalectomy for Cushing disease

2° Hypoadrenalism

PC: No pigmentation. Ix: ACTH ↓
Secondary: Late complication of hypopituitarism
Steroid therapy, during: Withdrawal, after several months of treatment
Intercurrent infection or trauma, when demand exceeds supply

PC

W².A.S.H.E.D. O.U.T.

Weakness/**W**eight loss and anorexia
Abdo pain ↓ ('acute abdomen'): Crisis often triggered by infection, trauma or surgery (i.e. high steroid demand)
Skin
  Hyperpigmentation of skin creases and buccal mucosa (1° hypoadrenalism) – due to high ACTH or melanocyte-stimulating hormone
  Hair loss: Bodily hair, esp. females
  Vitiligo
Hypotension, postural/shock
Eosinophilia: Wheeze, asthma attack
Diarrhoea + vomiting/constipation

O: hyp**O**glycaemia
U&Es: Urea ↑, Na^+ ↓, K^+ ↑, Ca^{2+} ↑ (thiazide-like ↓ Na resorption from distal convoluted tubule)
Thyroid: Hypothyroidism, responsive to steroids

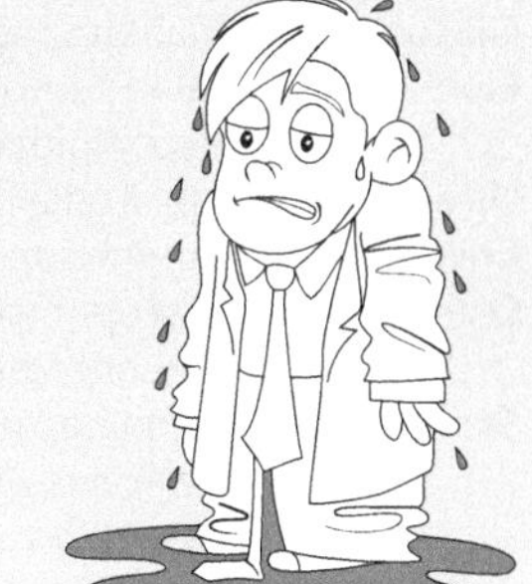

Ix

Plasma cortisol <200 nmol/l
Short Synacthen test (SST)
  Method: Synacthen 250 μg (IV or IM ACTH analogue) → measure cortisol at 0, 30, 60 min (ensure patient switched to dexamethasone or prednisolone first – not hydrocortisone)
  Result: Cortisol >550 nmol/l – normal
  Cortisol <550 nmol/l – adrenocortical insufficiency (1°, 2°)
Differentiation of 1° vs 2° hypoadrenalism
- ACTH – high in 1°, but not 2° hypoadrenalism
- Aldosterone at 30 min into SST: Rise in 2° but not 1° hypoadrenalism
- Depot Synacthen test: Give Synacthen 1 mg IM → measure cortisol at 0, 6 and 24 h
  - No cortisol rise — 1° hypoadrenalism
  - Cortisol peaks at 24 h — 2° hypoadrenalism
  - Cortisol peaks at 6 h (to 900 mmol) — normal

Rx

Acute
- Normal saline infusion; 50% dextrose if hypoglycaemic
- Hydrocortisone 100 mg 4 hrly

Chronic
- Hydrocortisone 20 mg mane + 10 mg evening
- Fludrocortisone 0.1 mg od (not required if on high-dose hydrocortisone, or if 2° hypoadrenalism)

Education: MedicAlert bracelet; double hydrocortisone dose if intercurrent illness

CUSHING SYNDROME

Glucocorticoids enhance breakdown of glycogen and protein to glucose and amino acids, respectively:

G.L.U.C.O.S.E.
A.M.I.N.O. A.C.I.D.s.

Glucose ↑	Diabetes mellitus; hyperphagia
Lipids	Fat redistributed centripetally: Buffalo hump; moon facies; supraclavicular fat pad Hyperlipidaemia
Ulcers, gastric	Esp. if taking NSAIDs
Children	Growth suppression
Osteo-	Osteoporosis esp. vertebral bodies; rib fractures with prominent callus formation Osteonecrosis: Avascular necrosis of bone, esp. femoral head (vasoconstriction)
Skin	Thinning, purple striae (>1 cm wide), bruises, telangiectasia, plethoric cheeks Acne; hirsutism, due to increased androgen secretion from adrenals Hyperpigmentation, due to ACTH excess Poor wound healing
Electrolytes	K^+ ↓; alkalosis, esp. when due to ectopic ACTH
ABP ↑	Diastolic hypertension, due to fluid retention and oedema
Myopathy	Proximal weakness, wasting, hoarseness (inhaled steroids – vocal fold myopathy)
Immunocompromise/**I**nfections	TB reactivation; *Aspergillus* Viruses – extensive disease: Measles; VZV; HSV (corneal dendritic ulcer – topical) Candidiasis, esp. oral with inhaled steroids
Neuropsychiatric	Fatigue Depression; psychosis; mania; emotional lability Primary intracranial hypertension
Ocular	Cataracts Glaucoma usually only from local steroid action (eye drops or nebulizer)
Abdomen	Acute pancreatitis
Coagulopathy	Hypercoagulability, e.g. DVT
Infertility	Amenorrhoea or impotence (pregnancy → fetal adrenal hypoplasia)
Dependence, steroid	Relative hypoadrenalism occurs during infection or trauma, necessitating an increase in steroid dose

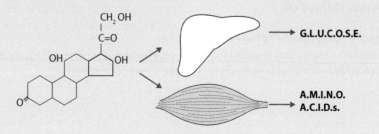

CH_2OH, C=O, OH, OH, O

→ **G.L.U.C.O.S.E.**

→ **A.M.I.N.O. A.C.I.D.s.**

Causes

Plasma cortisol suppressible by high-dose dexamethasone
Pituitary: 'Cushing disease' (60%)
Pituitary microadenoma (<1 cm) = 95% Cushing disease
Epi: Young females (age 25–35; F:M = 3:1)

Plasma cortisol insuppressible by high-dose dexamethasone
Adrenal adenoma/carcinoma/nodular hyperplasia (30%)
Ectopic ACTH or CRH (10%)
e.g. bronchial (small-cell carcinoma or adenoma); ovarian ca.; APUDomas
Epi: Elderly males

Steroid therapy (commonest overall cause)
'PseudoCushing: Alcoholism; depression; obesity; anorexia nervosa

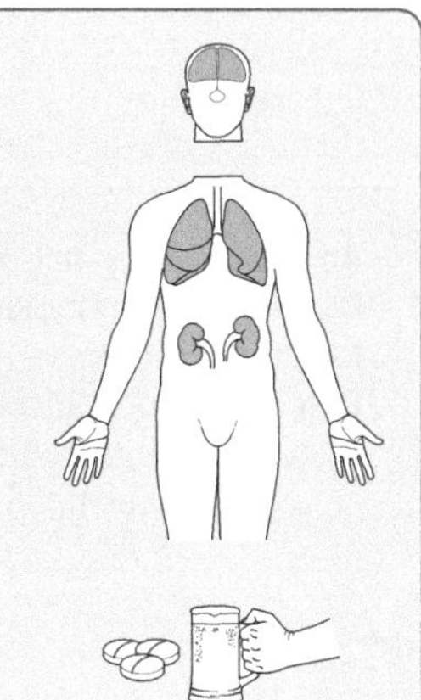

Ix

Bloods: Morning cortisol (normal <700 nmol/l) – screens for Cushing syndrome
ACTH ↑: Ectopic ACTH >> pituitary > adrenal cause
Na^+ ↑; K^+ ↓; Alkalosis – may be only abnormality in ectopic ACTH secretion
FBC: Neutrophilia, lymphopenia

Urine: 24-hour free cortisol: Normal <140 nmol/day
17-Hydroxycorticosteroid: ↑ in pituitary; ectopic ACTH
17-Ketosteroid: ↑ in adrenal carcinoma, ectopic ACTH

Radiol: Pituitary MRI – detects 60% microadenomas
CXR/Chest CT
Abdominal CT:
- Bilateral adrenal hyperplasia
- Adrenal nodules: small = adenoma; large, necrotic = carcinoma

Special: Low-dose dexamethasone (DXM) test
Method: 0.5 mg qds for 2 days (or 1 mg nocte) → measure plasma cortisol next morning
Result: Morning cortisol >140 nmol/l: Cushing syndrome (not 'PseudoCushing')
High-dose dexamethasone (DXM) test
Method: 2 mg qds for 2 days → measure plasma cortisol next morning
Result: Plasma cortisol ↓ to 50% baseline – pituitary (but not macroadenomas)
Plasma cortisol does not suppress – ectopic ACTH; adrenal; steroid Rx
Inferior-petrosal sinus sampling: IV CRH → 60 min sample of sinus and plasma
ACTH and cortisol: ↑ in pituitary cause (bilateral sampling enables localisation)

Rx

Pituitary
Trans-sphenoidal microadenectomy – 80% cure rate; ☠ Panhypopituitarism
Chemical adrenalectomy: Mitotane or 11β-hydroxylase inhibition with metyrapone or ketoconazole
Surgical adrenalectomy ☠ Addison syn; Nelson syn: pigmentation due to pituitary disinhibition

Adrenal
Adenoma: Resection: ☠ Addison due to previous contralateral adrenocortical atrophy
Carcinoma: Resection; mitotane; radiotherapy for bone mets. (overall 5-year SR = 20%)

Ectopic ACTH
Primary tumour: Resection/chemotherapy; Advanced – adrenalectomy as for Cushing disease

HYPERMINERALOCORTICOIDISM

1° Hyper-aldosteronism

Adenoma, adrenal (Conn syndrome) – 75% of primary hyperaldosteronism; esp. women in 30–50s
Bilateral nodular hyperplasia
Carcinoma, adrenal – rare
Defective gene: Glucocorticoid remediable aldosteronism (GRA) – chimeric gene of aldosterone synthase with 11β-hydroxylase-1 promoter, resulting in ACTH-sensitive secretion of aldosterone in zona fasciculata

PC

Hypertension (but no oedema, due to 'aldosterone escape')
Weakness, due to K^+ ↓

Ix

Bloods: K^+ ↓, Mg^{2+} ↓, metabolic alkalosis (Na^+ ↑ uncommon)
Aldosterone ↑↑; renin ↓; ratio of aldosterone (pg/ml):plasma-renin activity >400

- Stop diuretics for 2 weeks; correct K^+
- Prior salt-loading (NaCl 1.2 g od) increases sensitivity, but avoid if SBP >115 mmHg
- Effect of standing on aldosterone: Conn – paradoxical ↓ ; normal or BNH – ↑

Synacthen: Conn – aldosterone slight ↑; BNH – no effect; GRA – aldosterone ↑↑

Radiol: High-resolution CT: Adenomas >1 cm; BNH – bilateral adrenal cortex enlargement
Selective adrenal vein catheterisation: Compare aldosterone:cortisol ratio from each side
Radiolabelled cholesterol + dexamethasone (inhibits normal steroidogenesis): uni- vs bilateral

Rx

Adenoma or ca. – surgery; BNH – spironolactone, amiloride; GRA – dexamethasone (↓ACTH)

2° Hyper-aldosteronism

Primary hyper-reninism: Renin-secreting renal or ovarian tumour
Renovascular disease: Renal artery stenosis; malignant hypertension
Gitelman syndrome: ↓ NaCl resorption in distal convoluted tubule defect → thiazide-like diuresis
Bartter syndrome: ↓ NaCl resorption in ascending loop of Henle → frusemide-like diuresis
Hypovolaemia: Congestive cardiac failure, hypoalbuminaemia, profuse sweating

PC

Renovascular: Hypertension, weakness due to K^+ ↓
G/B/H: Hypotension, weakness due to K^+ ↓, Mg^{2+} ↓

Ix

Bloods: Na^+, Cl^-, K^+, Mg^{2+} – all ↓; renin ↑
Urine: Ca^{2+}: Gitelman – ↓ Bartter – ↑ (also, prostaglandins ↑)

Rx

Bartter – amiloride, ACE inhibitor, indomethacin (reverses juxtaglomerular hypertrophy)

Hypo-aldosteronism ('apparent hypermineralocorticoidism')

Adrenal hyperplasia, congenital – 11β-hydroxylase or 17α-hydroxylase deficiency (autosomal recessive)
Adrenal insuffiency, primary
Aldosterone synthase deficiency

NB: Hyporeninemic hypoaldosteronism is a common result of diabetic nephropathy (type 4 renal tubular acidosis)

PC

Virilisation of females – 11β-hydroxylase deficiency
Hypogonadism –17α-hydroxylase deficiency
Palpitations and arrythmia due to hyperkalaemia

Ix

Bloods: Hyperkalaemia
11-deoxycorticosterone ↑ in congenital adrenal hyperplasia and DOComas
Urine: Ratio of urine cortisol:cortisone ↑ in 11βHSD deficiency

Rx

Congenital adrenal hyperplasia, 11βHSD deficiency – dexamethasone

STEROID SYNTHESIS

The three main steroid types, mineralocorticoids (aldosterone), glucocorticoids (cortisol) and sex steroids are synthesized in the outer, middle and inner layers of the adrenal cortex, respectively

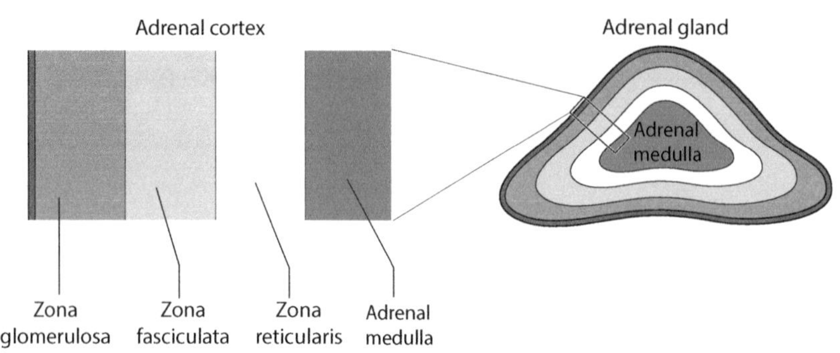

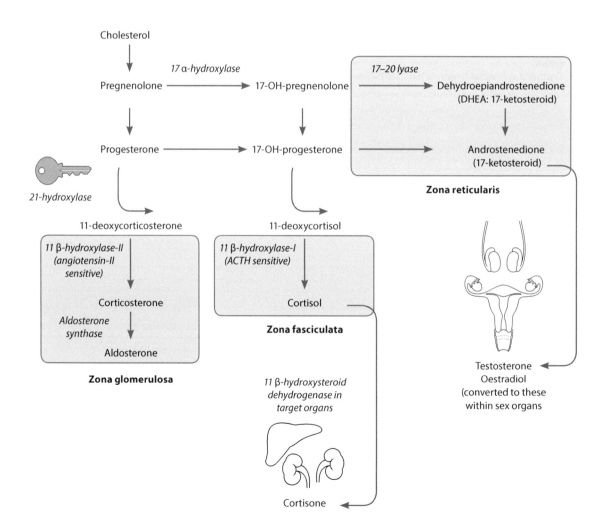

Cholesterol → Pregnenolone

Pregnenolone → (*17 α-hydroxylase*) → 17-OH-pregnenolone → (*17–20 lyase*) → Dehydroepiandrostenedione (DHEA: 17-ketosteroid)

Pregnenolone → Progesterone

17-OH-pregnenolone → 17-OH-progesterone

Dehydroepiandrostenedione (DHEA: 17-ketosteroid) → Androstenedione (17-ketosteroid)

Progesterone → 17-OH-progesterone → Androstenedione (17-ketosteroid)

Zona reticularis

21-hydroxylase

Progesterone → 11-deoxycorticosterone

17-OH-progesterone → 11-deoxycortisol

11-deoxycorticosterone → (*11 β-hydroxylase-II (angiotensin-II sensitive)*) → Corticosterone → (*Aldosterone synthase*) → Aldosterone

Zona glomerulosa

11-deoxycortisol → (*11 β-hydroxylase-I (ACTH sensitive)*) → Cortisol

Zona fasciculata

Cortisol → (*11 β-hydroxysteroid dehydrogenase in target organs*) → Cortisone

Androstenedione → Testosterone Oestradiol (converted to these within sex organs)

AMENORRHOEA – CAUSES

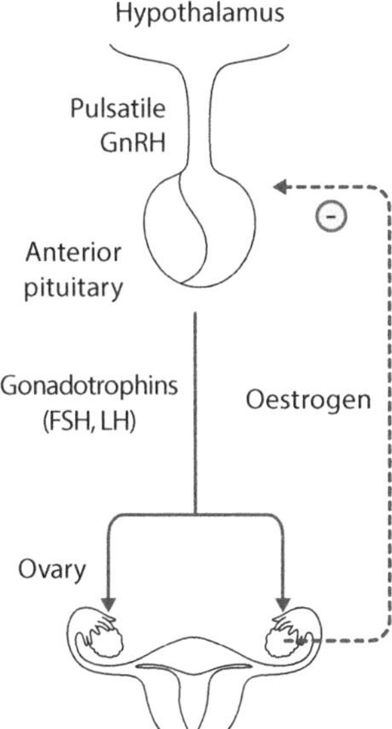

Hypothalamus–pituitary

Constitutional
Delayed puberty (inherited)
Anorexia, anxiety, exercise, severe illness

Hypothalamus–pituitary

D.I.V.I.N.I.T.Y.

Developmental: Kallman syndrome = failure of migration of GnRH cells from olfactory epithelium
Infection: TB, meningitis
Vascular: Infarction
Inflammation: Hypohysitis
Neoplasia:
- Craniopharyngioma, pinealoma
- Pituitary adenoma

Injury: Surgery, radiotherapy
Toxins, e.g. neuroleptics
Y: h**Y**drocephalus

Endocrine
Prolactin ↑
T4: ↑ or ↓
Cortisol: ↑ or ↓

Oestrogen excess

Mechanism: Excess, acyclical oestrogen switches off pituitary gonadotrophs; breakthrough bleeding may occur

Pregnancy; 'Pill'; post-pill

Ovarian tumour, oestrogen-secreting
Granulosa-theca cell
Mucinous
Brenner

Hyperandrogenism
Mechanism: Androgens are aromatized to oestrogen in adipose tissue

Causes:
Polycystic ovaries syndrome
Epi: 10% of women, esp. obese
PATH: Exaggerated adrenarche (adrenal androgens at puberty)
Ix: US ovaries
Androstendione and free testosterone ↑ ↑LH to FSH ratio
Cushing syndrome
Carcinoma: Adrenal, ovarian
Female pseudo-hermaphroditism

Amenorrhoea – Causes continued →

Amenorrhoea – Causes continued

Primary ovarian failure

Menopause

Congenital

Turner syn. (XO or mosaic with XX or XY)
17, 20-desmolase or 17α-hydroxylase deficiency
Galactosaemia – galactose toxic to ovaries

Acquired <40 years (premature ovarian failure)

T.A.I.N.T.

Toxins – chemotherapy, radiotherapy, smoking
Autoimmune – oophoritis
Schmidt syn.= oophoritis + thyroiditis + Addison
Infection – mumps, chlamydia, gonorrhoea (pelvic inflammatory disease)
Neoplasia, ovarian
Temporary resistant ovary syndrome: Normal oestrogen and follicles, but ovaries become FSH insensitive

Genital tract

Intersex

Androgen insensitivity syndrome: Male karyotype (XY), female phenotype (female external genitalia, no uterus)
5α reductase deficiency: XY karyotype, may be phenotypically female or male, tends to virilize at 12 years
Congenital adrenal hyperplasia:

- 21-hydroxylase deficiency (95% of cases)
- 11β-hydroxylase deficiency
- 3β-hydroxysteroid dehydrogenase deficiency

Congenital

Müllerian agenesis: Vaginal or uterine atresia
Imperforate hymen or vaginal septae
Extreme female genital mutilation, e.g. infibulation

Acquired

Cervical stenosis, e.g. 2° to electrocautery
Asherman syndrome: Intrauterine synechiae secondary to curettage
TB, trauma (incl. hysterectomy!)

AMENORRHOEA – PC

Types

Primary amenorrhoea: No menses by 15 years old
Secondary amenorrhoea: Failure of previously normal menses

Most causes of amenorrhoea may present in either way, including congenital causes that may present as secondary amenorrhoea

PC

The cause may be suggested by the patient's **S.H.A.P.E.**

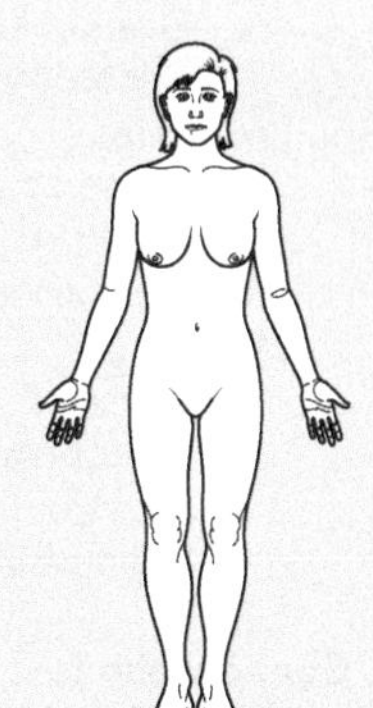

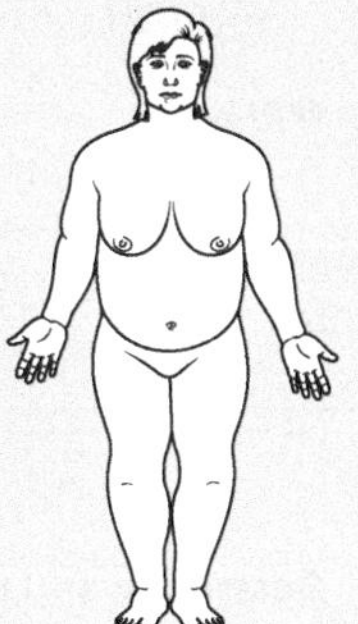

Syndrome, congenital

Turner syndrome (XO):
- Short stature, shield chest, wide-carrying angle
- Coarctation of aorta, ASD, mild learning disability, acalculia

Enzyme defect: Tall stature (failure of epiphyseal closure by oestrogen)
Kallman syndrome (X-linked): Puberty delay; anosmia, sensorineural deafness, colour blind; renal agenesis, short metacarpals, bimanual synkinesia

Hair

Hairy and obese – PCOS
- Acne, hirsutism on upper lip; subumbilical; thigh
- Associated acanthosis nigricans, diabetic retinopathy, etc.

Hairy and medium – other causes of virilisation and hirsutism:
- Congenital adrenal hyperplasia (21- or 11β-hydroxylase deficiency)
- Adrenal carcinoma

Hairy and thin – anorexia nervosa: Lanugo
Hairless (pubic hair absence):
- Androgen insensitivity syndrome
- Delayed puberty (small breasts)

ABP
- Hypertension: 17α or 11β-hydroxylase deficiency
- Hypotension: 21-hydroxylase deficiency; Addison

Private parts

Vagina:
- Haematocolpos: Imperforate hymen/vaginal septae – cyclical pain
- Blind-ending: Mullerian agenesis or androgen insensitivity
- Vulval atrophy: Ovarian failure

Cliteromegaly/labial enlargement or fusion:
- Polycystic ovaries syndrome
- Congenital adrenal hyperplasia (21- or 11β-hydroxylase deficiency)
- Adrenal carcinoma

Breasts:
- Enlargement: Oestrogen-secreting tumour
- Atrophy: Ovarian failure

Endocrine

Menopause (ovarian or hypothal–pit. failure): Hot flushes, night sweats, headaches, osteoporosis
Puberty: Precocious or delayed:
Addison: 21-hydroxylase deficiency or Schmidt syndrome (autoimmune) – latter also assoc. with hypothyroidism

AMENORRHOEA – IX

Hypothalamus–pituitary

Pituitary hormones

FSH:

Low:

- Pituitary failure
- Polycystic ovaries (elevated androgens)
- Genital tract defect (normal oestrogen levels)

High:

- Ovarian failure (as no –ve feedback)

Prolactin:

- Cause of amenorrhoea
- Also raised in PCOS

TSH, T4:

- Cause of amenorrhoea
- Also low in hypopituitarism

Gonadorelin test

Inject GnRH (IV or SC) →
FSH + LH ↑↑ in Kallman syn.
FSH + LH ↓ in hypopituitarism

MRI head

- Pituitary tumour, esp. prolactinoma
- Craniopharyngioma

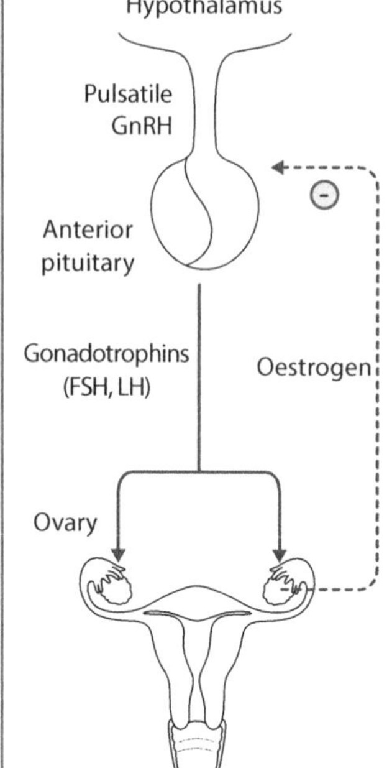

Oestrogen excess

Androgens

Serum testosterone ↑:

- DHEA ↑
- Androstenedione ↑ (principal circulating androgen)

Sex-hormone-binding globulin ↓ (binds testosterone preferentially)

Urine 17-ketosteroids ↑↑:

- PCOS
- Congenital adrenal hyperplasia
- Adrenal or ovarian carcinoma (dexamethasone suppresses 17-KS in PCOS and CAH, but not carcinoma)

Other bloods

β-HCG: pregnant?!
Glucose ↑: PCOS

Pelvic-abdominal USS

PCOS: Bilateral, multiple, small follicular cysts in 'necklace' around edge – stromal, endometrial hyperplasia
Adrenal or ovarian carcinoma

Ovaries

Oestrogen and progesterone

Low:

- Ovarian failure
- Pituitary failure
- Testicular feminisation

Variable: PCOS
Cyclical: Distinguishes vaginal obstruction (cyclical) from androgen insensitivity (acyclical)

Sex chromosome analysis

Turner syndrome (+ PCR of sex-determining region of Y)

Autoimmune cause:

AutoAbs: Anti-ovarian – thyroid; adrenal Abs
Glucose: Diabetes mellitus occurs as part of Schmidt syndrome

Genital tract

Cervical mucus analysis

Stretchiness
Ferning on microscopy

Progestagen withdrawal bleed

Method:

- Exclude pregnancy
- Give medroxyprogesterone for 5 days; then stop
- If no bleed then give oral conjugated oestrogen for 14 days prior (to prime uterus)

Results:

- Bleed: PCOS or other excess oestrogen
- Bleed after oestrogen: Pituitary or ovarian failure
- No bleed: Genital tract damage

Hysterosalpingogram or hysteroscopy

Cervical stenosis/Asherman syndrome

AMENORRHOEA – RX

Hypothalamus–pituitary

Gonadotrophins/GnRH

Human menopausal gonadotrophins (or purified FSH) + mid-cycle β-HCG (simulates LH)

Pulsatile GnRH in portable infusion pump: Improves efficacy of gonadotrophins

Clomiphene

Oestrogen partial agonist: FSH ↑

Ovary stimulant

Prolactinoma treatment

Dopamine agonists

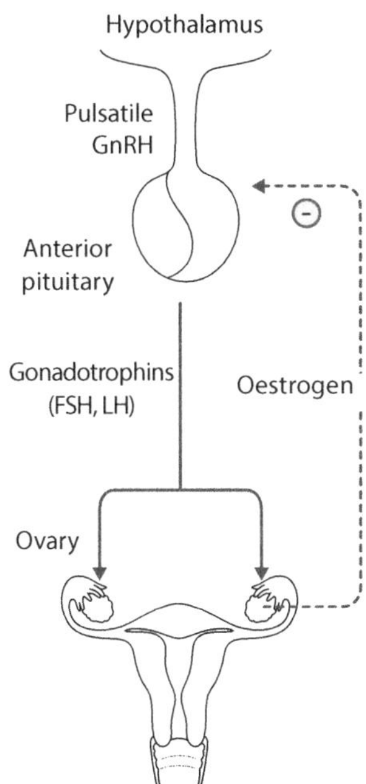

PCOS

Hormonal

Gonadotrophins/GnRH/clomiphene: ↑ fertility by ↑ FSH

Buserelin: ↓ LH

OCP: ↓ ovarian and adrenal androgen production

Obesity

Diet

Insulin sensitizers (metformin):

- ↓ ovarian androgen production by ↓ insulin secretion, as insulin has direct ovarian effect
- ↑ fertility, but stop drug in pregnancy

Hirsutism

Topical: Epilation, electrolysis, cover-up, H_2O_2 bleach

'Dianette'= cyproterone acetate (anti-androgen) + ethinylE2 (contraceptive, as cyproterone is teratogenic)

Electrocautery of cysts

Wedge resection of large cysts: ↓ ovarian androgen production and ovarian adhesions

Primary ovarian failure

If fertility desired: Ovum donation + cyclical gonadotrophins

If fertility not desired:

Combined OCP:

- Regularizes periods
- ↓ ovarian androgen production

HRT (conjugated oestrogens + progestagen): Used in ovarian or pituitary failure as prophylaxis against osteoporosis

Turner XY mosaic: Gonadectomy, as at risk of dysgerminoma

Genital tract

Surgery

Cervical stenosis/Asherman syndrome – dilatation

MALE SEXUAL PROBLEMS

Gynaecomastia

Causes

P.E.C.T.O.R.A.L.I.s.

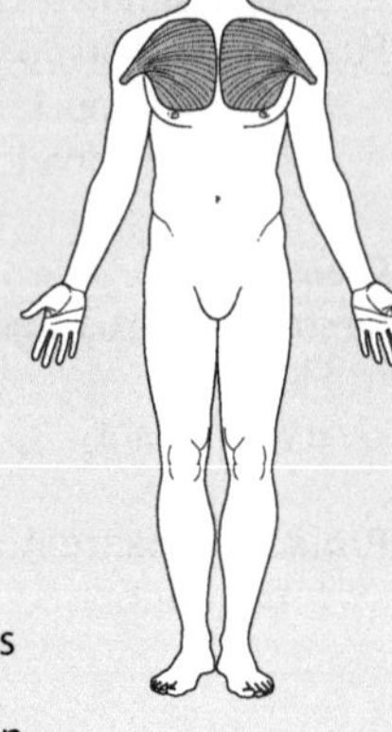

Physiological
  Neonatal, puberty (often unilateral; resolves within 1 year), elderly
Endocrine
  Hypogonadism:
  - Hypogonadotrophic: Kallman syn., hypopituitarism, hyperprolactinaemia
  - Hypergonadotrophic, e.g. Klinefelter, mumps orchitis, orchidectomy

  Other: Thyrotoxicosis, Cushing (both ↑aromatase activity), diabetes
Carcinoma
  Testis tumour
  Adrenal tumour
  Ectopic: Bronchial, liver, renal
Toxins – **C.U.P.S.**
  Cardiac: Spironolactone, digoxin, amiodarone, calcium antagonists
  Ulcer: Cimetidine, proton-pump inhibitors
  Psychiatric: Anti-dopaminergics, TCAs, opiates, cannabis, amphetamines
  Steroids: Goserelin, flutamide, ketoconazole, metronidazole, anabolic steroids
Organ failure
  Cirrhosis: Sex-hormone-binding globulin ↑, testis atrophy, alcohol ↑ oestrogen
  Chronic renal failure: Prolactin ↑; testicular failure
Refeeding syndrome – post-fast
Adrenal: Congenital adrenal hyperplasia (excess testosterone)
Local stimulation (via hyperprolactinaemia): Breast cancer, VZV, thoracotomy
Infection: TB, HIV

Rx

Medical: Testosterone, danazol, tamoxifen, stop causative drug
Surgical: Reduction mammoplasty + liposuction

Impotence

Causes

P.A.T.E.N.T.S.

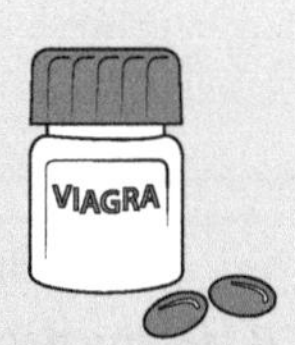

Psychological: Anxiety, depression
Arterial:
  Aorto-iliac thrombosis (Leriche syndrome)
  Sickle-cell anaemia
Toxins-1: Alcohol or drug abuse
Endocrine:
  Diabetes mellitus (autonomic neuropathy, arteriopathy)
  Hypogonadism; hyperprolactinaemia – dysthyroidism
Neurological: Autonomic neuropathy; cord disease, esp. MS; cauda equina lesion
Toxins-2 – as for gynaecomastia **(C.U.P.S.)**, e.g. spironolactone, digoxin, β-blockers, α_1-antagonists
Systemic: Liver, renal failure, carcinoma

Rx

Medical (oral): Phosphodiesterase-5 inhibitors (sildenafil, tadalafil)
Intra-urethral or intracavernosal alprostadil
Prosthesis or vacuum
Psychotherapy

MALE INFERTILITY

Hypothalamus–pituitary

Constitutional

Anorexia: Anxiety, severe illness, e.g. organ failure, carcinoma

Hypothalamus–pituitary

D.I.V.I.N.I.T.Y.

Developmental:

- Kallman syndrome
- Prader-Willi syndrome
- Spinocerebellar ataxia

Infection: TB, meningitis
Vascular: Infarction
Inflammation: Sarcoid
Neoplasia:

- Craniopharyngioma
- Pituitary adenoma

Injury: Surgery, radiotherapy
Toxins, e.g. neuroleptics
Y: h**Y**drocephalus

Endocrine

- GH ↑or ↓
- Prolactin ↑
- T4↑t or ↓

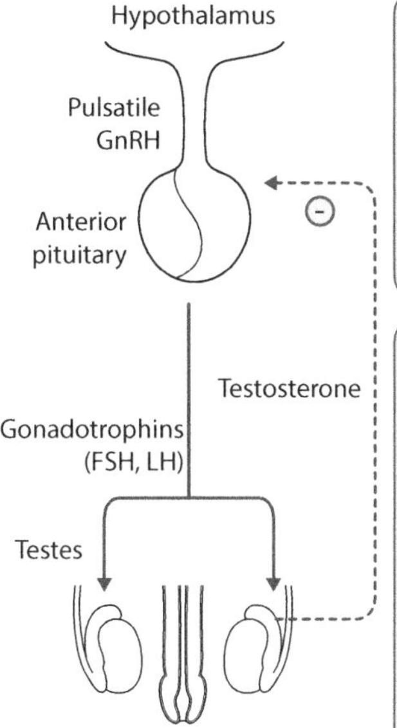

Oestrogen excess

Congential adrenal hyperplasia

Cushing syndrome (and Addison disease)

Anabolic steroids

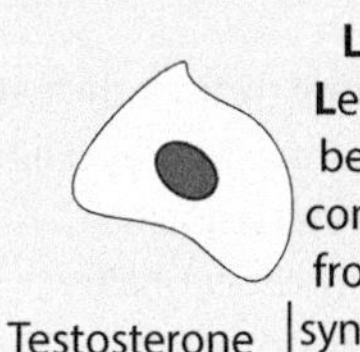

Leydig cells – **L**et testosterone be produced by converting DHEA from adrenals or synthesize *de novo* (**L**H-responsive)

Testosterone

Interstitium

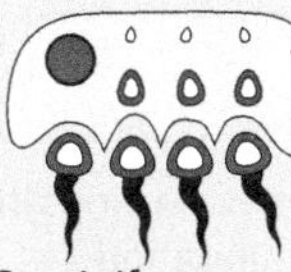

Sertoli cells – **S**uckle developing germ cells and spermatids (F**S**H-responsive)

Seminiferous tubule

Primary testicular failure

Congenital

Klinefelter syndrome (XXY):

- Small, firm testes, but potent
- Gynaecomastia, breast carcinoma
- Other: Gigantism, short spine, long limbs, high voice, learning disability, unemotional

Androgen resistance:

- 5α-reductase deficiency
- Myotonic dystrophy
- Spinobulbar muscular atrophy

Acquired

T.A.I.N.T³.

Toxins:

- Chemo-, radiotherapy, smoking, alcohol
- Digoxin, spironolactone
- Sulphasalazine, phenytoin, nitrofurantoin

Autoimmune: Polyarteritis nodosa orchitis
Infection: Mumps, mycoplasma, TB, STD (gonococcus, chlamydia)
Neoplasia, testis
Temperature ↑: Crytorchidism, varicocoele
Torsion/**T**rauma, incl. hernia repair

Spermatazoa defects

Genetic – 60% cases of male infertility!

Microdeletions Yq xsome, incl.:

- Azoospermia factor (AZF)
- Deleted in azoospermia (DAZ)

Germinal- or Leydig-cell aplasia

Autoimmune

Membrane-bound anti Ig-A (incl. vasectomy, infection, familial)

Immotility

Cystic fibrosis primary ciliary dysmotility

Kartagener syndrome: Associated dextrocardia, bronchiectasis, sinusitis

PRECOCIOUS PUBERTY

Def

Development of secondary sexual characteristics <8 years (in girls) or <9 years (boys)

True

Def: Premature activation of hypothalamo-pituitary-gonadal axis

Causes

D.I.V.I.N.E^2.

Developmental – idiopathic: Accounts for 2/3 of cases; girls > boys; often familial
Infection: Meningo-encephalitis, congenital infections
Vascular: Perinatal anoxia
Injury, head/hydrocephalus
Neoplasia – hypothalamic: Craniopharyngioma, hamartoma, neurofibroma
Epilepsy, idiopathic
Endocrine: Hypothyroidism → **FSH**↑

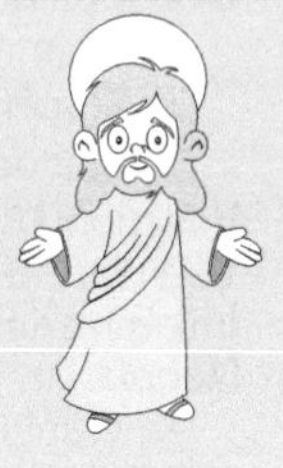
D.I.V.I.N.E.

PC

Boys: Spermatogenesis + virilisation
Girls: Periods + feminisation
i.e. appropriate sexual characteristics – isosexual
Growth spurt; eventual short stature (premature epiphyseal fusion)

Ix

Bloods: FSH ↑, LH ↓: Gonadorelin challenge → LH ↑ > FSH ↑

Rx

Long-acting gonadorelin analogue (goserelin): ↓ gonadotrophins

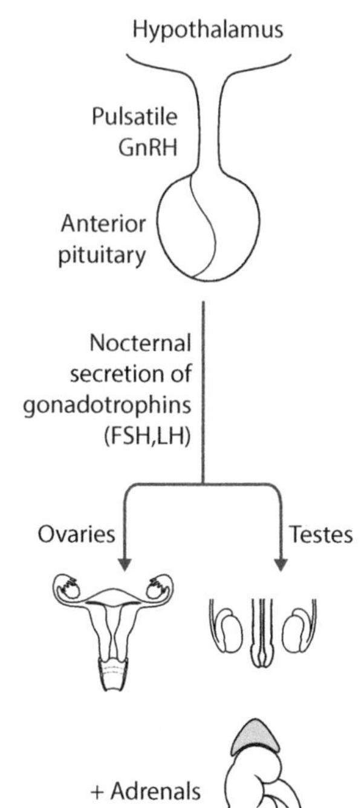

Pseudo

Def: Excess sex steroids or activation of steroid receptors, independent of HPA axis

Causes

G.A.M.E^2.S.

Gonadal tumour:
- Testis (teratoma, Leydig cell)
- Ovarian tumour (granulosa cell) or ovarian cysts

Adrenal:
- Congenital adrenal hyperplasia
- Adrenal tumour (suggested by >6 cm mass in adrenals)

McCune–Albright syndrome:
PATH: Autonomous LH receptor activity, via mutated Gsα
PC: Polyostotic fibrous dysplasia; café-au-lait spots

Exogenous sex steroids/**E**ctopic gonadotrophins:
Hepatoblastoma; pineal dysgerminoma → β-HCG, AFP

Syndrome – testotoxicosis: LH receptor mutation on Leydig cells, in boys only

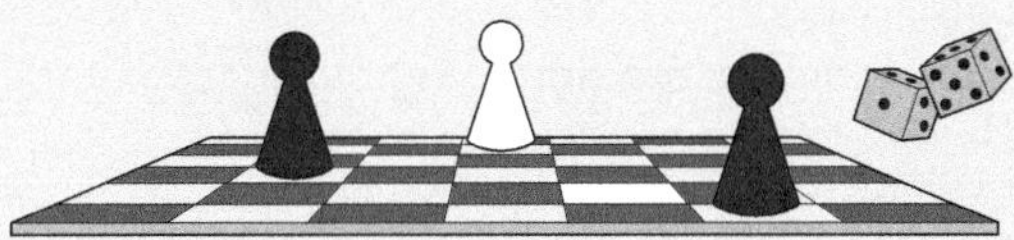

PC

Secondary sexual characteristics only

Ix

Bloods: FSH ↓, LH ↓; gonadorelin challenge → no response
Urine: 17-ketosteroids ↑: Gonadal or adrenal cause; dexamethasone → 17-KS ↓ in congenital adrenal hyperplasia
Radiol: MRI or CT adrenals; USS testes or pelvis

Rx

Medical
Medroxyprogesterone acetate, ketoconazole
Anti-androgens: Cyproterone acetate, spironolactone

DELAYED PUBERTY

Def

No development of secondary sexual characteristics by 14 years

Hypothalamic–pituitary failure

Causes

D.I.V.I.N.E.

Developmental:
- Idiopathic: Commonest cause in boys; often familial
- Kallman syndrome:
  - Anosmia, due to failure of GnRH cells to migrate from olfactory mucosa (also deaf occasionally)
  - Cryptorchidism, microphallus, renal agenesis
- Other syndromes:
  - Prader–Willi (hyperphagia, hypersomnolence, diabetes)
  - Lawrence–Moon–Biedl (retinitis pigmentosa, polydactyly, cardiac defects)

Infection: Meningo-encephalitis, TB
Very ill, incl. anorexia, anxiety, strenuous exercise
Inflammation: Sarcoid, SLE
Neoplasia: Hypothalamic craniopharyngioma, hamartoma
Endocrine:
- Hypopituitarism or 'isolated gonadotrophin deficiency'
- Hyperprolactinaemia
- Thyroid or cortisol abnormalities (high or low); diabetes

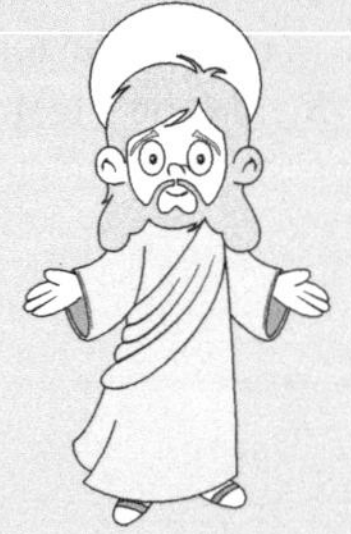

D.I.V.I.N.E.

Ix

Bloods: FSH ↓, LH ↑

Rx

Pulsatile gonadorelin or gonadotrophins

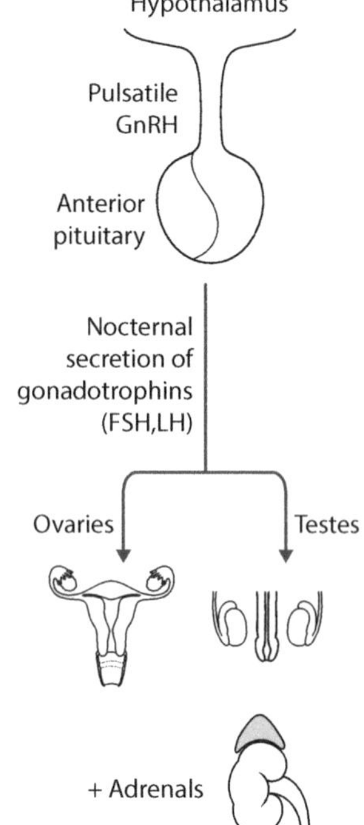

Gonadal failure

Causes

Congenital

Turner syndrome (XO or mosaic with XX or XY): Commonest cause in girls
PC: Webbed neck, wide-carrying angle, coarctation
Enzyme defect, e.g. 17α-hydroxylase deficiency
Klinefelter syndrome (XXY):

- Small, firm testes, azoospermia (but not impotent)
- Gynaecomastia, breast carcinoma
- Eunuchoidal: Gigantism (short spine, long limbs), high voice, learning disability, aggressive

Acquired

T.A.I.N.T.

Toxins: Chemotherapy, radiotherapy, surgery, smoking
Autoimmune, incl. Schmidt syndrome
Infection: Mumps, chlamydia (PID) oophoritis
Neoplasia, testis or ovarian
Trauma: Testis torsion

Ix

Bloods: FSH ↑, LH ↑
Karyotype/buccal smear for Barr body (sex chromatin)

Rx

Anabolic steroids; Ethinylestradiol + progestagen

NEUROENDOCRINE TUMOURS

Neuroendocrine tumours are mostly derived from neural-crest cells, and secrete amines or peptides. They are also known as APUDomas as they all exhibit 'amine precursor uptake and decarboxylation'

C.A.P.I.T.A.L.S.

APUD

Carcinoid tumours/syndrome – *see p. 370*
Adrenal phaeochromocytoma
Pancreatic endocrine tumours incl.:
  Islet-cell tumours
Thyroid medullary carcinoma
Additional – CNS ganglioblastoma, neuroblastoma, paragangliomas
Lung – small-cell carcinoma
Skin – melanoma

Ix

Most can be detected with an ^{131}I-MIBG scan

Adrenal phaeochromocytoma

Epi

10% Familial MEN-2a, b syndromes, neurofibromatosis 1, von Hippel–Lindau syn.
10% Bilateral (50% of familial are bilateral)
10% Malignant
10% Extra-adrenal, e.g.

- Organ of Zuckerkandl (sympathetic ganglia below inferior mesenteric artery)
- Bladder wall: Symptoms triggered by micturition!

PC

Paroxysmal hypertension: Weakness, anxiety, tremor, sweat, headache, N+V, for 15 min
Postural hypotension (due to decreased plasma volume)
Palpitations, ischaemic heart disease, cardiomyopathy
Pallor (not flushing)
Pain (chest, epigastric, abdominal due to constipation)

Ix

Bloods: Chromogranin A ↑
Glucose ↑
Urine: 24-hour acid urine collection: VMA, HMMA, metadrenaline, free catecholamines ↑
Radiol: CT, MRI abdo
^{131}I-MIBG scan
Special: Pentolinium suppression test

Rx

Crisis: IV phentolamine or labetalol
Surgery: Requires pre-operative phenoxybenzamine + β-blocker for 3 weeks
Metastases: ^{131}I-MIBG

PANCREATIC ENDOCRINE TUMOURS (PETS)

G.I.V.E²̣.S. GAS.

Glucagonoma (α-cells)
PC: Diarrhoea, loss of weight
Diabetes mellitus
Necrolytic migratory erythema, glossitis–stomatitis, nail dystrophy
Deep-vein thrombosis
Ix: Failure of glucose suppression following arginine stimulation
Insulinoma (β-cells) – *Most common*
PC: Fasting hypoglycaemia (see p. 330)
Ix: Proinsulin:insulin ratio increased, C-peptide raised
VLPoma = 'Werner–Morrison syn.' (δ1-cells: Vasoactive intestinal peptide)
PC: **W**atery **D**iarrhoea (>1 l/day) with **H**ypokalaemia and **A**chlorhydria (**W.D.H.A.**)
Ectopic endocrine secretions: GHRH – acromegaly; ACTH – Cushing; ADH – SIADH; PTH – hyperPTHism
Extra diarrhoea-causing secretions: PPoma (pancreatic polypeptide), neurotensinoma, calcitoninoma
Somatostatinoma (δ-cells)
PC: Diarrhoea, loss of weight, steatorrhoea
Gallstones (relaxes gallbladder)
Diabetes mellitus, hypertension

GAStrinoma = Zollinger–Ellison syndrome' – *2nd most common*
Epi: 30% MEN-I syndrome; 10% multiple
Site: Islet cells; duodenum or adjacent to (G-cells); ectopic (parathyroid, ovary)
PC: Peptic ulcers – multiple
Diarrhoea, malabsorption, steatorrhoea, vitamin B12 deficiency
Ix: Fasting serum gastrin (stop PPI/H2-antagonists for 1/52)
Secretin test (IV): Paradoxical ↑ in gastrin (normally gastrin suppressed)
CT abdomen, selective angiography of pancreas

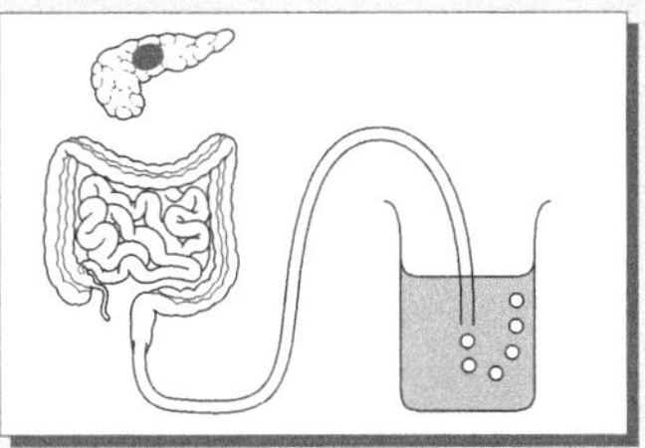

Rx

Somatostatin analogue (octreotide or lanreotide): Improves diarrhoea in all
Specific:

- Glucagonoma: Zinc, high-protein diet, aspirin (not warfarin)
- Insulinoma: Diazoxide, streptozocin
- Gastrinoma: High-dose omeprazole

Prog

About 2/3 of all islet-cell tumours metastasize (except insulinoma 10%; gastrinoma 30%)

CARCINOID TUMOURS

Def

Carcinoid tumours are one of the APUDomas, characterized by silver staining and the presence of cell markers chromogranin A, neuron-specific enolase and synaptophysin (on immunofluorescence), and somatostatin receptors

Carcinoid syndrome occurs when a carcinoid tumour secretes biologically active peptides that reach the systemic circulation. The main secreted products are 5-hydroxytryptamine (5-HT or serotonin), tachykinins (substance P) and prostaglandins

Carcinoid tumours – local

GIT

- Abdominal pain, GI bleeding, obstruction
- Peritoneal fibrosis (esp. midgut or ovarian carcinoid)

Bronchial

- Cough, haemoptysis, incidental finding on CXR

Carcinoid syndrome – systemic

F².I.V.E. H.T. A.M.i.N.E

Flushing/**F**acial oedema
    Acute paroxysms of flushing, wheals, pruritus, lacrimation, salivation, hypotension that last 5 min to days
    Triggered by alcohol, cheese, straining, salbutamol
    Causes of flushing: **M.A.M.A².**
        Menopause, **A**lcohol, **M**astocytosis, **A**PUDoma, **A**utonomic neuropathy
Intestinal – diarrhoea, weight loss
Valve fibrosis – right-sided lesions (e.g. pulmonary stenosis), except bronchial carcinoid (left side)
E – Wh**EE**ze (esp. foregut tumours)

Hypoglycaemia
Telangiectasia, facial cyanosis – due to repeated attacks of flushing

Arthritis
Metastases – liver (hepatosplenomegaly), bone (pain)
Nicotinamide deficiency ('pellagra') – dermatitis of sun-exposed areas
Endocrine – multiple endocrine neoplasia (MEN-1):
    Acromegaly (GHRH secreted by bronchial carcinoid)
    Cushing syndrome (thymic carcinoid)
    HyperPTHism

HO — $CH_2CH_2NH_2$ — N H

Epi

The proportion of **carcinoid tumours is:**

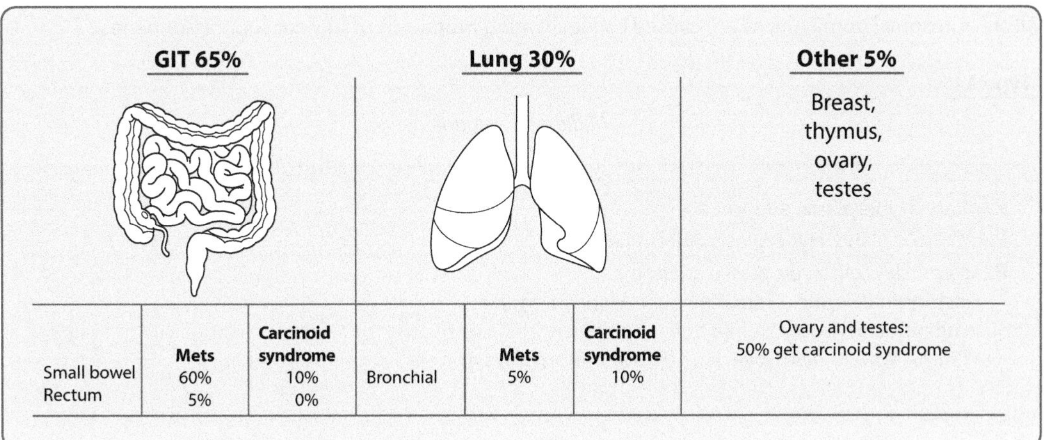

	Mets	Carcinoid syndrome		Mets	Carcinoid syndrome	
Small bowel	60%	10%	Bronchial	5%	10%	Ovary and testes: 50% get carcinoid syndrome
Rectum	5%	0%				

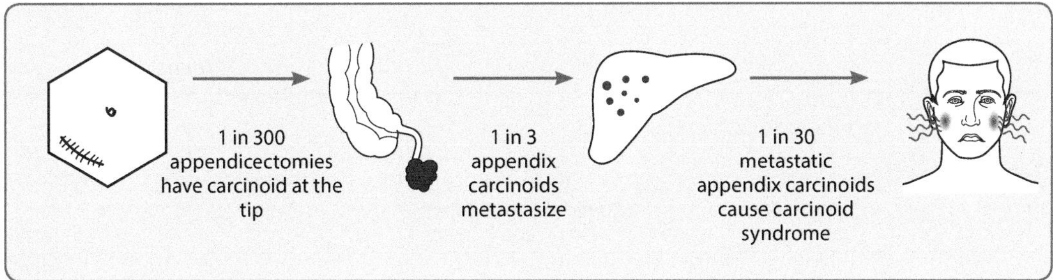

Ix

Bloods: 5-HT, 5-hydroxytryptophan (5-HTP), histamine, chromogranin A ↑

Urine: 5-hydroxyindoleacetic-acid (5-HIAA) ↑ – levels act as prognostic marker

- False +ve: Walnuts, bananas, paracetamol, aspirin, levodopa
- False −ve: Atypical foregut carcinoids (urine 5-HT or 5-HTP ↑ instead)

Radiol: CT/MRI
Selective angiography
Octreotide scintigraphy: Ligand for type 2 somatostatin receptors on tumour

Special: Provocative flushing with pentagastrin or adrenaline

Rx

Symptomatic:

Flushing: Somatostatin analogue (octreotide), diphenhydramine, ranitidine
Diarrhoea: Ketanserin, ondansetron
Wheeze: Aminophylline, steroids (avoid salbutamol!)

Curative:

Resection: Localized tumour or limited hepatic metastases
Hepatic artery embolisation
Chemotherapy/radiotherapy: Streptozocin, doxorubicin, interferon-α, ^{131}I-MIBG

Prog

5-year survival rate: Local, 95%; lymph nodes, 65%; hepatic, 20%
Tumours <1 cm – curable; >2 cm – frequently metastasize

MULTIPLE ENDOCRINE NEOPLASIA

All are autosomal dominant; all are caused by inactivating mutations of tumour suppressor genes

Type 1

Midline **'P'** *organs*

Pituitary: Hyperplasia, adenoma
Parathyroid gland: Hyperplasia, adenoma
Pancreas islet cell: Hyperplasia, adenoma
  Gastrinoma: Peptic ulcers (Zollinger–Ellinson syn.)
  Insulinoma: Hypoglycaemia
  VIPoma: Watery diarrhoea, $K^+ \downarrow$ (Werner–Morrison syn.)

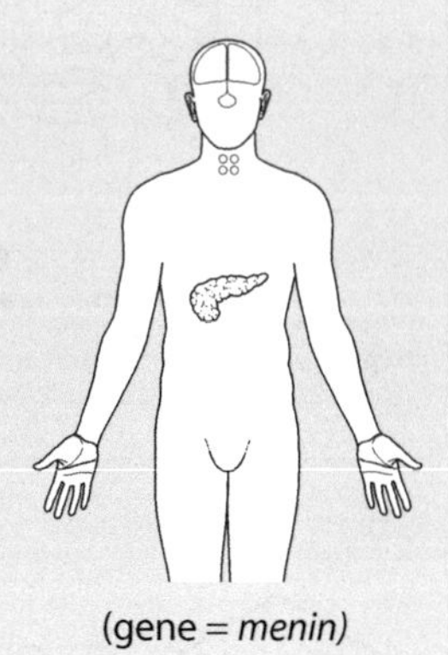

(gene = *menin)*

Type 2

Paired (i.e. 2) organs

Thyroid: Medullary carcinoma

Adrenals: Phaeochromocytoma

Type 2A
PAr**A**thyroid adenoma
Anus: Hirschsprung disease
Amyloid: Cutaneous lichen planus

Type 2B
Big: Marfanoid habitus
Big tumours: Mucosal, GIT neuromas

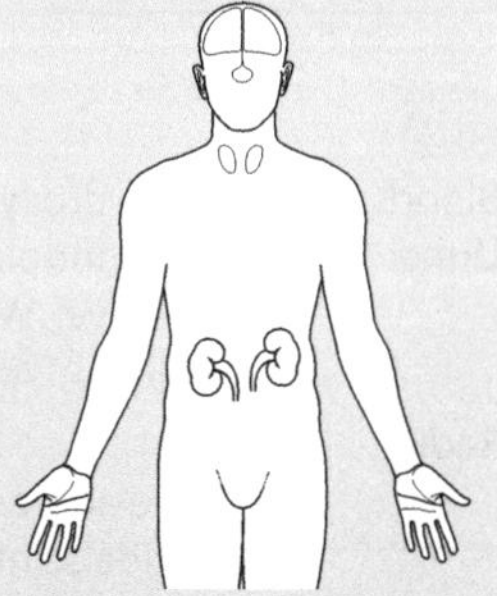

('**Re**arranged during **t**ransfection') = tyrosine kinase

Other

Carney's complex:
  Adrenal, testicular, pituitary adenomas
  Myxomas
  Spotty pigmentation
Von Hippel–Lindau syndrome:
  Phaeochromocytoma, pancreatic islet-cell neoplasms
  Renal tumours
  CNS tumours, esp. cerebellar haemangioblastoma

POLYGLANDULAR AUTOIMMUNE SYNDROMES

Two main types exist: type 1 – childhood onset and type 2 – adult onset

Type 1 PGAS

Inc: Rare
Age: Childhood
Sex: M = F
Aet: *APECED* gene = autoimmune polyendocrinopathy, candidiasis, ectodermal dystrophy
Autosomal recessive; chromosome 21

P.G.A.S.

Parathyroidism, hypo-
GIT:
- Mucocutaneous candidiasis (esp. oral)
- Malabsorption
- Pernicious anaemia
- Chronic active hepatitis

Addison disease
Skin:
- Dystrophy of teeth (enamel), nails, hair (alopecia)
- Vitiligo
- Otosclerosis

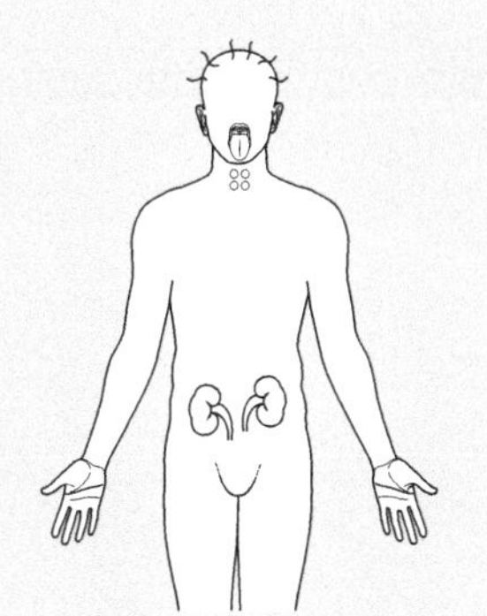

Type 2 PGAS (Schmidt syndrome)

Inc: Common
Age: Adulthood
Sex: F>M
Aet: Polygenic: HLA-DR3 and -DR4-associated
Autosomal dominant with incomplete penetrance

T.O^2.A.D. P.G.A.S.

Thyroidism, dys: Graves or Hashimoto disease
Oophoritis/**O**rchitis: Infertility
Addison disease
Diabetes, type 1

Pituitary: Lymphocytic hypophysitis
GIT:
- Coeliac disease
- Pernicious anaemia

Additional: Myasthenia gravis
Skin: Vitiligo

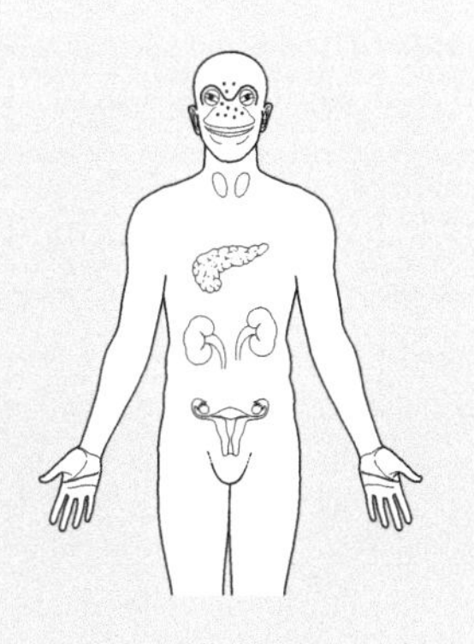

Clinical Chemistry

ACID–BASE BALANCE

Acidosis has two types of 1° cause, each being compensated by the other system:

- **Respiratory:** $PaCO_2$ ↑, due to ventilation ↓
  → renal compensation, via HCO_3^- resorption, and acid and NH_4^+ excretion
- **Metabolic**: HCO_3^- ↓ due to acid gain (high anion gap) or HCO_3^- loss (low anion gap)
  → respiratory compensation, by $PaCO_2$ ↓

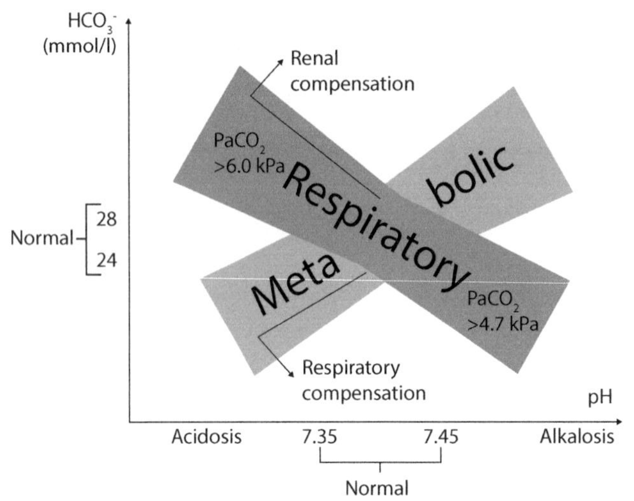

Normal compensation

$PaCO_2$ ↑ 1 kPa → HCO_3^- ↑ 3 mmol/l

HCO_3^- ↓ 6 mmol/l → $PaCO_2$ ↓ 1 kPa

(The opposite processes operate for alkalosis causes and compensations)

Respiratory

Acidosis

Failure of CO_2 excretion via lungs

Ventilatory failure:

- **Obstructive**: Small airways: COPD
  Intrathoracic: Cancer, lymph node
  Foreign body
- **Restrictive**: Pulmonary fibrosis
  Neuromuscular: Sedation, polio
  Skeletal: Spondylosis

Diffusion failure: Late pneumonia; ARDS

Alkalosis

Hyperventilation

Lung:

- Pulmonary embolism; atelectasis
- Pneumothorax; flail chest

CNS:

I.N.V.I.T.E. I.S. F.R.E.E.

- Intra-cranial:
  Infection (meningitis)
  Neoplasia
  Vascular
  Injury
  Toxin (aspirin, adrenaline)
  Extra – pain, anxiety
- Extra-cranial:
  Infection – septicaemia
  Systemic – anaemia, hypotension, high altitude
  Failure: Cardiac, liver
  Recovery from metabolic acidosis
  Endocrine-1 – thyrotoxicosis
  Endocrine-2 – pregnancy, progesterone

Iatrogenic: Mechanical ventilation, respiratory stimulants (e.g. doxapram)

Metabolic

Acidosis

Classified by size of anion gap = ($Na^+ + K^+$) – ($Cl^- + HCO_3^-$); normal = 8–18 mmol/l

K.I.L.L.E.R. T.R.I.G.G.E.R.

High anion gap: Organic acid gain

- **K**etoacidosis: DM, alcoholism (due to binge drinking, starvation)
- **I**ntake of organic acid: Aspirin overdose, methanol, ethylene glycol
  - High osmolar gap: Osmolality – (2 × Na^+ + glucose + urea) >15 mmol/l
- **L**actic acidosis, type A – tissue hypoxia:
  - Shock, hypoxia, poisoning: Carbon monoxide, cyanide, TCA overdose
- **L**actic acidosis, type B – metabolic abnormality:
  - Gluconeogenesis ↓: Liver failure; paracetamol overdose; metformin
  - Formation ↑: Neoplasia (e.g. leukaemia), infection (e.g. malaria, epilepsy)
- **E**nzyme mutation: Glycogen storage disease (G6Pase deficiency), mitochondrial disease, methylmalonic aciduria
- **R**enal failure (GFR <20 ml/min): Uraemic toxins, lactic acid

Low anion gap: Bicarbonate loss, failure of acid excretion, hyperchloraemia

- **T**oxins:
  - Cardiac: ACE inhibitors, A-II receptor blockers, K^+-sparing diuretics, acetazolamide
  - Other: Statins, trimethoprim, pentamidine, cyclosporin, cation-exchange resin
- **R**enal tubular acidosis:
  - K^+↓: RTA-1 = failure of acid excretion (severe – most tubulointerstitial nephropathies)
    RTA-2 = bicarbonate loss (isolated or part of Fanconi syndrome)
  - K^+↑: RTA-4 (hypoaldosteronism)
- **I**ntake of ammonium: Hyperalimentation (TPN), NH_4Cl
- **G**astrointestinal: Diarrhoea, esp. VIPoma
- **G**astrointestinal: Ureterosigmoidostomy, ileostomy, fistulae (pancreatic, biliary)
- '**E**xpansion acidosis' = rapid IV NaCl infusion
- **R**enal failure (GFR: 20–50 ml/min): Failure of acid excretion

NB:
- *Bicarbonate loss → high urine NH_4^+*
- *Failure of acid excretion → absent urine NH_4^+*

AlkalOsis

Mostly causes of hyp**O**kalaemia (p. 385)

C.a.R.D.I².ac.

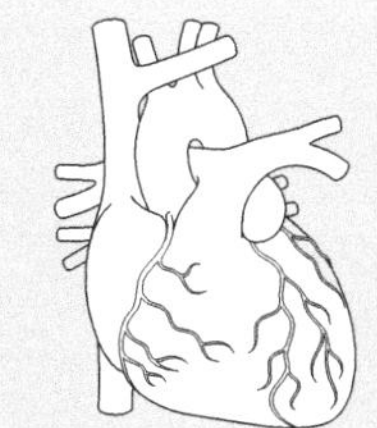

Corticosteroid excess:
- 1° Hyperaldosteronism: Adrenal adenoma, BNH or carcinoma; GRA
- 2° Hyperaldosteronism: Renin-secreting tumour, renal artery stenosis, Gitelman syn.

Renal: Osmotic diuresis

Drugs: Diuretics (e.g. thiazide, furosemide), penicillin, salbutamol

Intake of K^+ or Mg^{2+} ↓ (i.e. hypoMgaemia)

Intestinal loss: Vomiting, villous adenoma of rectum

HYPONATRAEMIA

Causes

Other solute

'Pseudohyponatraemia'

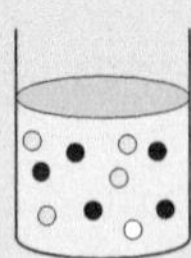

HOG (High osmolar gap)

Def:

- Osmolar gap = actual – estimated
- Estimated osmolality = 2× ($Na^+ + K^+$) + urea + glucose
- High osmolar gap >10 mmol/l

Causes:

- Hyperosmolality:
  - Hyperglycaemia, e.g. diabetes, TPN
  - Mannitol IV
- Normal osmolality:
  - Hyperlipidaemia, e.g. diabetes, nephrosis
  - Hyperproteinaemia, e.g. paraproteinaemia
  - NG-feed

Excess water

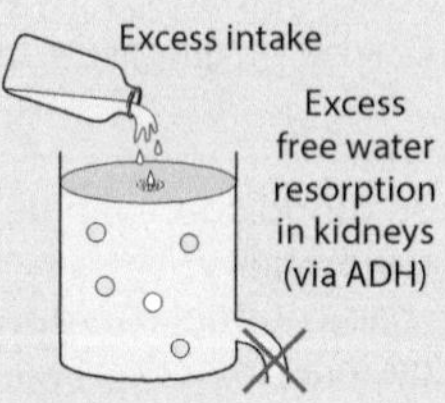

Polydipsia

Causes:

P.I.N.T.

- **P**sychogenic polydipsia; beer potomania = alcohol excess with inadequate solute in diet
- **I**atrogenic: Post-operative IVI
- **N**euro: Thalamus VMN lesion
- **T**URP (bladder instillation)

Chronic hypovolaemia (appropriate ADH excess)

Causes: Oedematous states (secondary hyperaldosteronism):

- CCF, nephrosis, cirrhosis
- Pregnancy

Mech:

- Hypovolaemia ↑ ADH release
- GFR ↓ impairs distal tubular diluting capacity
- 'Sick cell' syndrome = ↓ Na^+K^+ATPase; ↓ intracellular protein
- Hypothal. osmoreceptor resets

SIADH (inappropriate ADH excess)

Causes:

P.I.N.T.S. – *see opposite*

Mech: ADH causes free water resorption from distal convoluted tubule and medullary collecting duct

Sodium loss

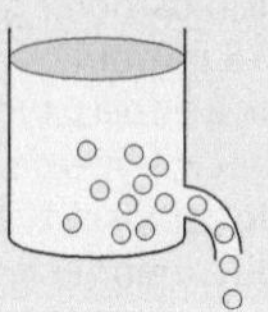

Renal

Causes:

- Diuretics (thiazide/loop)
- Tubulointerstitial nephritis
- Hypoaldosteronism (RTA type IV), e.g. Addison; DM

Extra-renal

- GIT, esp. villous adenoma, fistula, stoma
- Skin
- Blood

NB: Hyponatraemia never due to inadequate salt intake!

SIADH – Causes

P.I.N.T.S.

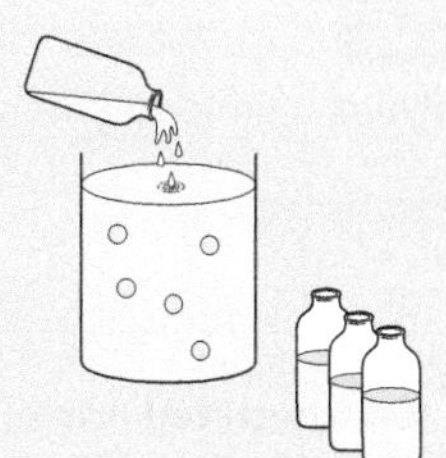

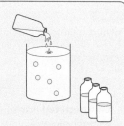

Pulmonary
- Infection esp. *Legionella*, TB (and rifampicin); bronchial carcinoma

Infection
- AIDS, pneumonia

Neurological
- CNS – meningo-encephalitis (esp. children):
  - Stroke, traumatic brain injury, tumour, dementia
  - Also causes 'cerebral salt-wasting syndrome'
- PNS – autonomic neuropathy: Acute intermittent porphyria, GBS pain (and NSAIDs)

Toxins
- CNS: Drugs of abuse – opiates, ecstasy
- Neuropsychiatric: Carbamazepine, chlorpromazine; TCA, SSRI
- Chemotherapy: Vincristine, cisplatin, cyclophosphamide

SLE
- Systemic:
  - Thyroid – hypothyroidism
  - Neoplasm – carcinoma of prostate, bladder, pancreas; carcinoid; lymphoma
  - Malnutrition

PC

Chronic: Asymptomatic, or lethargy
Acute (or late chronic):

- Headache/N+V
- Cerebral oedema: Confusion, fits, coma, death
- Weight gain: Due to intracellular swelling; but no oedema or hypertension (hypovolaemia with cerebral salt-wasting syndrome)

Ix

Bloods: Na^+ <135 mmol/l
Urea ↓; uric acid ↓ ADH ↑

Urine: Urine osmolality >300 mOsm/kg
Urine Na^+ >20 mmol/l: Due to hypervolaemia, inhibition of RAAS, and ↑ release of ANP

Special: Water load test: Ensure Na^+ >125; drink 1.5 l
Normal: >80% water excreted in 5 h; urine osmolality <100 mmol/l

Rx

Underlying cause
Fluid restrict: 500–1000 ml/day
Tolvaptan
Hypertonic saline IV**,** if CNS symptoms occur.

☠: Central pontine myelinolysis, if too rapid correction in chronic hyponatraemia (e.g. alcoholic)
PATH: Pontine, basal ganglia, cerebral demyelination
PC: Quadraparesis; pseudobulbar palsy or mutism; fits, 1–2 days after Na^+ correction

POLYURIA/POLYDIPSIA

Def

Polyuria = urine volume >3 l/24 h

Causes

Concentrated urine (urine osmolality >300 mOsm/kg)

Osmotic diuresis:

- Diabetes mellitus (glycosuria)
- TPN (urea)
- Mannitol

Tubulointerstitial disease:

- Resolving acute tubular necrosis, or post-obstructive uropathy
- Medullary cystic disease
- $K^+\downarrow$, $Ca^{2+}\uparrow$

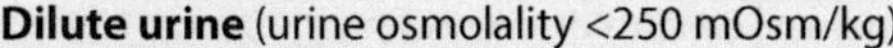

Dilute urine (urine osmolality <250 mOsm/kg)

Diabetes insipidus:

- Cranial
- Nephrogenic

Primary polydipsia:

- Psychiatric: Primary, anxiety, psychosis
- Neurological: Head injury, MS, sarcoid
- Toxins: Anti-psychotics, tricyclics, lithium, carbamazepine

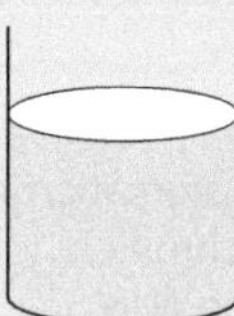

Ix

Bloods: Glucose
$K^+\downarrow$, $Ca^{2+}\uparrow$ (nephrogenic diabetes insipidus)
Osmolality

Urine: Osmolality

Special: Water-deprivation test|
ADH–osmolality plots, during water deprivation test or hypertonic saline challenges (p. 383)

HYPERNATRAEMIA

Causes

D.R.I.E.D. *out*

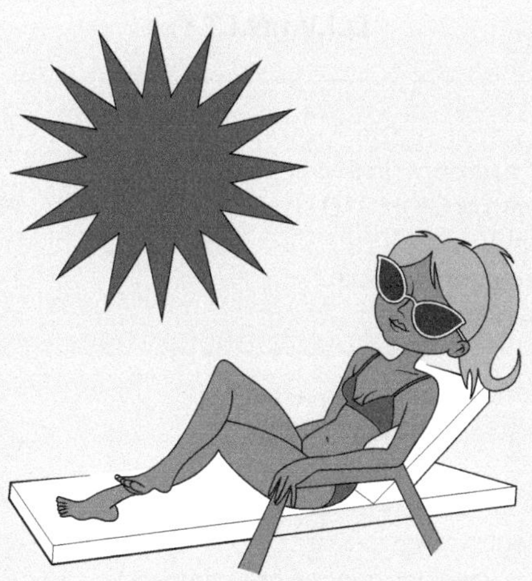

Deficiency – water restriction
- Debilitated, dementia, dysphagia, upper GI obstruction
- Hypothalamic disease may cause reduced thirst response (adipsic hypernatraemia)

Renal – water loss via osmotic diuresis
- Diabetes mellitus; TPN or NG feeding (high urea); IV mannitol

Intestinal or other water loss
- GIT: Infantile gastroenteritis, large solute load (e.g. NG feed)
- Skin: Acclimatisation to high temperature
- Lung: Hyperventilation (esp. in dry air), COPD

Excess salt
- Excess salt intake, e.g. seawater; excess IV normal saline
- Excess salt resorption, i.e. hypermineralocorticoidism

Diabetes insipidus *with* water deprivation
- Cranial: Insufficient ADH release to hypernatraemia
- Nephrogenic: Insufficient ADH sensitivity to hypernatraemia

DIABETES INSIPIDUS

Causes

Cranial

PATH: Hypothalamus, infundibulum or posterior pituitary lesion

D.I.V.I.N.I.T.Y.

Developmental/inherited:
- Autosomal dominant: AVP-neurophysin II gene
- Autosomal recessive: Wolfram or DIDMOAD syndrome (**DI**, **D**iabetes **M**ellitus, **O**ptic **a**trophy, **D**eafness + bladder atony)
- Congenital: Midline malformation (adipsia)

Infection: Basilar meningitis, e.g. TB

Vascular:
- Infarction: Sheehan syndrome, sickle cell anaemia
- Anterior communicating artery aneurysm

Inflammation:
- Lymphocytic infiltration of stalk – resolves in 3 y
- Sarcoid (also causes nephrogenic DI)
- SLE, granulomatosis with polyangiitis (midline granulomata)

Neoplasia:
- 1°: Pituitary adenoma **with** suprasellar extension; craniopharyngioma
- 2°: Metastases to pituitary or hypothalamus

Injury: Trauma or craniotomy – lasts 1 day to 3 weeks

Toxin: Alcohol

Pregnanc**Y**: Placental vasopressinase (remits post-partum)

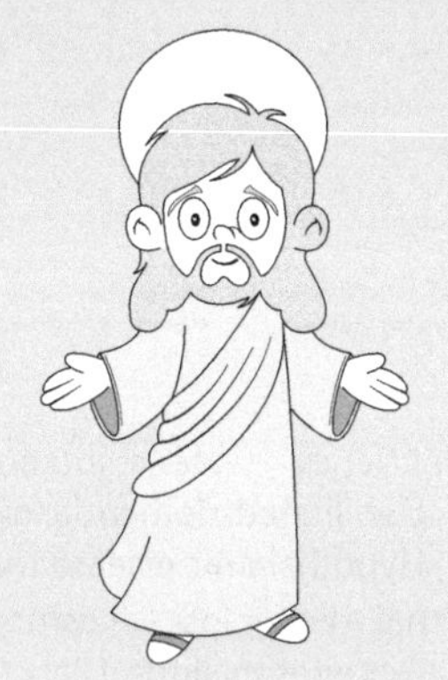

Nephrogenic

PATH: Collecting duct or tubulointerstitial disease

T.U.B.U.L.A.R. P.H.

Toxins: Lithium, amphotericin B, rifampicin, meflurane

Ureteric: Vesicoureteric reflux, obstruction

Blood vessel disease: Sickle cell, vasculitis, acute tubular necrosis

Uric acid ↑, calcium (plasma or urine) ↑, potassium ↓

Lymphoma, myeloma, amyloid

Autoimmune: SLE, Sjögren syndrome

Radiation

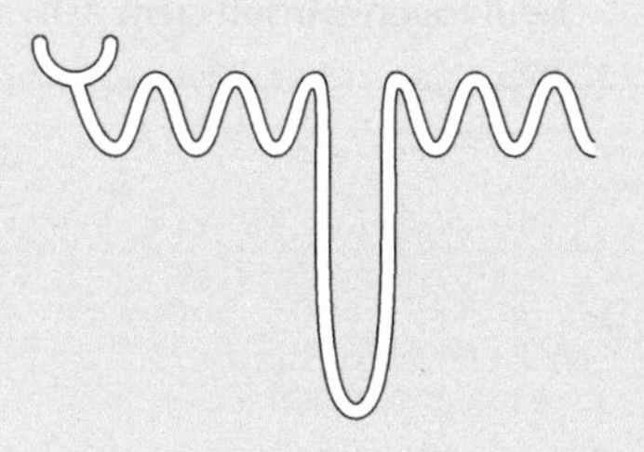

Papillary necrosis: Sickle cell, diabetes mellitus

Hereditary:
- X-linked recessive: *VR2* gene; results in cAMP ↓; presents in infancy
- Autosomal recessive: *aquaporin 2* gene

PC

Polyuria and polydispia

Fatigue: Due to nocturia, and volume depletion that only occurs if deprived of water

Symptoms may be masked by concomitant adrenal insufficiency due to equimolar Na^+ loss, and unmasked by steroid Rx

Ix

Bloods: Na^+ normal, or ↑ if patient is denied access to free water (↓ = primary polydipsia)
Osmolality >300 mOsm/kg

Urine: Osmolality <300 mOsm/kg, i.e. unable to concentrate urine

Special:

Water-deprivation test

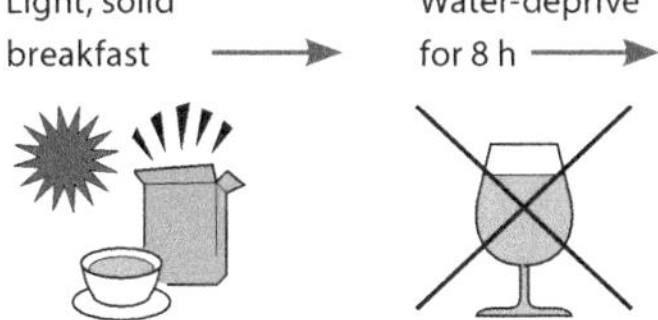

Criteria for diabetes insipidus
Weight loss >3%/h
Plasma osmolality >300 mOsm/kg
Urine osmolality <300 mOsm/kg
(partial DI: 300–600 mOsm/kg
primary polydipsia: >600)

NB 1: Co-existent hypocortisolism: Give pre-test dexamethasone if cortisol deficiency possible

NB 2: Cranial vs. nephrogenic DI: Give nasal desmopressin and allow free access to water:

- Cranial DI: Urine gets concentrated: ↓ urine volume + ↑ urine osmolality
- Nephrogenic DI: Urine can't be concentrated: ↑ urine volume + ↓ urine osmolality

ADH radioimmunoassay, plus hypertonic saline IV challenge
Right-sided shift patterns:

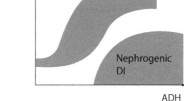

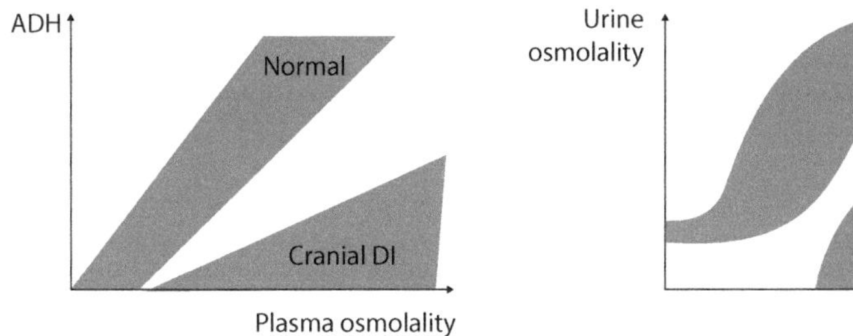

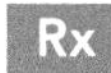

Rx

Cranial

Desmopressin (intra-nasal DDAVP); has advantage over AVP in having less pressor activity
Carbamazepine (induces SIADH)

Nephrogenic

Adequate water supply but Na^+ restrict; causes physiological ↓ urine output
Thiazide, e.g. hydrochlorothiazide: Causes physiological ↓ urine output
Indomethacin
High-dose intra-nasal desmopressin in partial nephrogenic diabetes insipidus

HYPERKALAEMIA

Causes

C.A.R.D.I^2.A.C^2.!

Plasma conc. >5 mmol/l

Corticosteroid deficiency:
- Addison disease
- Hyporeninaemic hypoaldosteronism (RTA type 4), e.g. diabetic nephropathy
- Aldosterone resistance, e.g. post-obstruction nephropathy

Acidosis, metabolic
- Poisoning with aspirin, ethylene glycol, methanol poisoning
- Diabetic ketoacidosis (not lactic acidosis due to free movement of anions into cells)

Renal failure – acute or chronic, **R**enal tubular acidosis type 4

Drugs:
- Cardiac:
  - ACE inhibitors, angiotensin-II receptor antagonists
  - Diuretics – spironolactone, amiloride, acetazolamide
  - Digoxin, beta-blockers (overdose)
- Nephrotoxic (tubulo-interstitial):
  - Cyclosporin, tacrolimus
  - NSAIDs, trimethoprim

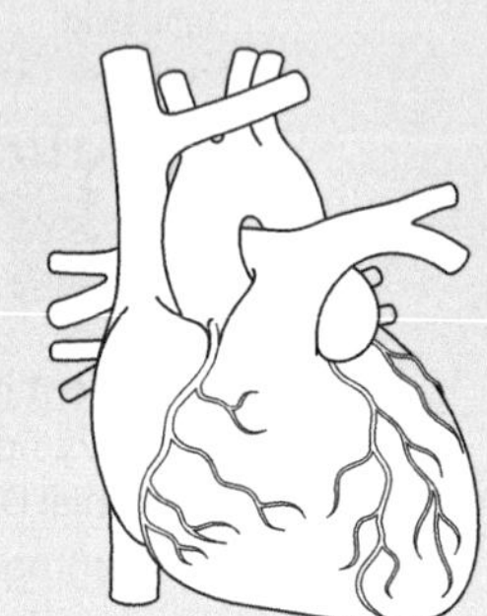

Intake ↑: citrus foods; IV fluids (iatrogenic)

Intestinal, gastro-: Haemorrhage

Artefactual:
- Haemolysis or blood clots, esp. prothrombotic states; Ix: PO_4 ↓, Ca^{2+} ↓, glucose ↓
- Hereditary stomatocytosis (autosomal dominant) – red-cells leak K^+ at room temperature

Cell-lysis:
- Catabolic states: Anorexia nervosa, trauma, chemotherapy
- Massive blood transfusion, esp. >7 days old

Channelopathy – hyperkalaemic periodic paralysis, due to Na^+-channel mutation (autosomal dominant)

PC

Dysrhythmias, e.g. VT, PEA arrest – but presents late (K^+ >6.5 mmol/l)! (Membrane potential decreases, resulting in shorter action potential and depolarisation)

ECG

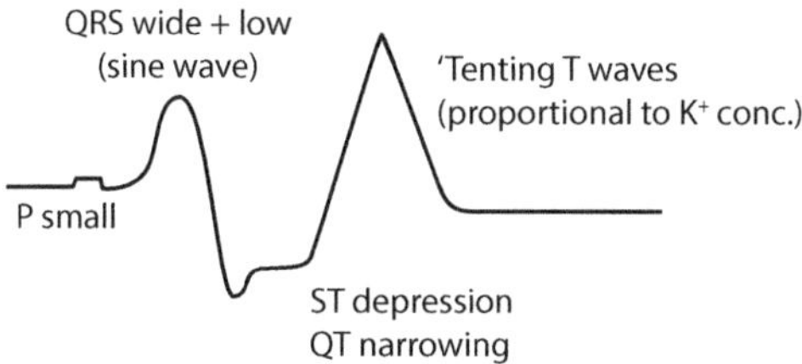

Rx

Cardioprotection: Calcium gluconate/chloride 10% IV 10 ml

Acute:
- Insulin (IV soluble 'Actrapid') + glucose (IV 50 g of 50% glucose), followed with sliding scale of soluble insulin and dextrose
- Salbutamol (high-dose nebulizer 10 mg)
- Dialysis

Chronic:
- Renal: Loop diuretic; dialysis
- GIT: K^+ restrict; resonium salts

HYPOKALAEMIA

Causes

C.A.R.D.I².A.C².!

Plasma conc. <3.5 mmol/l

Corticosteroid excess – hypermineralocorticoidism:
- 1° Hyperaldosteronism: Adrenal adenoma, BNH or carcinoma, glucocorticoid remediable aldosteronism
- 2° Hyperaldosteronism: Renin-secreting tumour, renal artery stenosis, Gitelman, Bartter syndromes, hypovolaemia
- Hypoaldosteronism: Liddle syn., 'apparent mineralocorticoid excess' syn.

Acidosis, renal-tubular, types 1 and 2

Renal – over-diuresis:
- Recovery phase of acute-tubular necrosis
- Osmotic diuresis, e.g. DM, TPN feeding

Drugs:
- Cardiac: Diuretics (thiazide, loop, osmotic)
- Nephrotoxic (tubulo-interstitial): Penicillins, amphotericin B
- β_2-agonists: Salbutamol, aminophylline (↑ Na^+K^+-ATPase)
- Insulin: Conjoint glucose–K^+ cell influx

Intake ↓ or Mg^{2+} deficiency, e.g. alcoholism, malabsorption, diuretics

Intestinal:
- Vomiting, naso-gastric tube suctioning
- Diarrhoea, esp. villous adenoma of rectum; purgative abuse
- Surgery: Fistula, ureterosigmoidostomy

Artefactual: Sample taken downstream from IV drip

Cell-proliferation: Anabolic states, e.g. convalescence from trauma, surgery, TPN feeding

Channelopathy: Hypokalaemic periodic paralysis, due to dihydropyridine Ca^{2+} channel mutation (autosomal dominant)

PC

Neurological: Weakness – skeletal muscle (hypotonia); smooth muscle (constipation/ileus) fatigue, confusion, depression

Nephrogenic diabetes insipidus

Dysrhythmias: Bradycardia, heart block, SVT, VT, digoxin toxicity potentiation

ECG

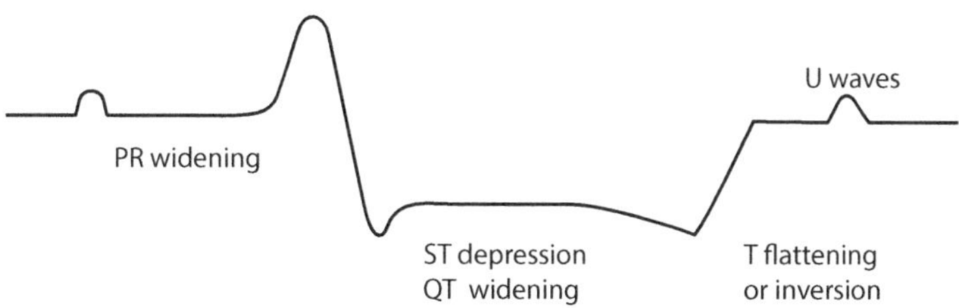

Rx

K^+ replacement: PO or IV
- Max conc. = 40 mmol/l; max rate over 4 hours via peripheral line
- Measure K^+ every few hours/ECG monitor

Mg^{2+} replacement (if VT): IV $MgSO_4$ 50% 8 ml

HYPOCALCAEMIA

Causes

Two-step process:

1. **Correct** for albumin: For every 4 g/l of albumin below 40 g/l allow 0.1 mmol/l from lower limit of Ca (2.2 mmol/l)
2. **Measure PTH** (parathyroid hormone), **ALP** (alkaline phosphatase) and **vitamin D**

PTH ↓

I. A.M.

Injury to parathyroid gland (commonest):
- Thyroidectomy, laryngeal carcinoma
- Parathyroidectomy (for ↑ Ca): 'Hungry bone syndrome' = rapid uptake of Ca, Mg + PO_4

Autoimmune – parathyroid inflammation:
- Thyroidectomy, laryngeal carcinoma
- Includes polyglandular autoimmune syndrome type 1 = PGAS: **P**TH, thyroid ↓; **G**IT (pernicious anaemia); **A**ddison; **S**kin (teeth, nail dystrophy, alopecia, candida)

Malignancy (carcinoma, lymphoma)/Metabolic (haemochromatosis, Wilson)

PTH ↑

V.I.B.R.A.T.I.N.'

Vitamin D deficiency/impaired activation = rickets (children) or osteomalacia (adults) (p. 390):
- Deficiency: Diet, malabsorption, e.g. coeliac
- Activation: Cirrhosis; chronic renal failure

Inherited: PseudohypoPTHism ('Albright osteodystrophy')

PATH: PTH-receptor insensitivity in proximal convoluted tubule → failure of Ca resorption and PO_4 excretion:
- Type 1: Renal adenylate cyclase, G protein *sα* subunit deficiency
- Type 2: Post-adenylate cyclase transduction abnormality

PC: Type 1 (autosomal dominant):
- Short: Height, 4th + 5th metacarpal and metatarsal length, IQ
- Oculocutaneous: Subcutaneous calcification, cataracts, blue sclera
- Endocrinopathy: Type 2 diabetes (and obese), hypogonadism, hypothyroidism (the presence of this phenotype, but normal calcium = 'pseudopseudohypoPTHism'!)

Burns, and other causes of cell lysis (infarction; haemolysis; sepsis; tumour lysis) :
- Due to hyperphosphataemia
- Also caused artefactually by delayed serum separation or haemolysis

Rhabdomyolysis: Releases phosphate

Acute pancreatitis (saponification)

Toxins:
- Citrate, e.g. blood transfusion, heparin, protamine, glucagon, fusidic acid
- Bisphosphonate

Infection: *Legionella pneumophila* pneumonia

Neoplasia: Prostate carcinoma

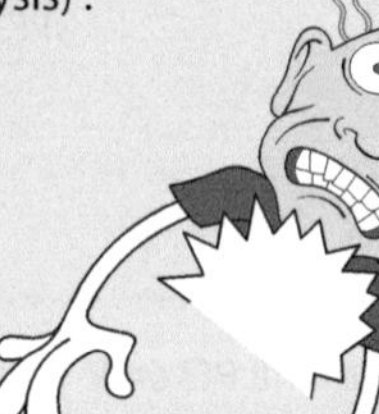

PC

General

Neurological:

- Sensory: Numbness, perioral paraesthesia
- Motor: Hyperexcitability – cramps, hyper-reflexia, tetany, stridor Chvostek Sx (tap facial nerve → twitching)/Trousseau Sx (carpopedal spasm)
- CNS: Seizures, depression, dementia, parkinsonism (basal ganglia calcification)

Oculocutaneous:

- Photophobia, papilloedema, subcapsular cataracts due to ectopic calcification
- Subcutaneous calcification (if PO_4↑)

Cardiac: Ventricular tachycardia (due to prolongation of QT), electromechanical dissociation

High PTH:

Osteomalacia, rickets (p. 390), bone pain and fractures; proximal myopathy; TB susceptibility
PseudohypoPTHism *(see opposite)*: Short; oculocutaneous, endocrinopathy

Ix

Bloods: Calcium – corrected total calcium <2.2 mmol/l
PTH – if normal, consider causes of hyperPTH-related hypocalcaemia (osteomalacia, etc.)
ALP ↑: Osteomalacia; rickets
ALP normal: HypoPTHism or pseudohypoPTHism
Vit. D: 25-HCC ↓ 1,25-DHCC ↓ – poor intake; liver failure
25-HCC ↑ 1,25-DHCC ↓ – chronic renal failure
25-HCC ↑ 1,25-DHCC ↑ – vitamin D resistance
PO_4↑ – hypoPTHism, pseudohypoPTHism or chronic renal failure
PO_4 ↓– osteomalacia; rickets (except that due to CKD)

Urine: PO_4 ↓: HypoPTHism or pseudoPTHism
cAMP, post-IV PTH – classifies pseudohypoPTHism

Micro: Throat/vaginal swab for candida

ECG: Hyp**O**calcaemia Pr**O**l**O**ngs QT interval

Radiol: X-rays

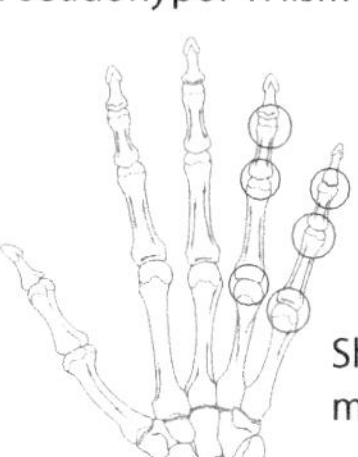

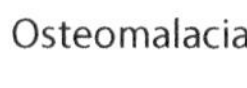

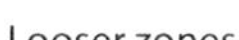

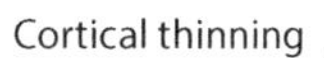

Rx

Calcium supplements:

- Calcium gluconate (IV) – use cardiac monitor
- Calcium carbonate (PO)

Vitamin D:

Ergocalciferol (D2) – non-hydroxylated
☠: Hypercalcaemia due to long half-life (must monitor for first few weeks)

Alfacalcidol (1α-HCC) or calcitriol (D3) – hypercalcaemia less likely

HYPERCALCAEMIA

Causes

Two-step process:

1. **Correct** for albumin, since physiologically inert, bound calcium increases with serum protein. Hence total calcium increases with hypergammaglobulinaemia, or dehydration (urea ↑)
2. **Measure PTH** (parathyroid hormone) and **ALP** (alkaline phosphatase)

PTH ↑ (ALP normal)

P.T.H.

Primary hyperPTHism – **commonest**
  Epi: Prevalence = 1% population; typically women in 30–50s
  Aet: Hyperplasia (15%), adenoma (80%), carcinoma (5%)
  Pre:
  - Hereditary, esp. when bilateral tumours present
  - **MEN** syndromes: I (pituitary, pancreatic islet-cell tumour) or IIA (thyroid ca., phaeochromocytoma)

  PC: Usually asymptomatic, unless additional cause occurs, e.g. carcinoma

Tertiary hyperPTHism: Following renal transplant in a patient with prior 2° hyperPTHism, vit. D and Ca rise, but parathyroid gland continues secreting autonomously

Hypocalciuric hypercalcaemia, familial (autosomal dominant, numerous mutations):
  PATH: Incorrectly set Ca sensor on parathyroid and renal tubules causes ↑ PTH secretion and ↑ Ca resorption in distal-convoluted tubule
  PC: Hypercalcaemic from birth (cf. primary PTH) – usually benign

PTH ↓

S.T.O².N.E.S.

Sarcoidosis; and TB (ALP ↑) due to 1α-hydroxylase activity in granulomas

Toxins (ALP normal):
- Vit. D or A, or antacids ('milk-alkali syndrome')
- Thiazide diuretics (also diuretic phase of acute tubular necrosis)
- Lithium: PTH is actually ↑ !

Osteoblast and **O**steoclast turnover increased (ALP ↑): Fracture, esp. with Paget, puberty or immobility

Neoplasia
  ALP ↑:
  - Bony metastases, e.g. breast, bronchial – **2nd commonest** (due to prostaglandin release causing osteoclast activation)
  - Lymphoma, leukaemia – due to 1α-hydroxylase activity

  ALP normal:
  - Myeloma
  - Carcinoma (PTH-related peptide): Squamous cell bronchial, renal, liver, pancreas

Endocrine:
  ALP ↑: Thyrotoxicosis
  ALP normal: Addison, acromegaly, androgen excess

Syndromes (ALP normal):
- Jansen syndrome: Autonomous PTH-receptor activity
  PC: Severe hyperPTHism-like bone disease in children, premature death
- William syndrome:
  PC: **WI**de mouth, **L**ow growth, **L**ow IQ, **A**ortic stenosis, **M**etabolic (Ca ↑)

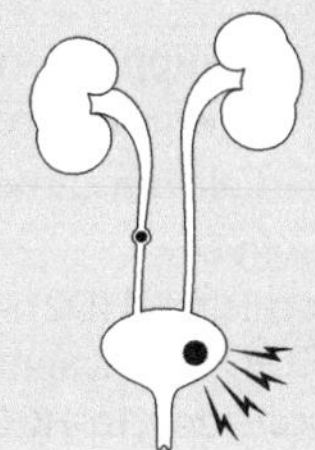

PC

'Bones'

- Bone pain, due to subperiosteal resorption
- Arthralgia (pseudogout; chondrocalcinosis)

'Stones'

- Renal stones
- Tubular dysfunction: Diabetes insipidus (polyuria, polydipsia), acidosis

Abdominal 'groans'

- Abdominal pain (incl. peptic ulcers, acute pancreatitis)
- N+V
- Constipation

Psychological 'moans'

- Fatigue, depression, psychosis, dementia

Ix

Bloods: Essential

Calcium: Corrected total calcium >2.6 mmol/l

PTH: If normal, consider causes of hyperPTHism

ALP

Auxillary:

PO_4 ↓ – hyperPTHism; lymphoma; PO_4 ↑ – carcinoma

Cl ↑, HCO_3 ↓: HyperPTHism

Other: Albumin ↓ – neoplasia; ESR ↑ – hyperPTHism or neoplasia; ACE ↑ – sarcoid

Urine: Calcium:

- Hypercalciuric (<99% tubular resorption) – all causes, except:
- Hypocalciuric (>99% tubular resorption) – familial hypocalciuric hypercalcaemia

Bence-Jones proteinuria: Myeloma

Micro: Consider TB (CXR, Mantoux, etc.)

ECG: Short QT interval (hyp**O**calcemia pr**OlO**ngs the QT)

Radiol: X-rays

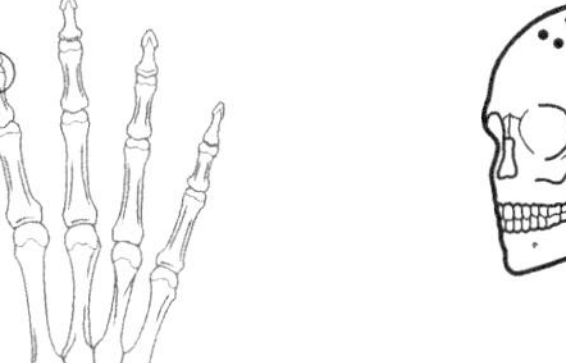

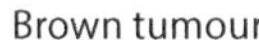

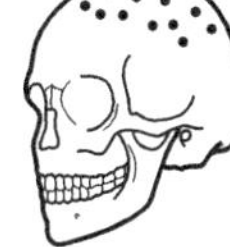

Radioisotopes:

- Parathyroid (pertechnetate – thallium or MIBI, to subtract out thyroid)
- Technetium bone scan: Bone metastases

Special: Selective neck venous catheterisation for hyperPTHism

Rx

General

High fluid intake (normal saline infusion) + furosemide (↑ Ca excretion)

Bisphosphonates: Pamiodronate IV, clodronate

Cytotoxins (IV mithramycin, gallium); calcitonin (IV or IM); cellulose phosphate resin

Dietary restrict, e.g. for hereditary causes

Specific

Prednisolone is indicated for:

- Sarcoid or TB
- Myeloma or lymphoma
- Addison
- Vit. D or A excess

HRT (oestrogen + progesterone): May obviate surgery in post-menopausal hyperPTHism

Surgery: For primary hyperPTHism, where Ca >3.0 mmol/l – neck exploration with adenoma resection or partial PTHectomy

OSTEOMALACIA AND RICKETS

Def

Defective mineralisation of osteoid, that leads to reductions in global skeletal mass and density. (Osteoid = composite of collagen type 1, glycosysaminoglycans and proteoglycan, secreted by osteoblasts)

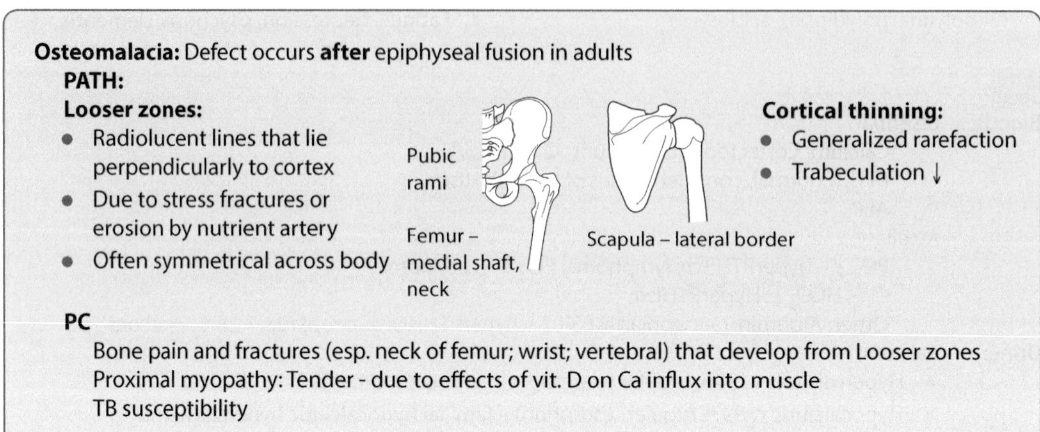

Osteomalacia: Defect occurs **after** epiphyseal fusion in adults
PATH:
Looser zones:
• Radiolucent lines that lie perpendicularly to cortex
• Due to stress fractures or erosion by nutrient artery
• Often symmetrical across body
Pubic rami
Femur – medial shaft, neck
Scapula – lateral border
Cortical thinning:
• Generalized rarefaction
• Trabeculation ↓
PC
Bone pain and fractures (esp. neck of femur; wrist; vertebral) that develop from Looser zones
Proximal myopathy: Tender - due to effects of vit. D on Ca influx into muscle
TB susceptibility

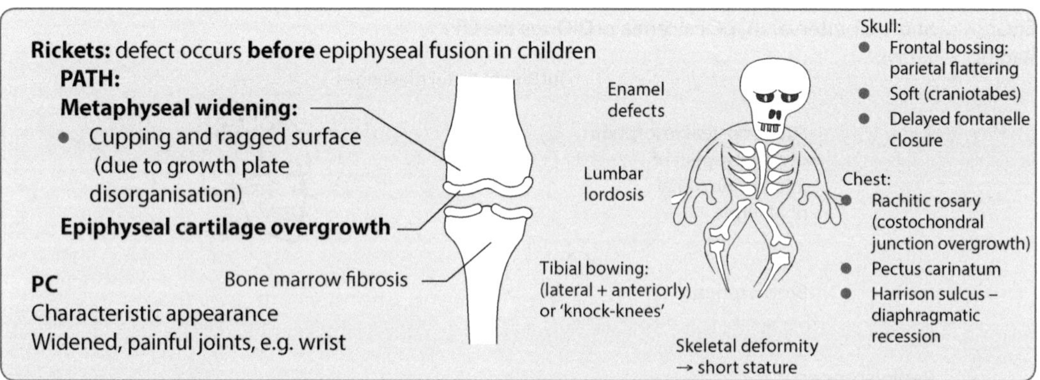

Rickets: defect occurs **before** epiphyseal fusion in children
PATH:
Metaphyseal widening:
• Cupping and ragged surface (due to growth plate disorganisation)
Epiphyseal cartilage overgrowth
Bone marrow fibrosis
PC
Characteristic appearance
Widened, painful joints, e.g. wrist
Enamel defects
Lumbar lordosis
Tibial bowing: (lateral + anteriorly) or 'knock-knees'
Skeletal deformity → short stature
Skull:
• Frontal bossing: parietal flattering
• Soft (craniotabes)
• Delayed fontanelle closure
Chest:
• Rachitic rosary (costochondral junction overgrowth)
• Pectus carinatum
• Harrison sulcus – diaphragmatic recession

Vitamin D physiology

Vitamin D is actually a hormone, because:

Endogenously produced: With adequate sunlight, no dietary fortification is required

Homeostatic control:

- Activated by ↓ Ca and ↓ PO_4
- Its action is to increase Ca and PO_4 via GIT (absorption) + bone (resorption)

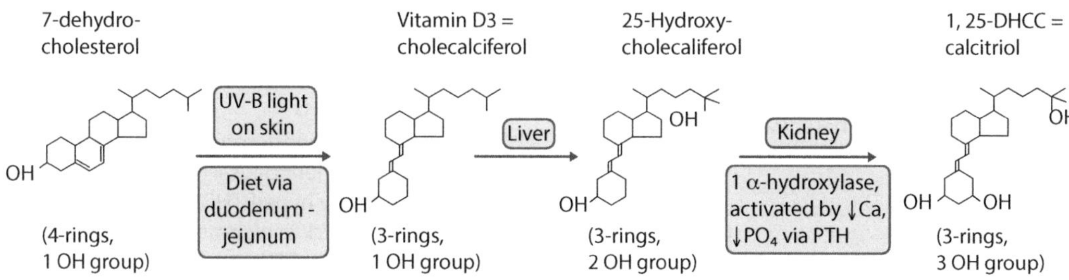

Causes

Due to either **vitamin D** or **phosphate** deficiency (but not calcium deficiency!)
Vitamin D deficiency causes:

- Decrease in GIT absorption of Ca and PO_4
- Secondary HyperPTHism with consequent increased Ca renal resorption and PO_4 renal loss

S.I.C.K. B.ON.E².

↓ Vitamin D

Supply
- Sunlight: Housebound, debilitated, elderly
- Diet: Vegans
- Fat malabsorption (vit. D = fat-soluble), e.g. coeliac; chronic pancreatitis

Inherited
- Renal 1*α*-hydroxylase deficiency ('vit. D-dependent rickets type 1'; auto. recessive)
- Resistance to vit. D ('vit. D-dependent rickets type 2'; auto. recessive)

Cirrhosis, esp. primary biliary cirrhosis, due to:
- 25-hydroxylase activity ↓
- Vit. D plasma-binding protein synthesis ↓
- Bile salt synthesis and circulation ↓

Kidney failure
- 1*α*-hydroxylase deficiency
- Nephrosis: Vit. D plasma-binding protein loss

Babies (pregnancy)/**B**reast feeding
- Due to increased demand (also trauma)

ONcogenic rickets
Endocrine: HypoPTHism or pseudohypoPTHism
Enzyme inducers, e.g. phenytoin

↓ PO_4

Supply
- Starvation/poor nutrition
- Malabsorption, e.g. coeliac, vomiting
- Antacids containing Mg or Al

Inherited: 'X-linked dominant hypophosphataemic rickets' = vit. D resistance in GIT and proximal convoluted tubule (Ix: Normal calcium levels!)

Cirrhosis, esp. alcohol bingers or post-glucose:
- Acetate displaces muscular PO_4
- Poor absorption of PO_4 from PCT

Kidney: Renal tubular acidosis
- Distal (type 1)
- Proximal (Fanconi syndrome), e.g. 2° to myeloma, Wilson

Binge alcohol drinking
ONcogenic rickets, esp. neurofibromatosis, cavernous haemangioma and giant-cell tumour of bone
Endocrine: Hyperaldosteronsim

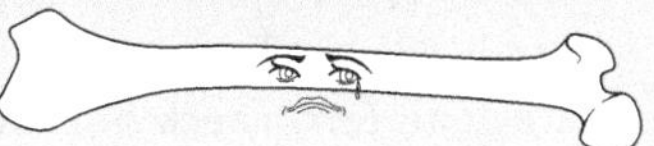

Ix

Bloods: Ca : Normal (initially, due to 2° hyperPTHism) → ↓ (severe hypovitaminosis D) (except in renal failure when ↑) PO_4 ↓
Alkaline phosphatase ↑
PTH ↑
Vit D:

- 25-HCC ↓
- 1,25-DHCC ↑ – supply ↓; demand ↑; cirrhosis (1,25-DHCC ↑ due to 2ndary ↑ PTH)
- 25-HCC ↑; 1,25-DHCC ↓ – chronic renal failure (1,25-DHCC ↓ in nephrosis)
- 25-HCC ↑; 1,25-DHCC ↑ – vit. D resistance

Urine: Renal tubular acidosis (pH >5.5)

Rx

Depends on cause:
Supply: Vit. D2 (ergocalciferol); vit. D3 (cholecalciferol) + UVB light
Malabsorption or resistance: High-dose or intramuscular vit. D + calcium
Liver/renal disease: Calcitriol or 1-α-calcidol (in renal failure) ☠ Hypercalcaemia
HypoPO_4aemia, e.g. RTA: Oral PO_4, but must correct Ca and vit. D first (or will worsen!)

OSTEOPOROSIS

Def

Bone mineral density< 2.5 standard deviations (−2.5 T) from normal young adult, adjusted for race and gender; in presence of normal bone composition

Due to imbalance between osteoblast synthesis vs. osteoclast resorption.

Localized (due to trauma, disuse, reflex sympathetic dystrophy) vs. generalized (see below).

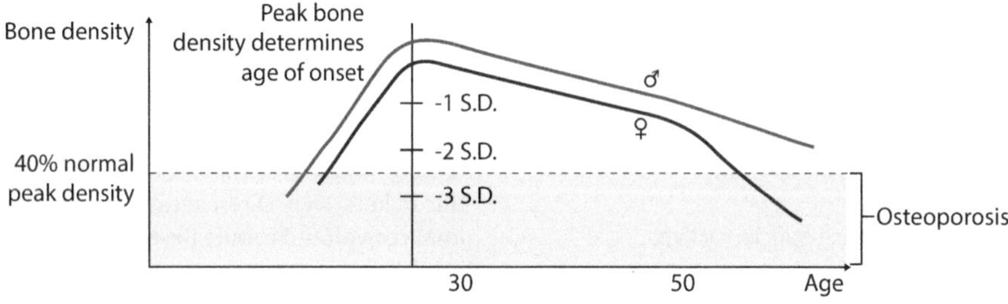

Causes

P.E.N.S².I.O.N.E.R.S.

Primary

Epi: 5% of population have, of which 10% get fractures every year

Predisposing: *White and Light* (i.e. Caucasian, low body mass index), genes, e.g. vit. D receptor gene inactivity, esp. in youth

Types:

Post-menopausal women (50–70 y)

- Site: Vertebral body; radius – trabecular bone
- Ix: Low PTH

Elderly (70+ y)

- Site: Femur neck, humerus, tibia – cortical bone
- Ix: High PTH

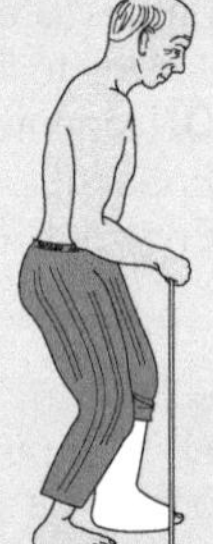

Endocrine: Steroid-related

Cushing

Hypogonadism, incl Turner or Klinefelter syn.

Addison disease

Neoplasia: Myeloma, lymphoma, carcinoma (PTH-related peptide)

Steroids/**S**moking, alcohol/other toxins

Heparin, warfarin

Anti-convulsants (also cause vit. D deficiency)

Lithium, buserelin, cyclosporin, thyroxine

NB : Must have annual DEXA scan if on steroids for >3 months

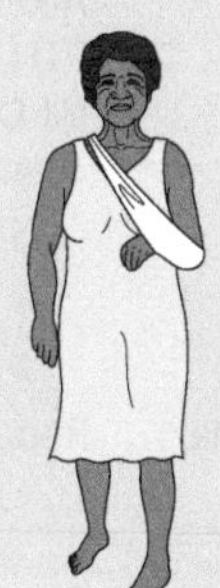

Intestine/nutrition

Malnutrition, anorexia nervosa,

Malabsorption (of Ca, vit. D, vit. C), TPN

Organ failure: Cirrhosis, esp. primary biliary cholangitis; haemochromatosis

Neurological: Dementia, MS, epilepsy

Endocrine: T4 ↑, PTH ↑, PRL ↑, acromegaly, type 1 DM (IDDM), pregnancy

Rheumatological: Rheumatoid arthritis; ankylosing spondylitis; TB arthritis

Syndromes: Osteogenesis imperfecta; Marfan; homocystinuria; Ehlers–Danlos

PC

Often asymptomatic and picked up by routine DEXA scanning

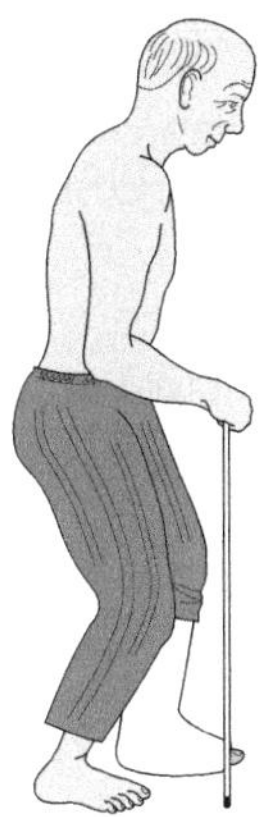

Ix

Assess bone mineral density (BMD) in all women >65 and men >75

Bloods: Ca: Normal, except for certain secondary causes: ↑ in malignancy; hyperPTHism; ↓ in malnutrition; malabsorption; osteomalacia
PO_4: Normal
ALP: Normal: or ↑ if fracture

Radiol: X-rays:
- Generalized osteopenia – thin cortex and trabeculae
- Fractures, esp. biconcave vertebral compression

DEXA (dual-energy X-ray absorptiometry)
- Generalized osteopenia – thin cortex and trabeculae
- Lumbar spine and femur neck 2D mineralisation area → estimates bone density
- T-scores relate individual result to normal young adult population (T <-2.0 to -2.5 = treat)
- Z-scores relate individual result to normal age-matched population

Quantitative CT: Advantage in estimating 3D mineralisation density

Rx

Avoid: Smoking, alcohol, steroids; Activity: Exercise in youth ↑ peak bone density
Bisphosphonates: Risedronate, alendronate
Mech: Inhibiting osteoclast ATP metabolism
☠: Poor absorption (take before breakfast); oesophagitis (stay upright for 30 min); ↓ Ca
Calcium (taken with bisphosphonates or calcitonin)/Mg/strontium
D, vitamin
O**E**strogens
Mech: ↑ osteoblast and ↓ osteoclast activity
HRT: Oestrogen ± progestagen (for protection against uterine ca.)
50% ↓ in fracture risk; ☠: Breast carcinoma
SERMs (selective oestrogen receptor modulators): Raloxifene, tamoxifen
40% ↓ in fracture risk; ☠: Uterine carcinoma (tamoxifen only)
Protective against breast ca., esp. oestrogen-dependent types
Fitness: Regular exercise improves bone mineral density

PAGET DISEASE

Def

Bone mineral density increased + disordered bone architecture + brittleness
Excessive osteoclastic activity, and overcompensatory osteoblastic remodelling and sclerosis

Epi

Inc: 4% of over-40s (although majority are asymptomatic)
Age: 50+: Inc. ↑
Sex: M > F
Geo: White Anglo-Saxons (W. Europe, Australia)
Aet: Paramyxovirus, e.g. canine dystemper virus (found in osteoclasts)
Genetic
Micro: Cycles of osteolysis and sclerosis occur in different parts of the same bone simultaneously

Osteolysis

- Osteoporosis circumscripta – V-shaped, sharply demarcated, advancing edge
- Vascularisation
- Deformable – bent and irregular cortex, with microfractures on convex surface

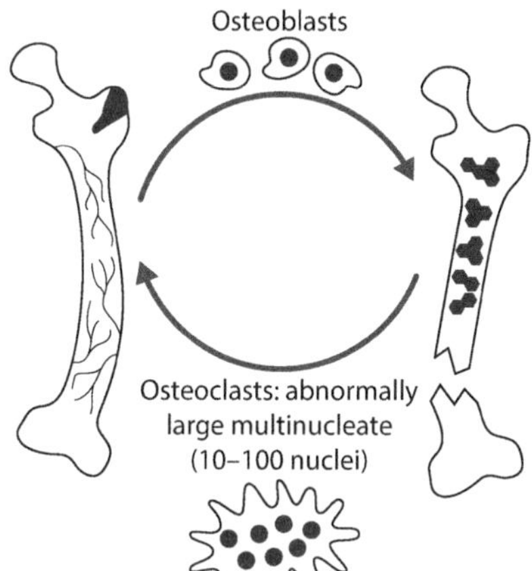

Sclerosis

- Coarse thickening of cortex and trabeculae (honeycomb radiolucencies)
- Brittle – mosaic pattern of lamellar bone

Sites

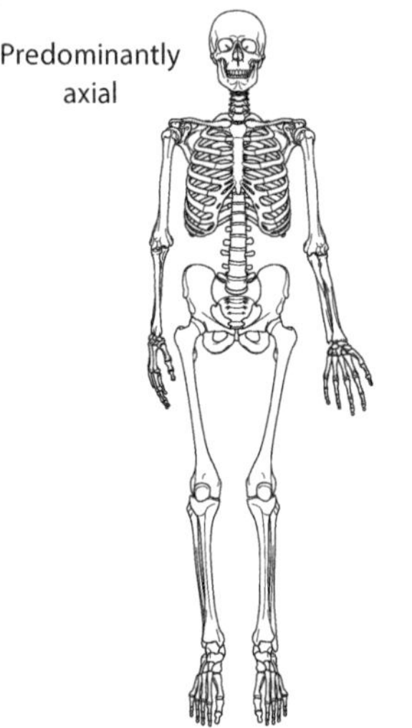

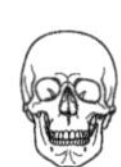

Skull

- Cotton-wool opacities in calvarium
- Platybasia – overgrowth of skull base
- Neural foramen stenosis

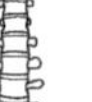

Vertebrae

- Sclerotic ('ivory') and enlarged (cf. Hodgkin lymphoma – = sclerotic, but same size)

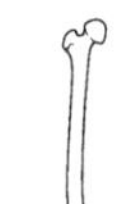

Femur/tibia

- Anterior bowing; 'sabre tibia' due to sclerosis

PC

Often asymptomatic, but picked up by X-rays + ALP ↑ ↑

P.V.C. B².O².N.E.S.

Pain
- Deep, boring pain
- ↑ at rest + night
- Not ↓by NSAIDs

Vascularity
- Warm bones, bruit, dilated superficial temporal arteries and external jugular vein

Cardiac
- High-output cardiac failure

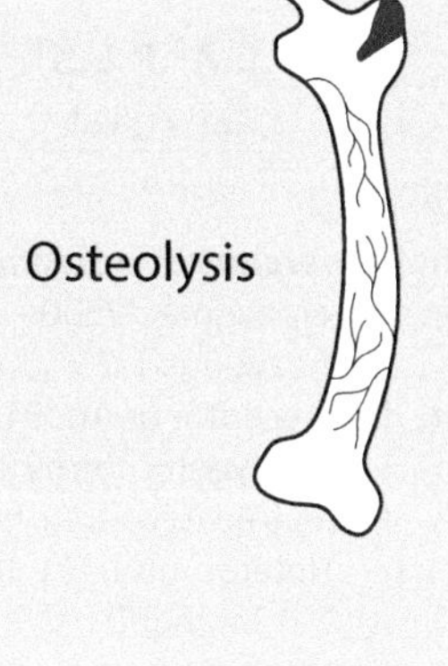

Bowing
- Deformable

Brittle
- Fractures, esp. femur neck or shaft

Orthopaedic deformity
- Skull enlargement; kyphosis

Osteoarthritis
- Secondary to misaligned bones

Neurological
- May be blind/deaf – due to nerve compression
  - Brainstem compression, hydrocephalus
  - Spinal stenosis, radicular compression

Electrolytes
- Gout
- Nephrocalcinosis (hypercalciuria)

Sarcoma, osteo
- In 1%
- Presents as ↑ in pain and ALP

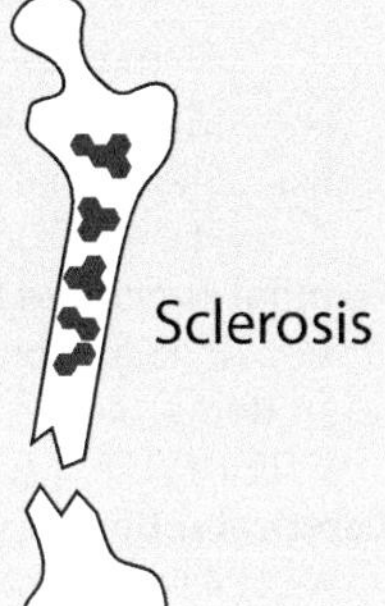

Ix

Bloods: Ca normal (but ↑ in immobility or fracture); PO_4 normal
ALP markedly ↑↑↑

Urine: Ca ↑
Bone resorption markers: Hydroxyproline:creatinine ratio or pyridinium crosslinks

Radiol: X-rays: Sclerosis and osteolysis *(see p. 394)*; used for Rx monitoring
^{99}Tc bone scan: Identifies 'hot-spots' of osteoblastic activity

Rx

Analgesics: NSAIDs only good for arthritis or fractures
Bisphosphonates: Alendronate, risedonate, pamidronate IV
Calcitonin, nasal: ☠: ↓Ca
Deformity: Osteotomy for bowed tibia; joint replacements for osteoarthritis

HYPERLIPIDAEMIA

Causes

P.E.A^2.R.L.S^2. and **P.E.A.R.L.S^4.**
(xanthomata are pearl-like papules)

P.E.A^2.R.L.S^2.
Cholesterol ↑

Primary (familial)
- **Familial hypercholesterolaemia**
  - Prev: Heterozygote: 1/500
    Homozygote: 1/250,000
  - Aet: LDL-receptor or ApoB100 mutations or polygenic forms (all auto. dom.)
  - PC: Premature ischaemic heart disease:
    - Heterozygous: By 40 (cholesterol 7–13 mmol/l)
    - Homozygous: By 20 (cholesterol >13 mmol/l)
    - Polygenic: By 40 (cholesterol 6–9 mmol/l)
  - Ix: LDL ↑= type IIa
  - Rx: Statins ineffective
    Plasmapharesis: Homozygous disease
- **Familial combined hyperlipidaemia**
  - Aet: ApoB overproduction in liver (auto. dom.)
  - Ix: LDL+VLDL ↑ (cholesterol+triglycerides↑)
- **Cerebrotendinous xanthomatosis**
  - Aet: Bile acid synthesis defect (auto. rec.)
  - PC: Progressive learning disability and ataxia
- **Familial causes of HDL ↓**
  - LCAT deficiency (corneal opacity)
  - Tangier disease (orange tonsils; neuropathy)

Endocrine
- Cushing (cholesterol + triglycerides ↑)
- Hypothyroidism

Anorexia nervosa/**A**cute intermittent porphyria
Renal: Nephrosis
Liver
- Cholestasis, e.g. primary biliary cirrhosis
- Hepatoma

Steroids/other toxins
- Glucocorticoids, progestagen
- Cylosporin
- Thiazide (cholesterol + triglycerides ↑)

Smoking: HDL ↓

P.E.A.R.L.S^4.
Triglycerides ↑

Primary (familial)
- **Familial hypertriglyceridaemia**
  - Prev: 1/600
  - Aet: Lipoprotein lipase mutation (auto. rec.)
    Apo-CII mutation (LPL activator)
  - Ix: **V**LDL↑ = type IV (auto. dom.)
    Chylmicrons↑ = type I (auto. rec.)
    esp. **C**hildren
    VLDL↑, Chylmicrons ↑, Triglyceride levels very high in types I and V = type V (auto rec)
- **Familial dysbetalipoproteinaemia**
  - Prev: 1/10,000
  - Aet: Accumulation of remnant lipoprotein due to impaired ApoE recognition by liver
    Apo E2/E2 homozygotes (1% pop.) plus obesity, diabetes or menopause
  - Ix: IDL ↑ (broad – β) = type III
- **Glycogen storage disease**
- **Lipodystrophy**

Endocrine
- Diabetes type 2 – also HDL ↓
- Acromegaly

Alcoholism – but HDL ↑/obesity – also HDL ↓
Renal: Chronic renal failure
Liver: Acute hepatitis
Steroids
Stress/**S**epsis/**S**urgery (ileal bypass)

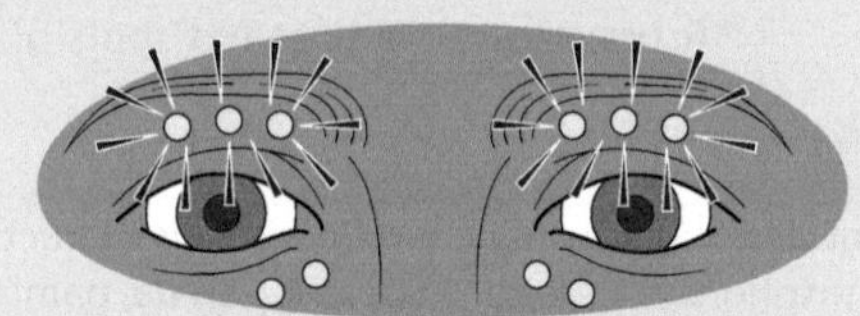

PC

O.X. C.H.O.P.S.

Ophthalmic
Cholesterol ↑: Xanthelasma palpebrum; corneal arcus (normal >50 y)
Triglycerides ↑: Lipaemia retinalis (white optic disc and vessels, when TG >10 mmol/l)

Xanthomata
Cholesterol ↑: Tendinous (normal skin colour as lie deep; Achilles, MCP, elbow)
Cutaneous: Homozygous FH only
Triglycerides ↑: Eruptive (pruritic, skin-colour papules, pustules; buttocks/elbows)
Striate palmar (orange–yellow papules on creases) – *Type III hyperlipidaemia*
Tuberous (large, pink-red nodules on bony prominences) – *Type III hyperlipidaemia*

Cardiac: Cholesterol ↑or type III triglycerides ↑ or diabetes – atherosclerosis (esp. coronary); aortic stenosis
Haematology: Cholesterol ↑ (esp. cholestasis or LCAT deficiency) – target cells
Organomegaly (hepatosplenomegaly): Triglycerides ↑
Pancreatitis, acute: Triglycerides ↑, when TG >10 mmol/l
Special: Arthritis – cholesterol ↑ (homozygous FH)

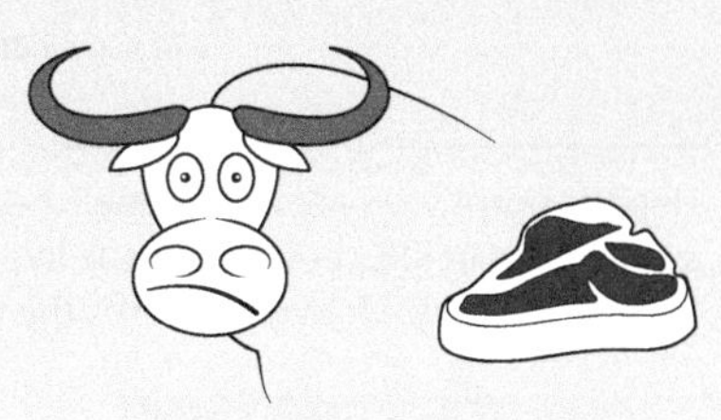

Ix

Cholesterol: Total >5.2 mmol/l: LDL >4.0; HDL <1.0; HDL/total cholesterol <0.25
Fasting triglyceride: Total >2.0 mmol/l (if >11, consider t chylomicrons)
Plasma appearance (after overnight storage at 4°C) – allows phenotype classification:

Clear	Turbid – milky	Creamy supernatant	Turbid + creamy supernatant	
LDL ↑ only **Type IIa**	VLDL ↑ **Type IIb or IV**	Chylomicrons ↑ **Type I**	VLDL ↑ + Chylomicrons ↑ **(Type V)**	IDL (broad-β) ↑ **(Type III)**

Rx

Conservative:
Diet – cholesterol ↓ by <10%
Exercise – HDL ↑
Alcohol, smoking, diabetes

Medical
Statins: Simva-, prava-, atorvastatin
HMG CoA reductase inhibitors cause upregulation of LDL receptors on liver
: Myositis; LFT Δ
Ezetimibe – GIT cholesterol absorption ↓

PORPHYRIA

Def

Hereditary or acquired defects along various steps of haem biosynthetic pathway
Causes one or combination of 3 clinical pictures, depending on step involved

Clinical	Biochemical abnormality	Organ
Neurological	Porphyrin precursor (ALA and PBG)↑↑	Hepatic
Cutaneous	Photosensitive porphyrins (tetrapyrolle ring) ↑↑	Hepatic/erythropoietic
Microcytic anaemia	Failure of haem synthesis	Erythropoietic

Hepatic porphyrias are commoner than erythropoietic porphyrias, even though 85% of body haem is synthesized in RBC, because in the liver, haem production is controlled by negative feedback, and so a failure to produce haem increases the rate of porphyrin production

Haem synthetic pathway

S.L.A.P → P.U.N.C.H

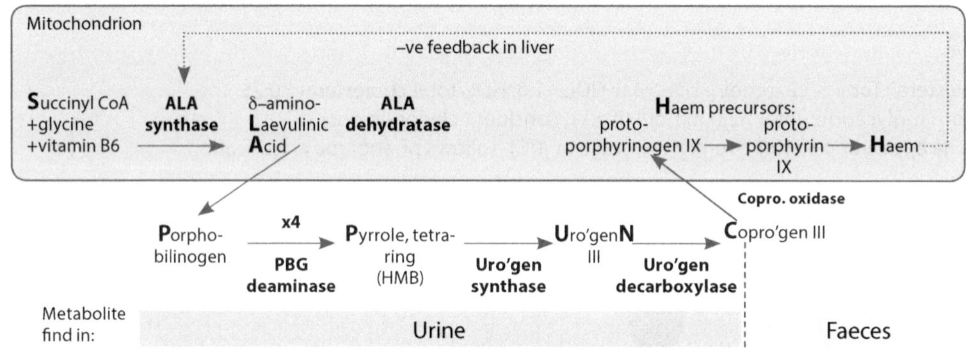

Types

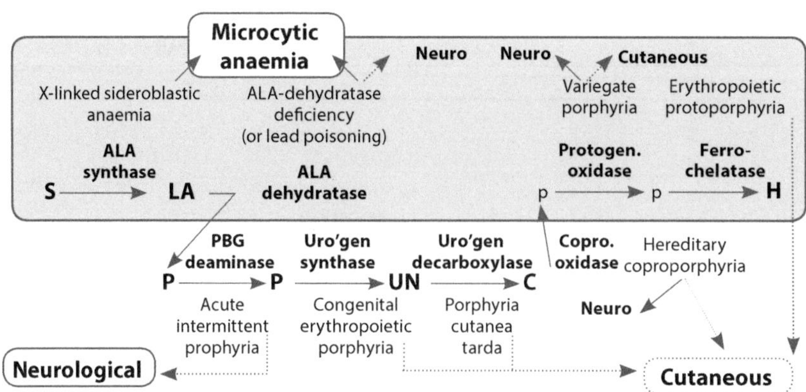

Key: copro'gen III, coporoporphyrinogen III oxidase; uro'gen, uroporphyrinogen

Acute intermittent porphyria

Epi

Inc: Commonest neurological porphyria (autosomal dominant)
Prev: 1/10,000 – PBG deaminase mutation; 1/100,000 – clinically affected (requires trigger)
Age: Onset in teens to 30s
Sex: F:M = 5:1, due to likely precipitants (pre-menstrual, pregnancy, 'pill', anorexia)
Pre: **A.I.P.** *is Asymptomatic until Induced by Precipitants* (esp. enzyme-inducers)
Alcohol, **A**nti-convulsants, **A**ntibiotics (sulphonamides, tetracyclines)
Intake ↓ (fasting), **I**nfection, **I**nhalation anaesthesia (halothane)
Pill (oestrogen), **P**ain-killers – opioids

PC

A.I.P².

Acute abdomen – constipation or diarrhoea; fever, N+V; dysuria; arthralgia
Ictus – fits, due to **I**CP rise and **I**nappropriate ADH secretion (Na ↓)
Peripheral and autonomic neuropathy:
PNS: Acute bulbar, limb and respiratory weakness (like Guillain–Barré syndrome)
ANS: Disproportionate tachycardia, hypertension; sweating, pallor; urinary retention
Psychiatric: Psychosis, mania, confusion, depression

Ix

Bloods: WCC ↑, Na ↓, Urea ↑, LFT ↑
Urine: Protein ↑, ALA and PBG (latter turns brown on standing, or pink with Ehrlich aldehyde)
Special: Fibroblast culture for enzyme assay

Rx

High-glucose drink or 20% dextrose IV – inhibits ALA synthase
Haematin (haem arginate IV) – inhibits ALA synthase
Symptomatic: Opioids; propranolol; diazepam or clonazepam ; fluid restrict (if SIADH); phenothiazine
Prophylactic: Avoid precipitants; screen relatives

Porphyria cutanea tarda

Epi

Inc: Commonest cutaneous porphyria; acquired in majority, or autosomal dominant.
Pre: Chronic liver disease, esp. alcohol, autoimmune hepatitis, haemochromatosis, oestrogen

PC

P².C³.T.

Photosensitivity (erythema, bullae, pigmentation); **P**itting oedema
Calcification of skin; **C**icatrix (scars); **C**irrhosis (cause)
Trichosis: Hypertrichosis or hirsutism

Ix

Bloods: LFTs deranged, Fe and ferritin ↑ (always raised), glucose ↑
Urine: Uroporphyrinogen ↑ (ALA and PBG not raised due to compensatory PBG deaminase activity)

Rx

Chloroquine – complexes porphyrins
Venesection – for Fe overload
Avoid sun, alcohol, oestrogens

Renal Medicine

ACUTE KIDNEY INJURY

Causes

Pre-renal

Due to decreased blood perfusion to the kidneys

C.R.A.S.H.

Cardiac failure
Renal artery stenosis
ABP ↓ (hypotension)
Sepsis
Hypovolaemia, due to loss of blood (haemorrhage) or fluid (dehydration)

Intrinsic Renal

Renovascular

V.A.N.

Vasculitis of renal vessels
ABP ↑ (malignant hypertension)
NSAIDS – decrease renal blood flow

Glomerulonephritis

P.A.I.N.T.

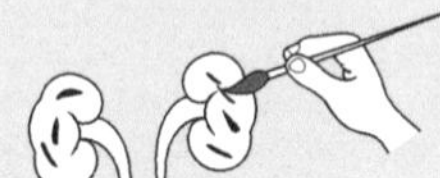

Primary: Proliferative, membranoproliferative
Autoimmune: SLE, vasculitis, anti-GBM, IgA nephropathy
Infection: Post-streptococcal, SBE, *Staphylococcus*, syphilis, HIV, HBV, HCV, malaria
Neoplasia: Myeloma, lymphoma
Toxins: Phenytoin, heroin (usually causes membranous GN)

Intrinsic Renal *continued*

Tubulo-interstitial nephritis

T.I.N.

Toxins:
- Allergic: Antibiotics, ACE-inhib., NSAID
- Tubular: Sulphonamides, acyclovir

Infection: Legionnaire, leptospirosis, brucellosis, CMV, candida
Neoplasia: Lymphoma; leukaemia

Acute tubular necrosis

Usually a consequence of untreated pre-renal AKI
Other causes:

A.T.N³.

ABP ↓: Patchy necrosis of tubules
Toxins: Aminoglycosides, cephalosporins, NSAIDs, cyclosporin, contrast, paracetamol overdose, paraquat, ethylene glycol (oxalate crystals)
Necrosis:
- Rhabdomyolysis (myoglobin)
- Intravascular haemolysis (Hb)

Neoplasia:
- Tumour lysis (uric acid)
- Myeloma (BJP)

Nephritis, pyelo-

Post-renal

Ureteric obstruction

Ureter or renal pelvis obstruction may cause AKI if bilateral involvement or unilateral with only one functioning kidney

S.N.I.P.P.I.N.G.

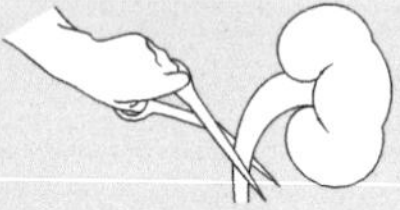

Stone
Neoplasia:
- Intrinsic: Transitional cell ca.
- Colorectal/gynaecological cancer
- Lymphoma

Infection: TB, schistosomiasis
Papillary necrosis
Pregnancy or other gynae.
Inflammation: Stricture/retroperitoneal fibrosis
Neurological
Genetic/congenital: PUJ or VUJ stenosis, ureterocoele

Urinary retention

S.N.I.P.P.I.N.G.

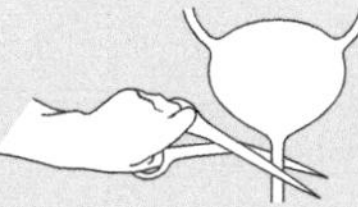

Stone
Neoplasia: Prostate, gynaecological
Infection: UTI
Papillary necrosis
Prostate: Hyperplasia or cancer
Inflammation: Stricture
Neurological:
- Neuropathy, cord lesion
- Toxins, post-operative atony
- Psychological

Genetic/congenital: Valves

PC

General
Anuria (or polyuria with ATN)
Fluid overload/hypertension
Electrolytes: K^+ – arrhythmia

Specific
Fever, arthralgia, rash – allergic TIN, autoimmune
Large tender kidneys – pyelonephritis, Hantavirus

Ix

Bloods: Biochem:
- K^+ ↑ (low in TIN), Mg^{2+}↑, Ca^{2+} ↓, PO_4 ↑, ABGs show metabolic acidosis
- Underlying causes: Ca^{2+} ↑, uric acid ↑

Haem:
- FBC (normocytic anaemia suggests chronic kidney disease – CKD)
- Eosinophils (TIN, vasculitis, cholesterol emboli), ESR, blood film

Immunol:
- ANA, dsDNA, ENA, ANCA, anti-GBM, Ig, cryoglobulinaemia, serum electrophoresis
- C3 ↓ only = post-streptococcal or membranoproliferative-II glomerulonephritis
- C3 and C4 ↓ = membranoproliferative-I glomerulonephritis, esp. SLE, HCV

Urine: Dipstick: Blood – nephritis; proteinuria; glycosuria – TIN
Cytology:
- RBC casts – GN; WBC casts – GN, pyelonephritis; eosinophiliuria – allergic TIN
- Epithelial casts, coarse granular casts – ATN
- Epithelial cells, hyaline casts, mildly granular casts – normal

Biochem:
- Na <20 mmol/l = pre-renal AKI
- Urea >10 × plasma urea = pre-renal AKI
- Osmolal. >1.5 × plasma osmolality = pre-renal AKI
- Protein: 30–300 mg/day or albumin:creatinine ratio >3 = microalbuminuria
- Protein: >3 g/day = nephrotic syndrome
- Protein electrophoresis: BJP

Micro: MSU
Serology: ASO, antiDNAse B; HBV, HCV (ELISA or PCR); parasite film; serology
Blood cultures × 3

Monitor: Fluid in and out
Daily weights (insensible losses)
Temperature

ECG

Radiol: USS: Large – obstruction; small – CKD; also stones, renal artery or vein duplex
CXR: Pulmonary oedema; bones may show signs of renal osteodystrophy if CKD
CT KUB stones, or other obstruction

Surgery: Biopsy:
- Linear Ig deposits: SLE, anti-GBM disease ('ribbons'), diabetes
- Subepithelial granular IgG: post-streptococcal GN
- Subepithelial spikes: Membranous GN
- Subendothelial IgG: Membranoproliferative GN

Cystoscopy

Rx

Underlying cause:
- Pre-renal – fluid challenge
- Renal – steroids, antibiotics, etc.
- Post-renal – removal or bypass of obstruction

Fluid management: CVP monitoring, haemodialysis
Electrolytes, esp. K^+; Ca gluconate, insulin infusion; haemodialysis

CHRONIC KIDNEY DISEASE – CAUSES

Def

Permanent ↓ in GFR to <50 ml/min (end-stage renal failure: <10 ml/min)

Causes

V.I.S.A.

Vascular disorders
Inflammation (i.e. vasculitis)
Stenosis of renal arteries
ABP ↑ (hypertension is commonest cause of CKD in UK)

G.L.A.D. G.R.A.C.E.

Glomerular disorders
Lupus nephritis
Auto-immune e.g. Goodpasture
Diabetic nephropathy

Glomerulonephritis **(P.A.I.N.T.)**
Retrovirus (i.e. HIV)
Ig**A** nephropathy
Collagen disease (Alport syndrome)
Endocarditis

Polycystic kidney disease

T.R.A.P. I.T.

Tubulo-intersitial disease
Reflux nephropathy
Amyloidosis
Plasma cell malignancy (i.e. myeloma)

Infection/abscess
Toxins

CHRONIC KIDNEY DISEASE – PC AND O/E

S.C.A.R.R.I.N.G T.U.B.E.S.

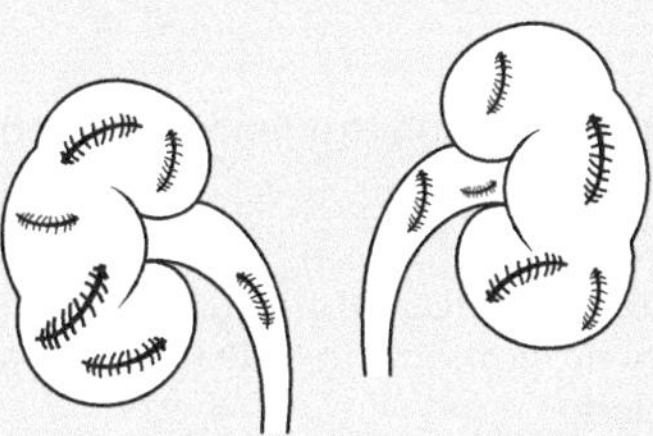

Skin:
- Uraemia: Pruritus (scratch marks), brown nails, hyperpigmented 'frost' or sallow, injected sclera
- Underlying cause: Vasculitis, scleroderma, amyloid, partial lipodystrophy, angiokeratoma
- Complications: Pallor (anaemia), subcutaneous or scleral calcification (↓ Ca^{2+}), tophi (gout)

Cardiac:
- Fluid overload: Pulmonary and peripheral oedema, JVP ↑ (or ↓ if salt-wasting)
- Pericarditis; tamponade (Kussmaul sign – paradoxical JVP ↑ on inspiration), chest pain
- Ischaemic heart disease, dilated cardiomyopathy – multifactorial, incl. hypertriglyceridaemia, hyperhomocystinaemia, low HDL, insulin resistance, vascular calcification

ABP↑: Fluid overload (less commonly; ↓: salt-wasting with tubular disease)
Respiratory: Pulmonary oedema (SOB), pleurisy (chest pain), pleural effusion, pulmonary fibrosis
Respiratory pattern: Hiccups, uraemic fetor, Kussmaul breathing (deep) due to metabolic acidosis
Immunocompromise, e.g. pneumonia
Neurological:
- Encephalopathy: Early – myoclonus, asterixis (hand flap); late – dementia, dysarthria, seizures
- Peripheral neuropathy, restless legs syndrome
- Myopathy: Due to uraemia and osteomalacia

GIT:
- Gastric ulcers due to gastrin ↑
- Haemorrhage, due to angiodysplasia and coagulopathy, impaired platelet function

Thrombocytopenia: Purpura, GIT haemorrhage (also due to impaired platelet function and coagulopathy)
Urine:
- Frequency or nocturia may occur with tubular disease
- Haematuria: IgA nephropathy, vasculitis or reflecting coagulopathy
- Loin pain, or renal mass – suggests renal cystic disease

Bones: Osteomalacia (vit. D deficiency), osteoporosis
Endocrine: Amenorrhoea, impotence, growth retardation (in children)
Systemic:
- Anaemia (depression, fatigue)
- Anorexia, weight loss, cachexia; hypothermia

CHRONIC KIDNEY DISEASE – IX

Bloods:

R.E.A.L.M.S.

Biochem:

Renal:

- Urea ↑: Endogenous and exogenous metabolite produced variably from amino acid degradation
- Creatinine ↑
  - Metabolite produced at constant rate from phosphocreatine in muscle
  - Inversely proportional to GFR: Plot inverse-creatinine over time and extrapolate
- Creatinine clearance = estimate of GFR

$$\text{Clearance} = \frac{U_{Cr} \times V}{P_{Cr}}$$

where P_{Cr} and U_{Cr} = plasma and urine concentration of creatinine and V = volume of urine over 24 h

Adjust for surface-area (standard = 1.73 m^2); age; sex; diet and drugs

Clearance <10 ml/min = end-stage renal failure

Electrolytes:

- Na^+ ↓, K^+ ↓
- Ca^{2+} ↓, PO_4 ↑, Mg^{2+} ↑, Vit D ↓, PTH ↑ due to – tubular Ca resorption ↓, PO_4 excretion ↓, 1α-hydroxylation of cholecalciferol ↓

ABGs: Metabolic acidosis and respiratory compensation

LFTs: ALP ↑ – osteomalacia; albumin ↓ – due to nephrosis, protein restriction,

Metabolic:

- Glucose: ↑ due to insulin resistance and decreased insulin release ↓ (in diabetes) due to ↓ insulin catabolism and ↓ gluconeogenesis
- Triglycerides, fasting ↑

Special: Uric acid ↑; T4 ↑ , T3 slightly ↓; serum and urine electrophoresis (myeloma, amyloid – cause of CKD)

Haem: Hb: Normochromic, normocytic anaemia (bone marrow suppression, EPO production ↓); film: Burr cells WCC, platelets, clotting – impaired function for all and thrombocytopenia

Immunol: ANA, rheumatoid factor, ANCA, cryoglobulins

Urine: Microscopy (early morning): Haematuria; RBC or WBC casts
Protein (24-hour): Glomerulonephritis
Amino acids, PO_4, glucose – tubular disease

Micro: MSU (UTI due to obstruction); *Schistosoma* urine microscopy
Hep B, C, HIV serology; malaria film

Monitor: ABP, fluid balance, weights: (oral + IV) vs. (urine + faeces + vomit + insensible losses [weight])
Glucose – insulin resistance

ECG: Sx of K^+ ↓
LVH 2° to hypertension

Radiol: CXR: Pulmonary oedema; CCF; AXR – calcification
USS:
- Small kidneys suggest CKD (except early diabetes, obstruction, amyloid)
- Renal tract obstruction (reversible!); cysts, tumour
- Functional: IVU/DMSA – scarring due to VuR; DTPA or MAG3 + captopril – renovascular disease

Special: Renal biopsy – if cause unclear and renal size normal (i.e. potentially reversible!)

CHRONIC KIDNEY DISEASE – RX

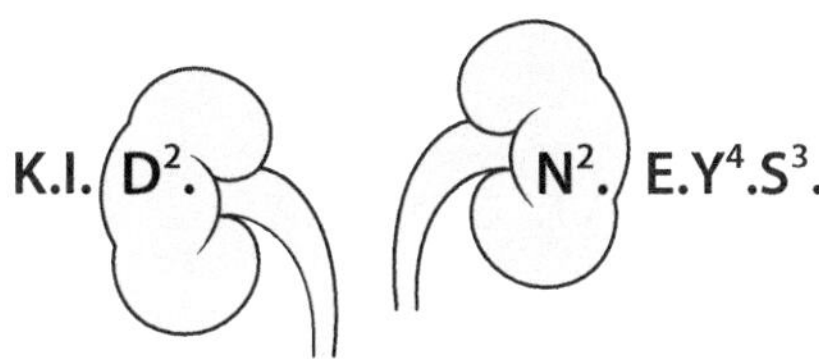

K.I.D²N².E.Y⁴.S³.

K+ correct:
- Particular concern during acute exacerbations
- Consider treating acidosis, but $NaHCO_3$ problematic due to high Na^+ content

Intake – salt/fluid:
- Fluid-overload: ↓ salt and fluid intake, until normal CVP or JVP obtained
- Fluid-depleted, e.g. post-ATN, post-obstruction, chronic TIN: ↑ salt and fluid intake, until UO > 2 l/day

Diuretics:
- High-dose loop diuretic, e.g. furosemide
- ACE inhibitors: Renoprotective in diabetes; contraindicated in renal artery stenosis

Dialysis:
- Haemodialysis:
  Method: 4 h/session; 3 sessions/week; 250 ml/min blood dialysed via forearm AV fistula
  Adv: Can vary dialysate composition; flow rate or pressure (therefore diffusion gradient)
  Disadv: Low creatinine clearance – 6 ml/min; loss of amino acids, vitamins; no vit. D; EPO
  ☠: **A**rterial injury: Haemorrhage, thrombosis, ischaemia ('steal') **A**BP: Postural hypotension
  Amyloid: β_2-microglobulin – carpal tunnel syndrome
  Aluminium toxicity: Brain (dementia); bone marrow (anaemia); bone (osteomalacia)
- Chronic ambulatory peritoneal dialysis (CAPD):
  Method: Introduce 2 l dialysate into peritoneum and replace 3–4 ×/day
  Adv: Slightly better creatinine clearance –7 ml/min, but still loses amino acids and vitamins
  ☠ **I**nfection of catheter, peritonitis; blockage, leakage
  Intake fluid – mechanical back pain, genital oedema, hernia, haemorrhoids, hydrothorax
  Insulin resistance due to glucose loading from dialysate, obesity

Nutrition:
- Low protein (0.5 g/kg/day – ↓ uraemic toxins and acidosis); high carbohydrate; low fat
- Haematinics (Fe, folate, vit. B12) and vit. C (as lost on dialysis)

NSAIDs – avoid; also avoid aminoglycosides

EPO (human recombinant erythropoeitin, slow-IV or subcut)
☠ ABP ↑; thrombocytosis; flu-like syndrome
May also require occasional blood transfusion with diuretic cover

Y: h**Y**perlipidaemia – simvastatin
h**Y**perglycaemia – avoid metformin, chlorpropamide; caution with insulins (due to risk of 'hypos')
h**Y**perPO_4aemia – **Rx first** to avoid ectopic calcification – PO_4 restriction; oral PO_4 binders – $MgCO_3$ or $CaCO_3$
h**Y**pocalcaemia – 1α-hydroxylated cholecalciferol; calcitriol; $CaCO_3$, high-dose: ↓ PTH and ↓ PO_4

Symptomatic:
- Hiccups or pruritus: Chlorpromazine
- Peptic ulcers: Omeprazole

Surgical – renal transplant
☠
- Rejection (immunological, ureteric anastomosis failure); immunosuppression (infections, neoplasia)
- Vascular: Polycythaemia, atherosclerosis, hypertension

Secondary renal failure: Treat underlying cause – diabetes, hypertension, SLE, etc.

HAEMATURIA – CAUSES

Pre-renal	Renal	Post-renal
M. S.P.A.C.E.	**S.T.I.G.M.A.T.A.**	**S.N.I.P.P.I.N.G.**
Malaria **S**ickle cell disease **P**NH **A**utoimmune haemolytic anaemia **C**oagulopathy **E**xercise	**S**tones – renal calculus **T**rauma – blunt trauma to flanks **I**nterstitial nephritis **G**lomerulonephritis **M**alignancy (RCC) **A**PCKD **T**hin membrane disease **A**lport syndrome	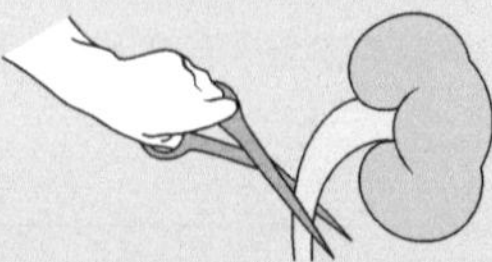 **S**chistosomiasis – commonest cause of haematuria worldwide, rare in UK **N**eoplasia: TCC **I**nfection: Urogenital TB, UTI **P**rostate: Cancer, prostatitis, BPH **P**igmented urine: Dye ingestion (beetroot; rifampicin, L-DOPA); porphyria **I**nflammation: Stricture/retroperitoneal fibrosis **N**ephrolithiasis **G**enetic/congenital: PUJ or VUJ stenosis, ureterocoele

IgA nephropathy

Epi

Inc: Commonest type of glomerulonephritis
Age: M:F = 3:1
Geo: Far East, SE Asia
Aet: Deposition of IgA in renal glomerulus, exacerbated by respiratory tract infections ('synpharyngitic')
Prog: Male, smoking, nephrotic syndrome, and older age favour poorer outcome

PC

Renal-limited (or Berger disease):

Haematuria – recurrent, macroscopic:	1/3
Proteinuria, incl. nephrotic syndrome:	1/3 (poor prognosis)
Hypertension; CKD:	1/3

Associations: **G.R.O.S.S. BLOOD**

GIT:
- Coeliac, Crohn, adenocarcinoma
- Biliary disease, chronic liver disease

Respiratory: Pneumonitis, obliterative bronchiolitis, adenocarcinoma
Ophthalmic: Anterior uveitis; episcleritis
Skin: IgA vasculitis (Henoch–Schönlein purpura)
Spondylitis, Sjögren syndrome, rheumatoid arthritis, ankylosing spondylosis

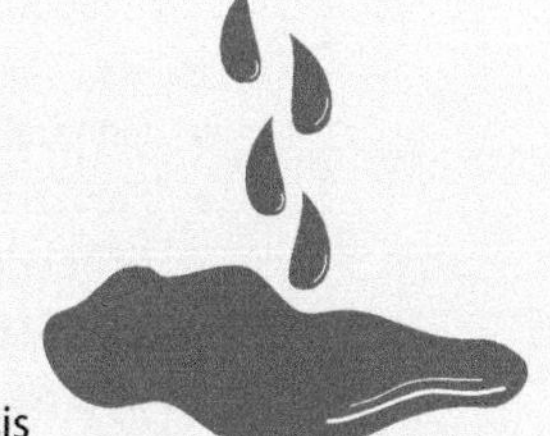

Blood: Monoclonal gammopathy of uncertain significance (IgA)

Ix

Serum IgA ↑ in 50%
Complement: Normal or ↑
Biopsy: Mesiangial proliferation and IgA deposits on immunofluorescence

Rx

Microscopic haematuria, no nephrotic syndrome and normal renal function – observation only
Steroids
Cyclophosphamide

Thin basement membrane disease

('Benign haematuria')

Epi

Inc: Commonest cause of asymptomatic haematuria
Aet: Sporadic or hereditary (autosomal dominant: collagen Type IV, α4 chain mutation)

PC

Haematuria post-URTI
Hypertension/proteinura – rare

Ix

Light microscopy + IF: Normal
Electron microscopy: Thin basement membrane (normal = 300–350 nm)

Rx

Follow-up only

NEPHROTIC SYNDROME

PC

N. E. P. H. R. O. T. I. C.

Nephritis: Nephrotic syndrome may occur alone or as part of a general nephritic syndrome

Nephrotic syndrome alone:

- Glomerulonephritis: Membranous GN, focal segmental glomerulosclerosis, minimal change disease, membranoproliferative GN
- Diabetic nephropathy
- Amyloidosis

Nephritic syndrome:

- IgA nephropathy
- Post-streptococcal GN
- Goodpasture syndrome

O**E**dema:

- Generalized, esp. peri-orbital
- Pleural effusion; ascites
- GIT oedema: Nausea, malabsorption, weight loss

Proteinuria: Frothy urine

Hypoalbuminaemia:

- Hypovolaemia
- Growth retardation
- Leukonychia

Raised lipids: LDL ↑, HDL ↓, triacylglycerides ↑
PC: Atherosclerosis; xanthoma; pseudohyponatraemia
Due to renal loss of apolipoprotein B

Osteomalacia: Due to renal-loss of vit. D-binding globulin, which results in Ca^{2+} ↓

Thrombosis: DVT; CVA; renal vein thrombosis; pulmonary embolism – due to renal loss of anti-thrombin-III; hypovolaemia; atherosclerosis

Infection, esp. pneumococcal peritonitis – loss of Igs + C3, C4

Chronic anaemia (hypochromic, but Fe-resistant): Renal loss of transferrin

Urine:

Protein:creatinine ratio

- 100 mg/mmol – moderate proteinuria
- ≥300 mg/mmol – heavy proteinuria = nephrotic syndrome

24-hour protein

- 150–500 mg/day – mild proteinuria (e.g. orthostatic; post-renal)
- 500 mg–3 g/day – moderate proteinuria (e.g. glomerulonephritides, hypertension, UTI)
- >3 g/day – heavy proteinuria, incl. nephrotic syndrome

Urine electrophoresis – establishes 'selectivity' of glomerular disease

- High (mid-molecular weight, e.g. albumin) – minimal-change glomerulonephritis
- Low (mid- and high-molecular weight, e.g. IgG) – membranous glomerulonephritis
- Low-molecular weight (e.g. β_2- microglobulin) – venous hypertension; proximal tubular disease
- Bence-Jones protein – myeloma

Rx

Treat underlying cause:

Diet: Protein (caution if incipient renal failure); calories (overcome GIT oedema)

Fluid balance: Salt and water intake; spironolactone or furosemide and amiloride; salt-free albumin 20%

Complications:

- Hypercholesterolaemia: Simvastatin
- Infection: Pneumococcal vaccine; IV benzylpenicillin
- DVT: LMW heparin; antithrombin III supplements

RENOVASCULAR DISEASE

Causes

S.T.E.N.T.A.B².L.E².

Stenosis, renal artery
Thrombosis, renal artery or vein
Embolus, renal artery:
- Cardiogenic: AF, endocarditis, paradoxical (DVT via patent foramen ovale)
- Cholesterol emboli: From aortic atheroma, esp. post-aortic surgery; arteriography – Ix: eosinophilia

NSAIDs: Vasodilate afferent and efferent arterioles, causing ↓ GFR
Toxins, other:
- Drugs: **A**CE inhibitors (and vasodilators); **A**mphotericin; **A**drenaline; cyclosporin
- Radiotherapy

Autoimmune:
- Scleroderma
- Vasculitides: Takayasu, PAN, granulomatosis with polyangiitis
  PATH: Intimal proliferation, medial thinning, fibrinoid necrosis of small arteries
  PC:
  - Microscopic haematuria, pyuria, cellular casts, mild proteinuria
  - Crisis: AKI, severe hypertension, microscopic angiopathic haemolytic anaemia (MAHA)

Blood pressure ↑:
- Hypertensive nephrosclerosis:
  PATH: Intimal hyaline arteriosclerosis, necrotising arteriolitis
  PC: Chronic kidney disease
- Malignant hypertension:
  PATH: Fibrinoid necrosis, 'onion-skinning', 'flea-bitten kidney'
  PC: AKI, haematuria, nephrosis, MAHA

Blood constituents:
- Disseminated intravascular coagulation (DIC)
- Haemolytic uraemic syndrome (HUS)
  Epi: Commonest cause of AKI in children
  Cause:
  - Children: Gastroenteritis, esp. verocytotoxicogenetic *E. coli* (VTEC), serotype O157, H7
  - Adults: Idiopathic, HIV, adenocarcinoma, SLE, post-partum, pre-eclampsia, genetic

  PC:
  - AKI: 'Flea-bitten kidney' = cortical haemorrhagic microinfarcts – MAHA (fragmented RBCs)
  - Platelets ↓
- Thrombotic thrombocytopenic purpura (TTP) – as for HUS, plus:
  - Fever; WCC ↑
  - Infarcts: Renal (AKI), brain–retina (focal neuro. Sx), bowel (mesenteric ischaemia)

Liver failure: Hepatorenal syndrome – hepatic toxins and prostaglandins induce vasoconstriction
Eclampsia, pre-
Electrolyte: Hypercalcaemia:
- Vasoconstrictor
- Also causes CKD via tubular and ureteric calcification

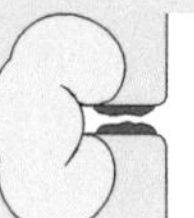
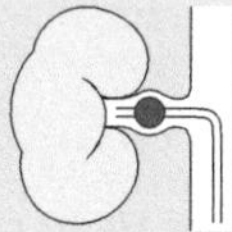
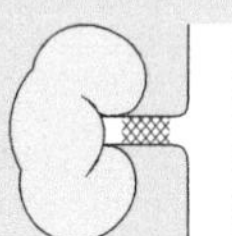

Stenosis, renal artery

Causes

Atherosclerosis:
- Epi: Elderly; hypertension; ACE inhibitors (dilate efferent arteriole and so oppose physiological response)
- Site: Proximal; bilateral in 50%

Fibromuscular dysplasia:
- Epi: Young women (30–40s; F:M = 4:1); smoking
- Site: Distal (dysplasia); right-sided or bilateral

PC

Hypertension ± renal failure
Bruit: High-pitched

Ix

Bloods: Creatinine ↑, K^+ ↓, metabolic alkalosis

Radiol: Digital subtraction angiogram, duplex or MRA: Fibromuscular dysplasia = 'string of beads'; smooth narrowing; local aneurysms; AVM; fistulae
Radionuclide scan (^{99m}Tc-DTPA or MAG3 scan ± captopril) – captopril dilates efferent arteriole → dramatic ↓ in GFR and ↓ uptake of tracer (DTPA)

Special: Captopril-induced hypotension: Causes exaggerated ↑ in plasma renin activity
Renal vein renin ratio of >1.5:1 between kidneys provides indication for surgery

Rx

Aspirin
Angioplasty
Surgery – better outcome

GLOMERULONEPHRITIS

Def

Glomerular inflammation

PC

Causes classified according to predominant clinical syndrome:

Nephritic syndrome

PATH: Capillary proliferation

PC:

- Oliguria
- Hypertension
- Haematuria and pyuria (presentation mimicked by renovascular disease, or acute tubulo-interstitial nephritis)

RPGN (rapidly progressive glomerulonephritis)

PATH: Glomerular 'crescents' = extreme form of capillary proliferation

PC:

- Anuria (glomerular effacement)
- As for nephritic syndrome

Nephrotic syndrome

PATH: Membrane disease

PC:

- Proteinuria
- Oedema
- Hypercholesterolaemia

Histology

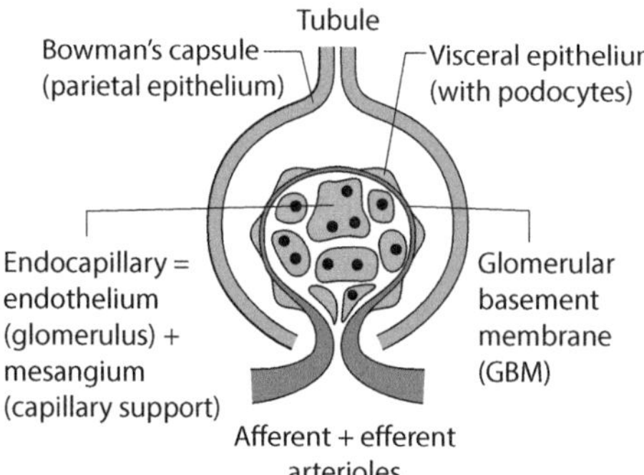

Segmental vs. Global: Glomerulus-level ascription
Focal vs. Diffuse: Kidney-level ascription

Nephritic syndrome and RPGN

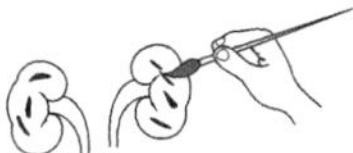

P.A.I.nts.

Primary: Proliferative glomerulonephritis:

Immune-complex:

- Proliferation of endocapillaries
- **P**roliferative = sube**P**ithelial granular deposits ('starry sky')

Ix: Low C3, C_H50

Pauci-immune:

- Proliferation of endocapillary and parietal cell epithelium ('crescents')
- Focal necrosis

Ix: Normal C3, 4, C_H50 but p-ANCA +ve, and ESR, CRP ↑ as associated with vasculitis

Autoimmune:

SLE, myositis – as for immune-complex GN

Vasculitides (e.g. PAN, granulomatosis with polyangiitis) – as for pauci-immune glomerulonephritis

Angiogram: Aneurysms, infarcts

Anti-GBM disease – linear immune-complex deposits on GBM and tubules ('ribbon-like'):

Epi: Smoking; hydrocarbons; flu; HLA DR-2, -4

PC: Haematuria; haemoptysis (Goodpasture syndrome)

Ix: Serology;

- Anti-GBM in 50% of Goodpasture = Ab against non-collagenous domain of collagen IV, a3-chain
- C3, 4 normal, ANCA +ve in 20%, respiratory function (KCO), bronchoscopy

Infection:

Streptococcus pyogenes:

Epi: 10–20 days post-pharyngitis/impetigo

PC: Smoky red urine (may persist for >6 years), headache, N+V (ABP ↑), flank pain, acute kidney injury that usually recovers within 1 month

Ix: Serology:

- Anti-DNAseB, ASO, Anti-NADase (throat), antihyaluronidase (skin)
- C3, C_H50 ↓, polyclonal IgG↑

Chronic bacterial:

- Bacterial endocarditis: C3, 4 ↓
- Visceral abscess: C3, C4 normal or ↑

Nephrotic syndrome

P.A.I.N.T.S^2.

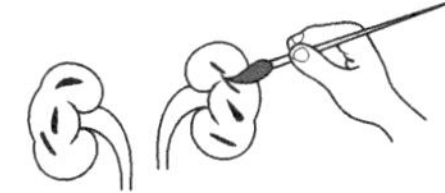

Nephritic and Nephrotic syn.

P.A.I.N.T.S.

Primary:
- **Membranous glomerulonephritis**
- Diffuse thickening of GBM
- Subepithelial immune-complex deposits ('silver spikes')
- Epi: 40% adult; <5% child nephrotic syndrome
  - 70% membranous GN are idiopathic
- Ix: C3, 4 normal
- **Minimal-change disease**
- No change/mild mesangial hypercellularity on light microscopy
- Diffuse effacement of podocyte foot processes on electron microscopy
- Epi: 20% adult; 80% child nephrotic syndrome
- **Focal segmental glomerulosclerosis:** Hyalinosis in parts of >50% glomerulus

Autoimmune:
- SLE, Sjögren, Hashimoto, Graves, PBC all cause membranous glomerulonephritis
- Atopy – associated with minimal-change GN

Infection:
- Hep B or C, malaria, enterococcal SBE, syphilis all cause membranous GN
- HIV, immunisation; URTI associated with minimal-change GN/FSGS

Neoplasia:
- Amyloid (1° and 2°: Congo red +ve); myeloma
- Lymphoma, renal-cell carcinoma – minimal-change
- Carcinoma, melanoma – membranous

Toxins:
- Captopril, penicillamine, NSAIDs – membranous
- Ampicillin, rifampicin – minimal-change
- Opioids – FSGS

Sclerosis (other FSGS causes):
- Diabetes mellitus – also causes membranous; minimal-change GN
- Sickle cell anaemia
- Glomerular capillary hypertension:
  - Renal ablation, e.g. contralateral renal agenesis or nephrectomy, renal artery thrombosis, diffuse renal disease, e.g. reflux nephropathy

Sarcoidosis

Primary
- **Membranoproliferative GN**
- Mesangial proliferation ('mesangiocapillary GN')
- Diffuse thickening of GBM
- Types:
  - Sube**N**dothelial and mesangial immune-complex deposits (mesa**N**gio)
    Ix: C3 + C4 ↓
    Course: Benign
  - Linear, intramembranous dense C3 deposits due to 'C3 nephritic factor', i.e. an IgG that stabilizes C3 convertase of the alternative complement pathway
    Ix: C3 ↓ only
    Course: End-stage renal failure in 5–10 y
- **Focal segmental proliferative:** Causes are same as for proliferative GN

Autoimmune:
- SLE, Sjögren, autoimmune hepatitis all cause membranoproliferative GN
- IgA nephropathy:
  - Epi: **Commonest glomerulonephritis** and cause of hypertension in young men
  - PC: Haematuria 3 days post-URTI
  - Types:
    - Renal-limited (Berger): 50% get CKD
    - Cutaneous vasculitis (Henoch–Schönlein purpura)
    - Systemic disease-associated

Infection:
- HBV, HCV (cryoglobulinaemia), HIV
- *Staphylococcus* – SBE, abscess, CSF 'shunt nephritis'
- Haemolytic uraemic syndrome all of these cause membranoproliferative GN

Neoplasia: Lymphoma, leukaemia

Toxins: Heroin

Syndromes:
- Thin-basement membrane disease:
  - Epi: Commonest cause of asymptomatic haematuria
  - Aet: Autosomal dominant or sporadic; collagen type IV, á4-chain mutation
- Alport disease
  - Epi: Commonest hereditary nephritis (X-linked)
  - Aet: Collagen type IV, α5-chain mutation
- Other: Nail–patella syn., partial lipodystrophy

RENAL TUBULAR DISEASE

The effects of tubular disease depend on whether proximal or distal convoluted tubules are affected

Proximal tubular disease

Types

B.A.N.G.'d. U.P.

Bicarbonaturia **(renal tubular acidosis – Type 2)**
Causes: Hereditary (autosomal recessive or autosomal dominant), or acetazolamide
PC:
- Weakness; failure to thrive (mild acidosis, hypokalaemia)
- Rickets or osteomalacia (but no renal stones due to ↓ citrate resorption)
- Polyuria, polydipsia (due to increased $NaHCO_3$ in distal tubule, and hypokalemia)

Ix:
- 'Normal anion gap' metabolic acidosis
  - Plasma HCO_3^- ↓, Cl^- ↑, K^+ ↓ ; urine HCO_3^- ↑
  - Aciduria: Minimum pH <5.5 (due to ↓ HCO_3^- filtration, ↑ distal H^+ excretion)
- Plasma PO_4 ↓, vit. D ↓; urine Ca^{2+} ↑

Rx: Bicarbonate

Amino aciduria (and low-molecular-weight proteinuria)
Causes:
- Overflow: Phenylketonuria, maple syrup urine, homocystinuria; acquired liver failure
- PCT resorption ↓:
  - Cystinuria: ↓ resorption of dibasic acids; PC: Renal stones
  - Hartnup disease: ↓ resorption of neutral amino acids; PC: Pellagra (tryptophan deficiency)

Na$^+$ and K$^+$ wasting
PC: Na^+ loss – hypovolaemia; K^+ loss – weakness

Glycosuria
Causes:
- Overflow (diabetes, stress)
- PCT resorption ↓ (hereditary, pregnancy)

PC: Polyuria, polydipsia

Uric aciduria

Phosphaturia
Causes:
- Overflow (paracetamol overdose)
- PCT resorption ↓ (X-linked dominant hypophosphataemic rickets)

'Fanconi syndrome'

Def: Generalized proximal tubule dysfunction of all or some of above defects
Causes:

F.A.N.C.O.N.I.

Familial: Autosomal dominant, autosomal recessive, X-linked
Autoimmune: Sjögren, autoimmune liver disease
Neoplasia: Myeloma, amyloid
Calcium ↑/↓: 1° or 2° hyperparathyroidism/chronic hypokalaemia
Other: Outdated tetracycline, lead, mercury, cadmium, cisplatin, aspirin, neomycin
Necrosis, acute tubular
Inherited: Wilson disease, cystinosis, Lowe oculocerebrorenal disease, tyrosinaemia

PC: As above + chronic kidney disease + vit. D deficiency + pyelonephritis
Rx: High fluid intake (sodium and water), $KHCO_3$, PO_4, α_1-calcidol

Distal tubular disease

H^+ excretion impairment (renal tubular acidosis – Type 1)

Causes:

T.U.B.U.L.A.R. P.H.

Toxins: NSAIDs, lithium, amphotericin
Ureteric-, vesico-, reflux: Chronic pyelonephritis, urinary obstruction
Blood pressure: Hypertension
Uric acid (gout)/Ca^{2+}↑ (hyperPTHism, vit. D toxicity)/K^+ ↓
Lymphoma, leukaemia, myeloma, amyloid
Autoimmune: Sjögren, SLE, autoimmune hepatitis
Radiation nephritis, renal transplant

Papillary necrosis: Diabetes mellitus, sickle cell anaemia
Hereditary: RTA-type 1 (autosomal dominant), medullary-sponge kidney

PC:

- Weakness; failure to thrive (acidosis, hypokalaemia)
- Rickets or osteomalacia, and renal stones
- Polyuria, polydipsia

Ix:

'Normal anion gap' metabolic acidosis: Plasma HCO_3^-↓, Cl^-↑, K^+↓

- Alkaluria: Minimum pH >5.5, and urine HCO_3^-↓ – cf. RTA type 2
- Low urine NH_4^+ (as estimated by urine cation gap) – cf. GIT cause of acidosis

Ca^{2+} ↓, vit. D ↓, PTH ↑; urine Ca^{2+} ↑
Acid load test: Loading with NH_4Cl fails to acidify urine (urine pH >6.5)

Rx: KCl, followed by bicarbonate

Aldosterone impairment (renal tubular acidosis – Type 4)

Causes:
Hyporeninism: Diabetes mellitus, hypertensive nephrosclerosis
Hypoaldosteronism: Addison, adrenalectomy
Aldosterone resistance: Obstructive nephropathy, spironolactone

Ix:
Bloods: Plasma: HCO_3^- ↓, Cl^- ↑, K^+ ↑ – cf. RTA types 1 and 2
Urine – as for RTA type 1: Alkaluria and urine HCO_3^-↓ (although minimum pH may be <5.5)

Rx: Fludrocortisone (high-dose if resistance)

Diabetes insipidus

Causes:
Cranial: **D.I.V.I.N.I.T.Y. –** e.g. hereditary, sarcoid, pituitary adenoma
Tubular: **T.U.B.U.L.A.R. P.H.** – e.g. toxins, ureteric reflux, blood pressure, uric acid ↑, Ca^{2+} ↑

Ix:
Plasma osmolality >300 mOsm/kg
Urine osmolality <300 mOsm/kg

URINARY OBSTRUCTION

Causes

The following cause obstruction in the renal pelvis, ureters, bladder or urethra

S.N.I.P.P.I.N.G.

Stones
Neoplasia:
- Intrinsic: Polyp/carcinoma – transitional cell (ureter/bladder) or squamous cell (urethra)
- Extrinsic: Colorectal, gynaecological or prostate carcinoma/lymphoma

Infection:
- TB: Intrinsic fibrosis, or para-aortic lymph nodes
- *Schistosoma haematobium* (Africa, Mediterranean)

Papillary necrosis:
- Diabetes mellitus/hypertension
- Sickle cell anaemia/vasculitis
- Acute tubular necrosis

Pregnancy (or other gynaecological)/**P**rostate:
- Pregnancy: Due to direct compression, oestrogen (smooth muscle relaxant)
- Other: Fibroids, ovarian cyst, haematocolpos, haematometria (occurs at menses)
- Prostate: Benign prostatic hyperplasia, carcinoma, prostatitis (all cause bladder-neck obstruction)

Inflammation – fibrosis:
- Stricture: Post-trauma, laparotomy (e.g. caesarian section – ureters), catheterisation (urethra)
- Retroperitoneal fibrosis, due to:
  - **P**rimary: Multifocal fibrosclerosis (66%); ESR ↑
  - **A**utoimmune: PAN
  - **I**nfection: TB
  - **N**eoplasia: Metastases, lymphoma, carcinoid
  - **T**oxins: Methysergide
  - **S**urrounding inflammation: Aortic aneurysm, pancreatitis, Crohn, diverticulitis

Neurological – failure of peristalsis, e.g. anticholinergics
Genetic/congenital – urinary tract anomalies:
- Stenosis: PUJ (pelvic-ureteric junction) or VUJ (vesico-ureteric junction)
- Ureter: Ureterocoele; retrocaval ureter
- Urethra: Valves (commonest cause of bilateral hydronephrosis in boys), phimosis

PC

Anuria/oliguria
Suprapubic pain
Abdominal distension

URINARY OBSTRUCTION

Causes

The following cause obstruction in the bladder neck or urethra

S.N.I.P.P.I.N.G^2.

Stones
Neoplasia: Carcinoma – bladder, prostate, colorectal, gynaecological
Infection: UTI, STD, abscess (e.g. bartholinitis, caruncle); PC: 'Holding on', strangury
Papillary necrosis
Pregnancy (or other gynaecological)/**P**rostate
  Pregnancy: Retroverted uterus/other – fibroids; ovarian cyst, haematocolpos, haematometria
  Prostate: Benign prostatic hyperplasia, carcinoma, prostatitis
Inflammation (fibrosis): Stricture post-trauma, catheterisation (urethra)
Neurological:
  LMN: Diabetic neuropathy, cauda equina; UMN: Multiple sclerosis, cord compression
  Atony: Overdistension, e.g. diuretics, post-operative, binge-drinking
  Toxins, e.g. anticholinergics
  Psychological
Genetic/congenital: Urethral valves; phimosis
GIT: Constipation (bladder neck obstruction)

Types

	Symptoms	Catheter residual volume	Renal function
Acute	Painful	<1 litre	Normal
Chronic	Painless	>1 litre	Renal failure
Acute-on-chronic (e.g. overfilling; UTI)	Painful	>1 litre (normal <600 ml)	Renal failure

Complications

Stones: Form in diverticulae that develop between hypertrophied trabeculations
Infection
Renal failure

Rx

Catheterize: Measure residual volume, and leave for 1–2 days
TWOC (trial without catheter): Perform at midnight to allow daytime observation
Indwelling catheterisation, if TWOC failure, chronic retention, or prostatism, prostate carcinoma

RENAL STONES

Epi

Inc: Lifetime risk = 1%
Age: 20–40s
Sex: M:F = 4:1 (opposite of gallstones)

Causes

Crystal formation depends on:
Chemical factors: Ca^{2+} ↑, oxalate ↑, alkali ↑, citrate ↓
Crystallisation factors: Stasis facilitates crystal nucleation

C.R.U.S.H.I.N.G.

Calcium – hypercalciuria
PATH: Ca oxalate or phosphate stones (hydroxyapatite or brushite) occur in 80% all cases
Causes:
Hypercalcaemia, esp. hyperparathyroidism
- PTH ↑ variant: Intestinal absorption ↑ and bone resorption ↑
- PTH ↓ variant: Renal PO_4 wasting and 2° intestinal absorption

Normocalcaemia: Hereditary hypercalciuria
Hypocitraturia: Idiopathic, or due to hypokalaemia, e.g. from chronic diarrhoea

Renal tubular acidosis, type 1
PATH: Encourages stones due to alkaline urine; hypercalciuria; hypocitraturia

Uric acid
PATH: Uric acid or sodium monourate occurs in 5% cases
Causes:
Hyperuricaemia (although only half of cases have gout)
Idiopathic, myeloproliferative states, chemotherapy, acidosis

Stasis: Renal cysts, bladder diverticulae, partial obstruction

Hereditary
Hyperoxaluria, due to hepatic oxalate synthesis ↑
Cystinosis: Cystine stones form due to failure of proximal tubule resorption
Hypouricaemia: Uric acid stones due to failure of proximal tubule resorption

Infection
Proteus mirabilis secretes urease that promotes alkaluria → struvite ($MgNH_4PO_4$ or $CaPO_4$)
Causes large, 'staghorn' calculi – makes up 10% cases
Assoc. women, chronic catheterisation, chronic UTI

Nutrition/Toxins
Nutrition:
- Hypercalciuria – high-salt diet
- Oxalic acid – rhubarb or strawberries, tea or coffee, nuts or spinach, vit. C
- Hyperuricaemia – purine-rich food, e.g. offal
- Hyperlipidaemia – high-fat diet

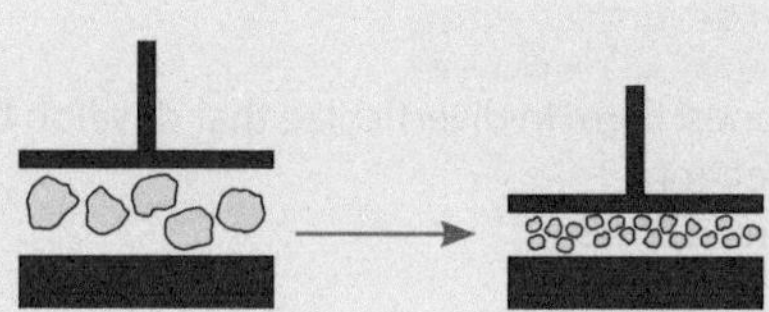

Toxins: Sulphonamide, aciclovir, indinavir, Mg trisilicate (antacid), loop diuretics

GIT – fat malabsorption
Causes: Crohn, coeliac, chronic pancreatitis, bacterial overgrowth
PATH: Ca^{2+} binds to intraluminal fatty acids, releasing oxalate that gets absorbed

PC

Colic: loin → flank → iliac fossa pain
Strangury (urethral spasm), dysuria, passage of stone or gravel
Haematuria: Micro- or macroscopic – essential!

Ix

Bloods: Renal: urea ↑ – volume depletion; creatinine ↑ – if only 1 functioning kidney/bilat. stones
Electrolytes: Ca^{2+}, PO_4, PTH, uric acid, acidosis
FBC: WCC ↑, ESR ↑

Urine: Dipstick: RBC (essential); WBC, nitrite (infection); pH; protein + glucose
24-h collection: Calcium, oxalate, citrate, uric acid
Sediment microscopy; birefringence (+ve = Ca^{2+} oxalate); chemical analysis

Calcium **Struvite** **Uric acid** **Crystine**

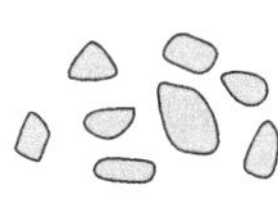

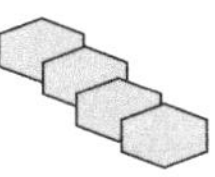

Dumb-bell Bipyramidal Staghorn Small, amorphous Yellow hexagons

Micro: MSU – *Proteus mirabilis* (cause) or other UTI due to urinary stasis

Radiol: PAXR: Opaque stones – 90%; lucent stones – 10% (*opposite of gallstones*) calcium, struvite – radio-opaque; cystine – slightly opaque; uric acid – radiolucent papillary nephrocalcinosis – medullary sponge kidney
IVU, USS

Special: RTA type 1: NH_4Cl loading test
Cystinuria: Na nitroprusside test – urine turns cherry-red

Rx

General

Fluid intake: Aim for > 2 l/day urine; look for stone passage
Analgesia: Morphine, indomethacin, propantheline
Stone removal**:**

- Lithotripsy – extracorporeal, percutaneous ultrasound, or ureteric laser
- Surgery: Nephro-/ureterolithotomy; cystoscopy with ureteric flexible-basket ensnarement

Type-specific

Calcium:
Hypercalcaemia: Treat accordingly
Normocalcaemic:
- Thiazides; low-salt, high-potassium diet (↑ tubular resorption of Ca^{2+})
- Na-cellulose PO_4 (↓ GIT absorption); oral PO_4 (urine PPi ↑ + Ca^{2+} ↓)

Renal tubular acidosis, type 1: KCl, bicarbonate
Uric acid: Low-purine diet; allopurinol; K citrate – alkalize urine
Stasis: Treat underlying cause
Hereditary:
Hyperoxaluria: Oral PO_4, pyridoxine, K citrate; liver + renal transplant
Cystinosis: Penicillamine (cystine chelator); K citrate – alkalize urine
Infection:
Antibiotics
Acidify urine – methananime mandelate; urease inhibitor – acetohydroxamic acid
Nutrition: Low-salt, high-potassium diet; low oxalic acid; low purines; low-fat diet
GIT:
Correct fat malabsorption – lipase supplements
Oxalate-binding resin – cholestyramine
Oxalate precipitate – calcium lactate

RENAL ENLARGEMENT

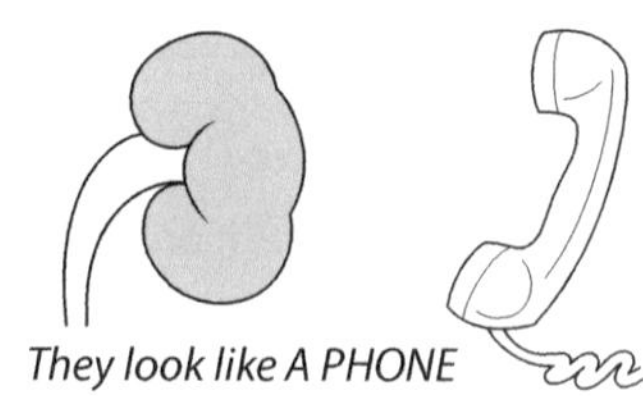

A. P.H.O^2.N.E.

Amyloidosis

Polycystic kidneys/simple cysts: Hereditary (APKD, IPKD, neurocutaneous)
Hypertrophy 2° to contralateral renal agenesis
Obstruction (hydronephrosis)/**O**cclusion (renal vein thrombosis)
Neoplasia:
  Renal cell carcinoma
  Myeloma, lymphoma
Endocrine: Early diabetes mellitus

Renal cysts

Large kidneys

Adult polycystic kidney disease
Infant polycystic kidney disease
Neurocutaneous syndromes
  Epi: Autosomal dominant
  PC: Similar to adult polycystic kidneys +
- Tuberous sclerosis: Hyperplastic nodules, angiomyolipomas
- Von Hippel–Lindau syndrome: Renal cell carcinoma

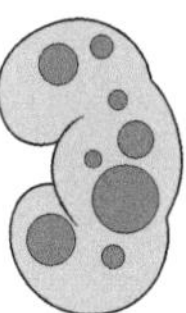

Normal size

Medullary-sponge kidneys
  Epi: Majority are sporadic and congenital; few are autosomal dominant
  PC:
- Incidental finding on AXR: Papillary nephrocalcinosis
- Stones, haematuria, infection

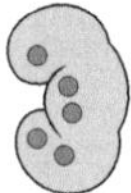

Small kidneys

Hereditary – nephronophthisis/ medullary-cystic disease
  Epi:
- Nephronophthisis – autosomal recessive, children
- Medullary-cystic disease – autosomal dominant; adult-onset

  PC:
- Renal failure, incl. polyuria
- Hepatic fibrosis, cerebellar ataxia (nephronophthisis)

Acquired – end-stage renal disease, dialysis
  PC:
- Stones, infection, haematuria
- Polycythaemia (EPO secretion)
- Renal cell carcinoma

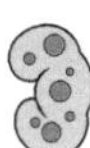

ADULT POLYCYSTIC KIDNEY DISEASE

Epi

Adults: Renal failure >20 y; usually 40–60 years
Autosomal dominant type (most common)
  PKD1 gene, polycystin-1 (80%): cell–cell and cell–matrix membrane receptor
  PKD2 gene, polycystin-2: Ca^{2+} channel that interacts with polycystin-1
Autosomal recessive type (less common)

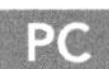

M.I.S.S.H.A.P.E^2.N.

Mass-effect: Abdominal mass; flank pain
Infection
Stones, esp. uric acid
Sensitivity (acute pain in flanks, especially if haemorrhage into a cyst)
Haematuria or haemorrhage into cyst
ABP ↑: Hypertension
Polyuria, nocturia:
  Impaired tubular concentration
  Renal failure
Extra-renal cysts: Liver, pancreas, lungs, ovaries
Extra: Colonic diverticulae, inguinal herniae
Neuro: Cerebral berry aneurysms/subarachnoid haemorrhage + mitral valve prolapse; aortic aneurysm

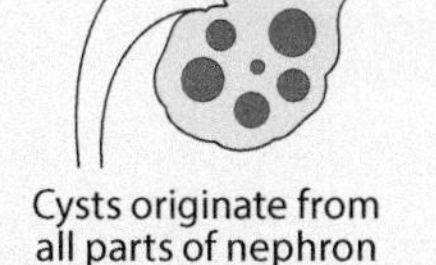

Cysts originate from all parts of nephron and become detached from parent nephron

INFANT POLYCYSTIC KIDNEY DISEASE

Epi

Autosomal recessive
  PKHD1 gene, fibrocystin

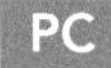

Kidney
  Abdominal masses in infant
  Hypertension/renal failure in childhood
Systemic
  Pulmonary hypoplasia
  Liver failure due to hepatic fibrosis

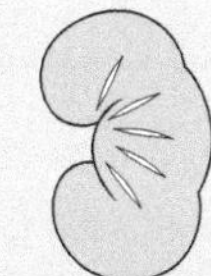

Cysts originate from distal tubule amd collecting tubule, and remain with nephron

RENAL CELL CARCINOMA

Def

Transformation of epithelial cells, predominantly from **proximal convoluted tubule**:

Clear cell	80%
Von Hippel–Lindau tumour suppressor gene inactivation (chromosome 3p)	
Chromophobic	10%
Oncocytic	5%
Collecting duct – medullary:	2%
Assoc: Young people, sickle cell anaemia	
Poor prognosis	

Epi

Inc: Increasing incidence – currently 5% of all cancers
Age: 50–70 years
Sex: M:F = 3:1

Causes

V.I.C.T.O.R.Y.

Von Hippel–Lindau (*VHL*) gene: Autosomal dominant
Inherited syndrome: Neurofibromatosis; tuberous sclerosis
Cystic disease: Adult polycystic kidney disease
Toxins: Smoking, cadmium, dry-cleaning; trichloroethylene
Obesity
Renal failure, end-stage, esp. on chronic dial**Y**sis, due to acquired renal cysts

PC

Pulmonary embolism 2° to renal vein thrombosis
Pulmonary metastases
Gynaecomastia (ectopic β-HCG secretion)

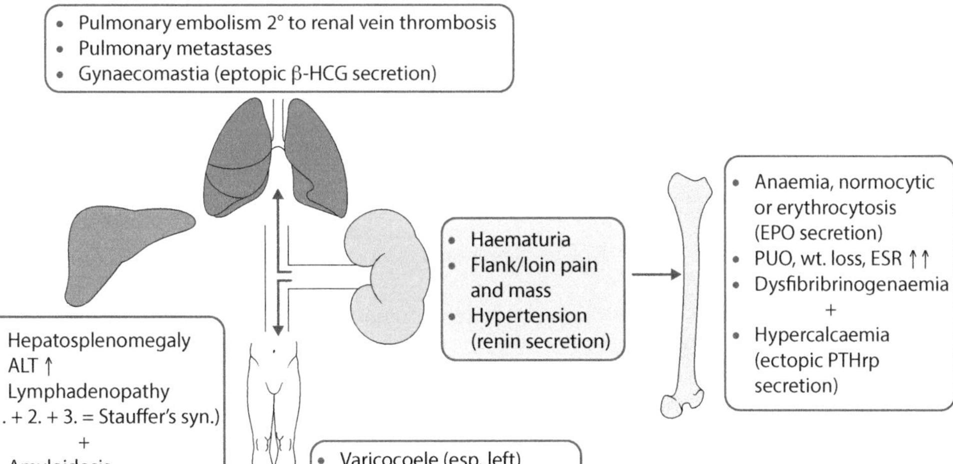

Ix

Urine: Cytology
Proteinuria – if heavy, may suggest renal vein thrombosis

Radiol: USS/IVU: Renal mass
– Differential diagnosis = cyst, abscess, benign neoplasm (adenoma; angiomyolipoma)
CT abdomen–pelvis–chest – staging
MRV: Inferior vena cava and renal vein thrombosis

Rx

Local disease: Radical nephrectomy
En bloc removal of Gerota fascia with adrenals, lymph nodes ± renal vein

Metastatic disease:
Cytotoxics
Hormonal therapy: Progestagens
Immunotherapy: Interferon-α, interleukin-2
(☠: Capillary leakage syndrome, fever, shock)
Surgery: Palliation of local signs

Prog

Poor, although some cases stabilize or even develop spontaneous regression

		5-year survival rate
Stage I	(renal-confined)	70%
Stage III	(renal vein thrombosis, lymphadenopathy)	40%
Stage IV	(metastases)	10%

TESTICULAR TUMOURS

Germ-cell tumours

Risk factors
Cryptorchidism:
- Risk is higher for abdominal than inguinal site
- Both testes at risk, even if one is in scrotum

Dysgenesis: Klinefelter syndrome, androgen insensitivity syndrome
Isochromosome 12p reduplication

Seminoma

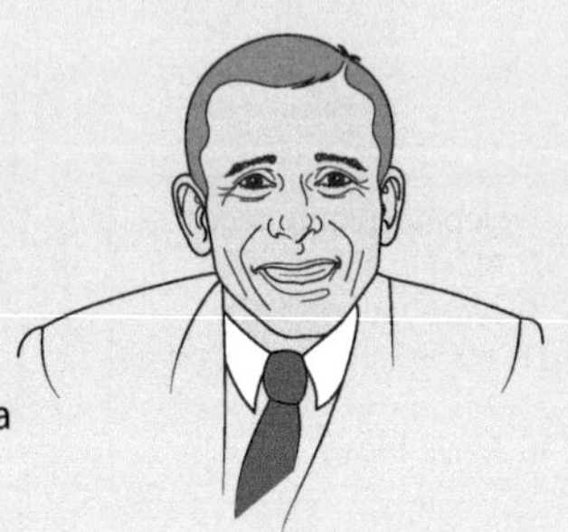

Epi: **S**emi, i.e. middle-aged (30–40s); commonest testis tumour
PATH:
- **S**heets of large, uniform, clear cells
- **S**permatic cord and epididymis infiltrated
- **S**ynctium in 10% that secretes β-HCG and causes gynaecomastia

Ix: Tumour markers: Placental alkaline phosphatase
Prog: **S**crotal involvement only (stage I) in 70%:
- Stage 1: 5-y survival rate 100%; stage II: 95%
- Good prognosis: Spermatocytic seminoma – doesn't metastasize (50s+)

Rx:
- Orchidectomy + retroperitoneal lymph-node dissection (RPLND)
- Radiotherapy to abdominal lymph nodes

Teratoma

Epi: **T**wenties: Prognosis worsens with age, as tumours are less differentiated
PATH: **T**otipotent tissue:
- Heterogeneous mix of differentiated cells
- Cartilage, bone, muscle, thyroid

Ix: **T**umour markers: AFP; β-HCG; hPL, LDH
NB: β-HCG and hPL may cause gynaecomastia
Prog: **T**errible prognosis (relative to seminoma):
- Rapid, disorderly growth: 60% present with lymph/vascular spread
- PC: Back pain (retroperitoneal mets.)/dyspnoea (pulmonary mets.)
- Worst prognosis: Undifferentiated 'embryonal carcinoma' or chorioca.
- Good prognosis: Yolk-sac tumour (Ix: AFP), usually <3 y old

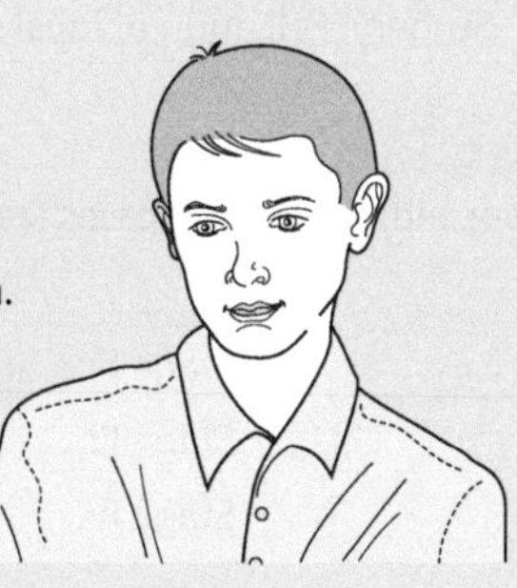

Rx:
- Orchidectomy + retroperitoneal lymph-node dissection (RPLND)
- Chemotherapy

Non-germ-cell tumours

Sex cord–**S**tromal

Epi: **S**emi, i.e. middle-aged (30–40s)

PATH:

Steroid-producing, esp. Leydig-cell tumour

PC:

- Gynaecomastia (oestrogen secretion)
- Precocious puberty (androgen or glucocorticoid secretion)

Sertoli–Leydig cell tumour/androblastoma – less hormone secretion spermatic cord and epididymis infiltrated ±

Synctium that secretes β-HCG and causes gynaecomastic (10%) – heterogeneous mix of differentiated cells (cartilage, bone, muscle, thyroid)

Prog: **S**crotal involvement only is usual good prognosis

Lymphoma

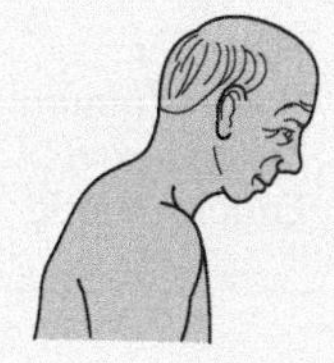

Epi: **L**ater life (50s+)

PATH: **L**arge-cell, diffuse, non-Hodgkin lymphoma

Prog: Poor

OVARIAN TUMOURS

Germ-cell tumours

Teratoma
Epi: **T**wenties
PATH: **T**otipotent tissue, due to unfertilized oocyte dividing and developing along 2 or 3 germ-cell lines (endo-, meso-, or ectoderm): Dermoid cyst (sebum, hair) + mamillary process (teeth, bone)
Ix:
Tumour markers – only in variants with poor prognosis:
- AFP – yolk-sac tumour; β-HCG – choriocarcinoma

Thyrotoxicosis ('struma ovarii')
Prog:
Not Terrible – unlike testis teratomas
- Usually benign and cystic
- Solid components may transform, e.g. skin – squamous cell carcinoma

20s–30s

Seminoma equivalent ('dysgerminoma')
Unlike testis seminomas, ovarian dysgerminomas are usually *aggressive* due to early spread via blood

Functional cysts (non-neoplastic)

Follicular	Resolve spontaneously
Corpus luteum	Unilateral pain; amenorrhoea
Theca-lutein	Large bilateral mass
Endometriotic	Pain; look like 'chocolate cysts' due to blood

Adenoma or adenocarcinoma (70%)

Aged (40s+); **A**bnormal ovarian function; **A**utosomal dominant – *See opposite*

Sex cord–stromal tumours

Granulosa-cell or theca-cell tumour:
PC: Secrete oestrogen:
- Amenorrhea (if pre-menopausal), menorrhagia, endometrial carcinoma
- Breast enlargement; precocious puberty (if in children)

Sertoli–Leydig cell tumour or androblastoma:
PC: Secrete androgen:
- Amenorrhea
- Virilisation, incl. cliteromegaly; breast atrophy

Fibroma:
PC:
- Torsion upon pedicle
- Ascites and pleural effusion (transudates) = 'Meig syndrome'

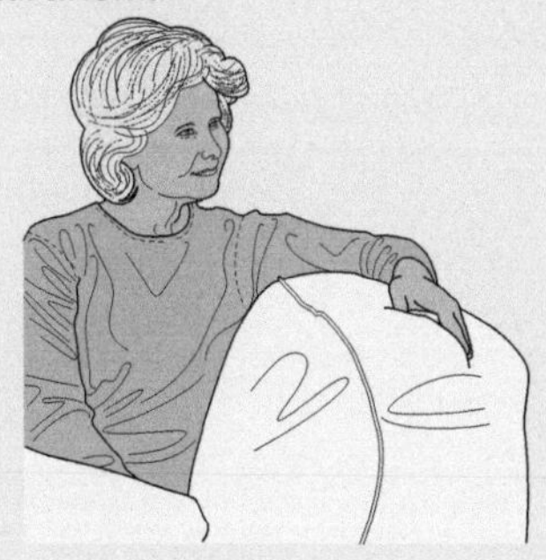

40s+

Metastases

Gynaecological: Endometrium, breast
GIT: Gastric; colon, via transcoelomic or lymph spread ('Krukenberg tumour') mucus-secreting, signet-ring cells; bilateral

OVARIAN ADENOCARCINOMA

Epi

Aged (40s+)

Aet

Abnormal ovarian function:

- Repeated ovulatory cycles induce epithelial trauma, repair and neoplasia – associated with nulliparity, early menarche, late menopause
- Persistent stimulation of ovaries by gonadotrophins – associated with clomiphene; protection offered by contraceptive pill

Autosomal dominant inheritance:

- *BRCA-1*, -2, hereditary non-polyposis colorectal carcinoma (Lynch syndrome)

PATH

Derived from surface-epithelium (origins indicated)

S.M^2.E.A.R.

Serous (Fallopian tube) – commonest adenocarcinoma:
- PATH:
  - Single cavity with **S**urface exophytic papillary growths
  - Prog: **SER**ious:
    - Rapid transcoelomic spread and bilateral in 50%
    - Metastases common, but may regress after 1° removal

Mucinous (endocervix):
- PATH: **M**ultilocular cyst – PC: Large **M**ass
- Prog: **M**ild – most are low-grade

Myxoma – 'pseudomyxoma peritonei': Cyst may rupture with peritoneal seeding and mucin release

Endometrioid (endometrium): Assoc: **E**ndometrial carcinoma, **E**ndometriosis

Author-named – **B**renner tumour: Assoc: **B**leeding, post-menopausally, due to oestrogen secretion

Renal-related = **C**lear-**C**ell tumour (like renal clear-cell carcinoma):
- Assoc: Calcium elevation (PTH-related peptide secretion)
- Commonly recur

PC

Local:

- Abdominal pain (chronic – mass effect; acute – bleed or torsion)
- Abdominal bloating (mass effect, ascites)
- Urinary frequency or constipation

Extra-abdominal: Pleural effusions – DVT; paraneoplastic: limbic encephalitis

Ix

CA125 tumour marker
CT abdomen

Rx

Surgery
Carboplatin + paclitaxel

Prog

		5-year survival rate
Stage I	Ovaries only	80%
Stage II	Pelvis extension	60%
Stage III	Peritoneal, retroperitoneal spread	30%
Stage IV	Metastases in liver, pleura, etc.	10%

Haematology

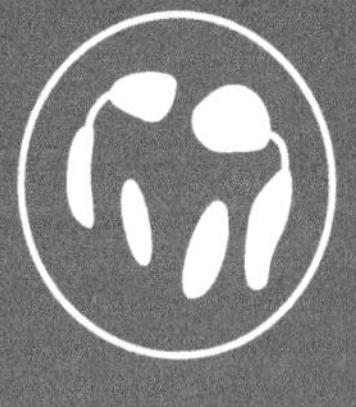

ANAEMIA

Def

Men:	Hb	<135 g/l
Women:	Hb	<115 g/l
Children:	Hb	<110 g/l
Newborn:	Hb	<150 g/l

NB: Allowances should be made for changes in plasma volume, in the absence of changes in total red cell mass. This can be approximated by inspecting packed cell volume (PCV):

Normal PCV (haematocrit):

Men:	40–50%
Women:	35–50%

PC

Fatigue, SOB
Cardiac: Palpitations; angina, CCF
Neuro: Headaches, TIAs, retinal bleeds
Other: Intermittent claudication

Presence of symptoms depend on:

- Severity, <10 g/dl = symptomatic
- Speed of onset: Acute more symptomatic, as not compensated
- Age: Reduced CVS compensation

O/E

Pale mucous membranes
Pruritus, koilonychia: Fe deficiency
Jaundice – haemolysis or megaloblastosis

Ix

Bloods: FBC, film, reticulocytes: Haematinics, transferrin saturation
Haemolysis tests, e.g. Coombs' test
Other: U&Es, LFTs, TFTs, ESR (↑ with Hb ↓)

Fine-needle aspirate and/or bone-marrow biopsy:
Marrow cellularity, myeloid:erythroid ratio (range 3–12)

Special: Ferrokinetics (^{59}Fe):

- Measures rate of Fe uptake from plasma = total erythropoiesis
- Sacrum, liver, spleen uptake?

RBC survival (^{51}Cr + RBC): Measure radioactivity over liver and spleen over 3 weeks

Microcytic
MCV <76 fl

Iron deficiency

Supply ↓: Diet, malabsorption
Demand ↑:
Physiological (pregnancy, periods)
Blood loss: GIT, urine, lung, haemolysis
Ix: Ferritin ↓, soluble transferrin receptor ↑

Haemoglobinopathy

Thalassaemia:

β: 1 gene on Chr 11 (100 mutations): β^0 = no globin; β^+ = ↓ globin
Major: β^0/β^0 or β^+/β^0 or β^+/**E**
Intermedia: mild β^+/β^+ or β^+/**D**
Minor or trait: β/β^++ or β/β^0

α: 2 genes on Chr 16
α = globin; – = no globin

Hydrops fetalis:	Hb Barts (γ_4)	––/––
Intermedia:	Hb H disease (β_4)	– – /α–
Minor or trait:	α–/α or ––/ αα	
Carrier:	α–/αα	

Hereditary spherocytosis:
Commonest hereditary haemolytic anaemia in Caucasians, due to spectrin deficiency (auto. dom.)

Bone marrow hypoproduction

Chronic disease, anaemia of:
Cause: Infection, autoimmunity, neoplasia
Ix: Ferritin ↑, soluble transferrin receptor normal

Hereditary sideroblastic anaemia: X-linked recessive; Rx: vitamin B_6

Poisoning:
Lead:
PC: Abdominal pain, motor neuropathy, hypertension, renal tubular acidosis
O/E: Blue line along gums
Ix: X-ray: Epiphyseal sclerosis
Film: Basophilic stippling
BM: Ringed sideroblasts
Aluminium, e.g. renal dialysate

Normocytic
MCV 76–96 fl

Acute haemorrhage
Restoration of plasma volume (over hours) is quicker than RBC ↑ (over days)

Haemolytic anaemias
Hereditary:
Haemoglobinopathy:
- Hb S (sickle cell)
- Unstable Hb or altered O_2 affinity

Membrane defect: Hereditary elliptocytosis
Enzyme defect: G6PD or pyruvate kinase deficiency

Acquired: S.P.L.I.T.T.I.N.G.
Spleen enlargement
PNH
Liver disease
Immune, e.g. SLE
Toxin, e.g. MeDOPA
Trauma to RBCs (MAHA)
Infection, e.g. malaria
Neoplasia, e.g. adenocarcinoma
Graft, arterial

Bone marrow hypoproduction
Aplastic anaemia: **A.P.L.A.S.T.I.C.**
Acquired mutation
PNH
Leukaemia
Autoimmune
Sniffing glue
Toxins
Infection
Congenital

Bone marrow replacement:
Myelofibrosis, myeloma, leukaemia
Malignancy: Osteoblastic metastases
Infection: Tb, *Brucella, Candida*

Chronic disease, anaemia of:
PATH: Failure of iron recycling
Cause: Infection, autoimmunity, malignancy
Diet: Malnutrition, malabsorption (protein ↓)
Endocrine: Addison, dysthyroidism

Macrocytic
MCV >96 fl

M.A.R.M².A.LA.D.E.

Megaloblastic
Vit. B_{12} deficiency
Intake ↓: vegetarian, e.g. Hindus
Absorption ↓:
- Stomach (IF and R protein synthesis): Pernicious anaemia, gastrectomy
- Duodenum, pancreas (R protein dissociation): Coeliac, chronic pancreatitis
- Small bowel (sequestration): Bacterial overgrowth, e.g. blind-loop
- Terminal ileum (absorption): Crohn, TB

Drugs: Metformin, colchicine, N_2O anaesthesia

Folate deficiency
Intake ↓: 'Tea + biscuits' diet – elderly
Absorption ↓: Coeliac, Crohn, AIDS
Drugs:
- **D**HFR inhibitor: Methotrexate, trimethoprim
- **D**ihydropteroate synthetase inhibitor: Dapsone, sulphonamides, nitrofurantoin
- **D**NA antagonist: AZT, azathioprine, hydroxyurea
  + Isoniazid, chloramphenicol
  + Malabsorption: Sulphasalazine, cholestyramine
  + Inducers: Phenytoin, phenobarbitone, OCP

Demand ↑:
- Physiological: Pregnancy, infancy
- Neoplasia: Myeloproliferative
- Haemolysis, erythroderma, autoimmune

Other: Orotic aciduria, transcobalamin-II deficiency

Alcoholic liver disease

Reticulocytosis: e.g. acute haemolysis or BM replacement

Myelodysplasia/Myeloma

Aplastic anaemia: Chronic idiopathic, or Fanconi

Leukaemia, Acute: Erythroleukaemia

Disordered iron ↑: Haemochromatosis or haemosiderosis

Endocrine: Hypothyroidism

BONE MARROW FAILURE

The following cause either a peripheral blood pancytopenia or anaemia due to failure of haematopoeisis

A.B.C.D.E.F.

Normocytic anaemia

- **A**plastic **A**naemia
  - **A.P.L.A.S.T.I.C.** – *see opposite*
  - Ix: Normocytic anaemia, but may be macrocytic in long-standing disease
- **B**one marrow replacement (myelophthisis)
  - Malignancy: Haematological – myelofibrosis, myeloma, leukaemia
  - Malignancy: Osteoblastic metastases
  - Infection: TB, *Brucella*, *Coxiella*, *Legionella*
  - Sarcoidosis
- **C**hronic disease, anaemia of
  - PATH: Failure of Fe recycling
  - Cause: Infection, autoimmunity, malignancy
  - Ix: Micro- or normocytic anaemia
- **D**iet
  - Malnutrition incl. anorexia nervosa
  - Malabsorption (protein ↓)
- **E**ndocrine
  - Addison
  - Dysthyroidism
  - Hypogonadism
- **F**ailure
  - Renal
  - Liver

Megaloblastic anaemia

- **F**olate or vit. B12 deficiency

APLASTIC ANAEMIA

Def

Haematopoeitic stem-cell failure, in presence of bone marrow hypocellularity, leading to peripheral blood pancytopenia

Causes

A.P^2.L.A.S.T.I.C.

Acquired mutation: Telomerase reverse transcriptase (*TERT*)
  Accounts for large proportion of 'idiopathic' cases
PNH (paroxysmal nocturnal haemoglobinuria) – recovery phase:
  Ix: Acid lysis test (Ham test); flow cytometry for GPI-linked proteins
Pregnancy
Leukaemia, acute; lymphoma or thymoma; myelodyplasia:
  Ix: Bone marrow shows abnormal cells; cytogenetic abnormalities
Autoimmune
  Accounts for large proportion of 'idiopathic' cases
  SLE, eosinophilic fasciitis
Sniffing glue; ecstasy; pesticides (DDT)
Toxins
  Dose-dependent: Chemotherapy, methotrexate, chloramphenicol
  Idiosyncratic: Chloramphenicol (1/50,000), tetracycline, sulphonamide
  Hypersensitivity: Any drug after repeated exposure
  Radiation
Infection – viruses
  Parvovirus B19 in hereditary haemolytic anaemia – causes pure red cell aplasia
  HAV, HBV, HCV (3 weeks to 8 months after)
  EBV, HIV
Congenital
  Fanconi's anaemia (AR):
    PATH: Chromosomal breaks and gaps due to failure of DNA repair mechanism
    PC: Skeletal hypoplasia; pigmented; heart or renal anomalies; AML
    Ix: Chromosome studies of peripheral blood cells
  Dyskeratosis congenita (AD):
    PATH: Premature ageing due to *TERT* mutation (no chromosome breaks or gaps)
    PC: Dementia, ectodermal dysplasia (alopecia, nail dystrophy)
  Diamond–Blackfan syndrome – pure red-cell aplasia:
    PC: Short stature, sunken nasal bridge; hepatosplenomegaly and CCF (iron overload)

Rx

Supportive care:
  Packed cell transfusions using leucocyte-depleted products or HLA-matched platelets
  Antibiotics, antifungals
Medical:
  Androgens
  Anti-thymocyte globulin (☠ Serum-sickness) ± cyclosporin
Bone marrow transplantation – allogeneic

HAEMOLYTIC ANAEMIA – CAUSES

Hereditary

Haemoglobinopathy

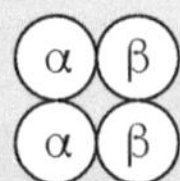

Microcytic: Thalassaemia: Ineffective erythropoiesis and haemolysis
Normocytic: HbS (sickle cell), C, D, E, M
Unstable Hb: Hb Koln, Hb Zurich
Altered O_2 affinity: Hb Yakima (↑), Hb Seattle (↓)

Membrane defect

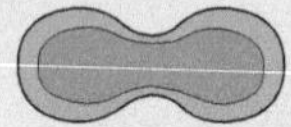

Microcytic: Hereditary spherocytosis (autosomal dominant) commonest hereditary haemolytic anaemia in Caucasians
PATH: Spectrin deficiency – spectrin is main structural unit of RBC membrane
Normocytic: Hereditary elliptocytosis (autosomal dominant)
PATH: Spectrin dimer or spectrin – ankyrin mutation → RBCs are squashed in capillaries
Hereditary stomatocytosis (autosomal dominant):
PATH: Na and K permeability ↑ → swollen or dehydrated RBCs

Enzyme defect

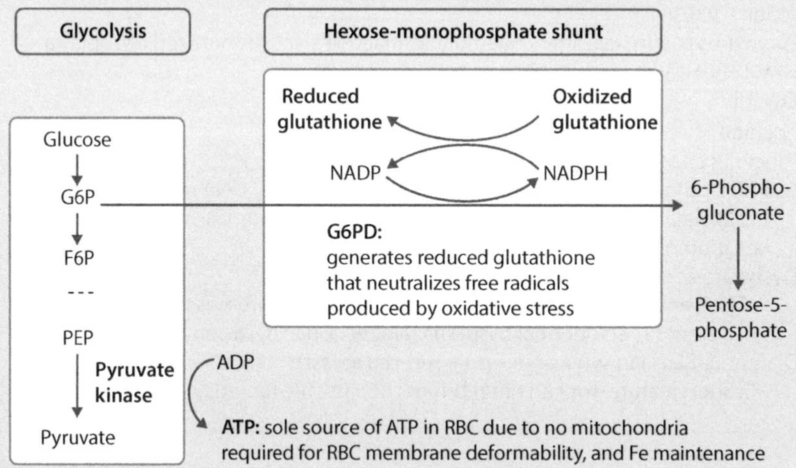

Normocytic:
Glucose-6-phosphate dehydrogenase (G6PD) deficiency (X-linked):
Common in pts. from Mediterranean (severe) and Africa
PC: Haemolytic crises and shock precipitated by oxidative stresses, viz. acute illness (e.g. infection, DKA); foods and drugs: B.A.N. M.E.
Broad beans (fava); **A**spirin (high dose); **N**itrofurantoin, sulphonamides, ciprofloxacin; **M**alaria (chloroquine, primaquine); dapsone; **E**xtra: probenecid, soluble vit. K
Pyruvate kinase deficiency (autosomal recessive)

NB: HbS, elliptocytosis, G6PD heterozygotes provide malaria protection

Acquired

Immune-mediated

Auto-immune:

Warm: **T.A.N.**:

Toxins: Methyldopa, L-DOPA (+ apomorphine), high-dose penicillin, quinidine, sulphonamides

Autoimmune: SLE, Evans syndrome (ITP + AIHA)

Neoplasia: Non-Hodgkin lymphoma, CLL

Cold: **N.I.P.PY**:

Neoplasia: Benign monoclonal gammopathy, lymphoma

Infection: EBV, mycoplasma

Paroxysmal cold haemoglobinuria: **P**rimary autoimmune, measles, VZV, 3° s**Y**philis

Allo-immune

Haemolytic disease of the newborn

ABO incompatibility

Antibiotic (and other drug) induced

Penicillin

Cephalosporins

Levofloxacin

Methyldopa

Non-immune mediated

Medications, e.g. ribavirin, dapsone, sulfasalazine

MAHA (microangiopathic haemolytic anaemia)

HUS, TTP, DIC, HELLP syndrome

Malaria and other infections, such streptococcal bacteraemia

Membrane disorders

Paroxysmal nocturnal haemoglobinuria (PNH):

PATH: Clonal inactivation of *pig-A* gene on X Chr → glycosyl phosphatidyl inositol (GPI) anchor deficiency

→ loss of RBC surface membrane complement inhibitors (e.g. decay accelerating factor)

→ haemolysis and platelet aggregation (arterial and venous thrombosis)

Liver:

Alcoholic cirrhosis: ↑ RBC cholesterol: Phospholipid ratio → ↓ membrane deformation (spur cells)

Wilson disease: Direct effect of copper

HAEMOLYTIC ANAEMIA – CLINICAL

PC

A.B.C.D.

Anaemia: Due to haemolysis or associated aplastic crises (e.g. sickle cell disease, PNH)
Breakdown products:
  Jaundice
  Pigment stones
  Haemoglobinuria
Compensation:
  Hepatosplenomegaly from erythropoietic hyperplasia (may also be *cause* of haemolysis if there is *hypersplenism*)
  Medullary hyperplasia, e.g. bossed skull, prominent maxillae in children
  Iron overload (p. 160) or *Yersinia* infections – due to many transfusions
Disease-specific:
  Sickle cell: Leg ulcers, dactylitis, chest crisis
  PNH: Venous or arterial thrombosis, pancytopenia due to myelofibrosis
  Cold autoimmune: Acrocyanosis; haemolysis on drinking cold liquids

Ix – General

Bloods: Reticulocytes >5%
MCV:
- Normocytic: Most chronic haemolytic anaemias
- Microcytic: Thalassaemia, spherocytes, secondary iron loss with chronic haemolysis
- Macrocytic: Acute haemolysis due to reticulocytosis

Film:
- Polychromasia, due to immature cells
- Specific red cell forms: Spherocytes (↓ surface area/volume); target cells (↑ s.a./vol.)

Bone marrow: erythroid hyperplasia

Chemistry:
LFTs:
- Unconjugated BR ↑ ('acholuric' – i.e. absent in urine)
- AST ↑ (but ALT normal)
- LDH ↑ (esp. intravascular haemolysis)

α_2-haptoglobin ↓: Binds to Hb and is cleared via reticuloendothelial system
Plasma haemoglobin (esp. intravascular haemolysis)

Urine:
Haemosiderin (intravascular haemolysis)
Haemoglobin (severe intravascular haemolysis)

Ix – Specific

Hereditary

Haemoglobinopathy

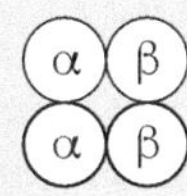

Thalassaemia: MCV, HbA2, genetics
Sickle cell: Film: drapanocytes, serum electrophoresis

Membrane defect

Hereditary spherocytosis:
Film: Microspherocytes (MCHC↑) osmotic fragility test; glucose incubation protects

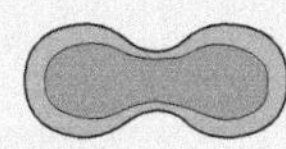

Enzyme defect

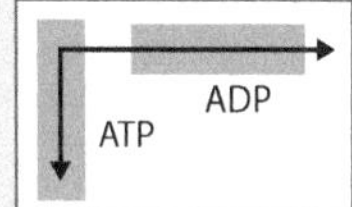

G6PD deficiency: Film – blister, bite cells; Heinz bodies (oxidized Hb) enzyme assay (reticulocytes have normal activity)
Pyruvate kinase deficiency: Film – poikilocytosis; prickle cells; enzyme assay

Acquired

S.P.L.I.T.

Spleen: Abdominal USS
Paroxysmal nocturnal haemoglobinuria (**PNH**):

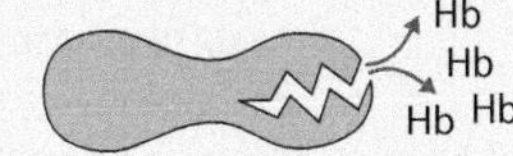

Complement-mediated lysis: Acidify (Ham test) or add sucrose
Flow cytometry for GPI-linked proteins, e.g. DAF, CD59

Liver: Film – spur cells
Immune, auto-:
Warm AIHA:
Direct Coombs' test: Mix pt's RBCs + specific anti-IgG or anti-C3
→ agglutination with anti-IgG (penicillin, methyldopa), C3 (other drugs), or both (SLE)

Cold AIHA:
Direct Coombs' test: Agglutination with anti-C3 only, and at T <30°C
Cold agglutinins test:
Cold agglutinin type:

- IgM anti-I (adult RBCs): Monoclonal gammopathy, mycoplasma
- IgM anti-i (fetal RBCs): Lymphoma, EBV
- IgG 'Donath–Landsteiner Ab': Cold paroxysmal haemoglobinuria (do syphilis serology)

Trauma to RBCs: Film – schistocytes (RBC fragments)

PNH:
Steroids
Androgens; anti-thymocyte globulin
Bone marrow transplant

AIHA:
Immunosuppressants: Steroids, azathioprine, cyclophosphamide, IVIg
Splenectomy
Blood transfusions, with prior adsorption of patient's 'panagglutinin antibodies', i.e. antibodies that cross-react with universal RBC antigens

SICKLE CELL ANAEMIA

Def

Defective synthesis of β-globin chain due to point mutation: Glu → hydrophobic Val
This results in less soluble HbS that tends to polymerize when deoxygenated

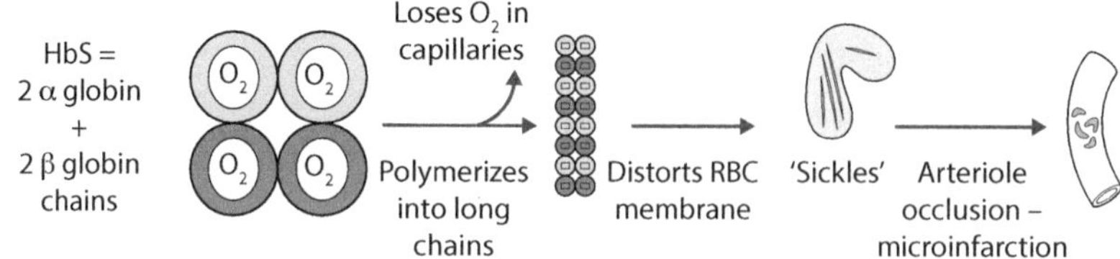

Epi

Black ethnicity, Greek ethnicity

PC

B.L.A.C.K.I.N.G. O.U.T.

Bone: Pain incl. dactylitis, finger shortening; *Salmonella* osteomyelitis
Avascular necrosis: Femoral, humeral head, vertebral end-plates – growth retardation
Reshaping – frontal bossing in children due to widened diploë

Liver: Pigmented gallstones

Anaemia: Hb 6–10 g/dl: not usually symptomatic

Crises:

S.H.A.R.P.

- **S**equestration: Spleen and liver venous occclusion – young children only
- **H**aemolytic anaemia
- **A**plastic anaemia: Triggered by parvovirus or hepatitis infection
- **R**espiratory ('chest crisis'): Chest pain, SOB, fever, hypoxia – due to pulmonary sickling leading to infarction, and pneumococcal infection
- **P**ainful, vaso-occlusive: Bones–joints–muscles, GIT, spleen – commonest crisis; triggered by infection, dehydration, sympathetic activation

Kidney: Medullary sickling: Hyposthenuria (diabetes insipidus); renal tubular acidosis
Papillary necrosis: Episodic haematuria, ureteric obstruction
Glomeruli: Focal segmental glomerulosclerosis; membranous glomerulonephritis

Infection – due to hyposplenism following repeated splenic microinfarcts

Neuro: Strokes: children – repeated infarcts; adults – haemorrhagic

Gonads: Infertility; recurrent miscarriage; pre-eclampsia
Priapism

Ophthalmological: Proliferative retinopathy, vitreous haemorrhage, retinal detachment

Ulcers: Leg, ankle – due to sluggish microcirculation

Thrombophilia: Deep-vein thrombosis, pulmonary embolism, pulmonary hypertension, coronary ischaemia (eventually cardiomyopathy)

Median age at death = 45 years, due to renal failure, pulmonary hypertension, cardiomyopathy

Bloods: FBC:

- Hb 7–10 g/dl; MCV normal
- Reticulocytes ↑
- Neutrophils ↑

Film:

- Drapanocytes ('sickle cells')

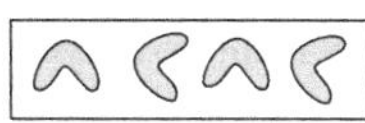

- Anisocytosis and poikilocytosis, incl. pencil cells

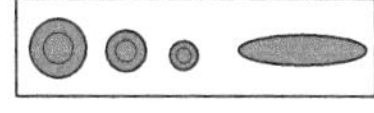

- Target cells

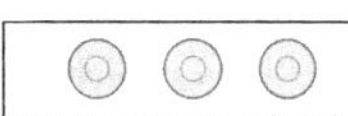

- Howell–Jolly bodies, due to hyposplenism

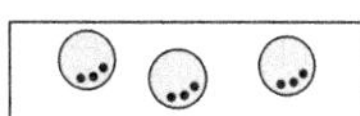

Electrophoresis:

- Hb S/S (homozygote) or Hb S/A (trait)
- Hb F ($\alpha_2\gamma_2$): ↑ 5–15%; higher levels correlate with less sickling and better prognosis

Sickling test: Reducing agent, e.g. Na metabisulphite, induces sickling by removing O_2

Prophylaxis:

Folic acid
Penicillin V
Vaccines: Pneumococcal, *Haemophilus influenzae* b, meningitis A, C (in endemic areas)

Disease-modifying:

Hydroxyurea: ↑ HbF levels, ↓ neutrophils; ↓ no. of crises (☠: Myelotoxic, carcinogenic)
Exchange transfusions: Given for pregnancy or frequent crises; recurrent CVA
Allogeneic bone-marrow transplant

Sickle crisis:

O_2 and IV hydration – both decrease further sickling
Opioids
Antibiotics
Exchange transfusion – reduces proportion of HbS to <30%

Variants

Sickle cell trait

Def: Heterozygotes, i.e. HbSA = 40% HbS, 60% HbA (co-dominant expression)
PC: Normal Hb level; development; life expectancy
Kidney: Papillary sloughing – episodic painless haematuria, or ureteric obstruction (esp. boys)
Crises: rare, but may be precipitated by high altitude; anaesthesia or pregnancy

Hb SC

Def: Hb C: Lysine amino-acid substitution at same position in β-globin chain as defect in HbS
PC: Anaemia less severe (Hb 10–14 g/dl) but vaso-occlusion more likely as more RBCs, e.g. sea-fan retinopathy
Ix: Film – target cells prominent

THALASSAEMIA

Def

Heterogeneous group of genetic disorders of Hb synthesis that result in:

- Ineffective erythropoeisis, due to decreased rate of globin synthesis
- Haemolytic anaemia, due to production of abnormal RBCs (nucleated; abnormal globin)

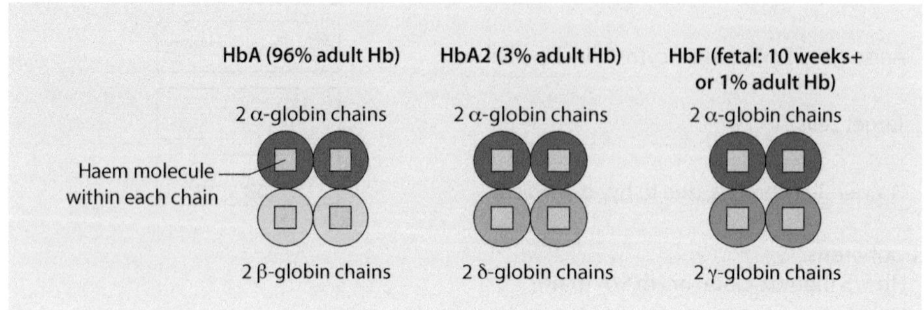

Epi

Mediterranean Basin – N+W Africa; Middle East; SE Asia; also occurs sporadically

Classification schemes

Globin chain mutation:

α: 2 genes on chromosome 16 (i.e. 4 genes per individual)
ß: 1 gene on chromosome 11 (i.e. 2 genes per individual)

Clinical severity:

Major	Hb <7 g/dl	Requires regular transfusion
Intermedia	Hb 7–10 g/dl	No regular transfusion; splenomegaly
Minor ('Trait')	Hb 10–14 g/dl	
Carrier	Anaemia only occurs at high altitudes or with general anaesthesia	

Types

α-Thalassaemia

No. of mutated genes	Name	Clinical
4 ––/––	**Hb Barts** γ_4	'Hydrops fetalis' – death in utero
3 α –/––	**Hb H** $ß_4$	Thalassaemia Intermedia
2 α –/α–	**Thalassaemia minor**	Mild anaemia or asymptomatic
αα/––		
1 αα/a –	**Carrier**	Asymptomatic

Key: α = normal gene; – = mutated gene; γ_4 or $ß_4$ represent alternative Hb type produced

ß-Thalassaemia

No. of mutated genes	Name	Clinical
2 ß°/ß°	**Thalassaemia major**	Regular transfusions
$ß^+/ß^+$ (different mutations)		
2 $ß^+/ß^+$ (mild mutations)	**Thalassaemia intermedia**	No regular transfusions
1 ß°/ß		
δß fusion gene (Hb Lepore)		
1 ß°/ß	**Thalassaemia minor**	
$ß^+/ß$		

Key: ß° = no ß globin; $ß^+$= ↓ ß globin (over 100 mutations recognized)

PC

Haemolytic anaemia from 3–6 months old, when fetal Hb → adult Hb
Anaemia: Fatigue, pallor; leg ulcers; congestive cardiac failure
Haemolysis: Mild jaundice (unconjugated bilirubin ↑); gallstones

Compensation of anaemia
Bones – medullary hyperplasia:

- Facies: Bossed skull (X-ray = 'hair on end')/enlarged maxilla ('chipmunk facies')
- Pathological fractures, growth retardation: due to cortical thinning

Extramedullary haemopoeisis: Hepatosplenomegaly, gingival hyperplasia

Therapy complications
Fe overload (see p. 160):
2° to repeated transfusions and ↑ GIT uptake (hence also present in thalassaemia intermedia), e.g. myocardial damage, diabetes, cirrhosis → death in 30s!!
Infections:
Yersinia enterocolitica: due to Fe overload and chelation therapy
Capsulated bacteria, due to splenectomy
Blood transfusion-associated

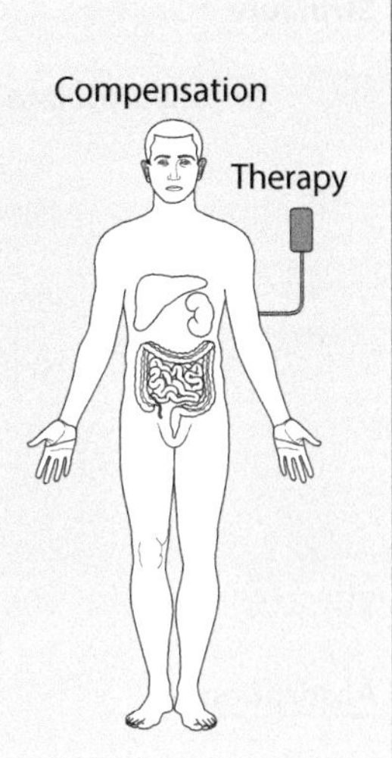

Ix

Bloods: FBC:

- Anaemia – microcytosis, hypochromia: Hb <7: major (ß-thal only); Hb 7–11: intermedia (α- or ß-thal); Hb 11–14: minor (α or ß-thal)
- Red cell count ↑
- Reticulocytes – normal/↓/↑; normal in thalassaemia intermedia

Film:

- 'Heinz bodies' due to oxidized Hb; 'golf ball cells' due to α_4 or β_4 precipitation in ß- or α-thalassaemia, respectively
- Nucleated RBCs: Normoblasts, reflect increased marrow turnover; nuclear remnants – Howell–Jolly bodies; basophilic stippling
- Other: Target cells (haemolysis); siderocytes (iron inclusions); poikilocytes (α-thalassaemia)

Electrophoresis:

- ß-thal major: Hb F ↑↑ (30–60%); Hb A absent!, Hb A2 variable
- ß-thal intermedia: Hb F ↑
- ß-thal minor: Hb F low; Hb A present, Hb A2 >3.5%
- α-thal intermedia: Hb H Hurries along, i.e. fast-moving band

Globin-chain synthesis studies or PCR or restriction-enzyme analyses for family screening/prenatal diagnosis via cord blood or amniocentesis

Rx

Blood transfusions plus desferrioxamine (Fe chelator)
Folic acid: Due to high RBC turnover predisposing to deficiency
Vit. C (ascorbic acid): Decreases Fe absorption
Splenectomy: Decreases haemolysis, but wait until >6 years old to reduce risk of infection
Bone marrow transplant

FOLATE AND VITAMIN B12 METABOLISM

Structure

Tetrahydrofolate polyglutamate

Pteridine ring
Para-amino-benzoic acid (PABA)
Polyglutamate
n

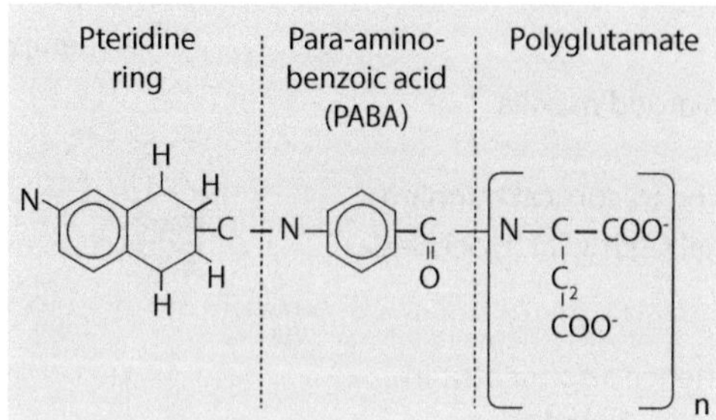

Vitamin B12 (cobalamin)

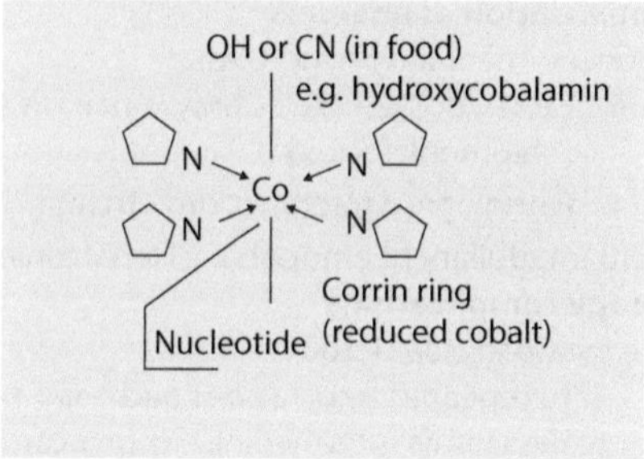

OH or CN (in food)
e.g. hydroxycobalamin
Co
Corrin ring (reduced cobalt)
Nucleotide

Absorption

Folic acid

Vitamin B12

Tetrahydrofolate polyglutamate
• Vegetables, meat, yeast
• RDA = 100–200 µg
Tetrahydro-
folate
polyglutamate
Duodenum
Poly-
glutamate
Mono-
glutamate
Pteroyl polyglutamate
hydrolase
Ileum
Addition of methylene group to form
active compound
Stores – lasts 4 months
Bone marrow stores –
lasts 3 years
Plasma – hydroxyl or
cyano group is replaced
with methyl or deoxyadenosyl
B12-TC-I or III
Recycled in
enterohepatic
circulation
B12 - TC-II
(transcobalamin)
Hydroxy- or cyanocobalamin
• Meat, fish, dairy, eggs
• ROA= 1–2µg
B12
R-
binding
protein
Intrinsic
Factor
Duodenum
B12
-R
Pancreatic
protease
B12
B12-
IF
B12-IF
Terminal ileum

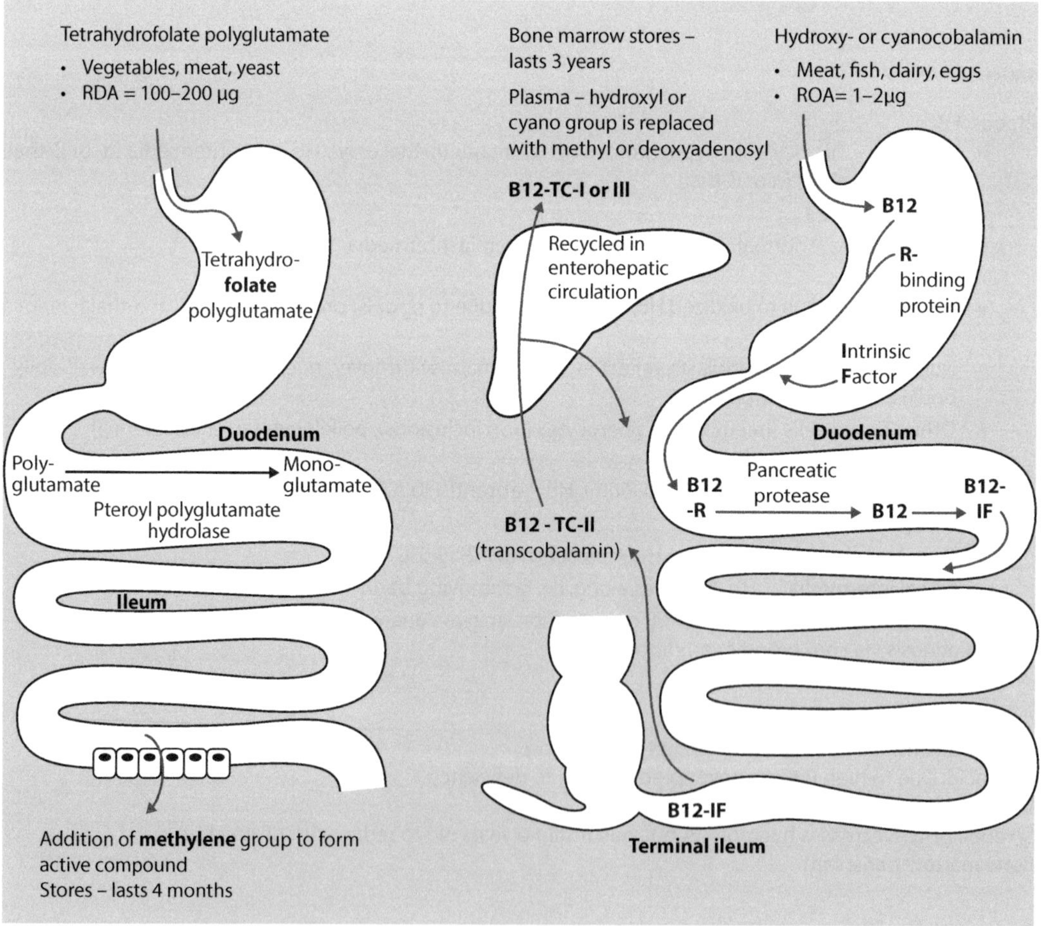

Metabolism

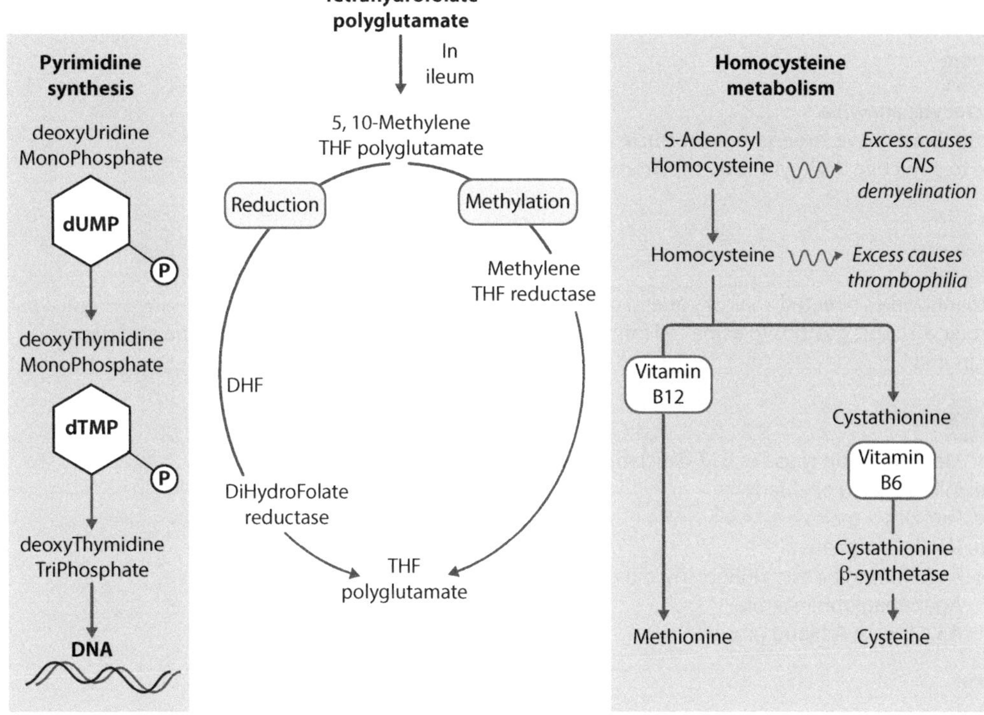

Other metabolic interactions

Folate: Purine synthesis, amino-acid interconversions, e.g. serine → glycine
Vit. B12: Methylmalonyl CoA → succinylCoA
NB: Deficiencies of DHF reductase, methylene THF reductase or cystathionine β-synthetase are responsible for homocystinuria

Bloods:

Serum B12/folate levels
Plasma homocysteine ↑ (folate or B12 deficiency)

MEGALOBLASTIC ANAEMIA

Def

Macrocytic anaemia
Erythroblasts have large, immature nuclei, reflecting diffuse, open chromatin structure
Due to defective DNA synthesis, esp. from vit. B12 or folate deficiency (see p. 433)

Pernicious anaemia

PATH

Autoantibodies directed against parietal cells (95%) and intrinsic factor (70%)
Chronic atrophic gastritis (plasma cell infiltrate of gastric lamina propria) → achlorhydria and gastric carcinoma

Epi

Inc: Most common cause of B12 deficiency in West
Age: Middle-aged or elderly
Sex: Females > males
Geo: North Europeans
Pre: **A**utoimmunity, esp. vitiligo, thyroid or parathyroid disease, Addison
Agammaglobulinaemia
A3 (HLA) or **A** blood group

PC

M.E².G.A.L.O.B.L.A.S.T.

Mucosal atrophy:
- Glossitis: Beefy red, sore, smooth tongue – due to papillae loss
- Angular cheilitis – due to decreased epithelial turnover
- Impaired healing, including fractures – due to decreased osteoblast activity

Eyes – blue, **E**arly greying of hair, wide-cheek bones (associations)
GIT: Indigestion, episodic diarrhoea
Anorexia
Loss of weight
Organomegaly: Splenomegaly
Bone marrow failure:
- Anaemia – pallor, cardiac failure
- Neutropenia – immunocompromise
- Thrombocytopenia – purpura

LFTs: Jaundiced, LDH ↑ due to haemolysis of abnormal RBCs
Autoimmune: Vitiligo, infertility, Addison, DM
Subacute combined degeneration of cord:
- PATH: Posterior column degeneration (vibration/JPSO, Rombergism, Charcot joints)
- PC: Sensory disturbance in feet; gait ataxia; Charcot joints; extensor plantars, areflexia + dementia, optic atrophy, peripheral neuropathy

Tumour: Gastric carcinoma in 4%

NB: Folate deficiency causes mucositis, anaemia, mild neuropath.

FBC

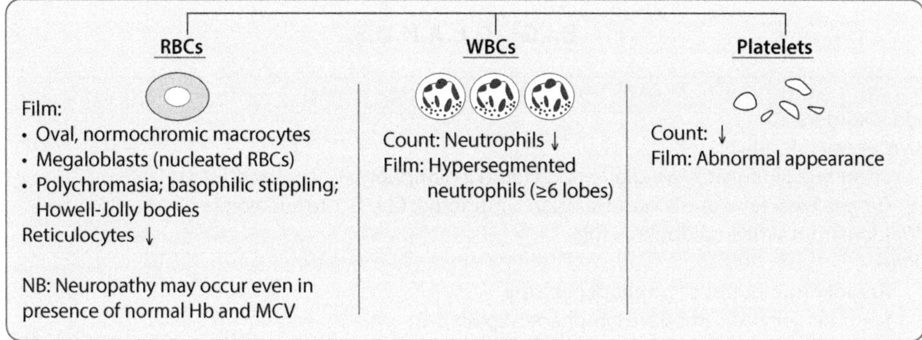

Bone marrow

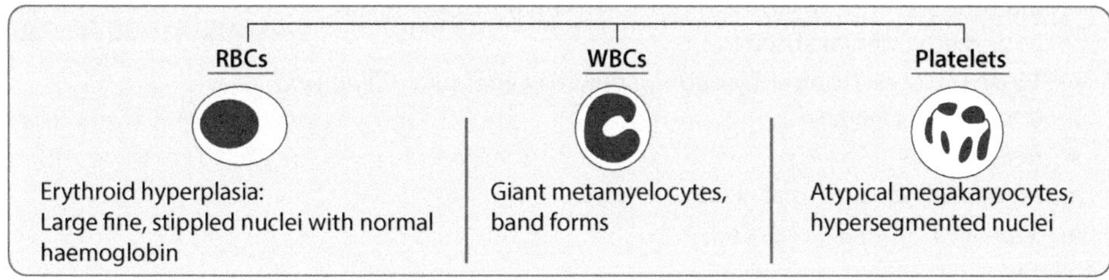

Chemistry

Haematinics:

- Serum vit. B12 ↓ (itself causes serum folate ↑ and red cell folate ↓)
- Red cell folate ↓ (reflects active THF polyglutamate form, cf. serum folate levels)
- Serum Fe and ferritin: ↑/↓ if co-existent malabsorption

Special tests to confirm vit. B12 deficiency:

- Urinary methylmalonyl CoA ↑ (B12 deficiency only)
- Deoxyuridine suppression test on bone marrow cells

LFT: Unconjugated BR ↑; LDH ↑

Identify underlying cause of vit. B12 or folate deficiency

Schilling test:

- Part 1: Give oral radiolabelled B12 (^{58}Co), and measure urinary radioactivity
- Part 2: Give oral intrinsic factor while repeating part 1 (corrects pernicious anaemia)
- Part 3: Give tetracycline + metronidazole for week prior to part 1 (corrects blind-loop syndrome)

Autoantibodies:

- Pernicious anaemia: Anti-parietal cell (95%); anti-intrinsic factor (70% +ve)
- Coeliac disease: Anti-endomysium or anti-tissue transglutaminase

Endoscopy:

- OGD: Pernicious anaemia, coeliac disease
- Colonoscopy: Crohn or other causes of terminal ileal disease

Malabsorption studies, e.g. faecal fat, ^{14}C-labelled–glycholate bile salt breath test

Vit. B12

Method: IM hydroxycobalamin 1 mg od on alt. days for 1–3 weeks, then 1 mg every 3 months
Monitor: Reticulocytes ↑; Hb ↑ 1g/dl per week; Platelets + WCC normalize in 10 days

Folic acid

Method: 5 mg od for 4 months – must correct B12 deficiency first to avoid neuropathy!

LYMPHOPROLIFERATIVE DISEASE

B.I.G^2. G.L.A.N.D.S.

Blood disorders
- Lymphoproliferative:
  - Localized: Hodgkin; high-grade non-Hodgkin lymphoma – localized
  - Generalized: Low-grade non-Hodgkin lymphoma; CLL; acute leukaemia
- Waldenström's macroglobulinaemia
- Rare:
  - Angioimmunoblastic lymphadenopathy
  - Sinus histiocytosis (massive lymphadenopathy)

Infection
- Localized – **S.T.A.B.S.**:
  - **S**treptococci or staphylococci, esp. URTI – pharyngo-tonsillitis; otitis media; dental abscess
  - **T**B (scrofula) or **T**ropical: Lymphogranuloma venereum (*Chlamydia trachomatis*), filariasis
  - ***A**ctinomyces*
  - ***B**artonella henselae* – cat-scratch fever
  - **S**yphilis, 1° (primary chancre)

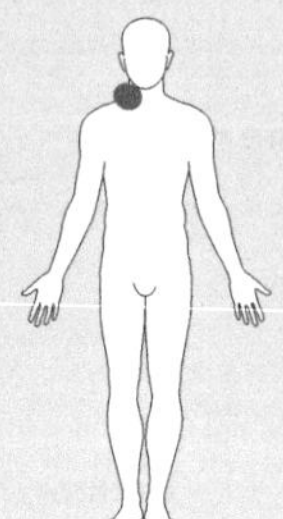

Generalized:
- Virus: EBV, CMV; hepatitis A–E; HIV; measles; rubella; pertussis
- Bacterial: Typhoid, septicaemia, esp. with streptococci or staphylococci
- Atypical bacteria: Secondary syphilis, TB, atypical mycobacteria, *Brucella*
- Toxoplasmosis
- Tropical: Schistosomiasis, *Echinoccocus*, leishmaniasis, trypanosomiasis

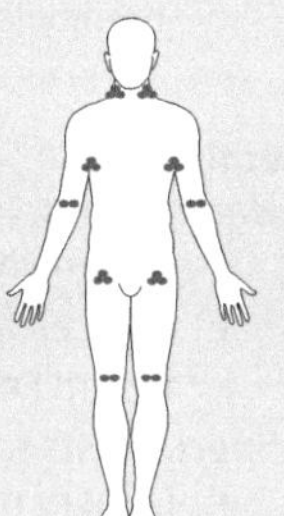

Granulomatous: Sarcoidosis

Generalized, e.g. CLL, HIV, toxoplasmosis
Localized, e.g. Hodgkin lymphoma, streptococci, TB, carcinoma
Autoimmune:
- SLE, rheumatoid arthritis (Still disease or Felty syndrome)
- Primary biliary cirrhosis
- Graves disease

Neoplasia:
- Squamous cell carcinoma, e.g. head–neck, bronchial – localized
- Adenocarcinoma, e.g. breast, gastric
- Melanoma, malignant

Drugs: Phenytoin
Special:
- Serum sickness, e.g. anti-lymphocyte globulin
- Berylliosis (granulomatous)

SPLENOMEGALY

B.I.G. S.P.A^2.N.

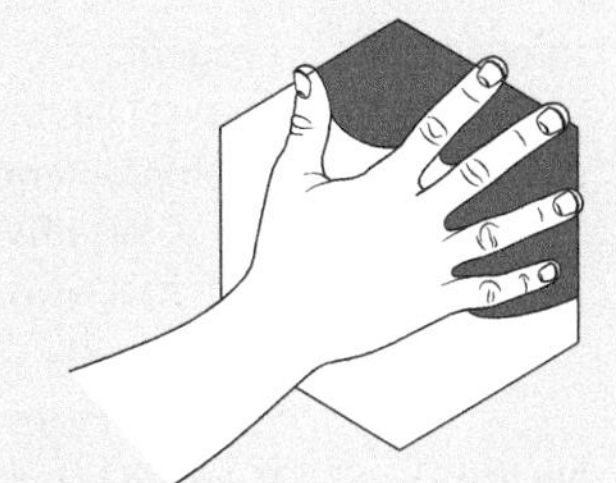

Blood disorders:

Neoplasia:

- Myeloproliferative:
  - Myelofibrosis, CML – massive
  - PRV, ET – medium
- Lymphoproliferative:
  - Prolymphocytic leukaemia ('hairy cell') – massive
  - CLL, lymphoma, acute leukaemia
- Other: Waldenström's macroglobulinaemia (but not myeloma), histiocytosis X – (massive)

Functional hyperplasia – removal of defective RBCs, and extramedullary haematopoiesis:

- Inherited haemolytic anaemia: Thalassaemia major or intermedia, hereditary spherocytosis
- Autoimmune: Autoimmune haemolytic anaemia, ITP, pernicious anaemia, PNH
- Other: Iron deficiency, aplastic anaemia

Infection:

Virus: EBV, CMV; hepatitis A–E; HIV

Bacterial: Endocarditis, typhoid, septicaemia with splenic abscess

Atypical bacteria: 2° syphilis, TB, atypical mycobacteria, *Brucella*

Toxoplasmosis

Tropical: Chronic malaria (massive), schistosomiasis, *Echinoccocus*, leishmaniasis, trypanosomiasis

Granulomatous: Sarcoid, primary biliary cirrhosis

Storage disease or other metabolic:

Lipid storage disease: Gaucher (massive splenomegaly), Niemann–Pick disease

Hyperlipidaemia

Portal vein hypertension:

Post-hepatic: Budd–Chiari syndrome, CCF

Hepatic, esp. cirrhosis

Pre-hepatic: Splenic vein; portal vein thrombosis

Pre-splenic: Splenic artery aneurysm

Autoimmune:

SLE, rheumatoid arthritis (Still disease or Felty syndrome)

Graves disease

Amyloid: AL or AA

Neoplasia:

Renal cell carcinoma (Stauffer syndrome)

Metastases, esp. melanoma

Cysts, incl. adult or infant polycystic kidney disease; hamartoma

LEUCOCYTOSIS

Neutrophilia

I.N.N.A.T.E^2.

Infection:	Pyogenic
	Atypical bacteria: Lyme, disseminated TB
Neoplasia:	Myeloproliferative:
	• CML, PRV, ET, myelofibrosis
	• AML, esp. M5 (Sweet disease – acute febrile neutrophilic dermatosis)
	Myelodysplasia: CMML
	Solid tumours: Carcinoma, melanoma, lymphoma
Necrosis:	Myocardial infarction (or even SVT)
	Pulmonary, or bowel, infarction
	Burns
Autoimmune:	Connective tissue disease, esp. myositis, rheumatoid arthritis (or acute gout)
	Vasculitis, esp. PAN, PMR, Behçet
Toxins:	Glucocorticoids (inhibits tissue margination); growth factors (G-CSF, GM-CSF)
	Digoxin; adrenaline (including stress, excitement, vigorous exercise)
	Poisoning: CO, mercury, lithium
Endocrine:	Diabetic ketoacidosis (or other acidotic states, e.g. uraemia)
	Pregnancy
Extra:	Acute haemorrhage or haemolysis
	Epileptic seizure
	Hyposplenism, incl. splenectomy – also causes eosinophilia

Eosinophilia

Infection	Helminths: Nematodes, cestodes, trematodes (also scabies)
	Bacteria: Rebound post-sepsis; Lyme
	Aspergillosis
Neoplasia:	Lymphoma: Hodgkin or T-cell non-Hodgkin (secretes IL-5)
	AML – eosinophilic leukaemia
	CML – hypereosinophilic syndrome
Nephrology:	Cholesterol emboli – acute renal failure
	Allergic tubulointerstitial nephritis
Autommune	Atopy: Food or drug allergy, eczema, acute asthma
	Vasculitis, esp. PAN; rheumatoid arthritis
	Addison
Toxins:	L-tryptophan
	Poisoning: Spanish toxic oil, nickel –cause eosinophilic-myalgia syndrome
Eosinophilia – myofasciitis: PC: Pain, swelling in both arms; erythema; carpal tunnel syndrome	
Extra:	Sarcoid
	Splenectomy

Lymphocytosis

Infection Viruses: EBV, CMV, hepatitis A–E (all may cause atypical lymphocytes), influenza, mumps, rubella
Bacteria: Post-sepsis, endocarditis, typhoid, pertussis
Atypical bacteria: TB, secondary syphilis, *Brucella*
Toxoplasmosis

Neoplasia: Lymphoproliferative:

- CLL, ALL
- Non-Hodgkin lymphoma

Myeloma
Carcinoma

Autoimmune – organ-based: Graves disease, myasthenia gravis, hypopituitarism

Monocytosis

Infection: Viruses: EBV
Bacteria: Septicaemia, endocarditis, typhoid, listeria
Atypical bacteria: TB, secondary syphilis, *Brucella*
Tropical: Rickettsia, malaria, leishmaniasis, trypanosomiasis

Neoplasia: Hodgkin lymphoma
AML – monocytic variant
Myelodysplasia

ACUTE LEUKAEMIA – 1

Def

Clonal proliferation of single abnormal progenitor, myeloid or lymphoid stem cell
Bone marrow infiltration >30% with blast cells (usually >50% at presentation)
Effects: Pancytopenia: Normal haematopoiesis is 'crowded out' and actively inhibited
Extreme leucocytosis: Spill-over of long-living immature cells into blood

Epi

Inc: 5/100,000 p.a. – most common childhood malignancy; 5% adult malignancies
Age: Commoner in children and elderly

Causes

T.R.I.G.G.ER.

Toxins: Alkylating agents, esp. with radiotherapy; smoking; benzene, esp. AML
Radiation: Atom bomb survivors – AML peaked at 5–7 years; or in children of exposed fathers
Infection: HTLV-I virus – adult T-cell leukaemia/lymphoma (West Indies, Japan)
Genetic: Chromosomal instability: Down syn. (ALL or AML), ataxia telangiectasia, Fanconi's anaemia
Translocations: AML-M3: t(15; 17): PML–RARA (promyelocytic leukaemia – retinoic acid receptor)
Genetic: Haematological transformation from myeloproliferative disease, esp. CML, PRV, myelofibrosis; myelodysplasia
ER: Electromagnetic radiation – pylons

PC

Bone pain, esp. children
Bone marrow failure:
Anaemia: Fatigue, LOW
Infections:
- Bacterial: PUO, mouth ulcers, *Strep. pneumoniae*
- Viral: HSV, VZV, CMV, measles
- Other: candida, aspergillosis

Thrombocytopenia: Purpura, excess bleeding time, cerebral or retinal bleeds
Clotting: DIC with AML-M3 (procoagulant release from granules with chemo Rx)

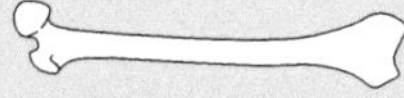

Hyperviscosity:
Fatigue, confusion
Seizures
Stroke, blindness

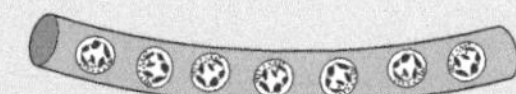

Organ infiltration:
Hepatosplenomegaly, lymphadenopathy, sternal pain
Meninges and eyes (esp. ALL, AML-M4, M5):
- Headaches, N+V
- Papilloedema, CNPs
- Fluid in anterior chamber

Other:
Spinal dura (AML-M2)
Gum hyperplasia, green skin, skin nodules (AML-M4, M5)
Renal failure, $K^+ \uparrow$ (AML-M5 due to lysozyme release from monocytes)

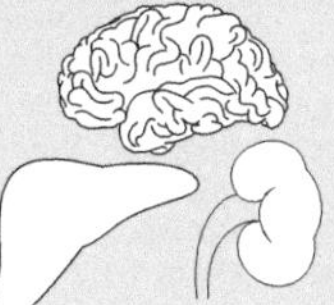

Ix

Bloods:

FBC:

- Normochromic, normocytic anaemia
- WBC: Often 100–300 × 10^9/l, esp. ALL and less differentiated AML, but can be normal, or even low ('aleukaemic leukaemia')
- Platelet ↑ (esp. AML; M3 also causes DIC)

U& E: Uric acid ↑; LDH ↑; calcium ↑

Radiol:

CXR:

- Infiltrates: due to leukaemia, infection or Rx, e.g. WBC transfusion
- Mediastinal lymph nodes, thymic enlargement

Bone: Lytic lesions (childhood ALL)

Brain MRI: Mass lesion: infiltrate or *Toxoplasma*; meningeal enhancement

Special:

Bone marrow aspirate and biopsy: Blast cell proportion:

30%	=	acute leukaemia
5–30%	=	myelodysplasia
<5%	=	remission (must also have normal FBC, no peripheral blasts or symptoms)
<0.001%	=	minimal residual disease: only identifiable with immune or genetic markers

Lumbar puncture: ICP ↑ or blast cells

Typing

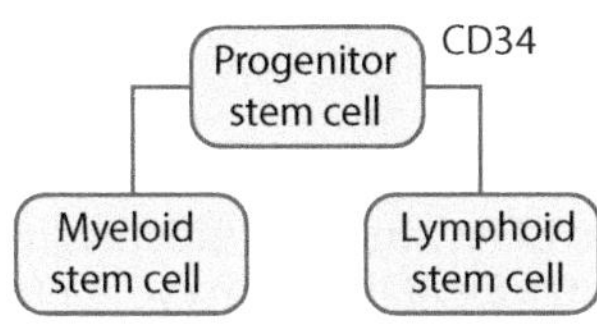

CD33
Persistent germ-line configuration of VDJ genes – not involved in myeloid cells

CD10
Terminal deoxynucleotidyl transferase (TdT) +ve – adds extra bases to DJ genes

Acute myeloid leukaemia (AML)

M0: Undifferentiated
M1, 2: Myeloblastic
M3: Promyelocytic: t(15;17) translocation
M4, 5: Monocytic – commonest extramedullary disease
M6: Erythroleukaemia – elderly, MCV ↑
M7: Megakaryocytic – bone marrow fibrosis

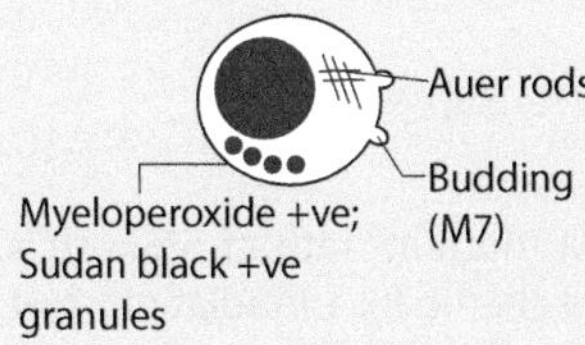

Acute lymphoblastic leukaemia (ALL)

Pre-B-ALL or T-ALL:
- **L1**: Small, uniform blasts, large nucleus:cytoplasm ratios
- **L2**: Large, heterogeneous blasts, small nucleus:cytoplasm ratios

B-ALL (leukaemic phase of lymphoma)
- **L3**: Blasts with vacuolated, basophilic cytoplasm; t(8;14) translocation

Pre-B-ALL and T-ALL can be differentiated by:
- CD type: B – CD19, 22; T – CD7
- VDJ gene clonal rearrangement pattern: B – Ig; T – T-cell receptor

ACUTE LEUKAEMIA – 2

Rx

Bone marrow failure

RBCs

Packed RBC transfusions

- If Hb <9 g/dl
- Use CMV –ve, if pt. is seronegative
- Use leucodepleted blood to avoid alloimmunisation
- ☠: Hyperviscosity (thrombi form in brain, lung, heart if WCC >100 $\times 10^9$); antibody formation with multiple transfusions

WBCs

Physical: Source isolate pasteurized food
Prophylaxis: Nystatin mouthwash, cotrimoxazole (PCP), VZV or measles Ig if exposed
Febrile neutropenic episode: Broad-spectrum, e.g. piperacillin, tazobactam, gentamicin; fluconazole; aciclovir
Granulocyte transfusion or GM-CSF or G-CSF

Platelets

Physical – avoid IM injections
Platelet concentrates

- If Plts. $<20 \times 10^9$/l
- ☠: Antibody formation with multiple transfusions

Tranexamic acid = anti-fibrinolytic

Leucopharesis – if hyperviscosity

Chemotherapy ± radiotherapy

Induction:

AML: Ca.D.Et. (cytarabine, daunorubicin)
ALL: D.O.P.A. (daunorubicin, vincristine [Oncovin], prednisolone, asparaginase)

- Consolidation therapy is essential for AML (repeat cycles of cytarabine), or
- Maintenance therapy required for ALL (out-patient Rx)

Sanctuary sites:

CNS: Indications: ALL, M4, M5 during remission
Rx: Systemic and intrathecal methotrexate + cranial irradiation (not children or elderly)
Testes: Irradiate

Alternative chemotherapy:

All-*trans*-retinoic acid used in promyelocytic AML (M3):
Induces differentiation of promyelocyte clone, but resistance may develop
Gemtuzumab (anti-CD33 monoclonal antibodies) used in relapsing AML; abs. are linked to calicheamicin (cytotoxic), but resistance common
Multi-drug resistance inhibitor, e.g. cyclosporin A – experimental

Supportive:

Venous access: Hickman line insertion – tunnelled subcutaneously into SVC
Nausea: Metoclopramide, ondansetron, nabilone, steroids
Gout: Prophylactic allopurinol, hydration (tumour lysis syndrome)
DIC: FFP and heparin used in M3 before chemotherapy

Bone marrow transplant

Indications: Remission from AML with high-risk karyotype, or 1st relapse (in AML)
Age <60, and match present (for allogeneic)

Allogeneic grafting is associated with more adverse events (10% mortality rate, cf. 5% with autologous), due to graft-versus-host disease and graft rejection (inadequate chemo Rx + irradiation), but is also more effective due to a graft-versus-leukaemia effect. Autologous transplants may also suffer from contamination with residual leukaemic cells. Both risk infection, esp. CMV

Prog

Poor prognostic factors

General

Age: Extremes: AML >60 y; ALL <2 y or >10 y
(partly due to intolerance of chemotherapy)

Sex: Boys – testes becomes sanctuary site in ALL

PMH: Preceding myelodysplasia, CML, alkylating chemotherapy (AML)

PC

Age: Extremes: AML >60 y
Extramedullary involvement, esp. CNS and hepatosplenomegaly

Ix

WCC $>50 \times 10^9$/l

Morphology: Undifferentiated or hybrid leukaemia
AML: M 0,5,6,7 (M3 best)
ALL: L3 (L1 best)

Immunophenotype:
ALL: B-ALL (surface Ig), or null-ALL (i.e. no B-cell markers) – worst T-ALL and c-ALL (common to B+T cells) have best prognosis

Genetics:
ALL: Philadelphia chromosome +ve (cf. CML where it's good!)
Hypodiploidy (cf. hyperdiploidy – best prognosis)
AML: Multiple complex chromosome abnormalities

Rx

Time to achieve remission >4 weeks

	AML	ALL
5-year disease-free survival	**40%** (20% in >60 y; 70% with M3)	**80%** (for children with c-ALL)
1st remission	**80%** (40% in >60 y)	**90%** (for children)

CHRONIC MYELOID LEUKAEMIA

Def

Clonal proliferation of the pluripotent stem cell, with predominance of granulocyte lineage at all stages of maturity
Medullary and extramedullary proliferation

Epi

Inc: 1/100,000 p.a.
Age: Middle age (40–60); childhood variants (e.g. juvenile Ph –)
Sex: M slightly > F
Geo: Factory workers – benzene
Nuclear fallout – Hiroshima, Nagasaki, Chernobyl
Aet: 95% exhibit the 'Philadelphia (Ph) chromosome' = t(9;22), found in all dividing progeny

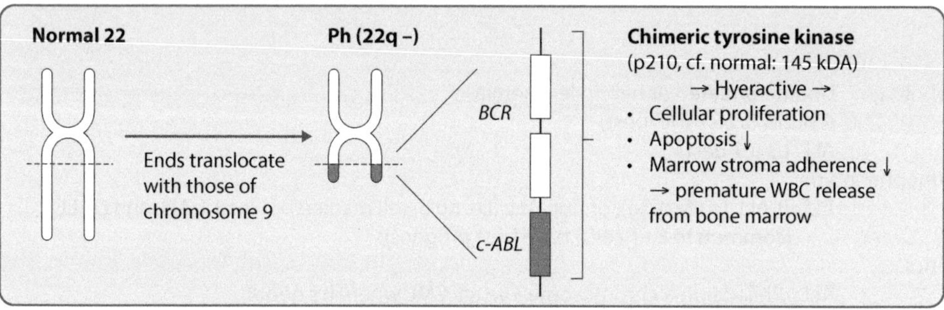

The Ph chromosome found in ALL has a short BCR component, resulting in a poorer prognosis
2.5% are Ph– (worse prognosis)
BCR–c-ABL rearrangement present, e.g. chronic monomyelocytic leukaemia
BCR–c-ABL rearrangement not present, e.g. *RAS* gene mutation – poor prognosis

PC

Can be **S.A.V.A^2.G.E**

Splenomegaly, ± hepatomegaly:
Left-upper quadrant pain or dragging sensation; dyspepsia; early satiety
Pleuritic, L shoulder pain, pleural rub – splenic infarction
Anaemia/infections/purpura
Viscosity, hyper- (WCC >500 × 10^9/l):
Neurological: Headache, confusion, TIA–CVA, retinopathy (blurred vision)
Other: Pulmonary infiltrates, skin nodules, priapism
Accelerated phase → **A**cute leukaemia
Accelerated phase: Pancytopenia, new cytogenetic abnormalities (cumulative transformation rate = 80%; annual rate = 20%)
Acute leukaemia: >30% blast cells in bone marrow; 80% develop AML (80% mortality); 20% develop ALL (50% mortality) (cumulative transformation rate = 70%; median occurence = 4 years)
Myelofibrosis: Alternative outcome following accelerated phase
Gout: Give rasburicase with chemotherapy
Extra:
'B symptoms': Fever, night sweats, weight loss, anorexia
Bone pain

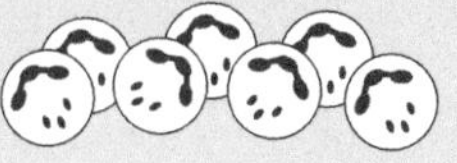
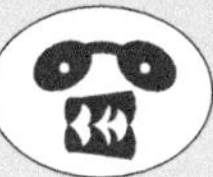
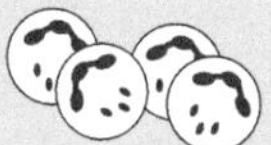

Bloods: FBC

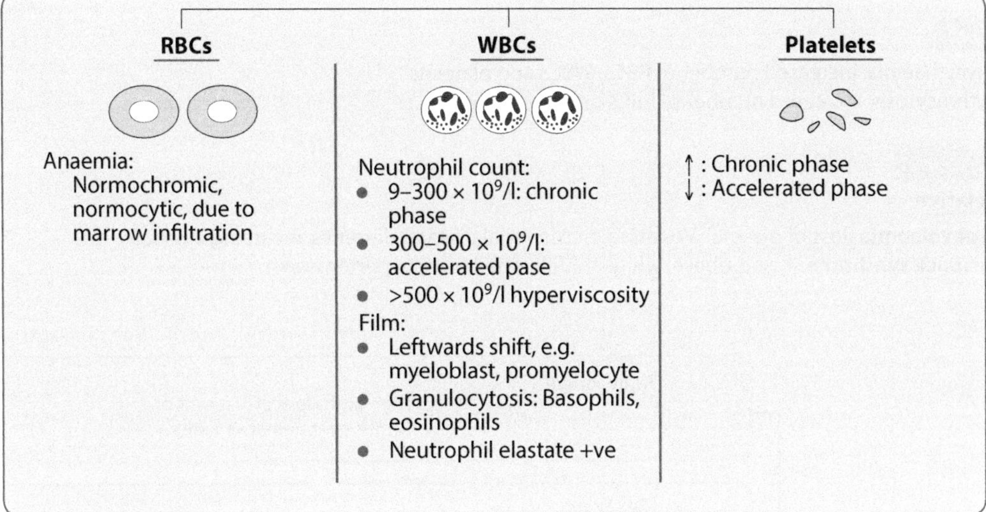

RBCs
WBCs
Platelets
Leucapharesis – for hyperviscocity
Splenectomy or splenic irradiation – for spleen pain or pancytopenia
Anaemia:
Normochromic, normocytic, due to marrow infiltration
Neutrophil count:
• 9–300 × 10⁹/l: chronic phase
• 300–500 × 10⁹/l: accelerated pase
• >500 × 10⁹/l hyperviscosity
Film:
• Leftwards shift, e.g. myeloblast, promyelocyte
• Granulocytosis: Basophils, eosinophils
• Neutrophil elastate +ve
↑ : Chronic phase
↓ : Accelerated phase

Other blood**s**

- Neutrophil alkaline phosphatase ↓ (cf. myeloproliferative disease, infection)
- ALP ↑
- Vit. B12 levels and vit. B12 binding capacity ↑; uric acid ↑

Special: Bone marrow biopsy: Hypercellularity of all haematopoietic lineages, esp. granulocyte precursors

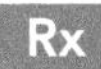

Supportive

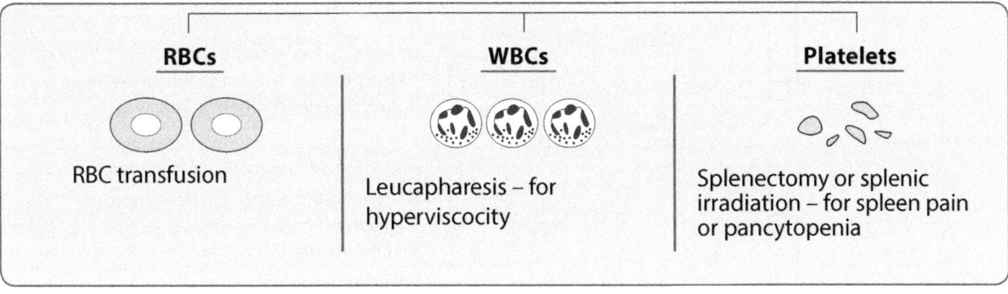

Medical:
Imatinib (oral tyrosine kinase inhibitor):

- Blocks ATP-binding site on p210 BCR–ABL fusion protein
- ☠: Fluid retention, nausea, cramps

Interferon-α: Direct anti-proliferative effect, RNase ↑, natural killer cells ↑ ☠: Lethargy, weight loss
Cytotoxics: Busulphan (☠ : Pulmonary fibrosis), hydroxyurea (better at ↓ platelets)
Allogeneic stem-cell transplant
Curative in 60%, providing <65 y old, compatible donor and early chronic phase

Prog

Median survival = 4 years; death due to acute leukaemia or bleeding

Poor prognostic factors
Ph –ve, e.g. elderly men, juvenile, CMML
Splenomegaly
FBC: Hb: Persistent anaemia
WBC: Peripheral blasts; basophils; eosinophils
Plt: Thrombocytopenia or thrombocytosis

POLYCYTHAEMIA

Def

Polycythaemia: Increased number of RBCs, WBCs and platelets
Erythrocytosis: Increased number of RBCs only

Causes

Relative

Hypovolaemia (loss of plasma): Vomiting, burns; renal disease; diuretics, including alcohol
Gaisbock syndrome: Assoc. obese, white, middle-aged men; hypertension

True

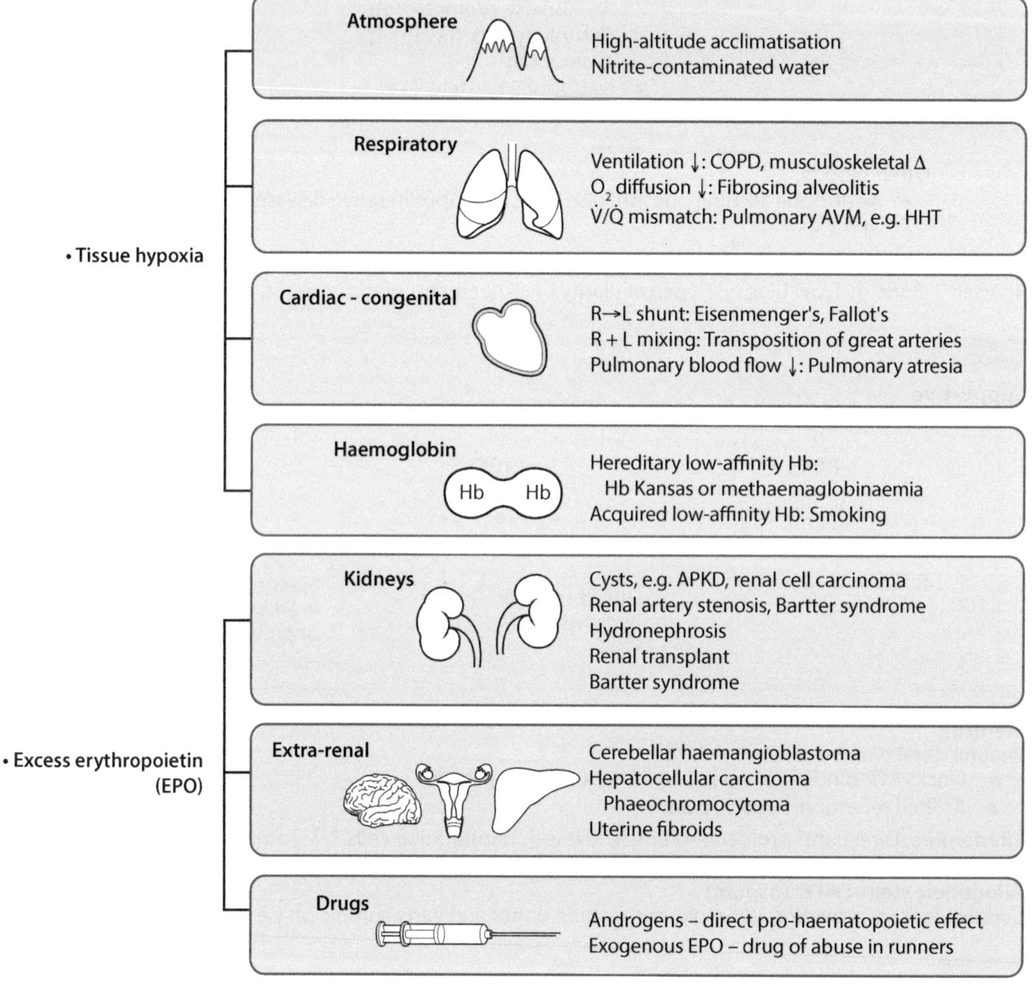

• Polycythaemia rubra vera (PRV)

POLYCYTHAEMIA RUBRA VERA (PRV)

Def

Red-cell count:

Hb >18 g/dl (may be masked by haemorrhage that is assoc. with disease)

Haematocrit >50%

RBC mass – high (ascertained by dilution method using ^{51}Cr-labelled RBCs and ^{125}I -labelled plasma)

Secondary causes excluded, including normal EPO levels

PC

P³.R.V. G.O.

Plethora: Including conjunctival suffusion; acne rosacea
Pruritus, esp. after hot bath: Due to histamine release from basophilia
Peptic ulcers: Due to histamine release
Retinopathy and neurological deficits:
Fundi: Venule engorgement, haemorrhages, papilloedema
Headaches ('fullness')
Dizziness; fatigue; confusion
Vascular:
Venous or arterial thrombosis – DVT, CVA
Haemorrhage, e.g. cerebral: Due to impaired platelet function
Hypertension, CCF

Gout: Due to hyperuricaemia
Organomegaly: Hepatosplenomegaly (in 90%)

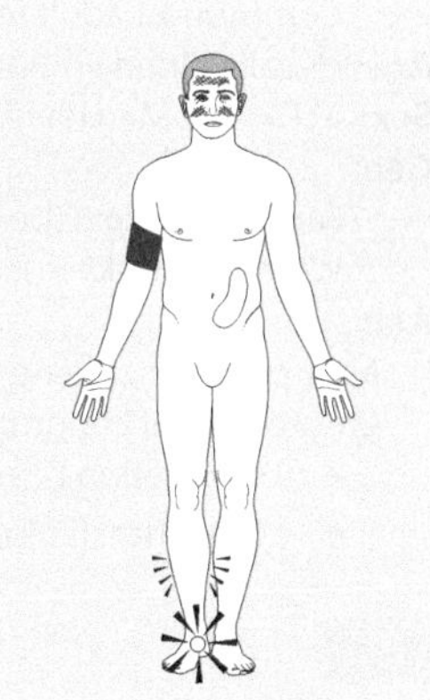

Ix

Bloods: FBC (other than as in definition):

- WCC ↑; neutrophil alkaline phosphatase (NAP) ↑, cf. CML, in which it is ↓
- Platelets ↑; but bleeding time ↑, due to abnormal platelet function
- ESR ↓

Chemistry:

- Vit. B12 ↑ and transcobalamin-I ↑
- LDH ↓, cf. myelofibrosis, in which it is ↑
- Ferritin ↑

Genetic testing: JAK2 mutation common

Special: Bone marrow biopsy:

- Erythropoiesis, granulopoiesis, megakaryocyte number and size – all increased
- Other: Reticulin fibres (Ag stain) increased; Fe stores decreased; blast, colony-forming units

Rx

Venesection: Decrease haematocrit to <46%, by venesecting 1 unit on alternate days

☠: DVT, tolerated poorly in elderly

Myelosuppression: Hydroxyurea, alkylating agents (e.g. chlorambucil, melphalan), radioactive ^{32}P – ☠: Malignant transformation

Low-dose aspirin may prevent thrombotic events

Prog

Median survival is 10 years if treated; but **transformation risk** to AML is 10%

CHRONIC LYMPHOCYTIC LEUKAEMIA

Def

Slow, indolent, clonal proliferation of lymphocytes in mantle zone of 2° lymphoid follicles
B lymphocytes (CD19+) with T-cell marker (CD5+)
Immunodeficiency due to:
- Lymphocyte immaturity; lymphopenia; Ig ↓
- Neutropenia, due to marrow infiltration and hypersplenism

Epi

Inc: Commonest adult leukaemia: 3/100,000 p.a.
Age: Usually elderly (>60). Middle-aged patients have aggressive variant
Sex: M:F = 2:1. Men have worse prognosis
Geo:
- Factory workers (benzene, asbestos); farmers (soya bean production, herbicide)
- Whites > Blacks > Japanese, Chinese

Aet:
- *bcl*-2 proto-oncogene over-expression
- Chromosomal abnormalities, esp.:
  - 13q deletion (75%) – good prognosis
  - 11 deletion (20%) – poor prognosis; bulky lymphadenopathy

PC

B.L.O.B.B.I.E.S.

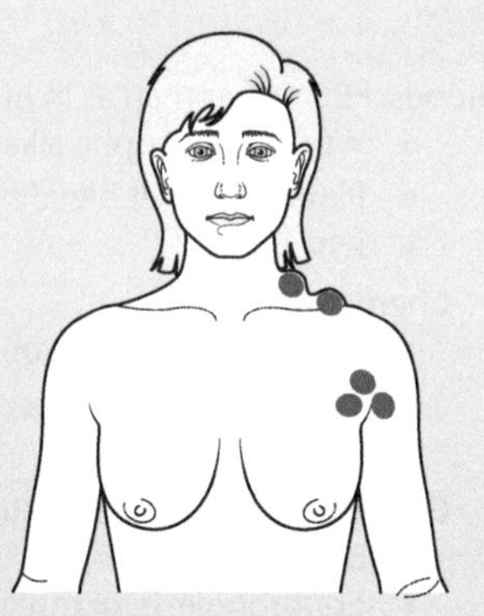

B symptoms (constitutional):
- Night sweats and weight loss
- Occur in late disease; or middle-aged aggressive variant, or Richter syn. (*see opposite*)

Lymphadenopathy: Painless, symmetrical, diffuse, rubbery
Organomegaly: Splenomegaly, hepatomegaly, esp. hairy cell or pro-lymphocytic variants
Bone marrow failure – anaemia (pallor)
Bone marrow failure – thrombocytopenia (purpura)
Immune dysfunction:
- Immunocompromised (cell-mediated immunity): Herpes, esp. zoster (disseminated in 20%); pneumonia – bacterial, fungal
- Autoimmune:
  - Mikulicz syndrome: Xerophthalmia, xerostomia, tonsil – salivary gland enlargement
  - Arthritis, effusions, vasculitis, esp. hairy cell, prolymphocytic or T-cell CLL
  - Hypersensitivity to insect bites or vaccinations ('vaccinia gangrenosum')

Excess
- Viscosity, esp. prolymphocytic CLL: WCC >400 × 10^9/l (poor prognosis)
- Uric acid: Gout, give prophylactic allopurinol if chemo Rx considered

Skin: Nodules; vesicles; bullae; pruritus – 'L'homme rouge' (T-cell CLL)

Ix

Bloods: FBC:

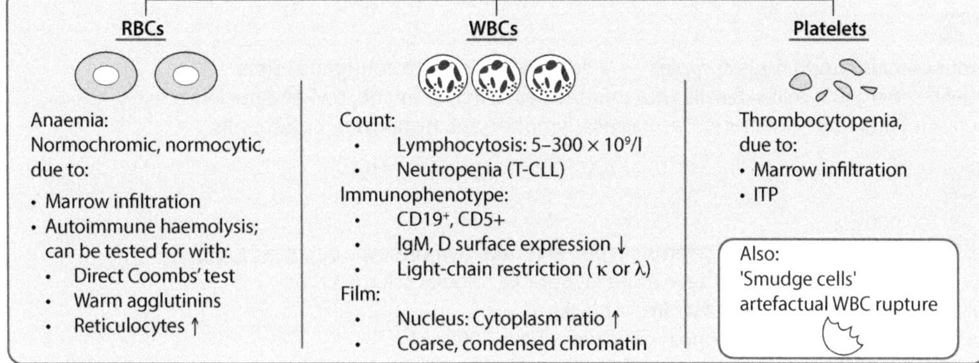

Other bloods:

Bilirubin (nodes at porta hepatis), ALT↑ (liver involvement), ALP ↑, albumin↓

IgG ↓ (paraproteinaemia in 5%); β_2-microglobulin ↑, LDH ↑ (poor prognosis)

Ca ↑, PO_4↓, uric acid ↑

Special: Lymph node or bone marrow biopsy:

- Lymphocytic replacement of >30% (poor prognosis)
- Richter syndrome: Rapid enlargement of lymph node by transformation into diffuse histiocytic lymphoma.

Rx

Supportive

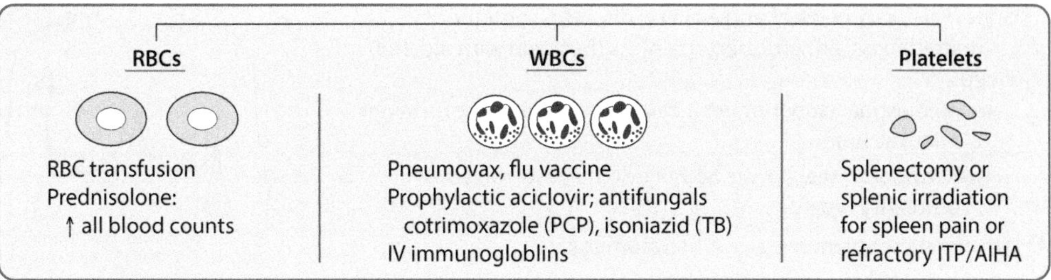

Medical:

Cytotoxics – in high-stage disease:

- Chlorambucil (alkylating agent) or fludarabine (purine analogues) ± cyclophosphamide
- Combination CHOP chemo Rx – for younger pts. to acheive ↑ response rate

Immunotherapy: Anti-CD52 (alemtuzumab) or anti-CD20 (rituximab)

Radiotherapy: Reduces lymph node and spleen size

Allogeneic therapies:

Allogeneic stem-cell transplant + intensive chemo Rx + TBI: if <55 years old

Allogeneic lymphocyte infusion + mild chemotherapy: Enables graft vs. leukaemia reaction

Prog

Rai staging	**Median survival**
0: WBC >15 × 10^9/l (worse if>5% prolymphocytes)	10 years
1: Lymph nodes (worse if >2 sites)	8 years
2: Splenomegaly	6 years
3: Hb <10 g/dl	5 years
4: Platelets <100 × 10^9/l	2 years

HODGKIN LYMPHOMA

Def

Tumour of main lymph node complex → orderly extension into contiguous sites
Reed–Sternberg (RS) cells = B cells with multinucleate, mirror-image, 'owl-eye' nuclei
Reactive inflammatory infiltrate: Plasma cells, lymphocytes, histiocytes, eosinophils

Epi

Inc: 3/100,000 p.a.
Age: Bimodal: 20–30s (nodular sclerosis type), and >60s (lymphocyte-depleted type)
Sex: M:F = 2:1. Women tend to have more favourable nodular sclerosis type
Geo: Low socioeconomic status; whites > blacks
Aet: Inherited: HLA-DPB-1 – monozygotic twins have 100× risk
Infection: EBV (genome present in RS cells in 40%) or HIV – mixed cellularity type
Toxins: Benzene, nitrous oxide, wood dust

PC

B.L.O.B.B.I.E.S.

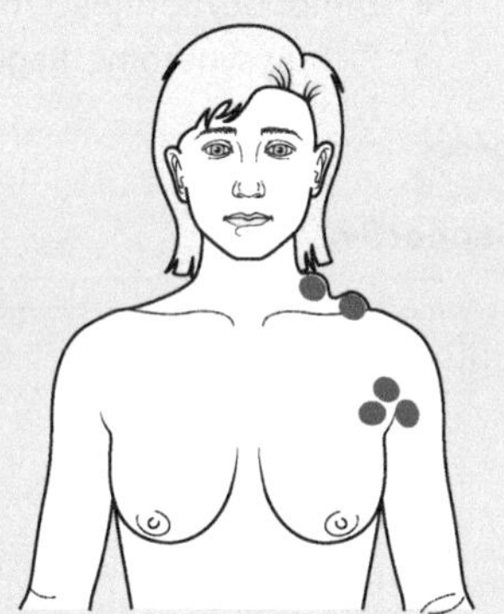

B symptoms (constitutional):
- Weight loss >10% in 6 months
- Fever/night sweats: Continuous or cyclical, high + swinging ('Pel–Ebstein'), or sepsis

Lymphadenopathy:
- Superficial, esp. cervical and axillary; discrete, continuous, matted mass; firm, rubbery, painless (but pain with alcohol)
- Deep:
  - Mediastinal (superior vena cava obstruction), esp. nodular sclerosis type
  - Retroperitoneal (lower body oedema), esp. mixed cellularity type

Organomegaly: Splenomegaly ± hepatomegaly
Bone marrow failure – pancytopenia
Bone pain – with alcohol
Immune dysfunction:
- Immunocompromised (cell-mediated immunity) herpes, esp. zoster, CMV; TB; *Candida*; *Cryptococcus*
- Autoimmune: Autoimmune haemolytic anaemia, ITP, paraneoplastic cerebellar degeneration

Extra: Nephrotic syndrome
Skin: Pruritus; erythema nodosum; ichthyosis

Bloods: FBC

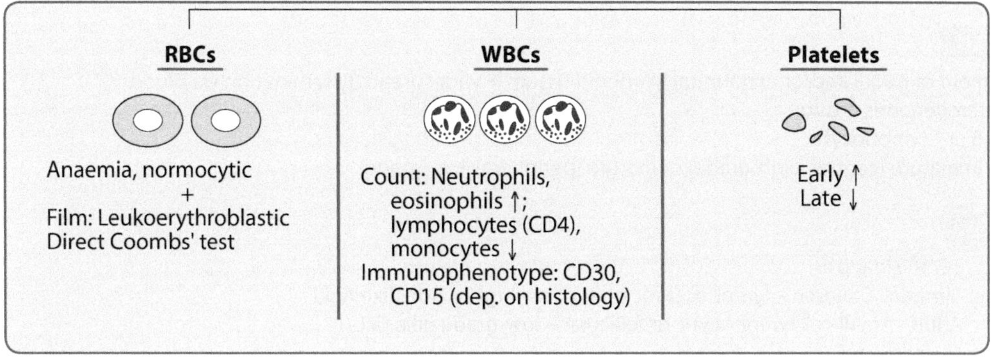

Other bloods

Bilirubin↑ (nodes at porta hepatis), ALT↑ (liver involvement), ALP ↑, albumin ↓

IgG normal; β_2-microglobulin ↑ and LDH ↑ (both suggest poor prognosis)

Ca ↑, PO_4, uric acid ↑

Special: Lymph node ± bone-marrow biopsy

Nodular sclerosis (50%): Fibrosis; lacunar variant of RS cell; eosinophilia; young women

Lymphocyte-predominant (10%): RS cells ↓; monoclonal B cells ↑; young men; good prognosis as ↑ inflammatory response

Mixed cellularity (30%): Intermediate between lymphocyte predominant and depleted

Lymphocyte-depleted (10%) : RS cells ↑; elderly men; poor prognosis

Radiol: Staging CT, PET

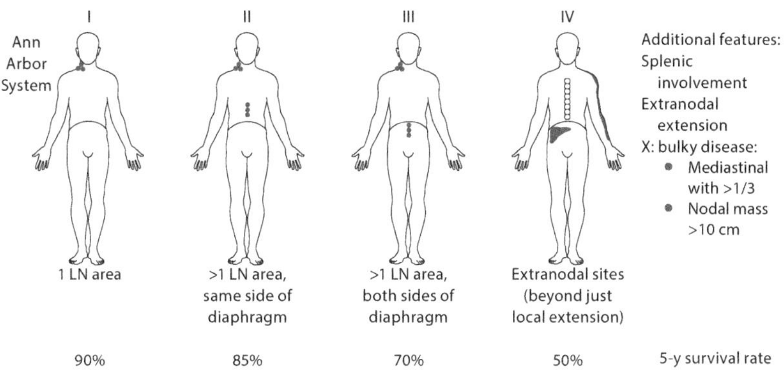

Rx

Supportive:

Blood products, prophylactic aciclovir, cotrimoxazole, vaccinate, sperm-oocyte bank

Medical:

Cytotoxics:

- MOPP (mustine, vincristine [Oncovin], procarbazine, prednisolone): ☠: Infertility; AML, solid tumour
- ABVD (doxorubicin [Adriamycin], bleomycin, vinblastine, dacarbazine): ☠: Cardiomyopathy; pulmo. fibrosis

Radiotherapy: Local; upper mantle (supra-diaphragmatic); inverted-Y (infra-diaphragmatic)

Autologous stem-cell transplant (+ intensive chemotherapy + total-body irradiation):

Reserved for patients after 1st relapse → 25% long-term disease-free survival

Prog

Poor prognosis suggested by:

Epi: Elderly, male

FBC: Hb <10 g/dl; WCC >15 × 10^9/l; lymphocytes <0.6 × 10^9/l

Other: ESR ↑, albumin ↓, β_2-microglobulin, LDH ↑

NON-HODGKIN LYMPHOMA

Def

Tumour of nodal and/or extranodal lymphoid tissue → widespread dissemination via blood
Heterogeneous group:
B or T lymphocyte
Immature (central, high-grade) or mature (peripheral, low-grade)

Epi

Inc: 10/100,000 p.a.
Age: Bimodal: Children – lymphoblastic or Burkitt – high-grade (like ALL)
Adult – small cell lymphocytic or follicular – low-grade (like CLL)
Sex: M slightly > F
Geo: Japan, Caribbean (HTLV-I); Africa (EBV, malaria, HIV –Burkitt)
Aet: Infection: EBV + immunodeficiency state, e.g. HIV, malaria, HTLV-I, *H. pylori*
Immunosuppression: Post-transplant, chemo Rx, radio Rx (e.g. Hodgkin lymphoma Rx)
Immunodeficiency – hereditary: ataxia telangiectasia, Wiskott–Aldrich syndrome
Autoimmune: Coeliac, Crohn, rheumatoid arthritis

PC

B.L.O.B.B.I.E.S.

B symptoms (constitutional): As for Hodgkin – but not prominent until advanced disease
Lymphadenopathy:
Superficial: Multiple, widespread, non-contiguous – suggests advanced disease
Deep: Mediastinal; retroperitoneal, esp. lymphoblastic
Mucosa-associated (MALTomas):

- Oral: Pharynx ('Waldeyer ring') – pharyngitis, dysphagia, stridor; mandible (Burkitt lymphoma); salivary glands – xerostomia, xerophthalmia
- Gastric: associated with *H. pylori*:
  - Bowel ('Peyer's patches'): Colic, D+V, clubbing, wasting – associated with T-cell lymphoma; coeliac; α- heavy chain disease
  - Respiratory tract: Cough, stridor

CNS: Associated with HIV, HTLV-I, lymphoblastic
Organomegaly: Splenomegaly ± hepatomegaly
Bone marrow failure – pancytopenia
Bone pain – with alcohol
Immune dysfunction: Autoimmune haemolytic anaemia, ITP
Endocrine: Thyroid or testes infiltration
Skin: T-cell lymphoma (mycosis fungoides); ichthyosis

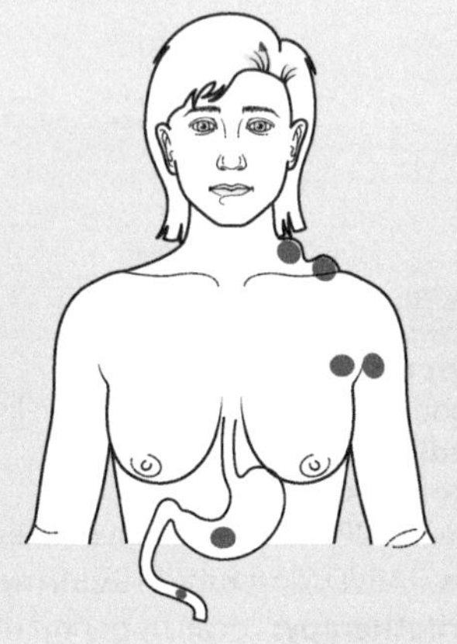

Ix

Bloods: FBC

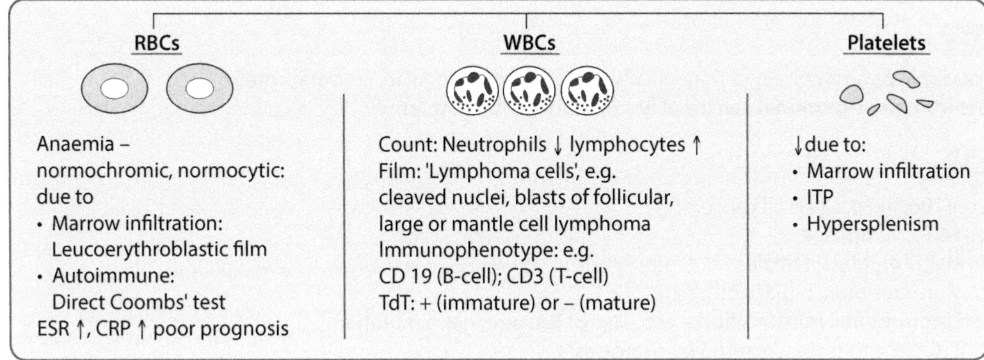

Other bloods Bilirubin ↑ (nodes at porta hepatis), ALT ↑ (liver involvement), ALP ↑, albumin↓
IgG – total ↓, but paraproteinaemia in 15% (esp. indolent lymphomas)
Ca ↑ (esp. adult T-cell leukaemia-lymphoma), PO_4↓, uric acid ↑

Special: Lymph node biopsy (or GIT, bronchial, brain, bone-marrow biopsy)

Grading: REAL classification (Revised European American Lymphoma)

(5-year survival rates)	**B cell**	**T cell**
Low-grade	MALToma (75%) Follicular (70%)	Mycosis fungoides (90%)
Intermediate-grade	Diffuse large cell (50%) Mantle cell (50%)	Anaplastic (75%) Peripheral (25%)
High-grade	Burkitt (50%) Lymphoblastic (50%)	Adult T-cell leukaemia-lymphoma (20%)

Staging: Whole-body CT, PET; CT brain and CSF; OGD; colonoscopy; ENT exam Ann Arbor System (see p. 463) – although staging less relevant to prognosis

Rx

Supportive: As for Hogkin lymphoma (p. 463)

Medical:

Cytotoxic: CHOP (cyclophosphamide, doxorubicin [hydroxydaunorubicin], vincristine [Oncovin], prednisolone)

Immunotherapy: Interferon-α; rituximab (anti-CD20), alemtuzimab (anti-CD52)

Radiotherapy:

Local – can be curative in stage I disease

Brain – CNS lymphoma

Autologous stem-cell transplant: (+ chemotherapy + total-body irradiation if pt. relapses)

Special:

Splenic lymphoma with villous lymphocytes – splenectomy (curative)

CNS lymphoma – brain irradiation; intrathecal (low-dose) and IV (high-dose) methotrexate

Prog

Poor prognosis suggested by grade and **International Prognostic Index:**

Epi: Age >60 y (also AIDS)

PC: Functional disability (Karnofsky score)

Bloods: LDH ↑ (also pancytopenia, ESR or CRP ↑, albumin ↓, β_2-microglobulin)

Staging: Ann Arbor stage 3 or 4; >1 extranodal site (also bulky disease of >10 cm)

MULTIPLE MYELOMA

Def

Monoclonal plasma cell clone that usually secretes monoclonal Ig, i.e. paraprotein
Arises from **post-germinal centre** of lymph node, or bone marrow

Epi

Inc: 5/100,000 p.a. (1% all cancers)
Age: >40 y, ↑ with age
Sex: Males slightly > females
Geo: More common in black ethnicity
Aet: Chromosomal translocation – esp. *Myc* or *Ras* oncogene mutation
IL-6: Growth factor secreted by osteoclasts

PC

P.O.P.U.L.A.T.I.O.N.

Plasma cells in >4% of bone marrow (usually >30% in myeloma)
Osteolytic lesions:
PATH: Osteoclasts activated (via IL-β, TNF-β); osteoblasts inhibited
PC: Bone pain, tenderness, worse with movement, during day, esp. back, shoulder, ribs
Pathological fractures, e.g. wedge vertebral-cord compression; radicular pain
Bony mass: Skull, sternum, clavicle
Paraproteinaemia: >30 g/l or rising
Def: Plasma: Monoclonal Ig and/or Urine: Bence Jones protein (κ or λ light-chain restriction)
Frequency: Plasma alone, 20%; BJP alone, 20%; both, 58%; none, 2% (esp. plasmacytomas)
PC: Hyperviscosity, esp. Ig M, A, D, IgG3, cryoglobulins → headache, visual blurring, Raynaud
Coagulopathy and impaired platelet function
U&Es:
Urine: Nephrotic syndrome; chronic renal failure (30%), due to:
- Deposition of Bence Jones protein; amyloid; infiltration of tumour
- Other: Calcium ↑, uric acid ↑; pyelonephritis (immunodeficient); NSAIDs

Electrolytes: Ca ↑ due to osteolysis → abdominal pain, N+V, polyuria, polydipsia
Uric acid ↑ due to cell turnover → gout
Light chain amyloid (AL or primary) → nephrosis, neuropathy, cardiac failure
Anaemia: Due to IL-1 myelosuppression
Thrombocytopenia
Immunodeficiency:
PATH: Due to polyclonal Ig ↓; cell-mediated immunity ↓; neutropenia; complement ↓
PC: Bacterial respiratory and urinary tract infections – streptococci, staphylococci, Klebsiella
Organomegaly: Hepatosplenomegaly
Neurological: Peripheral neuropathy, papilloedema, POEMS syndrome (peripheral neuropathy; osteosclerosis; endocrine [e.g. DM]; M-band; skin [e.g. hyperpigmentation])

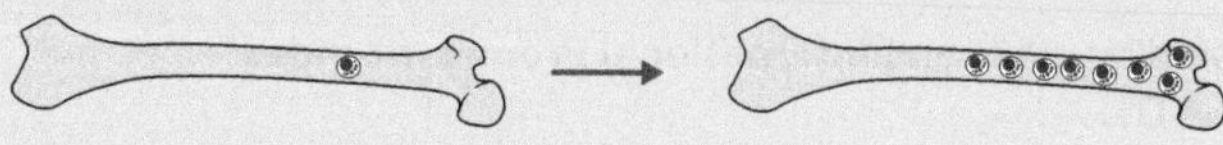

1st three features are essential for diagnosis

Ix

Bloods: FBC

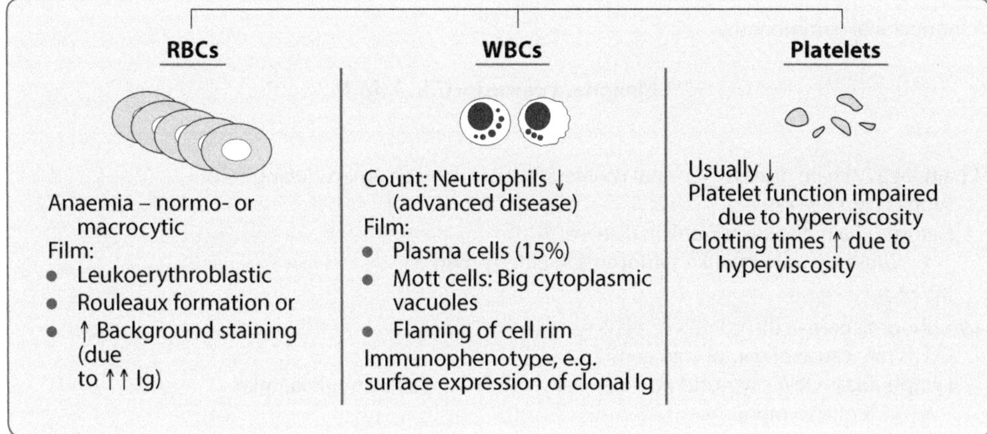

RBCs
WBCs
Platelets
Anaemia – normo- or macrocytic
Film:
• Leukoerythroblastic
• Rouleaux formation or
• ↑ Background staining (due to ↑↑ Ig)
Count: Neutrophils ↓ (advanced disease)
Film:
• Plasma cells (15%)
• Mott cells: Big cytoplasmic vacuoles
• Flaming of cell rim
Immunophenotype, e.g. surface expression of clonal Ig
Usually ↓
Platelet function impaired due to hyperviscosity
Clotting times ↑ due to hyperviscosity

Chemistry

Electrophoresis – serum and urine:

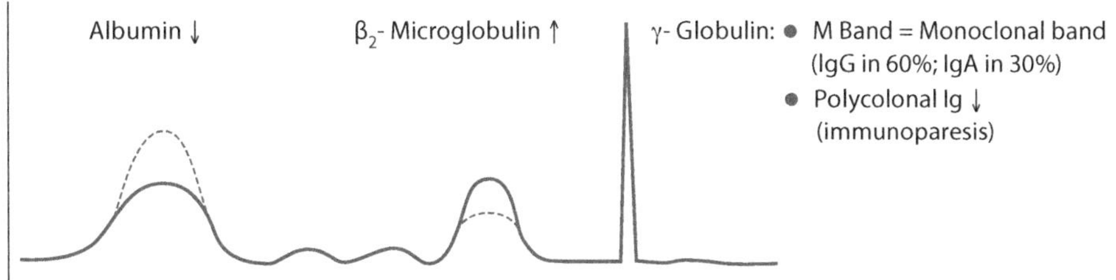

U&E: Urea ↑, creatinine ↑; Ca ↑, uric acid ↑, Na ↓ (real and pseudohyponatraemia due to Ig ↑), Cl ↑ (so anion gap ↓)

LFT: LDH ↑; albumin ↓; ALP normal as osteoblasts inactive

Urine: Proteinuria – suggests renal disease (Bence Jones protein is not detected by dipstick)
Glycosuria and aminoaciduria (Fanconi syndrome, due to tubular damage)

Radiol:

X-ray of limbs, spine, skull:

- Focal or generalized osteoporosis, e.g. 'punched-out' holes in skull
- Wedge fractures of spine

Tc bone scan: Silent due to osteoblastic inhibition (may be +ve if sclerotic reaction occurs)

Special: Bone-marrow biopsy

Rx

Supportive:

Bone marrow suppression: Blood products; antibiotics; IVIg

Bone lesions: Radiotherapy, surgery

Hyperviscosity: Plasmapharesis

Hypercalcaemia:- Hydration, bisphosphonates

Medical – cytotoxics:

Elderly: Single agent (melphalan or cyclophosphamide)

Young: VAD (vincristine, doxorubicin [Adriamycin], dexamethasone) ± IFN-α

Stem-cell transplant:

Autologous + high-dose melphalan: Increases survival time; decreases remission rate

Allogeneic: 50% curative or long-term remission, although 30% mortality rate from procedure

Prog

5-year survival rate = 20%, i.e. **B.A.D.** = poor prognostic markers:

β_2-microglobulin (albumin ↓, M-band ↑)

Bony lesions if extensive + symptomatic

Anaemia (ESR, CRP ↑↑)

Dehydration (urea >14; Ca ↑↑); L**D**H ↑

PARAPROTEINAEMIA

AKA monoclonal gammopathy

Malignant causes = C.L.A.M.P.

Chain (heavy chain disease) = clonal proliferation of heavy chain-producing cells:
- Alpha chain disease
- Gamma chain disease = Franklin disease:
  - Causes lymphoma-like symptoms in elderly men
- Mu chain disease

Lymphoproliferative disorder:
- CLL is rare cause of paraproteinaemia
- Lymphoplasmacytic lymphoma (AKA Waldenström's macroglobulinaemia):
  - 15% of all lymphomas
  - presents age 65
  - Lymphomatous infiltration of nodes, marrow, spleen
  - Usually IgM paraprotein >30 g/l
  - 10–30% have hyperviscosity

AL amyloidosis:
- Occurs in 15% cases of multiple myeloma
- May occur spontaneous (primary AL)
- Bence Jones proteins in urine

Multiple myeloma

Plasmacytoma = mass of plasma cells causing local symptoms, usually in bone

Non-malignant causes = M.A.I.L.

MGUS:
- 50% of paraproteinaemias
- <30 g/l paraprotein
- 1% cases per year progress to myeloma

Auto-immune disorders

Infections: SBE and mycoplasma

Liver cirrhosis

HYPERVISCOSITY

Causes

Cells	Polycythaemia: 1° (PRV) – commonest cause; 2° if severe Chronic myeloid leukaemia Acute leukaemia – if severe
Paraprotein	Waldenström's macroglobulinaemia: IgM Multiple myeloma: IgM or IgA Plasmacytoma
Latrogenic	Packed cell products Cryoprecipitate (given to haemophiliacs with circulating inhibitors): Causes hyperfibrinogenaemia IVIg therapy

PC

P^5.R.V. G.O.

Plethora, **P**ruritus, **P**eptic ulcers – all with PRV only

Purpura, **P**igmentation – reticulate, Raynaud phenomenon, necrosis – esp. with cryoglobulinaemia, due to paraproteinaemia

Retinopathy/neurological deficits:
- 'Slow-flow retinopathy':
  - PC: Visual disturbance – 'looking through a watery windscreen'
  - Fundi: Venule engorgement, constrictions – 'linked sausages'
    Flame haemorrhages, exudates, papilloedema
- CNS: Headaches ('fullness'); dizziness; encephalopathy – fatigue, confusion, seizures
- PNS: Peripheral neuropathy (demyelinating), due to anti-MAG Ab

Vascular:
- Venous or arterial thrombosis – DVT, CVA
- Haemorrhage, e.g. epistaxis, haematuria, cerebral: Due to impaired platelet function and coagulopathy
- Hypertension, CCF

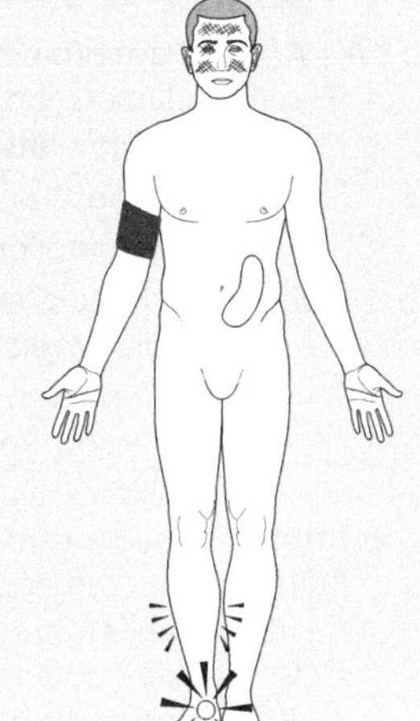

Gout: Due to hyperuricaemia, but only with cell proliferation cause

Organomegaly:
- Hepatosplenomegaly: PRV, CML, myeloma, lymphoma
- Lymphadenopathy: Waldenström's macroglobulinaemia

Ix

Bloods: FBC ↑: Myeloproliferative; ↓: Myeloma, Waldenström
ESR ↓: Myeloproliferative; ↑: Myeloma, Waldenström
Serum electrophoresis

Urine: Electrophoresis

Special: Biopsy: Bone marrow: Myeloproliferative, myeloma
Lymph node: Waldenström (lymphoplasmacytoid infiltrate)

Rx

Waldenström:

Supportive: Packed RBC transfusions; antibiotics

Plasmapharesis: Most effective for IgM as intravascularly confined

Chemotherapy: Cyclophosphamide + prednisolone if symptomatic or cytopenic

AMYLOIDOSIS

Def

Accumulation of any fibrillar protein that folds abnormally into β-pleated-sheets

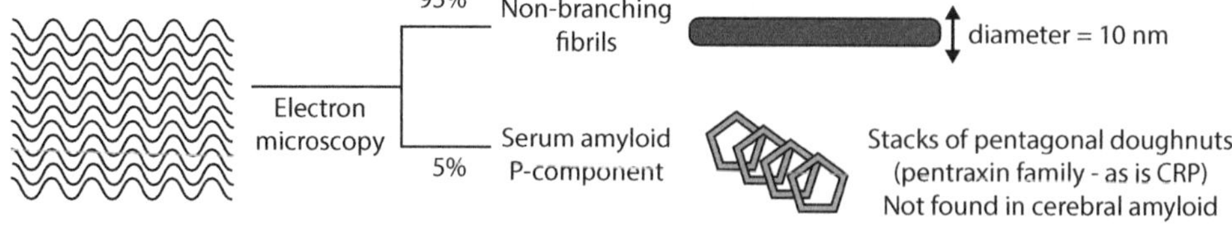

Types

Distinguished by type of protein that forms in excess:

Systemic

A**L** – **L**ight chain: Due to any cause of paraproteinaemia:
- Light-chain secretion only, esp. λVI, or N-terminus of V_L – commonest
- B-cell neoplasm, e.g. multiple myeloma, plasmacytoma, lymphoma
- MGUS

A**A** – **A**cute phase protein, protein A (breakdown product of serum amyloid A):
- Chronic inflammation (>2 y): IL-1, IL-6 cytokines → hepatocyte SAA secretion increases:
  - Autoimmunity: Rheumatoid arthritis (esp. Still), ankolysing spondylitis, ulcerative colitis
  - Infection: Bronchiectasis (staphylococci, TB), osteomyelitis, cellulitis
  - Neoplasm: Hodgkin, renal cell carcinoma
- Hereditary periodic fever:
  - Familial Mediterranean fever (autosomal recessive): Assoc: Sephardi Jews, Arabs
    - Type 1: Recurrent serositis (pleurisy, peritonitis, synovitis)
    - Type 2: Renal amyloid
  - Muckle–Wells syndrome

Autosomal dominant amyloidopathy:
- Transthyretin (carrier of thyroxine + retinol-binding protein; made in liver + choroid plexus)
  - PC: Lower limb and autonomic neuropathy, scalloped pupils, cardiac amyloid
- Gelsolin (actin modulator): Assoc: Finnish
  - PC: Cranial and autonomic neuropathy, corneal and vitreous dystrophy
- Other: Apolipoprotein AI, lysozyme, fibrinogen-α
  - PC: Renal, cardiac, GIT amyloid (not neuropathy)

Organ-based

Cerebral:
- Amyloid α_2: Dementia; cerebral lobar haemorrhage
- α-synuclein: Lewy body dementia, Parkinson disease
- Prion protein (PrP): Creutzfeldt–Jakob disease

Cardiac: Transthyretin plus atrial natriuretic peptide – causes LVF and IHD in elderly

Endocrine:
- Amylin (homology to calcitonin gene-related peptide): Type 2 DM/insulinoma
- Pro-calcitonin: Medullary carcinoma of thyroid + other APUDomas

Soft tissue, e.g. α_2-macroglobulin via haemodialysis: Arthritis, carpal tunnel syndrome

PC

O.R.G.A.N.i.S.E.D.

Organomegaly:
- Hepatosplenomegaly
- Lymphadenopathy – in AA amyloid and lymphoma

Renal:
- Proteinuria: Nephrotic syndrome, renal vein thrombosis
- Chronic renal failure: Glomerular + tubule – interstitial + vascular disease
- Renal enlargement

GIT:
- Macroglossia – dysphagia
- Bowel: Malabsorption, diarrhoea, obstruction
- Liver: Intrahepatic cholestasis; portal hypertension

Arthritis: Rheumatoid-pattern, or large-joint monoarthritis; shoulder-pad sign

Neurological:
- Neuropathy: Painful, sensory, autonomic, enlarged nerves
- Carpal tunnel syndrome
- 'Pseudomyopathy'

Skin:
- Waxy plaques and papules
- Purpura: 'Raccoon eyes' (factor X/fibrinogen deficiency)

Endocrine: Goitre; adrenal, pituitary, pancreas enlargement (rarely deficiency)

Death due to:
- Cardiac: Arrhythmias, heart block, digoxin hypersensitivity, restrictive cardiomyopathy, constrictive pericarditis, endocardial – valve disease
- Airway: Larynx or bronchial thickening – stridor, dysphonia

Ix

Myeloma Ix:
- FBC, film, BM biopsy; serum, urine electrophoresis, Ca, β_2-microglobulin; X-ray screen

Biopsy: Rectal; gingival; renal; abdominal fat pad aspirate
- Stain: H&E – hyaline, eosinophilic, amorphous, proteinaceous material; Congo red +ve; birefringent

SAP-scan: Radiolabelled serum amyloid P scintigram (^{99}Tc)

Rx

Treatment of underlying cause leads to regression of amyloid deposits, but prognosis poor for 1°

AL: Chemotherapy as for myeloma
- Serum amyloid P binding inhibitor: R-1-pyrrolidine carboxylic acid

AA: Immunosuppressants, e.g. chlorambucil in Still; or antibiotics for sepsis
- Colchicine for familial Mediterranean fever

Transthyretin: Liver transplant

β_2-**microglobulin:** Renal transplant (i.e. stopping haemodialysis)

HYPOSPLENISM

Causes

C.A.B.O.T.'S. *rings*

Congenital:
- Agenesis: Associated immunodeficiency, e.g. Fanconi's anaemia
- Congenital cyanotic heart disease

Autoimmune:
- SLE, rheumatoid arthritis (associated big spleen)
- GIT: Coeliac, inflammatory bowel disease, chronic active hepatitis (associated small spleen)
- Graves disease, Hashimoto's thyroiditis, hypopituitarism or growth hormone deficiency, glomerulonephritis (associated small spleen for all)

Blood disorder:
- Sickle cell: Big spleen in infancy, but numerous microinfarcts cause gradual fibrosis and contraction
- Thalassaemia; hereditary spherocytosis – often treated with elective splenectomy
- Lymphoma
  - Sezary syndrome (T cell)
  - Radiotherapy or graft-versus-host disease
- Amyloid

Occlusion: Splenic artery or vein thrombosis

Trauma/splenectomy

Indications for elective splenectomy:

Autoimmune ITP or autoimmune haemolytic anaemia: Both when steroid-resistant and chronic

Leukaemia or lymphoma:
- CML or myelofibrosis:
  - ↓ symptoms of massive splenomegaly
  - ↓ need for tranfusions
- CLL or lymphoma:
  - ↓ thrombocytopenia
- Thalassaemia major or intermedia; hereditary spherocytosis

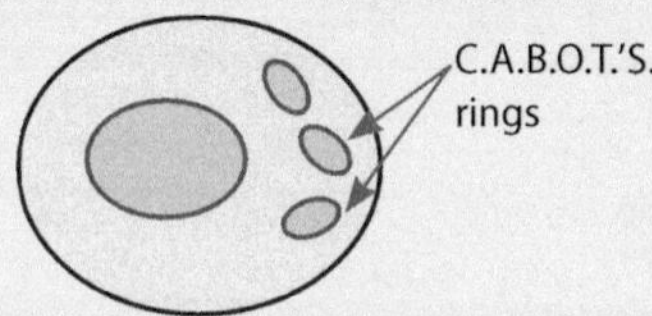

Sarcoid

PC

Infection: Due to decreased phagocytosis, chemotaxis, Ab production
Thrombocytosis: Ischaemic heart disease; CVA; peripheral vascular disease
Hypersplenism: From accessory spleen enlargement at hilum, mesentery, or pancreas tail
Autoimmunity: Due to impaired T cell suppression

Ix

Bloods: FBC and blood film: All cell counts ↑ due to less natural destruction

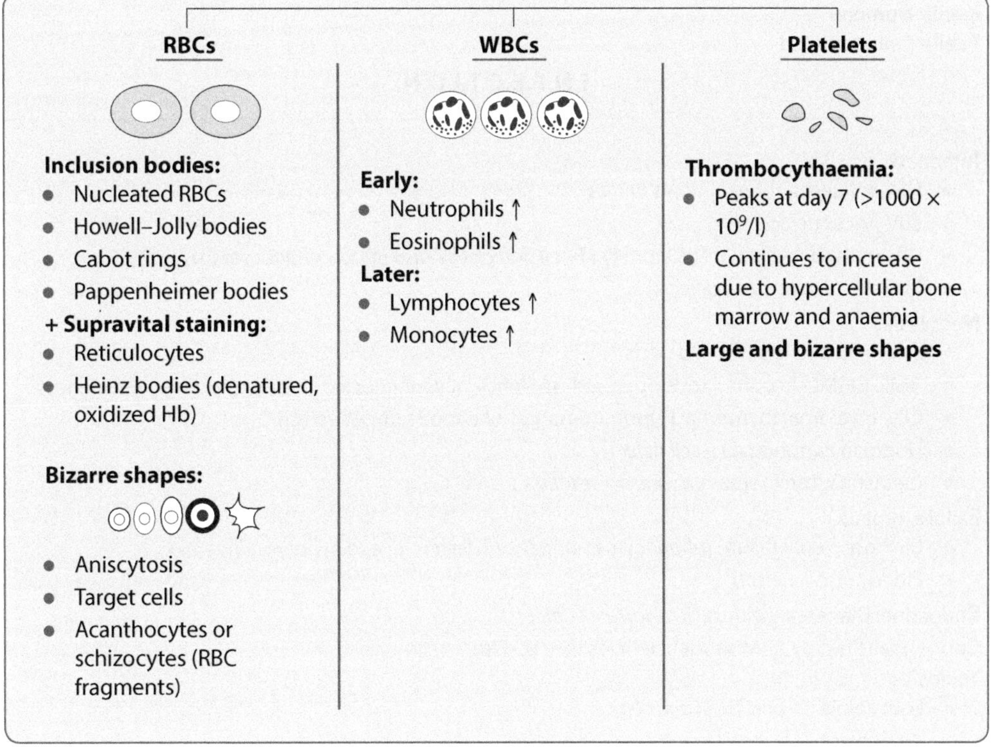

RBCs
Inclusion bodies:
Nucleated RBCs
Howell–Jolly bodies
Cabot rings
Pappenheimer bodies
+ Supravital staining:
Reticulocytes
Heinz bodies (denatured, oxidized Hb)
Bizarre shapes:
Aniscytosis
Target cells
Acanthocytes or schizocytes (RBC fragments)
WBCs
Early:
Neutrophils ↑
Eosinophils ↑
Later:
Lymphocytes ↑
Monocytes ↑
Platelets
Thrombocythaemia:
Peaks at day 7 (>1000 × 10⁹/l)
Continues to increase due to hypercellular bone marrow and anaemia
Large and bizarre shapes

Prophylaxis

Plan best time for splenectomy: Delay splenectomy, as <6 years old are most susceptible to infection
Vaccines:
- PneumoVax (from 1 month before operation)
- Hib *(Haemophilus influenzae* b)
- MeningoVax A + C (esp. if travelling abroad)

Antibiotics:
- Penicillin V/macrolide
- Anti-malarials (esp. if latent infection due to risk of reactivation or cerebral malaria)
- Salmonella infection

Anti-platelets: Aspirin

IMMUNODEFICIENCY – GENERAL

Causes

Causes can be categorized according to the part of the immune system affected:

Innate:

Mucosal defences:
- Neuromuscular weakness; recumbency; smoking
- Iatrogenic: Lines; cannulas; catheters; tracheostomy

Complement deficiency

Phagocytosis failure: respiratory viruses

B cells: Humoral

T cells: Cell-mediated

I.N.F.E.C.T.I.O.N.

Infection:
- HSV, influenza *(phagocytosis failure)*
- EBV *(B-cell defect)*
- HIV, malaria, lepromatous leprosy *(T-cell defect; HIV also affects phagocytosis)*
- Measles *(B- and T-cell defects)*

Neoplasia:
- Leukaemia *(B- and T-cell defects)*
- AML, CMML: Acquired myeloperoxidase deficiency *(phagocytosis failure)* and IgA deficiency
- CLL, myeloma, thymoma: Hypogammaglobulinaemia *(B-cell defect)*
- Hodgkin lymphoma *(T-cell defect)*
- Metastatic carcinoma *(phagocytosis failure)*

Failure, organ:
- Cirrhosis, renal failure *(phagocytosis and B-cell defects, due to hypoproteinaemia)*
- Elderly *(T-cell defect)*

Endocrine: Diabetes mellitus *(B- and T-cell defects)*

Congenital: Primary immunodeficiencies (see p. 476)

Toxins:
- Leukaemia *(B- and T-cell defects)*
- Alcohol *(phagocytosis failure)*
- Smoking *(cilia inhibition, phagocytosis failure)*
- Colchicine, NSAIDs *(phagocytosis failure)*
- Steroids *(phagocytosis failure; B-cell defect)*
- Chemotherapy, radiotherapy *(global immune effects)*

Immune:
- SLE, rheumatoid arthritis *(phagocytosis and complement deficiency – classical pathway)*
- Sarcoidosis *(T-cell defect)*

Organomegaly – hypersplenism *(due to neutropenia)*

Nutritional:
- Malnutrition, malabsorption *(global immune effects)*
- Protein deficiency, esp. burns, protein-losing enteropathy, nephrosis *(B-cell defect)*
- Zinc deficiency (acrodermatitis enteropathica) *(B- and T-cell defects)*
- Fe deficiency *(T-cell defect)*

PC

Innate

Infection:

Pyogenic

- Boils, bronchiectasis – staphylococci: Catalase +ve, and so can overcome peroxide-based defences when superoxide production is impaired in CGD
- Sinusitis, meningitis – streptococcus, *Haemophilus*

Fungi

B cell

Infection:

Pyogenic – esp. encapsulated bacteria: *Streptococcus pneumoniae*, *Haemophilus*, *Meningococcus*, *Salmonella*

Viruses:

- VZV, recurrent
- HBV, chronic
- Enterovirus meningoencephalitis
- Live vaccines may cause disease

Fungi: *Pneumocystis pneumoniae* (hyperIgM)

Protozoa:

- Giardia (Bruton agammaglobulinaemia)
- Malaria (splenectomy)

Autoimmunity:

Myositis (Bruton agammaglobulinaemia)
SLE, rheumatoid arthritis, coeliac (IgA deficiency)
Atopy (IgA deficiency, hyperIgM)

Neoplasia: Lymphoma (common variable immunodeficiency)

T cell

Infection:

Pyogenic, incl. TB
Viruses – herpes: HSV, VZV, EBV, HHV-8
Fungi: *Candida*, PCP, *Cryptococcus*
Protozoa: Cryptosporidia, toxoplasmosis

Autoimmunity: Sjögren-like sicca syndrome

Neoplasia: Non-Hodgkin lymphoma

IMMUNODEFICIENCY – PRIMARY

Causes

Innate

Mucosal defences

Muscular dystrophy, cystic fibrosis, Kartagener

Complement deficiencies

Classical pathway: C2, 1, 4 deficiency – causes SLE-like syndrome
Common pathway:
- Membrane-attack complex – *Neisseria meningitis*
- C3 deficiency – severe pyogenic infections

C1 esterase deficiency: Angioedema
GPI cell anchor (protects against complement): paroxysmal nocturnal haemoglobinuria

Phagocytosis dysfunction

CGD (chronic granulomatous disease):
Epi: X-linked – 60%; auto. recessive – 40%
PATH: NADPH oxidase deficiency → ↓ superoxide
PC: Staphylococcal sepsis (being catalase +ve, it can overcome peroxide-based defences)
Fungal sepsis
Ix: Nitrazolium blue test

Myeloperoxidase deficiency:
Epi: Autosomal recessive, 1/2000
PC: Mild, unless concomitant diabetes mellitus
Systemic candidiasis

G6P dehydrogenase deficiency:
Immunodeficiency if <5% G6PD activity

Chediak–Higashi syndrome:
PATH: Deficient cathepsin G and elastase → inhibits fusion of phagolysosomes
Ix: Blood film – large granules

Kostmann syndrome: G-CSF receptor defect, leading to decreased granulocyte number

B-cell disorders

Non-selective Ig deficiency

X-linked agammaglobulinaemia
Epi: 1/100,000; X-linked
PATH: Bruton tyrosine kinase mutation
B-cell count ↓; lymphoid hyperplasia
PC: Presents in 1st year:

A.G.A.M.M.A.G.LOB.

Autoimmune: Dermatomyositis
Gastroenteritis (giardia, enterovirus)
Arthritis: Mycoplasma (rheumatoid-pattern)
Malabsorption; lactose intolerance
Meningo-encephalitis (enterovirus)
Anaemia, pernicious
Growth hormone deficiency (X linkage)
LOBar pneumonia; bronchiectasis; sinusitis

Ix: Ig <2 g/l

Common variable immunodeficiency
Epi: 1/2000
PATH: Abnormalities in B- or Th-cell maturation
Germinal centre hyperplasia
PC: Presents in adulthood as for Bruton, plus:
Fever
Lymphadenopathy, hepatosplenomegaly, lymphoma, lymphocytosis, Hb↓ platelets ↓
Ix: Bone marrow: Pre-B cells (no surface Ig)
Rx: IVIg (for CVID and Bruton)

Selective Ig deficiency

IgA deficiency
Epi: 1/600 Caucasians
PATH: 1°, congenital infection, penicillamine, phenytoin
PC: **A**symptomatic, or immunodeficient (if ↓ IgG2, 4)
Allergies: Asthma, allergy to milk; blood transfusions (due to anti-IgA)
Autoimmune: coeliac, CAH, SLE, RA
Assoc: Ataxia telangiectasia
Absent vaccine response
Ix: B cells bear IgM
Rx: Use blood from IgA-deficient donor

IgG subclass or functional IgG deficiency
PC: Asymptomatic ↔ pneumococcal infection

Hypergammaglobulinaemia

Immunodeficiency with hyperimmunoglobulin M
PATH: Neutrophils, IgG, A ↓ ; IgM, D ↑
PC: Infections: Bacterial, PCP, cryptosporidiosis
Autoimmune liver disease
Neoplasia

Hyper IgE: Job syndrome

T-cell disorders

Hypoparathyroidism-associated

DiGeorge syndrome

PATH: Developmental defects of pharyngeal pouches 3+4

PC: **C.A.T.C.H. 22**

- **C**ardiac anomalies
- **A**rtery Δ
- **T**hymus aplasia: Immunodeficiency
- **C**raniofacial anomalies
- **H**ypocalcaemia
- **22** = chromosome affected

Chronic mucocutaneous candidiasis

PATH: Deficient migratory inhibitory factor

PC: Superficial candida only

Assoc: Polyglandular autoimmune syndrome-1

Fe deficiency

T-cell defects

Ataxia telangiectasia

Epi: Autosomal recessive

PATH: Deficient DNA repair

PC: Presents in early childhood with:

Ataxia **T.E.L.A.N.G.**

- **A**taxia; Apraxia of oculomotor system
- **T**elangiectasia on sclera, elbows, ears
- **E**ndocrine: DM, hypogonadism
- **L**iver: Fatty liver/AFP ↑↑
- **A**utoimmunity
- **N**eoplasia: ALL, CLL, lymphoma; CEA↑:
  - In early 20s
  - 10% heterozygotes affected
  - Radiosensitive: Risk of mammograms
- **G**lobulins: IgA deficiency

Wiskott–Aldrich syndrome:

Epi: X-linked

PATH: Non-specific T-cell receptor (CD43)

PC: Recurrent infections

Autoimmunity: ITP, AIHA/eczema/JCA

Lymphoma in 20s

Ix: IgM ↓

IgA ↑

B- and T-cell disorders

SCID – severe combined immunodeficiency

Epi: X-linked, autosomal recessive, Swiss-type

PATH: Numerous mutations, incl.:

- RAG 1+2: V (D)J recombination
- DNA-dependent tyrosine kinase
- Adenosine deaminase
- IL-receptor g chain (XL) → ↓T cells, ↓ NK cells, functionally defective B cells

Primary T-cell defects

(with 2° B-cell dysfunction)

- MHC-II deficiency
- TCR deficiency
- ZAP70 tyrosine kinase deficiency
- JAK3 protein kinase deficiency (similar to XL SCID)

Chromosomal defects

Aneuploidy: Down, Turner syndromes

Instability:

- Fanconi's anaemia
- Xeroderma pigmentosa
- Bloom syndrome

Other

Transcobalamin deficiency

PC: Megaloblastic anaemia

HAEMOSTASIS

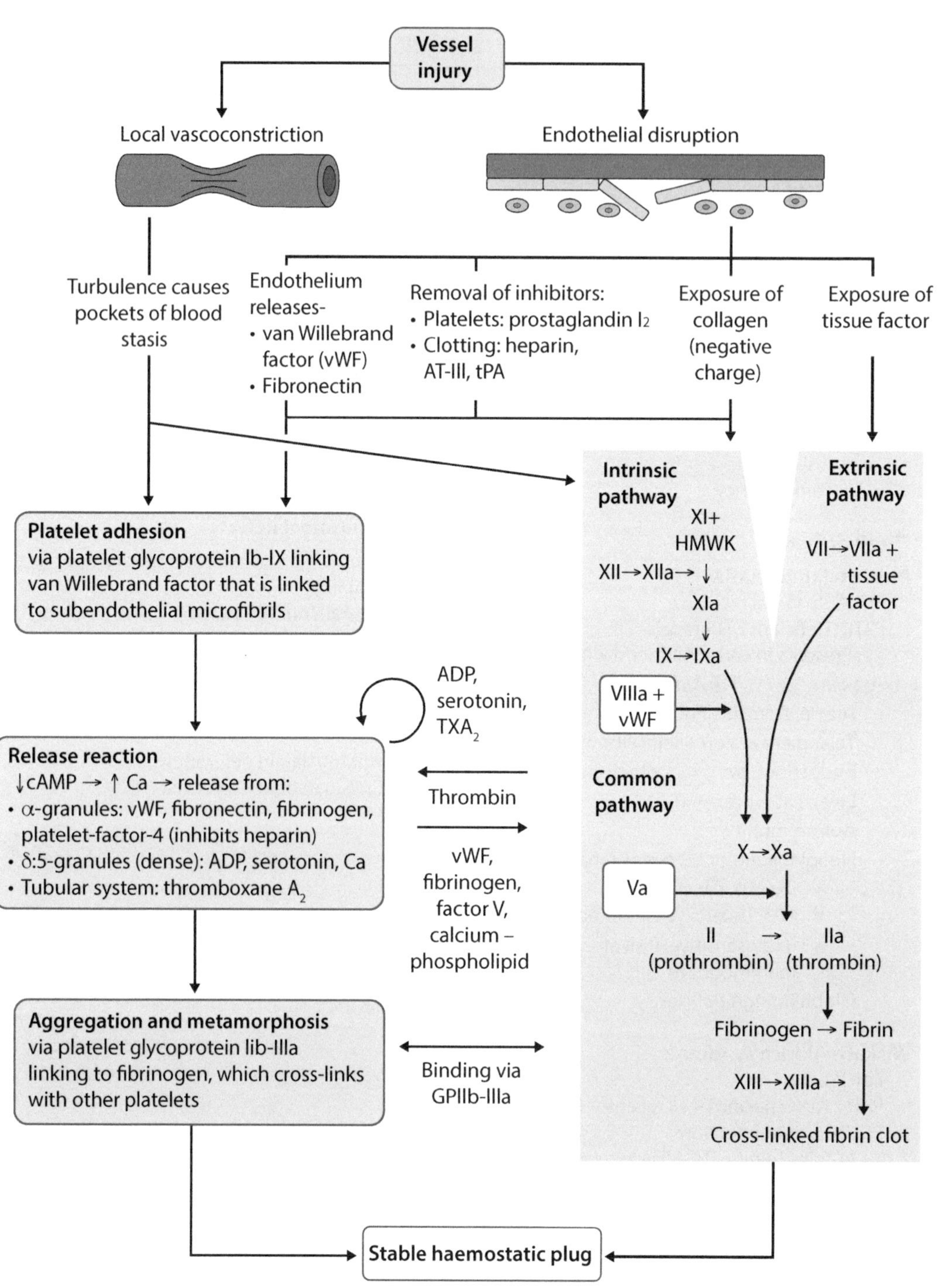

HAEMOSTASIS CONTROL

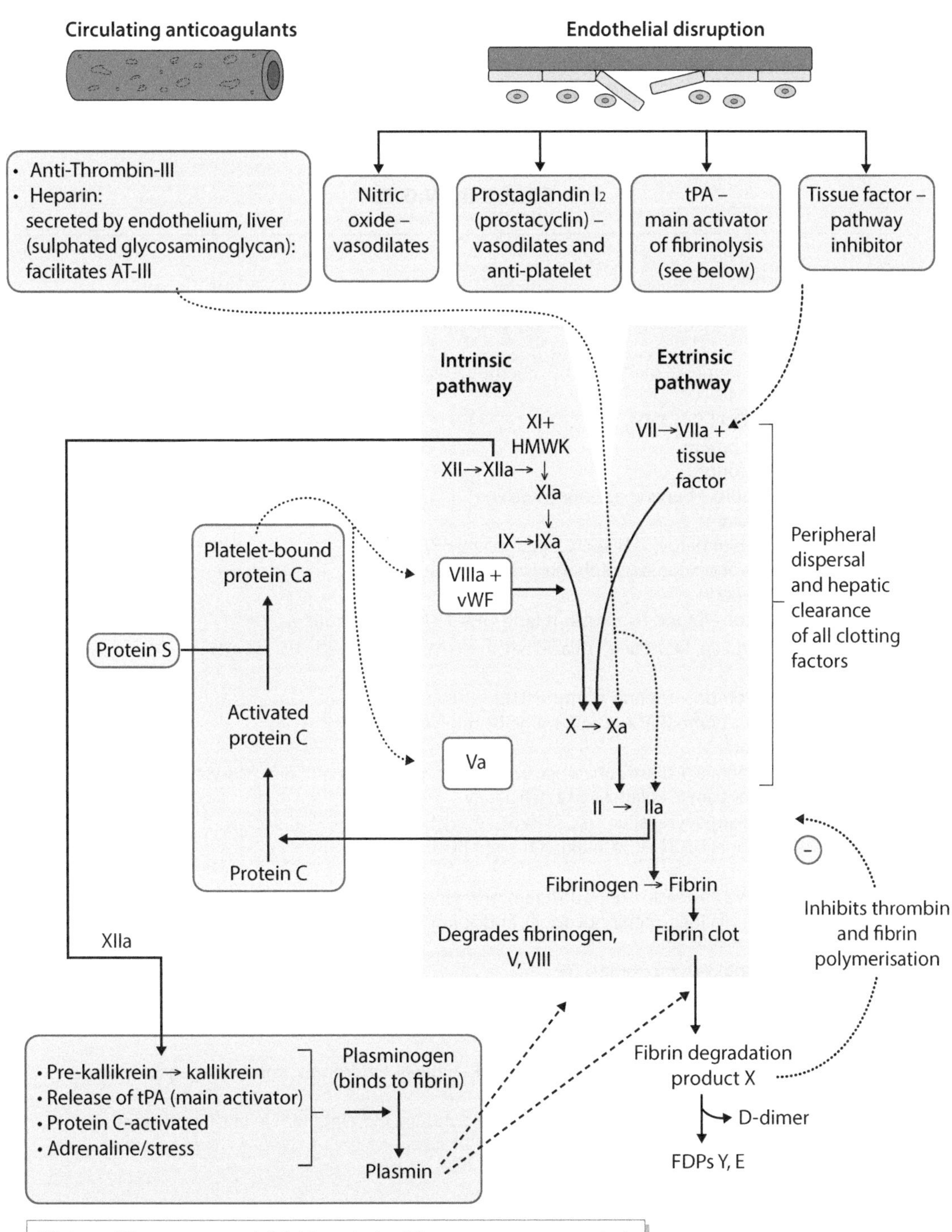

All dotted lines represent inhibition; dashed lines represent proteolysis

PLATELET DISORDERS

Causes

Platelet dysfunction may be caused by **thrombocytopenia or impaired platelet function**
Thrombocytopenia may be caused by:

- Spleen overactivity: Hypersplenism
- Peripheral destruction (immune) or consumption (non-immune)
- Bone marrow hypoproduction: Megakaryocyte failure

S.T.A.B.B.I.N.G.S.

Spleen: Hypersplenism
- PATH: Phagocytes remove platelets, and large spleen sequesters 60–90% platelets (normal = 30%)
- Causes: CML, portal hypertension, CCF (all cause pancytopenia)

Toxins
- PATH: Most are immune-mediated, but chemotherapy and alcohol have bone marrow suppressant effects
- Causes: **V.A.N.QU.I.S.H.E.D².**
  - **V**alproate
  - **A**lcohol
  - **N**euro – benzodiazepines, cocaine
  - **QU**inine
  - **I**nflammatory – NSAIDs inhibit platelet function
  - **S**ulphonylureas, sulphonamides (+ penicillins)
  - **H**eparin
  - **E**xtra – blood transfusions (anti-HPA-1a in multiparous women)
  - **D**igoxin, **D**iuretics – thiazides

Autoimmune
- 1°: Immune thrombocytopenic purpura (ITP)
- 2°: SLE, Evan syndrome (ITP + autoimmune haemolytic anaemia)

Bone marrow failure
- Normocytic anaemia: Aplastic anaemia, bone marrow replacement, diet (starvation)
- Megaloblastic anaemia: Folate or B12 deficiency
- Selective megakaryocyte failure, e.g. Wiskott–Aldrich syndrome, HIV, alcohol

Blood vessel damage: DIC, TTP, vasculitis, fat embolism

Infection:
- Virus: HIV, EBV, VZV, measles; dengue haemorrhagic fever
- Other: Septicaemia (esp. meningococcal), endocarditis, rickettsia, malaria

Neoplasia
- CLL (B-cell), Hodgkin lymphoma – ITP
- Myeloproliferative disease; paraproteinaemia, esp. Waldenström – causes impaired platelet function

Genetic
- Thrombocytopenia: Wiskott–Aldrich or Chediak–Higashi syndromes: Impaired megakaryocyte production
- Impaired function: von Willebrand disease; glycoprotein, platelet granule or thromboxane deficiency

Systemic
- Thrombocytopenia: Dilution, e.g. overhydration
- Impaired function: Uraemia, liver failure
- Artefactual: Clotted blood or anti-platelet antibodies

PC

General: Superficial: Skin purpura or petechiae
Mucous membranes: Epistaxis, gums, GIT, menorrhagia, haematuria
Deep: Intracerebral haemorrhage

ITP: Childhood: Acute, mild, self-limiting
Adult: Chronic, severe, relapsing–remitting

Bloods:

FBC, film, platelet size:

- Large platelets: ITP, myeloproliferative disease, grey platelet syn. (a-granule deficiency)
- Small platelets: CRF

Auto-antibodies:

- Anti-glycoprotein IIb-IIIa (IgG, M): ITP; anti-P1^{A1}: Post-transfusion purpura
- ANA
- Direct Coombs' test (Evans syndrome)

DIC tests: Film showing schistocytes, clotting, FDPs, D-dimers, circulating fibrin monomer

Micro: HIV, EBV serology

Radiol: Abdominal USS – splenomegaly

Special:

Bone marrow – fine-needle aspirate and biopsy:

- Megakaryocyte number ↓: Bone marrow failure
- Megakaryocyte number ↑: Peripheral destruction

Aggregation times impaired with:

- Adrenaline, ADP: d-granule or COX-deficiency (genetic or aspirin), ET
- Ristocetin: von Willebrand disease

Other platelet studies:

- Granule contents (↓ in storage pool diseases, myeloproliferative disease)
- Glycoprotein quantification, arachidonic acid metabolism, Ca flux studies

Rx

ITP

Supportive: Platelet transfusion (half-life = hours)
Severe: Prednisolone or IVIg
Chronic:
Immunosuppression: Steroids, azathioprine, cyclophosphamide, rituximab
Other drugs: Danazol, colchicine, IFN-a, high-dose vit. C
Splenectomy: If platelet count $<30 \times 10^9$/l, or intolerant of steroids, or young

PURPURA

Def

Purpura = pink-red macules <1 cm; petechiae = very fine macules
Non-blanching – due to intradermal bleeding

PC

The type of tissues in which bleeding occurs suggests the underlying cause:

Vascular: Petechiae, purpura, bruises
Platelets:
Petechiae, purpura, bruises
Mucous membrane bleeds: Epistaxis, gums, GIT, menorrhagia, urine
Deep: Intracerebral
Clotting:
Petechiae, purpura, bruises
Mucous membrane bleeds
Deep: Intracerebral, haemarthroses, subcutaneous (nerve palsies), teeth, tongue, trauma, bowel

Ix

Vascular:
FBC, film and clotting times are normal
Tourniquet Hess test: Blood pressure cuff inflated for 5 min; count petechiae within 2.5 cm diameter circle measured 4 cm below cubital fossa; if >20 petechiae = capillary fragility ↑
Platelets:
FBC: Platelets ↓ or normal:
- Platelet count↓: Film, bone marrow, autoAbs, FDP
- Platelet count normal: Platelet function times, incl. Duke method – small nick on the earlobe with a lancet; bleeding should stop after 2 min

Clotting:
Clotting times ↑
Dilution studies: Does normal serum correct?
Clotting factor, vWF assays; NB: Bleeding time normal

Causes

Vascular defect

V.I.G.I.L².A.N.T.

Vitamin C deficiency – scurvy:
PATH: Vit. C is required for collagen cross-linking
O/E: Perifollicular petechiae
Gum bleeding
Infection: Due to immune complexes:
Meningococcaemia
Rickettsia
Viruses: Measles, dengue haemorrhagic fever (all also associated with low platelet count)
Genetic:
Collagen disease: ED-IV, OI, Marfan
Pseudoxanthoma elasticum (AD/AR)
Hereditary haemorrhagic telangiectasia (AD): Endoglin mutation
Injury:
Mechanical
Thrombotic thrombocytopenic purpura
Leg purpura: Chronic venous stasis or venous hypertension:
DVT
Excessive standing
Right-sided heart failure
Excessive coughing or vomiting
Limiting, self:
Senile purpura
Painful bruising syndrome:
Epi: Women of child-bearing age
PC: Prodromal tingling under skin; bruising of limbs, trunk
Autoimmune:
Vasculitis: Henoch–Schonlein purpura, polyarteritis nodosa (men)
SLE, rheumatoid arthritis
Cryoglobulinaemia
Neoplasia: Amyloid, esp. facial purpura from AL amyloid
(Ix: Serum and urine electrophoresis)
Toxins:
Steroid
Anticoagulant therapy

Coagulopathy

V.I.G.I.L^2.A^2.N.T^3.

Vitamin K deficiency:
PATH: Vit. K epoxide reductase causes g-carboxylation of glutamate residue on clotting factors II, VII, IX, X → enables Ca binding → adsorption onto phospholipid surfaces
Malnutrition
Malabsorption – coeliac, chronic pancreatitis
Antibiotics
Haemorrhagic disease of newborn
Infection, due to DIC
Genetic:
Haemophilias: VIII C (A), IX (B), XI, VII – mild; XIII – severe
Von Willebrand disease, type 3
Injury due to DIC
Liver: Obstructive jaundice leads to ↓ vit. K absorption
Liver: Hepatocellular dysfunction due to ↓ clotting factor synthesis, ↓ tPA detoxification and DIC
Acute pancreatitis: Pancreatic proteases degrade clotting factors
PC: Bruising in flanks and umbilicus (Cullen sign)
Autoimmune: Circulating VIII inhibitors – complication of haemophilia
Neoplasia:
Paraproteinaemia; amyloid: Due to factor X and fibrinogen deficiency
Acute myeloid leukaemia M3
Metastatic carcinoma – hyperplasminaemia
Toxins:
Anticoagulants: Heparin, warfarin
Other: Asparaginase, isoniazid (blocks XIII activity)
Transfusion, massive: Dilutional effect
Thrombolysis:
tPA
Hyperplasminaemia: 1° or 2° to congenital cyanotic heart disease

Platelet defect (p. 480)

S.T.A.B.B.I.N.G.S.

All cause **thrombocytopenia**, except where indicated as causing **impaired platelet function**

Spleen: Hypersplenism, due to CML, portal hypertension, CCF
Toxins:

V.A.N.QUI.S.HE.D.

Valproate
Alcohol
Neuro – benzodiazepines, cocaine
QUInine; Inflammatory – indomethacin, gold
Sulphonylureas, sulphonamides (+ penicillins)
HEparin; Extra – blood transfusions (anti-P1^{A1})
Digoxin, Diuretics – thiazides + impaired function (NSAIDs)

Autoimmune:
1°: Immune thrombocytopenic purpura (ITP)
2°: SLE, Evans syndrome (ITP + haemolysis)
Bone marrow failure:
Normocytic anaemia:
- Aplastic anaemia
- Bone marrow replacement
- Diet (starvation)

Megaloblastic anaemia: Folate or B12 deficiency
Selective megakaryocyte failure, e.g. HIV, alcohol
Blood vessel damage: DIC, TTP, vasculitis, fat embolism
Infection:
Viruses: HIV; EBV, VZV
Other: Septicaemia, endocarditis; malaria
Neoplasia:
CLL (B cell), Hodgkin lymphoma: ITP
Myeloproliferative disease
Impaired function: Paraproteinaemia, esp. Waldenström (hyperviscosity syndrome)
Genetic:
Thrombocytopenia: Wiskott–Aldrich or Chediak–Higashi syndromes
Impaired function: von Willebrand disease; glycoprotein, granule, TXA2 deficiency
Systemic:
Thrombocytopenia: Dilution, e.g. overhydration
Impaired function: Uraemia, liver failure
Artefactual:
- Clotted blood
- Anti-platelet antibodies

THROMBOSIS

Prothrombotic states are summarized by Virchow's triad of pathological processes:

1. Endothelial injury: Arterial thrombosis
2. Stasis: Venous or cardiac thrombosis
3. Hypercoagulability: Venous > arterial thrombosis

Each pathology tends to be associated with thrombosis in particular parts of the circulation, as shown. However, all 3 processes are probably involved at each instance of thrombosis, e.g. an atherosclerotic plaque may rupture causing endothelial injury, exposure of procoagulants and turbulence with pockets of stasis.

Arterial thrombosis

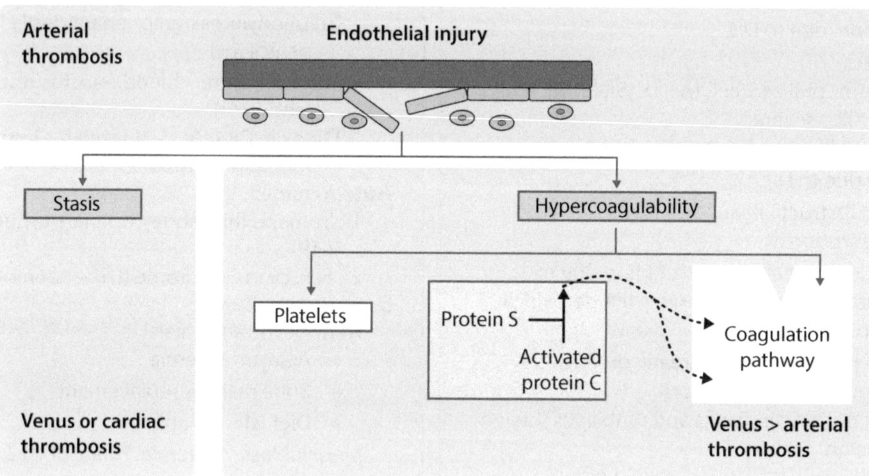

Causes

Endothelial injury

$(A.D.V.I.S.E.)^2$ $(O.R.)^2$ $H.E.P^3.A.R.I^2.N.I.S^2.E.$

Atherosclerosis: Hypertension, DM, cholesterol, smoking
Arteriosclerosis: Hypertension, DM
Dissection: Hypertension, connective tissue mutation – Ehlers–Danlos, Marfan
Dysplasia: Fibromuscular
Vasculitis:
* Autoimmune (e.g. polyarteritis nodosa, giant-cell arteritis, SLE)
* Infection (e.g. TB, syphilis, *Pneumococcus*, *Chlamydia*)

Valvulitis: Endocarditis, aortic stenosis
Injury: Trauma, catheterisation (angioplasty), indwelling central line
Injury: Radiation
Spasm: Migraine, variant angina
Sarcoidosis
External compression, e.g. tumour, cervical rib
Embolism: Should be considered as a mechanism in any case of arterial ischaemia

Stasis

Obesity
Operation, esp. hip or other orthopaedic, or for cancer
Recumbency, e.g. long-haul flight, peripartum, debilitated
Right-sided heart failure, or other venous hypertension, incl. varicose veins

Hypercoagulability

Hereditary:
- Prothrombin mutation
- Factor V Leiden mutation (activated protein C resistance); protein S or C deficiency; anti-thrombin-III deficiency
- Fibrinolysis defect: Fibrinogen/plasminogen mutation; tPA ↓/tPA inhibitor ↑
- Homocystinuria

Endocrine:
- Oestrogens:
  - Pregnancy: Phlegmasia alba dolens (3rd trimester/puerperium)
  - OCP: ↑ vit. K-dependent CFs, VIII; ↓ AT-III, tPA
  - HRT: Although ↓ LDL/HDL and hence ↓ IHD
- Androgens: Anabolic steroids, danazol (anti-oestrogen), oral contraceptive pill (anti-androgen)
- Diabetes mellitus, esp. due to HHS

Polycythaemia; **P**araproteinaemia; **P**NH (paroxysmal nocturnal haemoglobinuria):
- Polycythaemia, including myeloproliferative disease (hyperviscosity)
- Paraproteinaemia (hyperviscosity)
- Other haematological: PNH, sickle cell disease, Fe deficiency, DIC, TTP

Autoimmune:
- Antiphospholipid syndrome (primary or associated with SLE)
- Vasculitis: Behçet syndrome, PAN, granulomatosis with polyangiitis, Sjögren syndrome
- Ulcerative colitis + sarcoidosis

Renal:
- Nephrosis: Due to glomerular loss of AT-III
- Dehydration

Injury; **I**nfarction: Due to increased sympathetic response and CRP elevation

Neoplasia:
- Adenocarcinoma (mucin/protease-secreting), e.g. pancreas, bronchus, breast, bowel
  - PC: 'Trousseau phenomenon' = migratory thrombophlebitis
- Acute leukaemia (AML or ALL)
- Local:
  - Portal vein thrombosis, secondary to carcinoma of pancreas, liver, adrenal
  - Cerebral vein thrombosis, secondary to head–neck squamous cell carcinoma

Infection
- Systemic: Endotoxinaemia (lipopolysaccharide), TB, chlamydia
- Local: Cellulitis (DVT); otitis media, sinusitis (cerebral vein thrombosis)

Smoking; **S**enility (increasing age)

Exogenous: Chemotherapy (L-asparaginase, methotrexate); steroids; COX-2 inhibitors

DISSEMINATED INTRAVASCULAR COAGULATION (DIC)

Def

Run-away control of haemostasis

Triggered by: Extensive endothelial disruption, e.g. infection, trauma, AVM
Procoagulant release, e.g. neoplasia, placental disruption

Results in consumption, and consequently depletion, of platelets and clotting factors

Causes

Make sure you **N.O.T.I.C.E.** *it!!*

6th March	
Platelets	148
PT	13
APTT	40

7th March	
Platelets	80
PT	19
APTT	55

8th March	
Platelets	25
PT	26
APTT	84

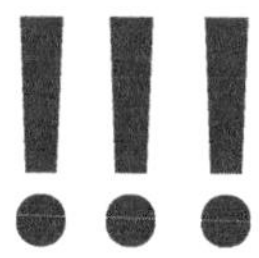

Neoplasia:
- Mucin-secreting adenocarcinoma: Pancreas, gastric, breast, bronchus
- AML: Acute promyelocytic leukaemia – M3

Obstetric:
- Abortion: Septic, missed, retained products of conception
- Peri-partum: Eclampsia; placental abruption; amniotic fluid embolism

Trauma:
- Crush injury, surgery, burns
- Hyperthermia or hypothermia
- Hypoxia (acute)

Infection:
- Bacterial: Meningococcaemia, coliforms (endotoxin), *Clostridium perfringens*, leptospirosis
- Viral: Purpura fulminans, esp. CMV, VZV, hepatitis
- Malaria: *Plasmodium falciparum* – large procoagulant release

Congenital: AVM, e.g. Kasabach–Merritt syndrome – giant haemangioma in infants

Extra:
- Acute anaphylaxis
- Blood transfusion reaction
- Liver failure

Prog

Large spectrum of severity, including asymptomatic cases
50% mortality rate (because of associated condition)

PATH

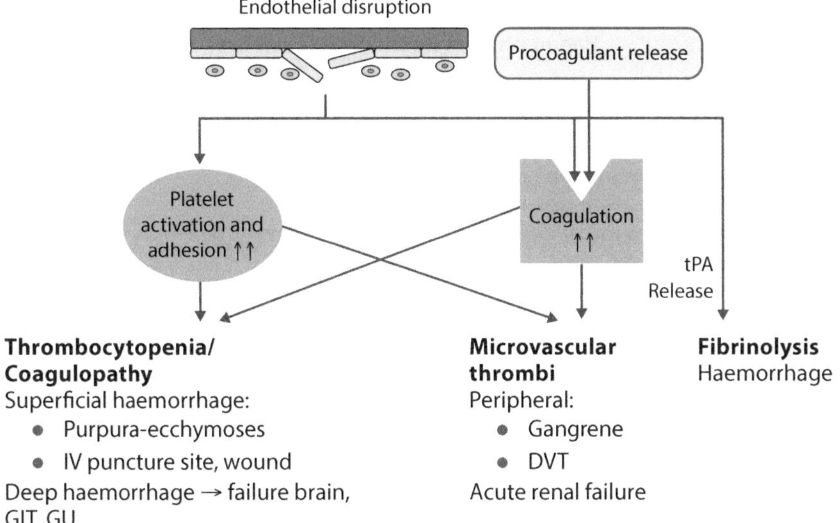

Thrombocytopenia/ Coagulopathy
Superficial haemorrhage:
- Purpura-ecchymoses
- IV puncture site, wound

Deep haemorrhage → failure brain, GIT, GU

Microvascular thrombi
Peripheral:
- Gangrene
- DVT

Acute renal failure

Fibrinolysis
Haemorrhage

Ix

Platelets ↓
Clotting: APTT ↑, PT ↑, TT ↑, fibrinogen ↓
NB: Clotting times may be normal in DIC, due to presence of activated clotting factors!

Film: Schistocytes, due to microangiopathic haemolytic anaemia (MAHA)
AT-III ↓

Fibrin degradation products, e.g. d-dimer ↑

Rx

Underlying condition +
Blood products
- Fresh frozen plasma (clotting factors)
- Platelet transfusion
- Cryoprecipitate (fibrinogen)
- Red blood cells

HAEMOPHILIA

Haemophilia A (factor VIII deficiency)

Inc: 1/10,000 males
Age: Presents in 1st year, e.g. cephalhaematoma, circumcision, crawling (bruising)
Sex: Males (X-linked), but female carriers may bleed after surgery/trauma due to 'lyonisation', i.e. if normal X-chromosome is disproportionately inactivated
Aet: Hereditary (75%): X-linked disease – numerous mutations on Xq
Sporadic (25%), i.e. new mutation or latent carriership for several generations
↓ Synthesis of VIII from liver, spleen, kidney + lymphoid tissue
Anti-VIII: C antibodies in 20%

PC

S^2.T^2.A.I.N^2.S.

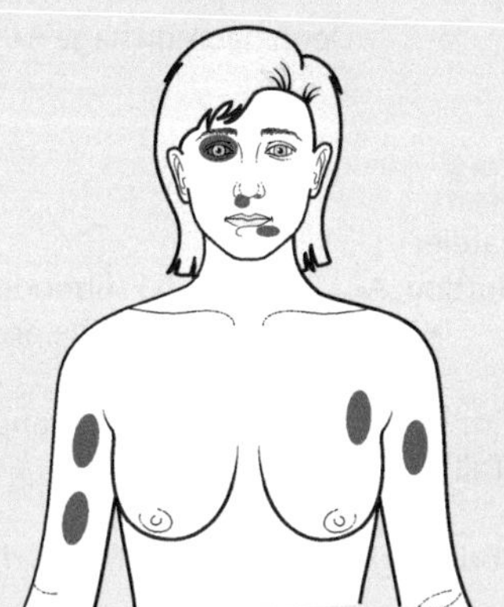

Skin – **S**ubcutaneous tissue: Bruising
Teeth (dental extraction)/**T**ongue (haematoma → stridor)
Arthritis:
- Acute haemarthroses, esp. hip, knee, ankle
- Osteoarthritis: Due to recurrent haemarthroses → ankylosis + muscle atrophy
- Bony pseudotumours/cysts: Due to subperiosteal bleeding → pathological fractures

Intestine/urinary haemorrhage:
- GIT haemorrhage: Due to coagulopathy/NSAIDs for arthritis/hepatitis C
- GU haemorrhage/ureteric colic, papillary necrosis due to antifibrinolytic use

Neurological:
- CVA (bleed): Commonest cause of death
- Femoral nerve compression – 2° to retroperitoneal-psoas sheath haematoma
- Compartment syndrome due to muscle/fascial haemorrhage

Nose: Epistaxis
Side-effects of Rx:
- Viral infections: Transfusions pre-1990s (HIV), pre-2000 (HCV)
- Factor VIII inhibitor in 20% of pts.
- Thrombosis, due to antifibrinolytics, DDAVP, prothrombin complex

Severity depends on % VIII activity:
- 20–5% – mild bleeding post-op. or trauma
- 5–1% – infrequent spontaneous bleeding
- <1% – frequent, severe spontaneous bleeds

Clotting times

APTT: ↑

If it normalizes with 50:50 mix with normal plasma suggests factor deficiency

If it does not normalize with 50:50 VIII-deficient plasma suggests an inhibitor

Immune assay of individual factors: VIII, IX, vWF

PT: Normal

TT: Normal

Genetic screening

Methods: RFLP; DNA hybridisation; PCR

Used to amplify chorionic villus sampled blood (10–12 weeks) or umbilical vein (18–20 weeks)

Conservative

Avoidance: Contact sports, unnecessary dental Rx; NSAIDs; IM injections

Vaccines: Hep B; regular LFTs

Haemarthrosis: Rest, splint, elevate; physiotherapy: prevents joint fibrosis

Factor VIII concentrate

Source: FFP, cryoprecipitate; immunoaffinity (adsorbed + eluted onto monoclonal Abs); recombinant DNA

Indications: Used to raise VIII activity to >30% activity in acute haemorrhage, or as prophylaxis, e.g. before sports or dental procedures

☠ Inhibitors, i.e. Anti VIII IgG

Rx:
- High-dose VIII; only if low Ig titre; porcine VIII
- Prothrombin complex concentrates = trace quantities of activated clotting factors
- Immunosuppression; immunodepletion

Autoimmune haemolytic anaemia – due to anti-A and -B in intermediate-purity concentrates

Allergy

DDAVP (desmopressin = ADH) – IVI or nasal snuff:

Releases VIII + vWF from endothelium; stabilizes VIII in plasma

Indications: Acute haemorrhage in mild disease, as endothelium contains only limited stores

☠: Thrombosis esp. in elderly; hyponatraemia

Antifibrinolytics – tranexamic acid or s-aminocaproic acid (IV, PO, mouth wash):

Inhibits plasmin formation by tPA (which is also released from endothelium by DDAVP!)

Indications: Acute haemorrhage or prophylaxis; as an adjunct to DDAVP

Haemophilia B (factor IX deficiency) or 'Xmas disease'

Epi: 1/3 as common as haemophilia A, but also X- linked

PC: As for haemophilia A

Ix: Immune assay reveals IX deficiency; otherwise as for haemophilia A

Rx: Factor IX concentrate – longer half-life than VIII (less frequent infusions); DDAVP is ineffective!

Factor XI deficiency

Mild bleeding disorder, tends to occur in Ashkenazi Jews, and is autosomal recessive

Factor XIII deficiency

Severe bleeding disorder with infertility and abortions. Rare and autosomal recessive

Ix: Urea-dissolution test (XIII assay)

BLOOD TRANSFUSION COMPLICATIONS

Incidence

Any reaction = 2%; death = 2/100,000

Early

Haemolytic reaction – Immediate (1/12,000 transfusions)

Causes:

Blood-group mismatch:
ABO – intravascular haemolysis: IgG, IgM, classical complement pathway
RhD, Kell – extravascular haemolysis: IgG, C3b, mononuclear phagocytic system
Mechanical: faulty blood warmer; pumps, tubes

PC: General: Fever, shock, acute renal failure
GIT symptoms: N+V, diarrhoea, abdominal–back pain
Chest symptoms: Chest pain, SOB, wheeze
Skin symptoms: Pruritus, jaundiced (haemolysis)
Ix: Sample donor and recipient blood: Serology, cross-match, direct Coombs' test, blood culture
Haemolysis tests: Unconjugated BR, AST, LDH; reticulocytes, α2-haptoglobin
Intravascular haemolysis: Haemoglobinuria, haemosiderinuria
Complications: Screen for DIC (FDPs and D-dimers) and MAHA (film: schistocytes)
Rx: Fluids, blood, FFP
Hydrocortisone, chlorpheniramine
'Renal' dopamine, adrenaline, haemodialysis

Immune reactions – Non-haemolytic

Non-haemolytic febrile transfusion reaction (NHFTR) (1/50 transfusions)
PATH: Anamnestic response to HLA-I and -II on WBCs, and platelets (HLA-I only), due to previous transfusion or pregnancies
PC: Fever at 30 min to 2 h; flushing; tachycardia
Prophylaxis: WBC-depleted products ('buffy-coat depleted'); in-line filters

Allergy – types (1/50 transfusions)
Atopy: Plasma proteins of donor, e.g. Igs, react in atopic pt. → mild urticaria (continue transfusion)
IgA deficiency: Reaction against donor IgA → anaphylactic shock
Inadvertent donor antigen, e.g. C4-albumin, penicillin, ethylene oxide

Pulmonary leucagglutinin reaction (1/5000 transfusions)
PATH: Donor or recipient has high anti-granulocyte Ab titre due to past transfusion or multiparity
PC: Non-cardiogenic pulmonary oedema due to agglutination and leucostasis in lungs
Neutropenia (cytotoxicity)
Shock (complement-driven vasodilation)

Overload – fluid: Presents as features of congestive cardiac failure

+ delivery problems: Thrombophlebitis; air embolism
+ massive transfusion complications:

- Hypothermia
- Ion toxicity (transfused citrate → Ca ↓; K ↑; acid–base disturbance)
- Clotting factor and platelet depletion/DIC (give platelets and FFPs after 4 units)

Late

Haemolytic reaction – Delayed (1/1000 transfusions)

Causes

Due to delayed, 2° immune response to RBC alloantigen other than those routinely screened for
Not detected pre-transfusion by cross-matching because of low recipient antibody levels
Risk increased by previous transfusions or in multiparous women
Extravascular haemolysis

PC: Occurs 1 day–2 weeks after transfusion
Hb fails to rise; jaundice (but may be life-threatening)
Ix: Direct Coombs' test
Indirect Coombs' test: Ab screen against wide RBC Ag assay; quantify by no. of units lysed
Type donor blood given

Immune reactions – Non-haemolytic

Alloantigen sensitisation = Abs generated to RBC or HLA antigens, without reaction; predisposes to future transfusion reactions, including haemolytic disease of the newborn
Post-transfusion purpura

Causes

Where recipient lacks platelet antigen HPA-1a (GPIIIa receptor), transfusion leads to development of anti-platelet antibodies to both donor and self platelets
2% population lack HPA-1A; Abs more likely in multiparous women

PC: Thrombocytopenia at 7–10 days post-transfusion

GVHD or immunosuppression
Immunocompromised patients may develop GVHD by donor T-cell activity
Lymphopenia may occur in post-surgery transfusion

Infection

Bacteria: Syphilis, *Salmonella*, *Brucella*
Viruses: Hepatitis B, C, E, G; HTLV-I; HIV; CMV (significant if recipient immunocompromised)
Parasites: Malaria, toxoplasmosis, microfilariasis
Other: Prion

Overload – Iron

At-risk groups = recurrent transfusions:
Congenital: Thalassaemia major or intermedia; pure red-cell aplasia (Diamond–Blackfan syndrome)
Acquired: Aplastic anaemia; myelodysplasia, myelofibrosis
Complications (as for 1° haemochromatosis – see p. 160

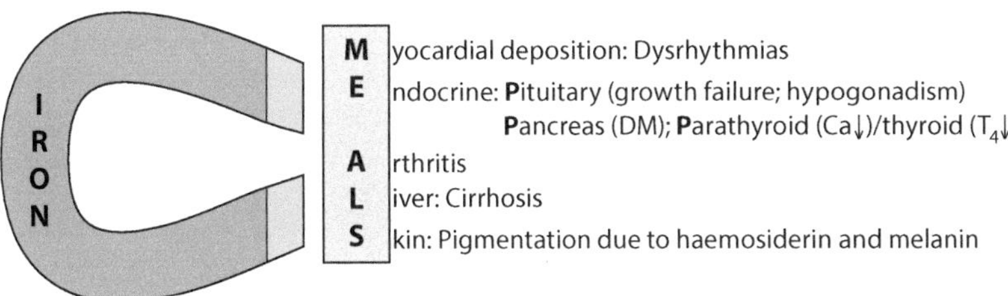

IRON
M yocardial deposition: Dysrhythmias
E ndocrine: **P**ituitary (growth failure; hypogonadism)
Pancreas (DM); **P**arathyroid (Ca↓)/thyroid (T_4↓)
A rthritis
L iver: Cirrhosis
S kin: Pigmentation due to haemosiderin and melanin

ABBREVIATONS

1,25-DHCC	1,25-dihydroxycholecalciferol
17-KS	17-ketosteroids
2,3-DPG	2,3-diphosphoglycerate
25-HCC	25-hydroxycholecalciferol
2-D	two-dimensional
3-D	three-dimensional
3TC	lamivudine
5-HIAA	5-hydroxyindoleacetic acid
5-HT	serotonin (5-hydroxytryptamine)
5-HT3	type 3 serotonin receptor
5-HTP	5-hydroxytryptophan
11BHSD	11 β-hydroxysteroid dehydrogenase
AA	amino acid(s)
AAA	abdominal aortic aneurysm
AAFB	alcohol- and acid-fast bacilli
Ab	antibody
ABG	arterial bypass graft, arterial blood gases
ABP	arterial blood pressure
ABPA	allergic bronchopulmonary aspergillosis
ABVD	doxorubicin (Adriamycin), bleomycin, vinblastine and dacarbazine
AcAc	acetoacetate
AcCoA	acetyl coenzyme A
ACE	angiotensin-converting enzyme
ACEI	ACE inhibitor
Ach	acetylcholine
AchR	acetylcholine receptor
ACS	acute coronary syndrome
ACTH	adrenocorticotrophic hormone
AD	autosomal dominant
ADEM	acute disseminated encephalomyelitis
ADH	antidiuretic hormone (= AVP)
ADHD	attention deficit hyperactivity disorder
ADP	adenosine diphosphate
AE	air entry or adverse effects
AED	anti-epileptic drug
AF	atrial fibrillation
AFB	acid-fast bacilli
AFP	α-fetoprotein
Ag	antigen
AICA	anterior inferior cerebellar artery
AIDP	acute inflammatory demyelinating polyneuropathy
AIDS	acquired immunodeficiency syndrome
AIHA	autoimmune haemolytic anaemia
A-II	angiotensin-II receptor
AION	anterior ischaemic optic neuropathy
$Al(OH)_3$	aluminium hydroxide
AKI	acute kidney injury
ALA	aminolaevulinic acid
Alb	albumin
Alk. Phos.	alkaline phosphatase
ALL	acute lymphoblastic leukaemia
ALP	alkaline phosphatase
α_1-AT	α_1-antitrypsin
ALS	amyotrophic lateral sclerosis
ALT	alanine aminotransferase (transaminase)
AMA	antimitochondrial antibody
AM(S)AN	acute motor (and sensory) axonal neuropathy
AML	acute myeloid leukaemia
AMML	acute myelomonocytic leukaemia
ANA	antinuclear antibodies
ANCA	antineutrophil cytoplasmic antibodies
Ank. Spond.	ankylosing spondylitis
ANP	atrial natriuretic peptide
Anti-LKM	antibodies to liver–kidney microsomes
AP	anteroposterior, abdominoperineal
APB	apex beat
APC	adenomatous polyposis coli
APKD	adult polycystic kidney disease
APSAC	anisoylated plasminogen streptokinase activator complex
APTT	activated partial thromboplastin time
APUD	amine precursor uptake and decarboxylation
AR	aortic regurgitation, autosomal recessive
ARAS	ascending reticular activating system
ARC	AIDS-related complex
ARDS	adult respiratory distress syndrome
AS	aortic stenosis
ASD	atrial septal defect
ASH	asymmetric septal hypertrophy
ASIS	anterior superior iliac spine
ASO	anti-streptolysin O
AST	aspartate aminotransferase (transaminase)
AT	antitrypsin
AT-III	anti-thrombin III
ATN	acute tubular necrosis
ATP	adenosine triphosphate
AV	aortic valve, arteriovenous, atrioventricular
A-V	atrioventricular

AVM	arteriovenous malformation
AVN	atrioventricular node
AVNRE	atrioventricular nodal re-entry (tachycardia)
AVP	arginine vasopressin (= ADH)
AVRE	atrioventricular re-entry (tachycardia)
AVRT	atrioventricular re-entry tachycardia
AXR	abdominal X-ray
Aza/AZA	azathioprine
AZT	azidothymidine (zidovudine)
Ba	barium
BAL	bronchoalveolar lavage
BCG	bacille Calmette-Guérin
β-B	beta-blockers
β-HCG	β-human chorionic gonadotrophin
BHB	β-hydroxybutyrate
BHC	benzene hexachloride
BHL	bihilar lymphadenopathy
BJP	Bence Jones protein
blk	block
BM	bone marrow or name of manufacturer of 'BM stick'
BMPR	bone morphogenetic protein receptor
BNH	bilateral nodular hyperplasia
BO	bowel opening
BP	blood pressure
bpm	beats per minute
BPPV	benign paroxysmal positional vertigo
BR	bilirubin
BSE	bovine spongiform encephalopathy
Bx	biopsy
BXO	balanitis xerotica obliterans
ca./Ca.	carcinoma
Ca/Ca^{2+}	calcium
CABG	coronary artery bypass graft
$CaCO_3$	calcium carbonate
CADASIL	cerebral autosomal dominant arteriopathy with subcortical infarcts and leucoencephalopathy
CAG	cytosine-adenine-guanine
CAH	congenital adrenal hyperplasia, chronic autoimmune hepatitis
cAMP	cyclic adenosine monophosphate
c-ANCA	cytoplasmic anti-neutrophil cytoplasmic antibodies
CAPD	chronic ambulatory peritoneal dialysis
CBD	corticobasal degeneration
CCF	congestive cardiac failure
CCHD	cyanotic congenital heart disease
CCK	cholecystokinin
CCl_4	carbon tetrachloride
CCU	coronary care unit
CD	cluster differentiation antigen
CEA	carcinoembryonic antigen
Cef	cefuroxime
CF	cystic fibrosis, clotting factor
CFA	cryptogenic fibrosing alveolitis
CFTR	cystic fibrosis transmembrane regulator
CGD	chronic granulomatous disease
cGMP	cyclic guanosine monophosphate
C_H50	complement functional assay
CHOP	cyclophosphamide, doxorubicin (hydroxydaunorubicin), vincristine (Oncovin) and prednisolone
Chr	chromosome
CI	contraindication
CIDP	chronic inflammatory demyelinating polyneuropathy
CJD	Creutzfeldt–Jakob disease
CK	creatine kinase
CKD	chronic kidney disease
Cl^-	chloride
CLL	chronic lymphocytic leukaemia
CMC	carpometacarpal
CMI	cell-mediated immunity
CML	chronic myeloid leukaemia
CMML	chronic myelomonocytic leukaemia
CMT	Charcot–Marie–Tooth (disease)
CMV	cytomegalovirus
CMZ	carbamazepine
CNS	central nervous system
CO	cardiac output, carbon monoxide
CO_2	carbon dioxide
CO_3	carbonate
CoA	coenzyme A
COMT	catechol-*O*-methyltransferase
COPD	chronic obstructive pulmonary disease
COX	cyclooxygenase
CPAP	continuous positive airway pressure
CPH	chronic persistent hepatitis
CPR	cardiopulmonary resuscitation
CPT	carnitine palmitoyltransferase
Cr	chromium, or creatinine
CRAG	cryptococcal antigen
CREST	calcinosis, Raynaud, oesophageal and gut dysmotility, sclerodactyly, and telangiectasia
CRH	corticotrophin-releasing hormone
CRION	chronic relapsing inflammatory optic neuropathy
CRP	C-reactive protein
CS	Churg–Strauss (syndrome)

CSF	cerebrospinal fluid
CSM	carotid sinus massage
CSU	catheter-specimen urine
CT	computed tomography
CTZ	chemoreceptor trigger zone
Cu	copper
CVA	cerebrovascular accident
CVID	common variable immunodeficiency
CVP	central venous pressure
CVS	cardiovascular system
CXR	chest X-ray
Cyt	cytochrome
Δ	disorder, difference
D+V	diarrhoea and vomiting
DA_2	type 2 dopamine receptor
DAF	decay accelerating factor (CD55)
DAG	diacylglyceride
DBP	diastolic blood pressure
DC	direct current
DCC	deleted in colon cancer gene
DDAVP®	desmopressin (1-deamino-8-D-arginine vasopressin)
ddC	zalcitabine (dideoxycytidine)
DDD	dual-chamber pacemaker
ddI	didanosine (dideoxyinosine)
DEET	diethyltoluamide
def.	deficiency
DEXA	dual-energy X-ray absorptiometry
DH	drug history
DHEA	dehydroepiandrostenedione
DHF	dihydrofolate
DHFR	dihydrofolate reductase
DI	diabetes insipidus
DIC	disseminated intravascular coagulation
DIDMOAD	diabetes insipidus, diabetes mellitus, optic atrophy, deafness + bladder atony
DIP	distal interphalangeal
DKA	diabetic ketoacidosis
DM	diabetes mellitus, dermatomyositis
DMARD	disease-modifying anti-rheumatoid drug
DMD	Duchenne muscular dystrophy
DMSA	dimercaptosuccinic acid
DMT-1	divalent metal transporter
DNA	deoxyribonucleic acid
DNase	deoxyribonuclease
DOC	11-deoxycorticosterone
DOTS	directly observed therapy
DRPLA	dentatorubral-pallidoluysian atrophy
dsDNA	double-stranded DNA
dTMP	deoxythymidine monophosphate
DTPA	diethylenetriamine pentaacetic acid
dUMP	deoxyuridine monophosphate
DVT	deep vein thrombosis
DXM	dexamethasone
DZ	dizygotic
E2	oestradiol
EBV	Epstein–Barr virus
ECC	ecchondroma
ECG	electrocardiography
ECHO	echocardiography
ED	Ehlers–Danlos (syndrome)
EDTA	ethylenediamine tetraacetic acid
EEG	electroencephalography
EF	ejection fraction
EGPA	eosinophilic granulomatosis with polyangiitis
ELISA	enzyme-linked immunosorbant assay
EMD	electromechanical dissociation, also termed pulseless electrical activity (PEA)
EMG	electromyography
EMU	early-morning urine
ENA	extractable nuclear antigen
ENC	enchondroma
ENT	ear, nose and throat
EPO	erythroporetin
ER	endoplasmic reticulum
ERCP	endoscopic retrograde cholangiopancreatography
ESM	ejection systolic murmur
ESR	erythrocyte sedimentation rate
ET	endotracheal
ET	essential thrombocythaemia
ethinylE2	ethinyloestradiol
F6P	fructose-6-phosphate
FAP	familial amyloid polyneuropathies
FB	foreign body
FBC	full blood count
FBPase	fructose-1,2-biphosphatase
FDP	fibrin degradation products
Fe	iron
FEV_1	forced expiratory volume in 1 second
FFA	free fatty acids
FFP	fresh frozen plasma
FH	family history, familial hyperlipidaemia
FiO_2	fractional concentration of oxygen in inspired air
FNA	fine-needle aspiration
FO	faeco-oral
FSGS	focal segmental glomerulosclerosis

FSH	facioscapulohumeral (dystrophy), follicle-stimulating hormone
fT3	free triiodothyronine
fT4	free thyroxine
FTA	fluorescent treponemal assay
FVC	forced vital capacity
G&S	Group and Save
G6Pase	glucose 6-phosphatase
G6PD	G6P dehydrogenase
GBM	glomerular basement membrane
GBS	Guillain–Barré syndrome
GCA	giant-cell arteritis
GCS	Glasgow Coma Scale
G-CSF	granulocyte colony-stimulating factor
GFR	glomerular filtration rate
GGP	glucose-6-phosphate
GGT	γ-glutamyl transpeptidase
GH	growth hormone
GHRH	growth hormone-releasing hormone
GI	gastrointestinal
GIT	gastrointestinal tract
Glu	glucose, glutamate
GLUT	glucose transporter
Gly	glycine
GM-CSF	granulocyte-macrophage colony-stimulating factor
GN	glomerulonephritis
GnRH	gonadotrophin-releasing hormone
G-O	gastro-oesophageal
GOR	gastro-oesophageal reflux
GP	glycoprotein
GPA	granulomatosis with polyangiitis
GPI	glycosylphosphatidylinositol
GRA	glucocorticoid-remediable aldosteronism
GTN	glyceryl trinitrate
GTP	guanosine triphosphate
GU	genitourinary
GVHD	graft-versus-host disease
H^+	hydrogen ion (proton)
H_1	type 1 histamine receptor
H_2	hydrogen, type 2 histamine receptor
H_2O_2	hydrogen peroxide
H_2S	hydrogen sulphide
HAART	highly active anti-retroviral therapy
HACEK	*Haemophilus* spp., *Actinobacillus actinomycetemcomitans, Cardiobacterium hominis, Eikenella corrodens* and *Kingella kingae*
HAV	hepatitis A virus
HB	heart block

Hb	haemoglobin
HBV	hepatitis B virus
HCC	hepatocellular carcinoma
HCG	human chorionic gonadotrophin
HCl	hydrochloric acid
HCO_3^-	bicarbonate
HCV	hepatitis C virus
HDL	high-density lipoprotein
HDV	hepatitis D virus
Hep	hepatitis
HFPEP	heart failure with preserved ejection fraction
HFREF	heart failure with reduced ejection fraction
HGPRT	hypoxanthine-guanine phosphoribosyl transferase
HHT	hereditary haemorrhagic telangiectasia
HHV	human herpesvirus
HIV	human immunodeficiency virus
HLA	human leucocyte antigen
HMG CoA	3-hydroxy-3-methylglutaryl coenzyme A
HMMA	4-hydroxy-3-methoxymandelic acid (= VMA)
HMWK	high-molecular-weight kininogen
HNPCC	hereditary non-polyposis colon cancer
HOCM	hypertrophic obstructive cardiomyopathy
HONK	hyperosmolar non-ketoacidosis
HPA	human platelet antigen
hPL	human placental lactogen
HPOA	hypertrophic pulmonary osteoarthropathy
HPV	human papillomavirus
HR	heart rate
HRT	hormone-replacement therapy
HS	heart sounds
HSAN	hereditary sensory and autonomic neuropathy
HSP	Henoch–Schönlein purpura
HSV	herpes simplex virus
HT	hypertension
HTLV	human T-cell lymphotrophic virus
HUS	haemolytic-uraemic syndrome
I/I^-	iodine/iodide
IBD	inflammatory bowel disease
IBM	inclusion body myositis
ICP	intracranial pressure
ICS	intercostal space
IDDM	insulin-dependent diabetes mellitus
IDL	intermediate-density lipoprotein
IF	immunofluorescence
IFN	interferon

Ig	immunoglobulin
IGF	insulin-like growth factor
IHD	ischaemic heart disease
IL-1 (etc.)	interleukin-1 (etc.)
IL-1R (etc.)	interleukin-1 receptor (etc.)
IM/im	intramuscular
IND	indication
INR	International Normalized Ratio
IP	interphalangeal (joint)
IPKD	infant polycystic kidney disease
IPPV	intermittent positive-pressure ventilator
IQ	intelligence quotient
IRMA	intraretinal microvascular abnormalities
ISMN	isosorbide mononitrate
ITP	idiopathic thrombocytopenic purpura
ITU	intensive therapy unit
IUCD	intrauterine contraceptive device
IUD	intrauterine (contraceptive) device
IV/iv	intravenous
IVC	inferior vena cava
IVDU	intravenous drug user
IVI	intravenous infusion
IVIg	intravenous immunoglobulin
IVU	intravenous urography
Ix	investigations
JCA	juvenile chronic arthritis
JPS	joint position sense
JVP	jugular venous pressure
K/K^+	potassium ion
KCl	potassium chloride
$KClO_4$	potassium perchlorate
KCO	gas transfer coefficient (diffusion rate) across alveoli
KI	potassium iodide
KOH	potassium hydroxide
L	left
LBBB	left bundle branch block
LA	left atrium
LAD	left atrial dilatation, left axis deviation
LADP	left atrial diastolic pressure
LAP	left atrial pressure
LATS	long-acting thyroid stimulator (anti-TSH-R stimulating antibodies)
LCAT	lecithin:cholesterol acyltransferase
LDH	lactate dehydrogenase
LDL	low-density lipoprotein
LE	lupus erythematosus
LEMS	Lambert–Eaton myasthemic syndrome
LFT	liver function tests
LH	luteinising hormone
LHOA	Leber's hereditary optic atrophy
LHRH	luteinising hormone-releasing hormone
LHS	left hand side
LIF	left iliac fossa
LKM	(antibodies to) liver kidney microsomes
LL	lepromatous leprosy
LMN	lower motor neurone
LMW	low-molecular-weight
LN	lymph node
LOC	loss of consciousness
LOS	lower oesophageal sphincter
LOW	loss of weight
LP	lumbar puncture
LPL	lipoprotein lipase
LSE	left sternal edge
LSH	left side of heart
LTB4	leukotriene B4
LV	left ventricle
LVEDP	left ventricular end-diastolic pressure
LVEDV	left ventricular end-diastolic volume
LVF	left ventricular failure
LVH	left ventricular hypertrophy
LVP	left ventricular pressure
Ly	lymphocyte
mAchR	muscarinic acetylcholine receptor
MAD	mandibular advancement device
MADSAM	multifocal acquired demyelinating sensory and motor (neuropathy)
MAG	myelin-associated glycoprotein
MAG3	mercaptoacetyl triglycine (technetium scan)
MAHA	microangiopathic haemolytic anaemia
MAI	Mycobacterium avium intracelluiare
MALT	mucosa-associated lymphoid tissue
MAO	monoamine oxidase
MAOI	MAO inhibitor
MAT	microscopic agglutination test
Mb	myoglobin
MCHC	mean corpuscular haemoglobin concentration
MCP	metacarpophalangeal
MCTD	mixed connective tissue disease
MOV	mean cell volume
MDI	metered-dose inhaler
MDR	multi-drug resistant
MECG	mixed essential cryoglobulinaemia
MELAS	mitochondrial encephalomyopathy, lactic acidosis and stroke-like episodes
MEN	multiple endocrine neoplasia
met	metastasis
Mg/Mg^{2+}	magnesium

$MgSiO_3$	magnesium silicate
$MgSO_4$	magnesium sulphate
MGUS	monoclonal gammopathy of uncertain significance
MHC-I	major histocompatability complex class 1 molecule
MI	myocardial infarction
MIBG	*m*-iodobenzylguanidine
MIP	maximum inspiratory pressure
MMN	multifocal motor neuropathy with conduction block
MMR	measles, mumps and rubella
MND	motor neurone disease
Mø	macrophage
MODY	maturity-onset diabetes of young
MOPP	mustine, vincristine (Oncovin), procarbazine and prednisolone
MPO	myeloperoxidase
MPTP	1-methyl-4-phenyl-1, 2, 5, 6-tetrahydropyridine
MR	mitral regurgitation, mortality rate
MRA	magnetic resonance angiography
MRI	magnetic resonance venography
mRNA	messenger RNA
MRSA	methicillin-resistant *Staphylococcus aureus*
MS	mitral stenosis, multiple sclerosis
MSA	multiple systems atrophy
MSU	midstream urine
MTP	metatarsophalangeal
MTX	methotrexate
MuSK	muscle-specific kinase
MV	mitral valve
MVP	mitral valve prolapse
MVR	mitral valve replacement
MZ	monozygotic
N	nerve
N. saline	normal saline
N+V (+D)	nausea and vomiting (and diarrhoea)
N_2	nitrogen
n_2o	nitrous oxide
Na	sodium
NABQI	*N*-acetyl-*p*-benzoquinoneimine
nAchR	nicotinic acetylcholine receptor
NaCl	sodium chloride
$NADH/NAD^+$	nicotinamide adenine dinucleotide (reduced/oxidized forms)
NADPH	nicotinamide adenine dinucleotide phosphate
NAG	*N*-acetylglucosamine
$NaHCO_3$	sodium bicarbonate
NAM	*N*-acetylmuramie acid
NAP	neutrophil alkaline phosphatase
NARTI	nucleoside analogue reverse transcriptase inhibitor
NBM	nil by mouth
N.chromic	normochromic
N.cytic	normocytic
Neutroø	neutrophil
NG	nasogastric
NGT	nasogastric tube
NH_4^+	ammonium
NIDDM	non-insulin-dependent diabetes mellitus
NK	neurokinin
NMJ	neuromuscular junction
NNARTI	non-nucleoside-analogue reverse transcriptase inhibitor
NO_2	nitrogen dioxide
NREM	non rapid eye movement
NSAID	non-steroidal anti-inflammatory drug
NSTEMI	non-ST-elevation myocardial infarction
O_2	oxygen
OA	osteoarthritis
OCP	oral contraceptive pill
OGD	oesophagogastroduedenoscopy
OGTT	oral glucose tolerance test
OI	osteogenesis imperfecta
OM	osteomalacia
OSA	obstructive sleep apnoea
OT	occupational therapy
P	phosphorus
P:S	pulmonary-to-systemic
P:SVR	ratio of pulmonary to systemic vascular resistance
PABA	*p*-aminobenzoic acid
$PaCO_2$	partial pressure of carbon dioxide in arterial blood
RAF	platelet activating factor
PAN	polyarteritis nodosa
p-ANCA	perinuclear anti-neutrophil cytoplasmic antibodies
PaO_2	partial pressure of oxygen in arterial blood
PAO_2	alveolar partial pressure of oxygen
PAS	periodic acid-Schiff (stain)
PAWP	pulmonary arterial wedge pressure
PAXR	plain abdominal X-ray
PBC	primary biliary cirrhosis
PBG	porphobilinogen
PC	presenting complaint (used in a loose sense to include signs and abnormal tests)
PCOS	polycystic ovarian syndrome

PCP	*Pneumocystis carinii* pneumonia
PCR	polymerase chain reaction
PCT	proximal convoluted tubule
PCV	packed cell volume
PD	Parkinson disease
PDA	patent ductus arteriosus
PDH	pyruvate dehydrogenase
PE	pulmonary embolism
PEEP	positive end-expiratory pressure
PEFR	peak expiratory flow rate
PEG	percutaneous endoscopic gastrostomy
PEP	phosphoenolpyruvate
PET	positron-emission tomography, pancreatic endocrine tumours
PFK	phosphofructokinase
PGAS	polyglandular autoimmune syndrome
PGE_1	prostaglandin E_1
PGL	persistent generalized lymphadenopathy
PH	personal history (e.g. smoking, alcohol, drugs)
Ph	Philadelphia chromosome
Phaeo.	phaeochromocytoma
PHT	pulmonary hypertension
PI	protease inhibitor
PICA	posterior inferior cerebellar artery
PID	pelvic inflammatory disease
PION	posterior ischaemic optic neuropathy
PIP	proximal interphalangeal
PIP	phosphatidylinositol phosphate
PKA	protein kinase A
PKU	phenylketonuria
Pits	platelets
PM	polymyositis
PMF	progressive massive fibrosis
PMH	past medical history
PML	progressive multifocal leucoencephalopathy
PML	promyelocytic leukaemia
PMP22	peripheral myelin protein 22 gene
PMR	polymyalgia rheumatica
PNET	primitive neuroectodermal tumour
PNH	paroxysmal nocturnal haemoglobinuria
PNS	peripheral nervous system
PO	*per os* (by mouth)
PO_2	partial pressure of oxygen
PO_4^{3-}	phosphate
POEMS	polpolyneuropathy, organomegaly, endocrinopathy, monoclonal gammopathy and skin changes
POTS	postural orthostatic tachycardia syndrome
PP	pancreatic polypeptide
PPD	purified protein derivative
PPI	proton-pump inhibitor
PPi	free (inorganic) pyrophosphate
PPM	permanent pacemaker
PPr	peroxisome proliferator-activated (receptor)
PR	*per rectum* (by/from rectum) and pulmonary regurgitation
PRL	prolactin
Prox.	prophylaxis
PrP	prion protein
PRPP	phosphoribosyl pyrophosphate
PRV	polycythaemia rubra vera
PS	pulmonary stenosis
PSC	primary sclerosing cholangitis
PSM	pansystolic murmur
PSM	progressive supranuclear palsy
pt	patient
PT	prothrombin time
PTH	parathyroid hormone
PTH-rp	parathyroid hormone-related peptide
PTT	partial thromboplastin time
PTU	propylthiouracil
PU	peptic ulcer
PUJ	pelvic-ureteric junction
PUO	pyrexia of unknown origin
PV	*per vaginam* (by/from vagina)
PVD	pulmonary venous dilatation
PXE	pseudoxanthoma elasticum
R	right
RBBB	right bundle branch block
RA	right atrium, rheumatoid arthritis
RAAS	renin–angiotensin–aldosterone system
RAD	right axis deviation
RARA	retinoic acid receptor α
RAST	radio-allergosorbent test
RBC	red blood cells
RCA	right coronary artery
REM	rapid eye movement
RF	radiofemoral
RFLP	restriction fragment length polymorphism
Rh	rhesus
RhF	rheumatoid factor
RHS	right hand side
RIF	right iliac fossa
RIPE	rifampicin, isoniazid, pyrazinamide and ethambutol
RNA	ribonucleic acid
RNase	ribonuclease

RNP	ribonucleoprotein
RPGN	rapidly progressive glomerulonephritis
RPLND	retroperitoneal lymph-node dissection
RPR	rapid plasma reagin
RR	respiratory rate
RS	Reed–Sternberg (cell)
RSE	right sternal edge
RSH	right-sided heart
RSV	respiratory syncytial virus
rT3	reverse triiodothyronine
RTA	renal tubular acidosis
RTI	respiratory tract infection
rtPA	recombinant tissue-type plasminogen activator
RUQ	right upper quadrant
RV	right ventricle, residual volume
RVEDP	right ventricular end-diastolic pressure
RVF	right ventricular failure
RVH	right ventricular hypertrophy
RVOTO	right ventricular outflow tract obstruction
Rx	treatments
SAA	serum amyloid A
SAH	subarachnoid haemorrhage
SALT	speech and language therapy
SAM	systolic anterior motion
SAN	sino-atrial node
SAP	radiolabelled serum amyloid P scintigram (^{99}Tc)
SARS	severe acute respiratory syndrome
SBE	subacute bacterial endocarditis
SBP	systolic blood pressure
SC/sc	subcutaneous
SCA	spinocerebellar ataxia
SCID	severe combined immunodeficiency
SE	side-effects
SEP	serum electrophoresis
SER	smooth endoplasmic reticulum
SERM	selective oestrogen receptor modulator
SH	social history
SHBG	sex hormone-binding globulin
SI	sacro-iliac
SIADH	syndrome of inappropriate antidiuretic hormone secretion
SK	streptokinase
SLA	(antibodies to) soluble liver antigen
SLE	systemic lupus erythematosus
SMA	spinal muscular atrophy
SNRI	serotonin and noradrenaline reuptake inhibitor
SO_2	sulphur dioxide
SOB	shortness of breath
SOBOE	shortness of breath on exercise
SOD	superoxide dismutase
SR	survival rate
SRP	signal recognition particle
SS-A	Sjögren syndrome antibodies A
SS-B	Sjögren syndrome antibodies B
ssDNA	single-stranded DNA
SSPE	subacute sclerosing panencephalitis
SSRI	selective serotonin reuptake inhibitor
SST	short Synacthen test
STD	sexually transmitted disease
STEMI	ST-elevation myocardial infarction
SUFE	slipped upper femoral epiphysis
SUNCT	short-lasting unilateral neuralgia with conjunctival injection and tearing
SV	supraventricular
SVC	superior vena cava
SVCO	superior vena cava obstruction
SVT	supraventricular tachycardia
Sx	symptoms, signs
syn.	syndrome
T4	thyroxine
TAC	trigeminal-autonomic cephalgia
TAG	triacylglyceride
TAPVD	total anomalous pulmonary venous drainage
TB	tuberculosis
TBB	transbronchial biopsy
TBG	thyroxine-binding globulin
Tc	technetium
TCA	tricyclic antidepressant
TCR	T-cell receptor
TdT	terminal deoxynucleotidyltransferase
TED	transverse elastic graduated
temp	temporary
TENS	transcutaneous electrical nerve stimulation
TERT	telomerase reverse transcriptase
TFTs	thyroid function tests
TG	thyroglobulin
TG	triglycerides
TGA	transposition of the great arteries
TGF	transforming growth factor
T_H	helper T (cell)
THF	tetrahydrofolate
TIA	transient ischaemic attack
TIBC	total iron-binding capacity
TIN	tubulo-intestinal nephritis
TIPSS	transjugular intrahepatic porto-systemic shunt

TLC	total lung capacity
TLCO	total lung diffusion coefficient
TMJ	temporomandibular joint
TNF	tumour necrosis factor
TnI	troponin I
TOE	transoesophageal echocardiography
top	topical
TORCH	toxoplasmosis, other (e.g. syphilis), rubella, cytomegalovirus, herpes (and hepatitis)
tPA	tissue-type plasminogen activator
TPHA	*Treponema pallidum* haemagglutination assay
TPI	*Treponema pallidum* immobilisation
TPN	total parenteral nutrition
TPR	temperature, pulse and respiration
TR	tricuspid regurgitation
TRH	thyrotrophin-releasing hormone
tRNA	transfer RNA
TSH	thyroid-stimulating hormone
TSH-R	TSH receptor
TT	tuberculoid leprosy
TTP	thrombotic thrombocytopenic purpura
TURP	transurethral resection of the prostate
TV	tricuspid valve
TVF	tactile vocal fremitus
TWOC	trial without catheter
TXA_2	thromboxane A_2
U&E	urea and electrolytes
UA	unstable angina
UC	ulcerative colitis
UDP	uridine diphosphate
UIP	usual interstitial pneumonitis
ULN	upper limit of normal
UMN	upper motor neurone
UO	urine output
URT	upper respiratory tract
URTI	upper respiratory tract infection
USS	ultrasound scan
UTI	urinary tract infection
UVA	ultraviolet A
V/Q	ventilation/perfusion
VAD	vincristine, doxorubicin (Adriamycin) and dexamethasone
Val	valine
VDRL	Venereal Diseases Research Laboratory (syphilis serological test)
VE	ventricular extrasystole
VF	ventricular fibrillation
VG	voltage-gated
VHL	von Hippel–Lindau (disease)
ViM	ventral intermediate
VIP	vasoactive intestinal peptide
Vit	vitamin
VLDL	very low-density lipoprotein
VMA	vanillylmandelic acid (= HMMA)
VMN	ventromedial nucleus (of thalamus)
VPB	ventricular premature beat
VRE	vancomycin-resistant enterococci
VSD	ventricular septal defect
VT	ventricular tachycardia
VTEC	verocytotoxicogenetic *Escherichia coli*
VUJ	vesico-ureteric junction
VUR	vesico-ureteric reflux
vWF	von Willebrand factor
VZV	varicella-zoster virus
WBC	white blood cell
WCC	white cell count
WG	Wegener's granulomatosis
WPW	Wolff–Parkinson–White (syndrome)
X-match	cross-match blood type
XL	X-linked
xsome	chromosome
xteristics or xters	characteristics
Zn	zinc
ZN	Ziehl–Neelsen (stain)

INDEX

D

E

H

I